105.00

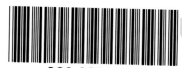

369 0289848

KU-627-866

This book is due for return on or before the last date shown below.

THERAPEUTIC DRUG MONITORING

Newer Drugs and Biomarkers

THERAPEUTIC DRUG MONITORING

Newer Drugs and Biomarkers

Edited by

AMITAVA DASGUPTA

University of Texas Health Sciences Center, Houston, Texas

AMSTERDAM • BOSTON • HEIDELBERG • LONDON • NEW YORK • OXFORD
PARIS • SAN DIEGO • SAN FRANCISCO • SINGAPORE • SYDNEY • TOKYO
Academic Press is an imprint of Elsevier

Academic Press is an imprint of Elsevier
32 Jamestown Road, London NW1 7BY, UK
225 Wyman Street, Waltham, MA 02451, USA
525 B Street, Suite 1800, San Diego, CA 92101-4495, USA

First edition 2012

British Library Cataloguing-in-Publication Data
A catalogue record for this book is available from the British Library

Library of Congress Cataloging-in-Publication Data
A catalog record for this book is available from the Library of Congress

ISBN : 978-0-12-385467-4

For information on all Academic Press publications
visit our website at elsevierdirect.com

Typeset by TNQ Books and Journals Pvt Ltd.
www.tnq.co.in

Printed and bound in United States of America

12 13 14 15 16   10 9 8 7 6 5 4 3 2 1

Dedicated to my wife Alice

Preface

Introduced in the 1970s in medical practice with monitoring of few classical anticonvulsants such as phenytoin and phenobarbital, therapeutic drug monitoring is capable of helping the clinician to personalize the dosage of medication in the individual patient. Therefore, although an indirect phenotype approach, therapeutic drug monitoring should be considered as an earlier attempt by laboratory professionals and healthcare professionals to personalize medicine. Therapeutic drug monitoring as a discipline has evolved from monitoring of a few classical anticonvulsant drugs in the 1970s into routine monitoring of over 25 drugs. In addition, therapy with additional 25-40 drugs may also benefit from therapeutic drug monitoring and such tests are available in large medical centers, academic medical centers and national reference laboratories. As more and more new drugs are being approved by the FDA (Federal Drug Administration), a few of the new drugs may be candidate for therapeutic drug monitoring. Examples include some new anticonvulsants, protease inhibitors used in HAART (highly active antiretroviral therapy) therapy, and the newly approved immunosuppressant agent everolimus. Moreover, with the completion of the human genome project, our understanding of drug response in an individual patient is growing and pharmacogenomics testing is gaining acceptance as a valuable tool in individualizing certain drug therapy to obtain maximum efficacy and at the same time minimizing adverse drug reaction. Because pharmacogenomics testing can predict behavior of a drug based on polymorphism of various drug metabolizing enzymes in individual patients, such testing is a proactive approach to personalizing drug therapy rather than adjusting dosage based on the result of therapeutic drug monitoring, which is a reactive approach. Therefore, various polymorphisms of drug metabolizing enzyme are biomarkers which can provide valuable insight into metabolism and efficacy of a drug in a particular patient before initiation of therapy. It is also possible to predict if a drug can be useful in a particular patient. Calcineurin activity has been demonstrated to be useful as a biomarker to assess the efficacy of different calcineurin inhibitor-based regimens using cyclosporine and tacrolimus in transplant recipients. Inosine monophosphate dehydrogenase (IMPDH) activity in peripheral blood mononuclear cells or $CD4^+$ cells has been proposed to be an excellent biomarker to assess mycophenolic acid pharmacodynamics.

The focus of this book is to discuss the utility of therapeutic drug monitoring of newer drugs but at the same time cover therapeutic drug monitoring of more common drugs so the readers can have access to up-to-date information on the current practices of therapeutic drug monitoring. In addition, emphasis is only placed on discussing appropriate biomarkers and also future research trends in the field. Specialized topics such as clinical utility of monitoring free drug concentration, dosage adjustments based on computerized models using pharmacokinetic and pharmacodynamic data, application of pharmacogenomics warfarin therapy and cancer chemotherapy with certain anticancer agents have been covered along with more traditional topics such as challenges in therapeutic drug monitoring of digoxin, monitoring of tricyclic antidepressants and guidelines for monitoring of aminoglycosides and vancomycin. In addition, emerging topics in therapeutic drug monitoring such as application of therapeutic drug monitoring in antiretroviral therapy, drug testing in pain management and how therapeutic drug monitoring can be utilized to identify a clinically significant drug-herb interaction have also been addressed in this book.

I would like to thank all contributors for taking time from their busy schedule to write excellent chapters for this book. All contributors are experts in their respective field and without their dedication and concerted effort, it would be impossible for me to complete this book project. I would like to thank Professor Robert L. Hunter, Chairman of Department of Pathology and Laboratory Medicine for his support to work on this book project. Last but not least I would like to thank my wife Alice for tolerating my long hours of work on this book project during evenings and weekend. I hope both practicing clinicians, pathologists and laboratory professionals will find this book useful. Finally readers are the judge for the success of this book. If they find this book useful, efforts of all contributors and this editor will be well rewarded.

Amitava Dasgupta
Professor of Pathology and Laboratory Medicine, University of Texas Health Sciences Center, Houston, Texas

Contributors

Leland B. Baskin MD   Calgary Laboratory Services, Calgary, AB, Canada

Roger L. Bertholf PhD   University of Florida College of Medicine, Jacksonville, FL

Joshua Bornhorst PhD   University of Arkansas for Medical Sciences, School of Medicine, Little Rock, AR

Gunnar Brandhorst MD   George-August University, Goettingen, Germany

Valerie Bush PhD   Bassett Medical Center, Cooperstown, New York, NY

Anthony W. Butch PhD   University of California, Los Angeles, CA

Jill Butterfield PharmD   Albany College of Pharmacy, Albany, NY

Alex C. Chin PhD   Calgary Laboratory Services, Calgary, AB, Canada

Amitava Dasgupta PhD   University of Texas-Houston, Houston, TX

Angela Ferguson PhD   Children's Mercy Hospitals and Clinics, University of Missouri, Kansas City, MO

Uttam Garg PhD   Children's Mercy Hospitals and Clinics, University of Missouri, Kansas City, MO

Gary Hardiman PhD   University of California at San Diego, San Diego, CA

Kathleen A. Kelly PhD   University of California, Los Angeles, CA

Charles J.L. la Porte PharmD, PhD   Ottawa Hospital Research Institute and University of Ottawa, Ottawa, ON, Canada

Thomas P. Lodise, Jr. PharmD   Albany College of Pharmacy, Albany, NY

Matthew Luke MD   University of New Mexico, Albuquerque, NM

Jennifer Martin PhD, FRACP   Queensland, Brisbane, Austral

Ronald W. McLawhon MD, PhD   California, San Diego, School La Jolla, CA

Michael C. Milone MD, PhD   Pennsylvania, Philadelphia, P/

Marcel Musteata PhD   Albany Pharmacy and Health Services

Michael Oellerich MD   George University, Goettingen, Germa

Manjunath P. Pai PharmD   Alb Pharmacy, Albany, NY

Natella Y. Rakhmanina MD, Ph Washington University School and Children's National Medi Washington, DC

Gary M. Reisfield MD   Univers College of Medicine, Gainesvi

Franck Saint-Marcoux PhD   De Pharmacology and Toxicology University Hospital, Limoges,

Maria Shipkova MD   Central I Clinical Chemistry and Labor: Klinikum Stuttgart, Stuttgart,

Andrew Somogyi PhD   Univers Adelaide, Australia

Annjanette Stone BS   Central / Veterans Healthcare System (F Laboratory Medicine, Researcl Little Rock, AR

Eberhard Wieland MD   Centra Clinical Chemistry and Labor: Klinikum Stuttgart, Stuttgart,

1

Introduction to Therapeutic Drug Monitoring
Frequently and Less Frequently Monitored Drugs

Amitava Dasgupta

Department of Pathology and Laboratory Medicine,
University of Texas-Houston, Houston, TX

OUTLINE

DOI: 10.1016/B978-0-12-385467-4.00001-4

INTRODUCTION

There are over 6000 prescription and non-prescription (often termed as over-the-counter) drugs approved by the FDA (Federal Drug Administration of the United States government) for clinical use. The spending for prescription drugs was US$234.1 billion in 2008, which was more than double the amount of money spent in 1999. The percentage of Americans who had used at least one prescription drug in the past month increased from 44% in 1999–2000 to 48% in 2007–2008, and, as expected, the percentage of Americans using five or more drugs also increased steadily during this period (Fig. 1.1). People aged over 60 years required more prescription drugs than younger people: only 7.9% of Americans between the ages of 20 and 59 used five or more drugs, but 36.7% of Americans aged over 60 years used five or more medications. The most commonly used drugs, based on drug use in the 2007–2008 survey, are as follows: children (age up to 11 years), bronchodilators; adolescents (12–19 years), central nervous system stimulants; adults (20–59 years), antidepressants; and elderly patients, cholesterol-lowering medications. The percentages of the most often used prescription drugs in various age groups of the American population are shown in Fig. 1.2. Diuretics and beta-blockers are also commonly used by adults and older Americans. People without a regular place for health care, health insurance, or prescription drug benefits had lower use of prescription drugs [1].

Many patients, especially the elderly, take drugs for controlling chronic conditions. Although none of the non-prescription drugs requires therapeutic drug monitoring, except for salicylate and acetaminophen in cases of overdose or attempted suicide, some prescription medications require routine therapeutic drug monitoring. Fortunately, the number of such drugs requiring routine monitoring is relatively low. Approximately 26 prescription drugs are frequently monitored in a majority of hospital-based laboratories using

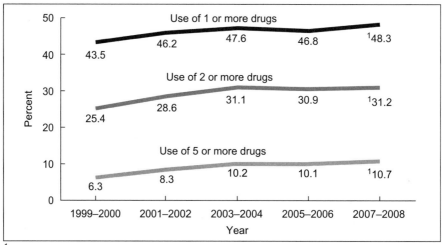

[1]Significant linear trend from 1999–2000 through 2007–2008.

FIGURE 1.1 Trend in use of prescription drugs among Americans. (*Source: Reference 1: US Government Document*).

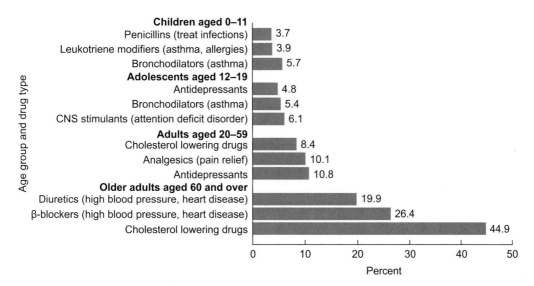

FIGURE 1.2 Percentage of prescription drugs used most often in various age groups of American population. *(Source: Reference 1: US Government Document).*

commercially available immunoassays and automated analyzers. In addition, approximately 25–30 drugs are subjected to therapeutic drug monitoring less frequently, and immunoassays are available for only a few such drugs. Therefore, chromatographic techniques are used for monitoring of these drugs, and such tests are only available in clinical laboratories of major medical centers and academic centers as well as reference laboratories. The most sophisticated method for therapeutic drug monitoring is liquid chromatography combined with mass spectrometry or tandem mass spectrometry (see Chapter 3 for a detailed discussion on this topic).

Therapeutic drug monitoring not only consists of measuring the concentration of a drug in a biological matrix but also involves the proper interpretation of the value using pharmacokinetic parameters, drawing appropriate conclusions regarding the drug concentration and dose adjustment. The International Association for Therapeutic Drug Monitoring and Clinical Toxicology adopted the following definition for drug monitoring [2]:

> Therapeutic drug monitoring is defined as the measurement made in the laboratory of a parameter that, with appropriate interpretation, will directly influence prescribing procedures. Commonly, the measurement is in a biological matrix of a prescribed xenobiotic, but it may also be of an endogenous compound prescribed as a replacement therapy in an individual who is physiologically or pathologically deficient in that compound.

Therapeutic drug monitoring has been used in clinical practice to individualize drug therapy since the beginning of the 1970s. The goal of such monitoring is to optimize the pharmacological responses of a drug while avoiding adverse effects. Traditionally, therapeutic drug monitoring involves measuring drug concentration in a biological matrix — most commonly serum or plasma — and interpreting these concentrations in terms of relevant clinical parameters. Whole blood is the preferred matrix for therapeutic drug monitoring of immunosuppressants except for mycophenolic acid. For success of a therapeutic drug monitoring program, good communication between clinicians, laboratory professionals and pharmacists is essential. In one report, the authors clearly documented that the intervention of pharmacists significantly improved the appropriateness of therapeutic drug monitoring use and significantly reduced unnecessary costs. In addition, the authors commented that using a screening checklist including the indication for therapeutic drug monitoring, specimen collection time and data needed for proper interpretation of the drug level can improve appropriateness of utilization of the therapeutic drug monitoring service [3].

DRUGS THAT REQUIRE THERAPEUTIC DRUG MONITORING

As stated earlier, only a small fraction of prescription drugs require therapeutic drug monitoring because for most prescription drugs there is a wider difference between therapeutic and toxic concentrations. For example, the therapeutic range of acetaminophen found in many over-the-counter drugs is $10-30\,\mu g/mL$, while toxicity is encountered at serum or plasma concentrations over $200\,\mu g/mL$. Because of the more than six-fold difference between the upper end of the therapeutic and lower end of the toxic concentration, acetaminophen is not monitored except in the case of a suspected overdose. In contrast, the therapeutic range of phenytoin is $10-20\,\mu/mL$ while toxicity may be encountered at a concentration of $30\,\mu g/mL$. Genetic polymorphism can precipitate phenytoin toxicity after a therapeutic dose. Ramasamy *et al.* described a case where a female developed phenytoin toxicity after administration of a therapeutic dosage of 300 mg per day of phenytoin. Her serum phenytoin level was $33\,\mu g/mL$. She was homozygous for a CYP2C9*3*3 mutation that led to a marked decrease in enzymatic activity of CYP2C9, which is responsible for metabolism of phenytoin [4]. Situations where therapeutic drug monitoring is beneficial include the following:

1. Where there is difficulty in interpreting therapeutic or low toxicity levels of a drug based on clinical evidence alone and there is no clearly defined clinical parameter for dose adjustment.
2. Where correlation between serum or whole blood drug concentration and dosage is poor.
3. Where there is a narrow therapeutic range, so the dose of a drug which produces the desired therapeutic concentrations in one patient may cause toxicity in another patient.
4. Where toxicity of a drug may lead to hospitalization, irreversible organ damage and even death, but an adverse drug reaction may be avoided by therapeutic drug monitoring.
5. Where there is a correlation between serum or whole blood concentration of the drug and its therapeutic response or toxicity.
6. Where there are clinical indications for therapeutic drug monitoring — for example, poor response to the drug, suspected treatment failure due to non-compliance, or signs of toxicity despite no dosage adjustment.

For strongly protein-bound drugs (protein binding $> 80\%$), a better correlation may be observed between unbound (free) drug concentration (rather than traditionally monitored total drug concentration) and clinical outcome, because it is only the unbound drug that is responsible for the drug's pharmacological action. For example, adjusting phenytoin dosage in patients based on their serum phenytoin concentrations rather than seizure frequencies not only decreases morbidity but also prevents phenytoin toxicity in these patients. Peterson *et al.* reported that, in their study involving 114 patients, free phenytoin concentrations correlated better with clinical picture than did total phenytoin concentrations [5] (see Chapter 4 for further details).

Usually, anticonvulsants, cardioactive drugs, immunosuppressants, anti-asthmatic drugs, antidepressants, antiretroviral drugs, antineoplastic drugs and antibiotics with narrow therapeutic windows, such as vancomycin and aminoglycosides, require routine therapeutic drug monitoring. In most instances the trough blood level (15–30 minutes prior to the next dosage) is the preferred specimen for therapeutic drug monitoring except for certain antibiotics (vancomycin and aminoglycosides), where both peak and trough drug levels are monitored. Vancomycin and aminoglycoside can produce serious nephrotoxicity and ototoxicity. Suggested therapeutic ranges for commonly monitored drugs as well as less commonly monitored drugs are listed in Table 1.1.

BENEFITS OF THERAPEUTIC DRUG MONITORING

Benefits of therapeutic drug monitoring are listed in Table 1.2. In general, many drugs are used as a prophylactic to prevent clinical symptoms — for example, phenytoin is given to a patient in order to prevent an episode of seizure. However, non-compliance has serious clinical consequences, and therapeutic drug monitoring is very useful in identifying such non-compliance. Mattson *et al.* commented that a zero drug level, subtherapeutic levels or variable drug levels are indicators of non-compliance in a medication where therapeutic drug monitoring is available. In the authors' experience, 93% of their patients showed good adherence to the treatment protocol, as determined by therapeutic drug monitoring [6]. In contrast, in another report the authors used routine therapeutic drug monitoring to study compliance with theophylline and phenytoin therapy in a group of 80 outpatients and observed that only 37% of patients studied were complaint. The most interesting finding by the authors was that approximately half of the non-compliant patients were unaware of the necessity for taking their medication on a continuous basis [7]. Chandra *et al.* commented that poor patient compliance is one of the major causes of non-responsiveness to anti-epileptic drug therapy. Compliance is mostly assessed by self-reporting, therapeutic drug monitoring and pill-counting, but therapeutic drug monitoring is superior to other approaches for determining patient compliance with therapy. The authors determined that an adult patient receiving a dosage of 300 mg or more of phenytoin a day and showing plasma phenytoin levels of less than 5 µg/mL should be investigated for potential non-compliance [8]. Reis *et al.* determined partial compliance with sertraline therapy in depressed patients by determining plasma levels of sertraline and its metabolite [9]. Stieffenhofer and Hiemke commented that lack of or an insufficient response to a drug may be due to non-compliance of the patient or reduced absorption of the drug, or to ultra-rapid metabolism of the drug due to the genetic makeup of the patient. Therefore, to identify the reason(s) for a poor response to a drug, suboptimal plasma concentrations should be investigated further to identify non-compliance of a patient and pharmacogenetic testing considered in order to identify a rapid metabolizer [10].

TABLE 1.1 Frequently and Less Frequently Monitored Therapeutic Drugs

Drug class/Drug	Recommended therapeutic range	
	Trough concentration	Peak concentration
ANTICONVULSANTS		
Frequently monitored		
Phenytoin	10–20 µg/mL	Not required
Carbamazepine	4–12 µg/mL	Not required
Phenobarbital	15–40 µg/mL	Not required
Primidone	5–12 µg/mL	Not required
Valproic acid	50–100 µg/mL	Not required
Clonazepam	10–75 ng/mL[#]	Not required
Less frequently monitored		
Gabapentin	2–10 µg/mL[#]	Not required
Lamotrigine	3–14 µg/mL[#]	Not required
CARDIOACTIVE DRUGS		
Frequently monitored		
Digoxin	0.8–1.8 ng/mL	Not required
Procainamide	4–10 µg/mL	Not required
N-Acetylprocainamide	4–8 µg/mL	Not required
Quinidine	2–5 µg/mL	Not required
Lidocaine	1.5–5.0 µg/mL	Not required
Less frequently monitored		
Amiodarone	1.0–2.5 µg/mL	Not required
Flecainide	0.2–1.0 µg/mL	Not required
Mexiletine	0.5–2.0 µg/mL	Not required
Propranolol	50–100 ng/mL	Not required
Verapamil	50–200 ng/mL	Not required
Tocainide	5–12 µg/mL	Not required
ANTI-ASTHMATIC		
Frequently monitored		
Theophylline	10–20 µg/mL	Not required
Caffeine	5–15 µg/mL	Not required

TABLE 1.1 Frequently and Less Frequently Monitored Therapeutic Drugs—cont'd

Drug class/Drug	Recommended therapeutic range	
	Trough concentration	Peak concentration
ANTIDEPRESSANTS		
Frequently monitored		
Amitriptyline + nortriptyline	120—250 ng/mL	Not required
Nortriptyline	50—150 ng/mL	Not required
Doxepin + nordoxepin	150—250 ng/mL	Not required
Imipramine + desipramine	150—250 ng/mL	Not required
Lithium	0.8—1.2 mEq/L	Not required
Less frequently monitored		
Amoxapine	200—400 ng/mL	Not required
Fluoxetine + norfluoxetine	300—1000 ng/mL	Not required
Sertraline	30—200 ng/mL	Not required
Paroxetine	20—200 ng/mL	Not required
IMMUNOSUPPRESSANTS		
Frequently monitored		
Cyclosporine*	100—400 ng/mL	Not required
Tacrolimus*	5—15 ng/mL	Not required
Sirolimus*	4—20 ng/mL	Not required
Everolimus*	3—8 ng/mL	Not required
Mycophenolic acid	1—3.5 μg/mL	Not required
ANTINEOPLASTIC		
Frequently monitored		
Methotrexate	Varies with therapy type	Varies with therapy type
Less frequently monitored		
Busulfan	600—920 ng/mL	Not required
5-Fluorouracil	2—3 μg/mL	Not required
ANTIBIOTICS		
Frequently monitored		
Amikacin	20—35 μg/mL	4—8 μg/mL
Gentamicin	5—10 μg/mL	< 2 μg/mL
Tobramycin	5—10 μg/mL	< 2 μg/mL

Continued

TABLE 1.1 Frequently and Less Frequently Monitored Therapeutic Drugs—cont'd

Drug class/Drug	Recommended therapeutic range	
	Trough concentration	Peak concentration
Vancomycin	20–40 µg/mL	5–15 µg/mL
Less frequently monitored		
Ciprofloxacin	3–5 µg/mL	0.5–3 µg/mL
Chloramphenicol	5–20 µg/mL	Not required
Isoniazid	May not be monitored	3–6 µg/mL
Rifampin	May not be monitored	8–24 µg/mL
Ethambutol	May not be monitored	2–6 µg/mL

Monitored in whole blood instead of serum or plasma.
#*Reference range recommend by the ARUP reference laboratory, Salt Lake City, UT.*
Therapeutic ranges based on published literature, books as well as ranges adopted by reputed national reference laboratories such as Mayo Medical Laboratories and ARUP laboratories. However, therapeutic ranges vary widely among different patient populations and each institute should establish their own guidelines. These values are for the purpose of providing examples only.

TABLE 1.2 Benefits of Therapeutic Drug Monitoring (TDM)

Benefits	Comments
Identification of non-compliant patient	Zero or subtherapeutic drug level/highly variable drug level are indications of total or partial non-compliance. However, subtherapeutic level may also be observed in ultra-rapid metabolizers.
Personalization of dosage	Metabolism and elimination of certain drugs depend on various pathophysiological conditions such as uremia and liver disease. Elderly patients, children and pregnant women require dosage adjustments of certain drugs based on TDM.
Avoidance of adverse drug event/drug toxicity	TDM is very useful in preventing an adverse drug event. TDM is also useful in avoiding drug toxicity.
Improvement in patient safety/ decreased hospital stay	TDM can greatly improve patient's safety and decrease hospital stay, thus saving health care cost.
Investigation of non-response	If a patient does not respond to a drug it may also be due to poor absorption or genetic variation in drug metabolism. TDM is useful to identify such patients. If drug is within therapeutic range then a patient may not respond to that drug.

Other than non-compliance, a patient's response to a particular drug depends on many factors, including bioavailability, drug clearance, drug protein binding and the pathophysiological condition of the patient, as well as many other factors such as whether the medication is taken with food, whether the patient is a smoker, etc. The genetic makeup of an individual is also very important in determining whether a person will respond to a particular drug and how well the drug, if effective, exerts its pharmacological action. Pharmacotherapy could in many cases be ineffective, because as many as 30–60% of patients may be non-responders to a particular drug due to these factors [11]. Therapeutic drug monitoring can greatly reduce the chance of treatment failure by personalizing the drug dosage based on the results of therapeutic drug monitoring. Personalized drug therapy based on the genetic makeup of a patient has gained importance in the past decade, especially since the complete characterization of the human genome. This topic is addressed in Chapter 6. In addition, life-threatening adverse drug reactions are responsible for 6–7% of all hospitalization in the US and account for over 100 000 deaths annually [12]. Therapeutic drug monitoring helps to avoid adverse drug reactions due to drug–drug interaction and can also reduce the toxicity of an individual drug where therapeutic drug monitoring is available. Billaud *et al.* reported a case of a 54-year-old male renal transplant recipient who received antifungal treatment in combination with the immunosuppressant drug everolimus in order to prevent post-transplant reactivation of aspergillosis. Voriconazole was withdrawn after 1 month due to elevated trough concentrations (5 mg/L) and hepatotoxicity, and posaconazole was substituted. However, both voriconazole and posaconazole interacted with everolimus, causing 7.5- and 3.8-fold increases in the trough everolimus level, respectively, due to inhibition of everolimus metabolism by CYP3A4. The authors were successful in avoiding drug toxicity by careful therapeutic drug monitoring of both the antifungal drug and everolimus, and subsequent dosage adjustment to keep the everolimus concentration within the therapeutic range [13]. Gulbis *et al.* described a clinically significant drug interaction between busulfan and metronidazole where an adverse reaction was avoided by therapeutic drug monitoring of busulfan. A 7-year-old boy with a history of myelodysplasias that progressed to myeloid leukemia was treated with busulfan, clofarabine and thiotepa as a pretransplant conditioning regime for a cord blood transplant, and after receiving metronidazole his clearance of busulfan decreased by 46% as determined by therapeutic drug monitoring of busulfan. Busulfan was eventually discontinued to avoid drug toxicity [14].

Therapeutic drug monitoring is useful in minimizing adverse drug effects due to drug toxicity. In one report, the authors concluded that therapeutic drug monitoring in pain management using opioids can minimize adverse drug events while maximizing efficacy of the therapy [15]. Patel *et al.* studied the benefits of therapeutic drug monitoring of olanzapine in 3207 patients and observed that in patients aged 17 years or younger, median plasma olanzapine was higher than in adult patients at all olanzapine dosages. In addition, smoking status, age, sex and body weight together explained 24% of the variance in plasma olanzapine concentrations. The degree of adherence, drug–drug interactions and pharmacogenetic factors also contributed to wide variance in the olanzapine drug level in plasma specimens. Interestingly, female non-smokers had higher plasma olanzapine concentrations for a given dosage than did male smokers. The authors concluded that therapeutic drug monitoring of olanzapine may have a role in limiting olanzapine dosage to minimize the risk of long-term toxicity [16]. Slaughter *et al.* reported that therapeutic drug monitoring of aminoglycoside can significantly reduce incidences of nephrotoxicity from therapy with aminoglycosides. The authors further concluded that, from the pharmacoeconomic point of view, therapeutic drug monitoring of aminoglycosides is beneficial because therapeutic drug monitoring for an individual patient during therapy cost approximately US$301 while each case of nephrotoxicity cost the hospital US$4583 [17]. Crist *et al.* evaluated the impact of therapeutic drug monitoring of aminoglycoside (gentamicin and tobramycin) in 221 patients on the length of hospital stay, cost-effectiveness and related factors. The mean length of hospital stay was 8.4 days in the patient group that received individualized aminoglycoside doses (study group) versus 11.8 days in the control group. In addition, the hospital cost was lower by US$725 per patient in the study group, which would produce an annual saving of US$640 000 at the author's institution [18]. In another report, the authors concluded that therapeutic drug monitoring of beta-lactam antibiotics in critically ill patients twice a week and dosage adjustments based on blood level resulted in prevention of drug toxicity and a positive outcome in 87.3% of the patients studied [19]. Reduced drug-related toxicities are not only beneficial for patients, but also diminish the liability of physicians and improve the quality of patient care as well as patient safety. Ried *et al.* evaluated the effectiveness of therapeutic drug monitoring in reducing toxic drug reactions by meta-analysis of 14 studies. The authors concluded that patients monitored for appropriate drugs suffered fewer toxic drug reactions than patients where therapeutic drug monitoring was not undertaken [20]. Another study reported that determination of serum drug concentrations and evaluation of such results by clinical pharmacists resulted in significant cost savings [21].

Routine therapeutic drug monitoring is also very useful in investigating non-response to a drug. Apart from non-compliance, various other factors may contribute to non-response to a drug. Muller *et al.* observed that patients not responding to the antipsychotic drug amisulpride had significantly lower plasma levels than patients who showed moderate improvement despite comparable dosage. Moreover, the daily amisulpride dosage did not predict non-response or response. The authors also established the optimal plasma concentration of amisulpride to avoid non-response to be 100 ng/mL. The authors concluded that therapeutic drug monitoring of amisulpride is very useful for clinical decision-making [22]. Babalik *et al.* commented that low levels of antituberculosis drugs may be responsible for a poor treatment outcome because monitoring of these drugs is not routinely performed. The authors studied 20 patients, and observed that the majority of them (17 patients) had at least one low serum level of an antituberculosis drug. The authors concluded that therapeutic drug monitoring is potentially useful in improving outcome when treating these patients [23]. Sometimes a higher serum drug level may be needed to achieve optimal therapeutic benefit from a drug in a particular ethnic group. Wang *et al.* reported that among Chinese patients with HIV infection the therapeutic trough concentration of nevirapine was 3.9 μg/mL − significantly higher than the recommended drug concentration of 3.0 μg/mL. The authors commented that the correlation between nevirapine concentrations and efficacy as well as hepatotoxicity suggests benefits of dosage adjustment of nevirapine based on therapeutic drug monitoring in Chinese patients infected with HIV in order to optimize antiretroviral therapy [24].

PATHOPHYSIOLOGICAL CONDITIONS AND OTHER FACTORS THAT AFFECT DRUG CONCENTRATIONS

The serum concentration of a particular drug is determined by absorption, distribution, metabolism and excretion of a drug. Major characteristics that affect serum drug concentrations include genetic makeup, pathophysiological condition and various other factors. Hepatic disease may alter the metabolism of a drug, where a patient with renal failure may clear a drug in urine more slowly than a patient with normal renal function. Pregnancy alters the metabolism of several drugs, while drug–drug interactions may also significantly alter serum drug concentrations.

Basic Pharmacokinetics

When a drug is administered orally it undergoes several steps in the body that determine the concentration of that drug in serum/plasma or whole blood. These steps include:

1. *Liberation* — the release of a drug from the dosage form (tablet, capsule, extended-release formulation).
2. *Absorption* — movement of the drug from the site of administration (for drugs taken orally) to the blood circulation. Many factors affect this stage, including gastric pH and presence of food particles, as well as the efflux mechanism if present in the gut. First-pass metabolism plays an important role in determining the bioavailability of a drug given orally.
3. *Distribution and protein binding* — movement of a drug from the blood circulation to tissues/target organs. Drugs may also be bound to serum proteins, ranging from no protein binding to 99% protein binding.
4. *Metabolism* — chemical transformation of a drug to the active and inactive metabolites. The liver is responsible for metabolism of many drugs, although drugs may also be metabolized by a non-hepatic path or be subjected to minimal metabolism.
5. *Excretion* — elimination of the drug from the body via renal, biliary or pulmonary mechanisms.

Basic pharmacokinetics is discussed in detail in pharmacology textbooks, and therefore only a brief discussion of this important topic is presented in this chapter. Liberation of a drug after oral administration depends on the formulation of the dosage. An immediate-release formulation releases the drugs at once from the dosage form when administered, while the same drug may also be available in a sustained-release formulation. Absorption of a drug depends on the route of administration. Generally oral administration is the route of choice, but under certain circumstances (nausea, vomiting and convulsions) the rectal route may present a practical alternative for delivering anticonvulsants, non-narcotic and narcotic analgesics, theophylline, and antibacterial and anti-emetic agents. This route can also be used for inducing anesthesia in children. Although the rate of drug absorption is usually lower after rectal administration compared to oral administration, for certain drugs rectal absorption is higher compared to oral absorption due to avoidance of the hepatic first-pass metabolism. These drugs include lidocaine, morphine, metoclopramide, ergotamine and propranolol. Local irritation is a possible complication of rectal drug delivery [25]. When a drug is administered by direct injection, it enters the blood circulation immediately.

When a drug enters the blood circulation it is distributed throughout the body into various tissues, and the pharmacokinetic parameter is called the volume of distribution (V_d). This is the hypothetical volume to account for all drugs in the body, and is also termed the apparent volume of distribution:

$$V_d = \frac{\text{Dose}}{\text{Plasma concentration of drug}}$$

The amount of a drug that interacts with the receptor or target site is usually a small fraction of the total drug administered. Muscle and fat tissues may serve as a reservoir for lipophilic drugs. For neurotherapeutics, penetration of the blood—brain barrier is essential. Drugs usually undergo chemical transformation (metabolism) before elimination. Drug metabolism may occur in any tissue, including the blood — for example, plasma butylcholinesterase metabolizes drugs such as succinylcholine. The role of metabolism is to convert lipophilic non-polar molecules to water-soluble polar compounds for excretion in urine. Many drugs are metabolized in the liver in two phases by various enzymes, but cytochrome P450, a mixed function oxidase, is the major liver enzyme responsible for the metabolism of a majority of drugs in the Phase I step that involves manipulation of a functional group of a drug molecule in order to make the molecule more polar. The Phase II step may involve acetylation, sulfation, methylation, amino acid conjugation or glucuronidation in order to increase the polarity of the drug metabolite.

The half-life of a drug is the time required for the serum concentration to be reduced by 50%. The fraction of a drug remaining in the body after five half-lives is approximately 0.03% for administration of a single dosage of the drug, while for repeated dosages of a drug a steady state is reached after five to seven half-lives. Therapeutic drug monitoring is recommended when a drug reaches a steady state. The half-life of a drug can be calculated from the elimination rate constant (K) of a drug:

$$\text{Half-life} = 0.693/K$$

The elimination rate constant can be easily calculated from the serum concentrations of a drug at two different time points using the formula

$$K = \frac{\ln Ct_1 - \ln Ct_2}{t_2 - t_1}$$

where Ct_1 is the concentration of drug at time point t_1 and Ct_2 is the concentration of the same drug at a later time point t_2.

A drug may also undergo extensive metabolism before fully entering the blood circulation. This process is called first-pass metabolism. If a drug undergoes significant first-pass metabolism, then the drug may not be delivered orally — for example, lidocaine. Renal excretion is a major pathway for the elimination of drugs and their metabolites; therefore impaired renal function may cause accumulation of drugs and metabolites in serum, thus increasing the risk of adverse drug effects. Moreover, other pathological conditions such as liver disease, congestive heart failure and hypothyroidism may also decrease the clearance of drugs. Drugs may also be excreted via other routes, such as via the biliary tract. The factors which determine biliary elimination of a drug include chemical structure, polarity and molecular weight, as well as active transport sites within the liver cell membranes for that particular drug. A drug excreted in bile may also be reabsorbed from the gastrointestinal tract or a drug conjugate may be hydrolyzed by the bacteria of the gut, liberating the original drug, which can return to the blood circulation. Enterohepatic circulation may prolong the effects of a drug. Cholestatic disease, where normal bile flow is reduced, may reduce bile clearance of the drug, causing drug toxicity.

Genetic Variations in Drug Metabolism and Therapeutic Drug Monitoring

Genetic differences between patients may significantly alter drug metabolism. Drugs are metabolized by various enzymes in the body, including serum butylcholinesterase, thiopurine methyltransferase and *N*-acetyltransferase, but, most notably, by liver cytochrome P450 mixed-function oxidase, also known as the cytochrome P450 family of drug-metabolizing enzymes. The cytochrome P450 proteins (CYPs) comprise a large group of heme-containing monooxygenase proteins that are localized to the endoplasmic reticulum and mitochondrial membrane. NADPH (nicotinamide adenine dinucleotide phosphate) is a required cofactor for CYP-mediated biotransformation, and oxygen serves as a substrate. The CYP superfamily is found in many organisms, with over 7700 known members across all species studied. At present, 57 human genes are known to encode CYP isoforms; of these, at least 15 are associated with xenobiotic metabolism. The major CYP isoforms responsible for metabolism of drugs include CYP1A2, CYP2B6, CYP2C8, CYP2C9, CYP2C19, CYP2D6, CYP2E1 and CYP3A4/CYP3A5. However, CYP3A4 is the predominant isoform of the CYP family (almost 30%) usually responsible for the metabolism of approximately 37% of drugs, followed by CYP2C9 (17%), CYP2D6 (15%), CYP2C19 (10%), CYP1A2 (9%), CYP2C8 (6%) and CYP2B6 (4%). In addition to liver, CYP3A4 isoenzyme is also present in significant amounts in the epithelium of the gut. Therefore, orally administered drugs which are substrates of CYP3A4 may undergo significant metabolism before entering circulation. Examples of representative drugs that are metabolized by various isoforms of the cytochrome P450 family of enzymes are given in Table 1.3. These cytochrome enzymes show marked variation in different people. Some of these enzymes also exhibit genetic polymorphism (CYP2C19, CYP2D6), and a subset of the population may be deficient in enzyme activity (poor metabolizers). Therefore, if a drug is administered to a patient who is a poor metabolizer, drug

TABLE 1.3 Example of Representative Drugs that are Metabolized by Various Isoforms of the Cytochrome P450 Family of Enzymes

Isoform of cytochrome P450	Representative drugs metabolized by the enzyme
CYP3A4*	Alprazolam, atorvastatin, carbamazepine, clarithromycin, cyclosporine, diazepam, erythromycin, fentanyl, indinavir, ketoconazole, lidocaine, lovastatin, quinidine, ritonavir, tacrolimus, tamoxifen, verapamil
CYP1A1	Acetaminophen, clomipramine, clozapine, olanzapine, theophylline
CYP2C9	Glipizide, ibuprofen, nelfinavir, phenytoin, tolbutamide, warfarin
CYP2C19	Citalopram, imipramine, lansoprazole, omeprazole
CYP2D6	Clomipramine, codeine, desipramine, dextromethorphan, flecainide, fluoxetine, haloperidol, hydrocodone, imipramine, metoprolol, paroxetine
CYP2E1	Chlorzoxazone, halothane and variety of industrial toxins such as aniline and benzene; in alcohol abusers, CYP2E1 is also involved in metabolism of alcohol

Isoform represents highest amount of isoform in the cytochrome P450 family of drug-metabolizing enzymes and responsible for metabolism of majority of drugs metabolized via the cytochrome P450 family of enzymes.

toxicity may be observed even with a standard dose of the drug. Mutation of CYP2D6 affects the analgesic effect of codeine and tramadol [26]. Knowledge of the polymorphism of various cytochrome P450 enzymes is important for the management of patients receiving various anticancer drugs, including tamoxifen, docetaxel, paclitaxel, cyclophosphamide, ifosfamide, imatinib, irinotecan, etoposide, teniposide, thalidomide and vincristine [27].

Therapeutic drug monitoring is a phenotyping procedure and can be used to identify slow as well as fast metabolizers. However, a superior approach is pharmacogenomics testing, which is based on the utilization of genetic information data in pharmacotherapy and drug delivery, thus ensuring better drug efficacy and safety in patient management. The AmpliChip CYP450, which is capable of genotyping cytochrome P450 (CYP2D6 and CYP2C19) and predicts phenotypes for 27 CYP2D6 alleles, is the first FDA approved pharmacogenomics test [28]. This important topic is addressed in Chapter 6.

Effect of Gender Difference and Pregnancy on Drug Response and Metabolism

Men and women may show both pharmacokinetic and pharmacodynamic differences in response to certain drugs due to anatomical variation and different metabolism rates of specific drugs. Pregnancy may also significantly alter the disposition of a limited number of drugs. Gender difference affects bioavailability, distribution, metabolism and elimination of drugs due to variations between men and women in body weight, blood volume, gastric emptying time, drug protein binding, activities of drug-metabolizing enzymes, drug transporter function and excretion activity [29]. In general, the average male has higher body-weight, greater body surface area and total water content (both extracellular and intracellular) compared to the average female, causing differences in volumes of distribution of certain drugs − most notably lipophilic drugs. Although absorption of a drug is not different between the two genders, the absorption rate may be slightly slower in females. Hepatic metabolism of drugs by Phase I (via CYP1A2 and CYP2E1) and Phase II (by glucuronyl transferase, methyltransferases and dehydrogenases) reactions appears to be faster in males than females, although metabolism of drugs by CYP2C9, CYP2C19 and N-acetyltransferase, or clearance of drugs which are substrates for P-glycoprotein, appear to be similar in both males and females. Women usually have higher activity of CYP3A4 [30]. Gallagher *et al.* reported gender difference in UDP-glucuronosyltransferase (UGT) activity, where men exhibited a fourfold higher level of expression of the UGT2B family of genes, especially UGT2B17, than women. Therefore, men have a higher amount of UGT2B17 glucuronidation activity than women, which may lead to significant gender variation in metabolism of steroid hormones, carcinogens, cancer chemotherapy agents and addictive agents found in cigarettes [31]. Women also have high levels of sex hormones, and may take oral contraceptives which usually contain progesterone alone or in combination with estrogen (natural or synthetic). Both natural and synthetic estrogens and progesterones (including common ethinyl estradiol) are metabolized by CYP3A4 and may affect metabolism of certain drugs. Ethinyl estradiol in combination with other components of oral contraceptive preparations can reduce serum lamotrigine concentration by 50% [32]. Soldin and Mattison reviewed sex differences in the pharmacokinetics and pharmacodynamics of many commonly used drugs [33].

In general, women are also more susceptible to adverse effects of than men. Women are at increased risk of QT prolongation with many anti-arrhythmic drugs, which may even lead to critical conditions such as torsade de pointes compared to men even at the same levels of serum drug concentrations [34]. Other classes of drugs that may cause more adverse drug reactions in women compared to men include anesthetics, and antiretrovirals. Hormonal effects may be one of the underlying causes in the majority of adverse drug reactions observed in women [35]. Women are also more vulnerable to drug abuse than men, and gonadal hormone estrogen may facilitate drug abuse in women. In addition, phases of the menstrual cycle when estrogen levels are high are associated with enhanced effects of both cocaine and amphetamine [36]. Increased age and female gender are well-known risk factors for the development of desmopressin-induced hyponatremia. Juul et al. observed that at a dosage of 100 µg the decrease in serum sodium was more significant in women aged over 50 than men, and recommended a lower dosage (25 µg) in women compared to men (50–100 µg) [37]. However, women gain a greater effect of analgesia in pain management from opioid analgesics [38]. In addition, certain psychotropic drugs such as chlorpromazine, fluspirilene and various antipsychotic drugs appear to be more effective in women than in men for the same dosage [39].

Epidemiologic surveys have indicated that between one-third and two-thirds of all pregnant women will take at least one medication during pregnancy. Drug therapy in pregnant women usually focuses on potential teratogenic effects of drugs, and therapeutic drug monitoring during pregnancy aims to improve individual dosage, taking into account pregnancy-related changes in drug disposition [40]. Gastrointestinal absorption and bioavailability of many drugs vary in pregnancy due to changes in gastric secretion and small intestine motility. In addition, various pregnancy-related hemodynamic changes, such as an increase in cardiac output, blood volume, renal perfusion and glomerular filtration rate, may affect drug disposition and elimination of several drugs [41]. Elevated concentrations of various hormones in pregnancy, such as estrogen, progesterone, placental growth hormone and prolactin, could be related to altered drug metabolism observed in pregnant women [42]. The renal excretion of unchanged drugs is increased in pregnancy. In addition, the metabolism of drugs catalyzed by isoenzymes of cytochrome P450 (CYP3A4, CYP2D6 and CYP2C9) and uridine diphosphate glucuronosyltransferase (UGT1A4 and UFT2B7) are increased in pregnancy. Therefore, dosages of drugs that are metabolized by these enzymes may need to be increased during pregnancy in order to avoid loss of efficacy. In contrast, activities of some isoenzymes (CYP1A2 and CYP2C19) are reduced in pregnancy. Therefore, dosage reduction may be needed for drugs that are metabolized via these isoenzymes [43]. Increases in clearance of lamotrigine have been reported in pregnancy. Apparent clearance seems to increase steadily during pregnancy until it peaks at approximately week 32, when 330% increases in clearance from base line values can be observed [44]. Lower serum concentrations of lithium have been reported in pregnancy, and this may be related to an increase in the glomerular filtration rate. Reduced plasma concentration of both the antimalarial drug chloroquine and its active metabolite desethyl-chloroquine in pregnancy could compromise the curative efficacy and post-treatment prophylactic property of chloroquine in pregnant women [45]. In general, dosage adjustments are required for anticonvulsants, lithium, digoxin, certain beta blockers, ampicillin, cefuroxime and certain antidepressants in pregnant women. In addition, certain drugs such as tetracycline, antithyroid medications, coumarin anticoagulants, aspirin, indomethacin, opioids, barbiturates and phenothiazine may have unwanted effects in the fetus despite careful adjustment of maternal dosage of these drugs

TABLE 1.4   Gender Differences in the Effects of Some Representative Drugs

Drug	Comments
Acebutolol	Greater therapeutic effect in women due to higher blood levels, but women are also more susceptible to adverse drug reactions
Aspirin	Rate of absorption and clearance higher in women
Atenolol	Lower clearance in women than men
Cefazolin	Clearance increases in pregnancy
Ciprofloxacin	Clearance is lower in women
Clozapine	For similar dose, serum concentration higher in women than men
Diazepam	Plasma protein binding decreases during pregnancy
Digoxin	Clearance increases in pregnancy requiring more frequent administration
Erythromycin	Oral bioavailability may decrease in pregnant women
Lithium	Clearance increases during pregnancy
Metoprolol	Oral bioavailability decreases in pregnancy
Ofloxacin	Clearance in lower in women compared to men
Phenobarbital	Clearance increases during pregnancy
Prednisolone	Oral clearance and volume of distribution lower in women than men
Quinidine	Reduced plasma protein binding during pregnancy
Theophylline	Plasma protein binding decreases in pregnancy
Valproic acid	Plasma protein binding decreases during pregnancy
Warfarin	Free fraction higher in women than men

Source of data: Soldin and Mattison [33].

[46, 47]. Gender differences and the effect of pregnancy on metabolism of common drugs are listed in Table 1.4.

Effect of Age on Drug Response and Metabolism

In the fetus CYP3A7 is the major hepatic enzyme of the cytochrome P450 family of enzymes, but CYP3A5 may also present at significant levels in half of children. However, in adults CYP3A4 is the major functional cytochrome P450 enzyme responsible for metabolism of many drugs. CYP1A1 is also present during organogenesis, while CYP2E1 may be present in some second-trimester fetuses. After birth, hepatic CYP2D6, CYP2C8/9 and CYP2C18/19 are activated. CYP1A2 becomes active during the fourth to fifth months after birth [48]. Neonates and infants have increased total body water to body fat ratio compared to adults, whereas the reverse is observed in elderly people. These factors may affect the volume of distribution of drugs depending on their lipophilic character. Moreover, altered plasma binding of drugs may be observed in both neonates and some elderly people due to low albumin, thus increasing the fraction of pharmacologically active free drug. In general, the drug-metabolizing capacity of liver enzymes is reduced in newborns, particularly in premature babies, but increases rapidly during the first few weeks and months of life to reach values which are generally higher than adult metabolizing rates and then decline with old age. Renal function at the time of birth is reduced by more than 50% compared with adults but then increases rapidly in the first 2—3 years of life; it does, however, start declining with advanced age. Oral clearance of lamotrigine, topiramate, levetiracetam, oxcarbazepine, gabapentin, tiagabine, zonisamide, vigabatrin and felbamate is significantly higher (by 20—120%) in children compared to adults, depending on the drug and the age distribution of the patients. On the other hand, clearance of these drugs is reduced (by 10—50%) in the elderly population compared to middle-aged adults [49]. Zakrzewski-Jakubiak *et al.* reported that elderly patients are at higher risk of adverse drug reactions because most elderly patients receive multiple drugs and thus have an increased risk of pharmacokinetic drug interactions. The authors demonstrated the utility of InterMED-Rx software, a new cytochrome P450-based software that is capable of identifying elderly patients who are at risk of pharmacokinetic drug interactions as well as facilitating interventions aimed at reducing adverse drug events [50].

Premature infants may also metabolize a drug differently to adults; for example, only unchanged theophylline and caffeine is found in the urine of premature neonates, indicating the oxidative pathways for theophylline metabolism. In contrast, in children and adults 3-methylxanthine and 1,3-dimethyl uric acid are the major metabolites of theophylline recovered in the urine [51].

Drug Disposition in Uremia

Renal disease causes impairment in the clearance of many drugs by the kidney. Correlations have been established between creatinine clearance and clearance of digoxin, lithium, procainamide, aminoglycoside and several other drugs, but creatinine clearance does not always predict renal excretion of all drugs. Moreover, elderly patients may have unrecognized renal impairment, and thus caution should be exercised when prescribing medications to these patients. Serum creatinine remains normal until the GFR (glomerular filtration rate) has fallen by at least 50%. Nearly half of older patients have normal serum creatinine but reduced renal function. Dose adjustments based on renal function are recommended for many medications in elderly patients, even for medications that exhibit large therapeutic windows [52]. Renal disease also causes impairment of drug protein binding because uremic toxins compete with drugs for binding to albumin. Such interaction leads to increases in pharmacologically active free drug concentration, especially for classical anticonvulsants such as phenytoin, carbamazepine and valproic acid. Therefore, monitoring of free phenytoin, free valproic acid and to some extent free carbamazepine is recommended in uremic patients in order to avoid drug toxicity [53]. However, chronic renal failure can also significantly reduce non-renal clearance of many drugs, and drugs that are metabolized by Phase II reactions and drug transporter proteins such as P-glycoprotein and organic anion transporting polypeptide. High amounts of circulating uremic toxins, cytokines and parathyroid hormones are probably responsible for such reductions in clearance of these drugs, thus increasing the possibility of adverse drug reactions in uremic patients [54]. Animal studies have demonstrated significant downregulation (40−85%) of hepatic and intestinal metabolism mediated by cytochrome P450 enzymes in chronic renal failure [55]. Nolin *et al.* demonstrated that in patients with uremia, non-renal clearance of fexofenadine can be decreased up to 63% compared to controls. Moreover, there was a 2.8-fold increase in the area under the plasma concentration curve of fexofenadine in uremic patients compared to healthy subjects used as the control group. However, clearance of midazolam was not affected, indicating that function of CYP3A4 was not altered in patients with uremia. The authors further observed that the changes in hepatocytes and enterocyte protein expression were consistent with reduced clearance of fexofenadine, which is cleared through the activity of drug transport protein [56].

Drug Disposition in Hepatic Disease

Liver dysfunction not only reduces clearance of a drug metabolized through hepatic enzymes or the biliary mechanism but also affects plasm protein binding due to reduced synthesis of albumin and other drug-binding proteins. Even mild to moderate hepatic disease may cause an unpredictable effect on drug metabolism. Portal-systemic shunting present in patients with advanced liver cirrhosis may cause a significant reduction in first-pass metabolism of high extraction drugs, thus increasing bioavailability as well as the risk of drug overdose and toxicity [57]. In addition, activities of several isoenzymes of cytochrome P450 enzymes (CYP1A1, CYP2C19 and CYP3A4/5) are reduced due to liver dysfunction while activities of other isoenzymes such as CYP2D6, CYP2C9 and CYP2E1 may not be affected significantly. Therefore, drugs that are metabolized by CYP1A1, CYP3A4/5 and CYP2C19 may show increased blood levels in patients with hepatic dysfunction requiring dosage adjustment in order to avoid toxicity [58]. Although the Phase I reaction involving cytochrome P450 enzymes may be impaired in liver disease the Phase II reaction (glucuronidation) seems to be affected to a lesser extent, although both Phase I and Phase II reactions in drug metabolism are substantially impaired in patients with advanced cirrhosis. At this point there is no universally accepted endogenous marker to access hepatic impairment and a semi-quantitative Child-Pugh score is frequently used to determine the severity of hepatic dysfunction and thus dosage adjustments, although there are limitations to this approach [57]. Non-alcoholic fatty liver disease is the most common chronic liver disease. This type of liver disease also affects the activity of drug metabolizing enzymes in the liver, with the potential to produce adverse drug reactions from standard dosage [59].

Mild to moderate hepatitis infection may also alter the clearance of drugs. Trotter *et al.* reported that the total mean tacrolimus dose in year one after transplant was lower by 39% in patients with hepatitis C compared to patients with no hepatitis C infection [60]. Zimmermann *et al.* reported that the oral dose clearance of sirolimus was significantly decreased in subjects with mild to moderate hepatic impairment compared to controls, and the authors stressed the need for careful monitoring of trough whole blood sirolimus concentrations in renal transplant recipients exhibiting mild to moderate hepatic impairment [61]. Wyles and Gerber reviewed the effect of hepatitis with hepatic dysfunction on antiretroviral therapy, especially HAART (highly active antiretroviral therapy) in patients suffering from AIDS, and commented that the dosage of protease inhibitors indinavir, lopinavir, ritonavir, amprenavir and atazanavir may require reduction in patients with liver disease although hepatic dysfunction does not affect pharmacokinetics of nucleoside-reverse transcriptase inhibitors (NRTI) because these drugs are not metabolized by liver enzymes [62]. Ho *et al.* reported two novel genetic variations in the promotor sequence of CYP2D6 gene 1822A→G and 1740C→T in patients infected with hepatitis C that are associated with a lower activity of the CYP2D6 enzyme which is responsible for the metabolism of many drugs. Therefore, patients infected with the hepatis C virus may be at risk of drug toxicity and adverse drug reactions from drugs that are metabolized via CYP2D6 [63].

Hypoalbuminemia is often observed in patients with hepatic dysfunction which impairs the protein binding of many drugs. Because free (unbound) drugs are responsible for pharmacological action, careful monitoring of free concentrations of strongly albumin-bound anti-epileptic drugs such as phenytoin, carbamazepine and valproic acid is recommended in patients with hepatic dysfunction in order to avoid drug toxicity [53] (see Chapter 4 for more detail).

Cardiovascular Disease and Drug Disposition

Cardiac failure is often associated with disturbances in cardiac output, influencing the extent and pattern of tissue perfusion, sodium and water metabolism and gastrointestinal motility that eventually may affect the absorption and disposition of many drugs. Hepatic elimination of drugs via oxidative Phase I metabolism is impaired in patients with congestive heart failure due to decreased blood supply in the liver [64]. Theophylline metabolism is reduced in patients with severe cardiac failure, and dose reduction is strongly recommended. Digoxin clearance is also decreased. Quinidine plasma level may also be high in these patients due to a lower volume of distribution [65]. Therefore, therapeutic drug monitoring is crucial in avoiding drug toxicity in these patients. Physiological changes in critically ill patients can significantly affect the pharmacokinetics of many drugs. These changes include absorption, distribution, metabolism and excretion of drugs in critically ill patients. Understanding these changes in pharmacokinetic parameters is essential for optimizing drug therapy in critically ill patients. Norgard and Prescott commented that genetic biomarkers may play an important role in predicting a heart-failure patient's response to therapy, as well as susceptibility to an adverse drug reaction [66].

Thyroid Dysfunction and Drug Disposition

Patients with thyroid disease may have an altered drug disposition because thyroxine is a potent activator of the cytochrome P450 enzyme system. Therefore, lower levels of drugs may result from high thyroxine levels due to induction of the hepatic oxidative metabolism pathway. In contrast, hypothyroidism is associated with inhibition of hepatic oxidative metabolism of many drugs. Hypothyroidism also affects the metabolism of immunosuppressants. Haas *et al.* reported a case where a patient developed hypothyroidism 6 months after single lung transplantation and was admitted to the hospital for anuric renal failure. The patient showed a toxic blood level of tacrolimus, which was resolved with the initiation of thyroxine replacement therapy and dose reduction of tacrolimus [67]. Therapeutic drug monitoring of immunosuppressants can thus aid in avoiding such drug toxicity. Amiodarone is a potent anti-arrhythmic drug associated with thyroid dysfunction because, due to high iodine content, amiodarone inhibits 5-deiodinase activity. Although most patients treated with amiodarone remain euthyroid, amiodarone-induced thyrotoxicosis or amiodarone-induced hypothyroidism may occur depending on the iodine status of the patient as well as the history of prior thyroid disease. Screening for thyroid disease before amiodarone therapy and periodic monitoring of thyroid functions are recommended for patients treated with amiodarone [68]. Burk *et al.* reported that thyroid abnormalities can exert significant effects on the expression of P-glycoprotein, thereby altering the disposition and efficacy of drugs that are substrates for it. In hypothyroidism, digoxin clearance was significantly reduced, whereas bioavailability, volume of distribution, half-life and protein binding were unaltered, as reported by these investigators [69].

THERAPEUTIC DRUG MONITORING OF VARIOUS DRUG CLASSES

Usually, the concentration of a therapeutic drug is measured in the serum or plasma. However, whole blood concentrations of immunosuppressant drugs such as cyclosporine and tacrolimus are usually measured for therapeutic drug monitoring. Obtaining blood for measurement of a drug during the absorption or the distribution phase may lead to misleading information. Moreover, in order to measure the peak concentration of a drug, timing of the sample should depend on the route of administration. After intravenous administration, the peak concentration of a drug may be achieved in a few minutes. The trough concentration is clinically defined as the serum drug concentration just prior to the next dose. Usually trough concentrations are monitored for most drugs, but for aminoglycosides and vancomycin both peak and trough concentrations are monitored. For a meaningful interpretation of a serum drug concentration, time of specimen collection should be noted along with the time and date of the last dose and route of administration of the drug. This is particularly important for aminoglycoside because without knowing the time of specimen collection, the serum drug concentration cannot be interpreted. Information needed for the proper interpretation of drug levels for the purpose of therapeutic drug monitoring is listed in Table 1.5.

Usually, therapeutic drug monitoring is useful after a drug reaches its steady state. It generally takes at least five half-lives after initiation of drug therapy to reach the steady state. For example, the half-life of digoxin is 1.6 days. A steady state of digoxin is reached after 7 days of therapy with digoxin, but it may take 3 weeks to reach the steady state for a renally compromised patient. However, for a drug with a shorter half-life than digoxin, such as valproic acid (half-life 11—17 hours), it takes only 3 days to reach the steady state. Collection of specimens for digoxin monitoring is difficult because digoxin exhibits a long distribution phase as well as a lag in the time between dosing and pharmacological response to digoxin. Therefore, specimens for digoxin measurement should be collected no earlier than 6—8 hours after dosing, and preferably after 12 hours. Specimens collected before the distribution phase is complete often demonstrate elevated digoxin concentrations that may confuse clinicians, as digoxin toxicity may not be experienced at such elevated concentrations because these concentrations represent peak rather than trough concentrations. In one extensive study involving 666 institutions and 18 675 toxic digoxin results, the authors demonstrated that

TABLE 1.5 Information Required for Interpretation of Results of Therapeutic Drug Monitoring

Patient-related information required on the request:

Name of patient

Hospital identification number

Age

Gender (if female, pregnant?*)

Ethnicity*

Other essential information:

Time of last dosage

Duration of the therapy*

Type of and number of specimen (serum, whole blood, urine, saliva, other body fluid)

Identification of peak versus trough specimen (for aminoglycosides and vancomycin only)

Special request (such as free phenytoin)

Reason to request therapeutic drug monitoring* (routine monitoring, lack of response, suspected toxicity)

Essential information needed for interpretation of result:

Dosage regimen

Other drugs the patient is receiving

Concentration of the drug as determined by the laboratory, and type of assay used (immunoassay versus chromatography)

Pharmacokinetic parameters of the drug

Is the patient critically ill or suffering from hepatic, cardiovascular or renal disease?

Albumin level, creatinine clearance

Optional information.

for every five specimens for which toxic concentrations were obtained, three were inappropriately collected with respect to the dosing interval [70].

Pre-analytical errors can contribute significantly to an erroneous result for therapeutic drug monitoring. For example, although most drugs can be monitored in serum or plasma, for cyclosporine, tacrolimus, sirolimus and everolimus EDTA (ethylenediamine tetraacetic acid) whole blood is the preferred specimen. Collecting the specimen in a serum separator tube may affect the concentration of a few therapeutic drugs. The effect of pre-analytical variables on therapeutic drug monitoring is addressed in Chapter 2.

Frequently and Less Frequently Monitored Anticonvulsants

Phenytoin, phenobarbital, primidone, ethosuximide, valproic acid and carbamazepine are considered to be conventional anticonvulsant drugs. All of these anti-epileptic drugs have a narrow therapeutic range. Phenytoin, carbamazepine and valproic acid are strongly bound to serum proteins. Therapeutic monitoring of all classical anticonvulsants is essential for optimal patient management. In addition, for selected patient populations monitoring of free phenytoin, free valproic acid and free carbamazepine is clinically useful. However, free phenobarbital monitoring is not required because this drug is only moderately bound to serum protein. For routine therapeutic drug monitoring of classical immunoassays there are many commercially available immunoassays which can be easily adopted on various automated analyzers. Fourteen new AED drugs have been approved since 1993 – eslicarbazepine acetate, felbamate, gabapentin, lacosamide, lamotrigine, levetiracetam, oxcarbazepine, pregabalin, rufinamide, stiripentol, tiagabine, topiramate, vigabatrin and zonisamide. In general, these anti-epileptic drugs have better pharmacokinetic profiles and improved tolerability in patients, and are less involved in drug interactions compared to traditional anticonvulsants; however, felbamate is a very toxic drug which may cause fatal aplastic anemia and its use is reserved for the few patients where the benefit may override the risk. Therapeutic drug monitoring of some of these new anticonvulsants is not needed, although some of these drugs are less frequently monitored and such tests are mostly available in large medical centers, academic medical centers and large national reference laboratories. In addition, reference ranges for many of these newer anticonvulsants have not been established clearly. In general, gabapentin, pregabalin, tiagabine and vigabatrin are not good candidates for therapeutic drug monitoring. Therapeutic drug monitoring of levetiracetam and pregabalin is justified in patients with renal impairment. Monitoring the active metabolite of oxcarbazepine (10-hydroxycarbazepine) has some justification. Usually, chromatographic techniques are employed for therapeutic drug monitoring of these newer anticonvulsants. These methods are generally free from interference. However, there are commercially available immunoassays for lamotrigine, zonisamide and topiramate. See Chapter 10 for a more in-depth discussion of therapeutic drug monitoring of classical and newer anticonvulsants.

Frequently and Less Frequently Monitored Cardioactive Drugs

Therapeutic drug monitoring of several cardioactive drugs, including digoxin, lidocaine, procainamide and quinidine, is routinely performed in clinical laboratories due to the established correlation between serum drug concentrations and pharmacological response of these drugs. Moreover, drug toxicity can mostly be avoided by therapeutic drug monitoring. Digoxin is one of the most frequently ordered drugs among all cardioactive drugs in the clinical laboratory. This drug has a narrow therapeutic window, and immunoassays employed in monitoring serum digoxin concentration are subjected to interference from both exogenous and endogenous compounds. Less frequently monitored cardioactive drugs include tocainide, flecainide, mexiletine, verapamil, propranolol and amiodarone. Tocainide was developed as an oral analog of lidocaine because lidocaine cannot be administered orally due to high first-pass metabolism, but tocainide and lidocaine have similar electrophysiological properties. Challenges in therapeutic drug monitoring of digoxin and other cardioactive drugs are discussed in Chapter 11.

Frequently Monitored Anti-Asthmatic Drugs

Theophylline and caffeine are two anti-asthmatic drugs that require therapeutic drug monitoring. Theophylline is a bronchodilator and respiratory stimulant effective in the treatment of acute and chronic asthma. The drug is readily absorbed after oral absorption, but peak concentration may be observed much later with sustained-release tablets. The therapeutic range of theophylline is 10–20 µg/mL, and adverse reactions may be observed at concentrations exceeding 20 µg/mL [71]. Theophylline is metabolized by hepatic cytochrome P450, and altered pharmacokinetics of theophylline in disease states has been reported. Clearance of theophylline is slow in neonates compared to adults, while theophylline metabolism is also altered in hepatic disease. Acute viral illness associated with fever may prolong the half-life of theophylline [72]. Patients with pneumonia and episodes of severe airways obstruction also may metabolize theophylline slowly [73]. Theophylline is metabolized by CYP1A2, and smoking induces theophylline metabolism. In one study, the half-life of theophylline was reduced by almost two-fold in smokers compared to non-smokers [74]. Lee *et al.* reported that theophylline clearance was increased by 51.1% and steady state serum concentrations were reduced by 24.5% in children who were exposed to passive smoking [75]. Because the half-life of theophylline varies from 3 to 12 hours a steady state can be quickly reached in 2–3 days after initiation of therapy, when therapeutic drug monitoring can be conducted. Protein binding of theophylline varies from 55–65%; therefore, free drug monitoring is not required. Although trough specimens are recommended for therapeutic drug monitoring, a specimen can be drawn 1–4 hours after administration or immediately if toxic symptoms such as seizure are observed. Theophylline toxicity may be encountered just above the upper end of the therapeutic concentration of 20 µg/mL [76].

Apnea with or without bradycardia is a common medical problem in premature infants. Caffeine is effective in treating apnea in neonates. Because effectiveness of caffeine therapy can readily be observed clinically, therapeutic drug monitoring of caffeine is only indicated when caffeine toxicity is apparent from clinical symptoms, including tachycardia, gastrointestinal intolerance and jitteriness. In addition, therapeutic drug monitoring of caffeine is also indicated if a neonate is unresponsive to caffeine therapy despite a high dose. Caffeine can be administered once daily in neonates due to its long half-life. Caffeine can be monitored either in serum or plasma, using an immunoassay or a chromatographic method. Caffeine has a wider therapeutic index, and although some investigators suggested a therapeutic range of caffeine as high as 26–40 µg/mL, severe life-threatening toxicity usually occurs at concentrations of 346 µg/mL or higher although a caffeine serum level exceeding 50 µg/mL should be considered as a critical value [76]. Natarajan *et al.* commented that a majority of preterm babies attain plasma caffeine levels of 5–15 µg/mL independent of gestation, and therapeutic drug monitoring of caffeine in neonates is not necessary [77].

Frequently and Less Frequently Monitored Antidepressants

Tricyclic antidepressants (TCAs), including amitriptyline, doxepin, nortriptyline, imipramine, desipramine, protriptyline, trimipramine and clomipramine, were introduced in the 1950s and 1960s. These drugs have a narrow therapeutic window, and therapeutic drug monitoring is essential for their efficacy as well as to avoid drug toxicity. The efficacy of lithium in acute mania and for prophylaxis against recurrent episodes of mania has been well established. Blood concentrations of lithium have been shown to parallel total body water and brain concentrations of lithium. Therapeutic drug monitoring of lithium is essential for efficacy as well as to avoid lithium toxicity. More recently introduced antidepressants are selective serotonin reuptake inhibitors (SSRIs) — for example, citalopram, fluoxetine, fluvoxamine, paroxetine and sertraline. This class of drugs has a wide therapeutic index. Usually most of these drugs do not require routine therapeutic drug monitoring, but some drugs may benefit from infrequent monitoring especially in certain patient populations. Hiemke *et al.* commented that patient populations that may benefit from therapeutic drug monitoring in psychiatry include children, pregnant women, elderly patients, individuals with intelligence disabilities, forensic patients, and patients with known or suspected genetically determined pharmacokinetic abnormalities [78]. Challenges in therapeutic drug monitoring of classical antidepressants and newer antidepressants are discussed in Chapter 13.

Frequently Monitored Immunosuppressants

Whole blood concentrations of cyclosporine, tacrolimus, sirolimus and everolimus and serum or plasma concentrations of mycophenolic acid are routinely determined in clinical laboratories in order to avoid drug toxicity as well as subtherapeutic levels of these drugs that may lead to organ rejection. Although immunoassays are commercially available for therapeutic drug monitoring of these drugs, the immunoassays are subject to various interferences, most notably from metabolites of individual immunosuppressants. Therefore, chromatographic methods, especially liquid chromatography combined with mass spectrometry or tandem mass spectrometry, are considered the gold standard for therapeutic drug monitoring of immunosuppressants. Therapeutic drug monitoring of immunosuppressant drugs is discussed in detail in Chapter 15.

Frequently and Less Frequently Monitored Antibiotics

The aminoglycoside antibiotics consist of two or more amino sugars joined by a glycosidic linkage to a hexose or aminocyclitol. Streptomycin was the first aminoglycoside discovered, in 1914. These drugs are used in the treatment of serious and often life-threatening systemic infections. However, aminoglycoside can produce serious nephrotoxicity and ototoxicity. Aminoglycosides are poorly absorbed from the gastrointestinal tract, and these drugs are administered intravenously or intramuscularly. Children have a higher clearance of aminoglycosides. Patients with cystic fibrosis usually exhibit altered pharmacokinetics of antibiotics. After a conventional dose of an aminoglycoside, a patient with cystic fibrosis shows a lower serum concentration compared to a patient not suffering from cystic fibrosis. For these reasons, therapeutic drug monitoring of aminoglycosides is essential. Therapeutic drug monitoring is also frequently employed during vancomycin therapy. The drug is excreted in the urine with no metabolism. However, there are other antibiotics which are monitored infrequently. Examples of less frequently monitored antibiotics include ciprofloxacin, chloramphenicol, isoniazid, rifampin and rifabutin. Roberts *et al.* commented that although to date the clinical outcome benefits of systematic therapeutic drug monitoring of antimicrobials have only been demonstrated for aminoglycosides, the increasing cost of pharmaceuticals as well as emerging data on pharmacokinetic variabilities of antimicrobials suggest that benefits of therapeutic drug monitoring are likely for some other antimicrobial agents [79]. Therapeutic drug monitoring of aminoglycosides, vancomycin and other antibiotics is discussed in Chapter 12.

Less Frequently Monitored Drugs: Antiretroviral Agents

Human immunodeficiency virus (HIV) is the virus that causes AIDS (Acquired Immunodeficiency Syndrome). Six classes of drugs are used today to treat people with AIDS: nucleoside reverse transcriptase inhibitors (NRTIs) such as zidovudine; non-nucleoside reverse transcriptase inhibitors (NNRTIs), which include nevirapine, delavirdine, and efavirenz; protease inhibitors (PIs) saquinavir, ritonavir, indinavir, nelfinavir, amprenavir, lopinavir and atazanavir; entry inhibitors such as maraviroc; fusion inhibitors such as enfuvirtide; and integrase inhibitors such as raltegravir. Although some antiretroviral agents do not require therapeutic drug monitoring, patients receiving protease inhibitors and certain other retroviral agents may benefit from therapeutic drug monitoring. Currently, there is no commercially available immunoassay for any antiretroviral agent. Therefore, therapeutic drug monitoring for these drugs is only available in major academic medical centers and reference laboratories. See Chapter 16 for discussion on therapeutic drug monitoring of these drugs.

Frequently and Less Frequently Monitored Antineoplastic Drugs

Methotrexate is a competitive inhibitor of dihydrofolate reductase, a key enzyme for the biosynthesis of nucleic acid. The cytotoxic activity of this drug was discovered in 1955. The use of leucovorin to rescue normal host cells has permitted higher doses of methotrexate therapy in clinical practice. Methotrexate is used in the treatment of acute lymphoblastic leukemia (ALL), brain tumors, carcinomas of the lung and other cancers. Most toxicities of this drug are related to serum concentrations and pharmacokinetic parameters. Methotrexate is also approved for the treatment of refractory rheumatoid arthritis. Usually, low doses of methotrexate are used for treating rheumatoid arthritis (5−25 mg once weekly). Although therapeutic drug monitoring of methotrexate is not indicated in patients receiving low-dose methotrexate for rheumatoid arthritis, such monitoring is essential during high-dose treatment with methotrexate because of frequent adverse reactions leading to leukopenia and thrombocytopenia.

Pharmacokinetic studies showed that clinical response as well as toxicity of 5-fluorouracil are related to AUC (area under the curve). Individual dosage adjustments based on pharmacokinetic monitoring lead to a higher response rate of this drug as well as survival rates associated with tolerability. Although it is less frequently monitored than methotrexate, there are benefits of therapeutic drug monitoring of 5-fluorouracil. Sedar *et al.* described a liquid chromatography combined with tandem mass spectrometric method for determination of 5-fluorouracil and its metabolite dihydrofluorouracil, to ascertain the activity of dihydropyrimidine dehydrogenase which determines toxicity from 5-fluorouracil. Patients who are deficient in this enzyme, which is responsible for catabolism of 5-fluorouracil, are at increased risk of toxicity from this drug [80].

There is a wide interpatient variability in drug response and toxicity to standard doses of many anticancer medications due to polymorphism of genes encoding drug-metabolizing enzymes, receptors and drug transporters. The potential for applying pharmacogenetic screening before cancer chemotherapy may have applications with several anticancer agents. The goal of pharmacogenomics testing in patients receiving anticancer drugs is to identify genetic polymorphisms that predispose patients to an adverse drug reaction or non-response [81]. This topic is discussed in Chapter 14.

CONCLUSIONS

Therapeutic drug monitoring is required for a small fraction of drugs used in pharmacotherapy, but for these drugs such monitoring is essential in order to achieve maximum efficacy of the drug as well as to avoid drug toxicity. Therapeutic drug monitoring is also useful in avoiding adverse drug events. Currently, the old approach of therapeutic drug monitoring for avoiding drug toxicity needs to be revised due to new developments in information technology, new analytical procedures for less frequently monitored drugs, and new clinical pharmacological expert opinions in the presentation of laboratory medicine results. Today, therapeutic drug monitoring can be used to prevent an adverse drug reaction rather than confirming the cause of an existing adverse drug reaction. Therefore, blood should be drawn for therapeutic drug monitoring after the pharmacokinetic steady state has been reached (five times the elimination half-life of the drug) after administration of low to moderate dosage under the intended poly-medication if the patient is considered not to belong to the normal patient population. The benefits of therapeutic drug monitoring include significant cost saving because hospitalization will be shortened for the patient, and avoidance of expensive diagnosis and treatment of an adverse drug event [82].

References

[1] Gu Q, Fillon CF, Burt VL. Prescription Drug Use Continues to Increase: US Prescription Drug Data for 2007—2008. NCHS data brief no 42, September 2010. Atlanta, GA: US Department of Health and Human Services, Center for Disease Control and Prevention National Center for Health Statistics; 2010.
[2] Watson I, Potter J, Yatscoff R, et al. Editorial. Ther Drug Monit 1997;19:125.
[3] Ratanajamit C, Kaewpibal P, Setthawacharavanich S, Faroongsarng D. Effect of pharmacist participation in the health care team on therapeutic drug monitoring utilization for antiepileptic drugs. J Med Assoc Thai 2009;92:1500—7.
[4] Ramasamy K, Narayan SK, Chanolean S, Chandrasekaran A. Severe phenytoin toxicity in a CYP2C9*3*3 homozygous mutant in India. Neurol India 2007;55:408—9.
[5] Peterson GM, Khoo BH, von Witt RJ. Clinical response in epilepsy in relation to total and free serum levels of phenytoin. Ther Drug Monit 1991;13:415—9.
[6] Mattson RH, Cramer JA, Collins JF. Aspects of compliance: taking drugs and keeping clinic appointments. Epilepsy Res (Suppl) 1988;1:111—7.
[7] Dowser R, Futter WT. Outpatient compliance with theophylline and phenytoin therapy. S Afr Med J 1991;80:550—3.
[8] Chandra RS, Dalvi SS, Karnad PD, et al. Compliance monitoring in epileptic patients. J Assoc Physicians India 1993;41:431—2.

[9] Reis M, Akerblad AC, Ekselius L, von Knorring L. Partial compliance as determined from plasma levels of sertraline and its metabolite in depressed patients in primary care. J Clin Psychopharmacol 2010;30:746–8.

[10] Stieffenhofer V, Hiemke C. Pharmacogenetics, therapeutic drug monitoring and non-compliance [in German]. Ther Umsch 2010;67:309–15.

[11] Spear BB, Health-Chiozzi M, Huff J. Clinical application of pharmacogenetics. Trends Mol Med 2001;7:201–4.

[12] Lazarou J, Pomeranz BH, Corey PN. Incidence of adverse drug reactions in hospitalized patients: a meta-analysis of prospective studies. J Am Med Assoc 1998;279:1200–5.

[13] Billaud EM, Antoine C, Berge M, et al. Management of metabolic cytochrome P450 3A4 drug–drug interaction between everolimus and azole antifungals in a renal transplant patient. Clin Drug Investig 2009;29:481–6.

[14] Gulbis AM, Culotta KS, Jones RB, Andersson BS. Busulfan and metronidazole: an often forgotten but significant drug intearction. Ann Pharmacother 2011;45:e39.

[15] Jannetto PJ, Bratanow NC. Pain managemnt in the 21st century: utilization of pharamcogenomics and therapeutic drug monitoring. Expert Opin Drug Metab Toxicol 2011;7:745–52.

[16] Patel MX, Bowskill S, Couchman L, et al. Plasma olanzapine in relation to prescribed dose and other factors: data from a therapeutic drug monitoring service. J Clin Psychopharmacol 1999–2009;31:411–7.

[17] Slaughter RL, Cappelletty DM. Economic impact of aminoglycoside toxicity and its prevention through therapeutic drug monitoring. Pharmacoeconomics 1998;14:385–94.

[18] Crist KD, Nahata MC, Ety J. Positive impact of a therapeutic drug monitoring program on total aminoglycoside dose and cost of hospitalization. Ther Drug Monit 1987;9:306–10.

[19] Roberts JA, Ulldemolins M, Roberts MS, et al. Therapeutic drug monitoring of beta-lactams in crtitically ill patients: proof of concept. Intl J Antimicrob Agents 2010;36:332–9.

[20] Ried LD, Horn JR, McKenna DA. Therapeutic drug monitoring reduces toxic drug reactions; a meta-analysis. Ther Drug Monit 1990;12:72–8.

[21] Levine B, Cohen SS, Birmingham PH. Effect of pharmacist intervention on the use of serum drug assays. Am J Hosp Pharm 1981;38:845–51.

[22] Muller MJ, Regenbogen B, Hartter S, et al. Therapeutic drug monitoring for optimizing amisulpride therapy in patients with schizophrenia. J Psychiatr Res 2007;41:673–9.

[23] Babalik A, Babalik A, Mannix S, et al. Therapeutic drug monitoring in the treatment of active tuberculosis. Can Respir J 2011;18:225–9.

[24] Wang J, Kou H, Fu Q, et al. Nevirapine plasma concentrations are associated with virologic response and hepatotoxicity in Chinese patients with HIV infection. PLoS One 2011;6:e26739.

[25] van Hoogdalem E, de Boer AG, Breimer DD. Pharmacokinetics of rectal drug administration, Part I: General considerations and clinical applications of centrally active drugs. Clin Pharmacokinet 1991;21:11–26.

[26] Rollason V, Samer C, Piguet V, et al. Pharmacogenomics of analgesics: toward the individualization of prescription. Pharmacogenomics 2008;9:905–33.

[27] van Schaik RH. CYP450 pharmacogenetics for personalized cancer therapy. Drug Resist Update 2008;11:77–98.

[28] de Leon J. Amplichip CYP450 test: personalized medicine has arrived in psychiatry. Expert Rev Mol Diagn 1006;6:277–286.

[29] Gandhi M, Aweeka F, Greenblatt RM, Blaschke TE. Sex difference in pharmacokinetics and pharmacodynamics. Annu Rev Pharmacol Toxicol 2004;44:499–523.

[30] Schwartz JB. The influence of sex on pharmacokinetics. Clin Pharmacokinet 2003;42:107–21.

[31] Gallagher CJ, Balliet RM, Sun D, et al. Sex difference in UDP-glucuronosyltransferase 2B17 expression and activity. Drug Metab Dispos 2010;38:2204–9.

[32] Noe KH. Gender specific challenges in the management of epilepsy in women. Semin Neurol 2007;27:331–9.

[33] Soldin OP, Mattison DR. Sex differences in pharmacokinetics and pharmacodynamics. Clin Pharmacokinet 2009;48:143–57.

[34] Makkar RR, Fromm BS, Steinman RT, et al. Female gender as a risk factor for torsade de pointes associated with cardiovascular drugs. J Am Med Assoc 1993;270:2590–7.

[35] Nicolson TJ, Mellor HR, Roberts RR. Gender difference in drug toxicity. Trends Pharmacol Sci 2010;31:108–14.

[36] Anker JJ, Caroll ME. Females are more vulnerable to drug abuse than males: evidence from preclinical studies and the role of ovarian hormones. Curr Top Behav Neurosci 2011;8:73–96.

[37] Juul KV, Klein BM, Sandstrom R, et al. Gender difference in antidiuretic response to desmopressin. Am J Physiol Renal Physiol 2011;300:F1116–1122.

[38] Dillingim RB, Gear RW. Sex difference in opioid analgesia: clinical and experimental findings. Eur J Pain 2004;8:413—25.

[39] Rademaker M. Do women have more adverse drug reactions? Am J Clin Dermatol 2001;2:349—51.

[40] Loebstein R, Koren G. Clinical relevance of therapeutic drug monitoring during pregnancy. Ther Drug Monit 2002;24:15—22.

[41] Pavek P, Ceckova M, Staud F. Variation of drug kinetics in pregnancy. Curr Drug Metab 2009;10:520—9.

[42] Jeong H. Altered drug metabolism during pregnancy: hormonal regulation of drug metabolizing enzymes. Expert Opin Drug Metab Toxicol 2010;6:689—99.

[43] Anderson GD. Pregnancy induced changes in pharmacokinetics: a mechanistic based approach. Clin Pharmacokinet 2005;44:989—1008.

[44] Pennell PB, Newport DJ, Stowe ZN, et al. The impact of pregnancy and childbirth on the metabolism of lamotrigine. Neurology 2004;27:292—5.

[45] Karunajeewa HA, Salman S, Muller I, et al. Pharmacokinetics of chloroquine and desethylchloroquine in pregnancy. Antimicrob Agents Chemother 2010;54:1186—92.

[46] Hodge LS, Tracey TS. Alterations in drug disposition during pregnancy: implications for drug therapy. Expert Opin Drug Metab Toxicol 2007;3:557—71.

[47] Mucklow JC. The fate of drugs in pregnancy. Clin Obstet Gynecol 1986;13:161—75.

[48] Oesterheld JR. A review of developmental aspects of cytochrome P450. J Child Adolesc Psychopharmacol 1998;8:161—74.

[49] Perucca E. Pharmacokinetics variability of new antiepileptic drugs at different ages. Ther Drug Monit 2005;27:714—7.

[50] Zakrzewski-Jakubiak H, Doan J, Lamoureux P, et al. Detection and prevention of drug—drug interactions in the hospitalized elderly: utility of new cytochrome P450 based software. Am J Geriatr Pharmacother 2011 October 20 [e-pub ahead of print].

[51] Grygiel JJ, Birkett DJ. Effect of age on patterns of theophylline metabolism. Clin Pharmacol Ther 1980;28:456—62.

[52] Terrell KM, Heard K, Miller DK. Prescribing to older ED patients. Am J Emerg Med 2006;24:468—78.

[53] Dasgupta A. Usefulness of monitoring free (unbound) concentrations of therapeutic drugs in patient management. Clin Chim Acta 2007;377:1—13 [Review].

[54] Dreisbach AW. The influence of chronic renal failure on drug metabolism and transport. Clin Pharmacol Ther 2009;86:553—6.

[55] Dreisbach AW, Lertora JJ. The effect of chronic renal failure on drug metabolism and transport. Expert Opin Drug Metab Toxicol 2008;4. 1—65—1074.

[56] Nolin TD, Frye RF, Le P, et al. ESRD impairs nonrenal clearance of fexofenadine but not midazolam. J Am Soc Nephrol 2009;20:2269—76.

[57] Verbeeck RK. Pharmacokinetics and dosage adjustment in patients with hepatic dysfunction. Eur J Clin Pharmacol 2008;64:1147—61.

[58] Villeneuve JP, Pichette V. Cytochrome P450 and liver disease. Curr Drug Metab 2004;5:273—82.

[59] Merrell MD, Cherrington NJ. Drug metabolism alterations in nonalcoholic fatty liver disease. Drug Metab Rev 2011;43:317—34.

[60] Trotter JF, Osborne JC, Heller N, Christians U. Effect of hepatitis C infection on tacrolimus dose and blood levels in liver transplant recipients. Aliment Pharmacol Ther 2005;22:37—44.

[61] Zimmermann JJ, Lasseter KC, Lim HK, et al. Pharmacokinetics of sirolimus (rapamycin) in subjects with mild to moderate hepatic impairment. J Clin Pharmacol 2005;45:1368—72.

[62] Wyles DL, Gerber JG. Antiretroviral drug pharmacokinetics in hepatitis with hepatic dysfunction. Clin Infect Dis 2005;40:174—81.

[63] Ho MT, Kelly EJ, Bodor M, et al. Novel cytochrome P450-2D6 promotor sequence variations in hepatitis C positive and negative subjects. Ann Hepatol 2011;10:327—32.

[64] Ng CY, Ghabrial H, Morgan DJ, et al. Impaired elimination of propranolol due to right heart failure: drug clearance in the isolated liver and its relationship to intrinsic metabolic capacity. Drug Metab Dispos 2000;28:1217—21.

[65] Benowitz NL, Meister W. Pharmacokinetics in patients with cardiac failure. Clin Pharmacokinet 1976;1:389—405.

[66] Norgard NB, Prescott GM. Future of personalized pharmacotherapy in chronic heart failure patients. Future Cardiol 2011;7:357—79.

[67] Haas M, Kletzmayer J, Staudinger T, et al. Hypothyroidism as a cause of tacrolimus intoxication and acute renal failure: a case report. Wien Klin Wochenschr 2000;112:939—41.

[68] Padmanabhan H. Amiodarone and thyroid dysfunction. South Med J 2010;103:922—30.

[69] Burk O, Brenner SS, Hofmann U, et al. The impact of thyroid disease on the regulation, expression and function of ACB1 (MDR1/P-glycoprotein) and consequences for the disposition of digoxin. Clin Pharmacol Ther 2010;88:685—94.

[70] Howanitz PJ, Steindel SJ. Digoxin therapeutic drug monitoring practices. A College of American Pathologists Q-Probes study of 666 institutions and 18,679 toxic levels. Arch Pathol Lab Med 1993;117:684—90.

[71] Zeildman A, Gardyn J, Frandin Z, et al. Therapeutic and toxic theophylline levels in asthma attacks—is there a need for additional theophylline? [in Hebrew]. Harefuah 1997;133:3—5.

[72] Chang K, Bell TD, Lauer B, Chai H. Altered theophylline pharmacokinetics during acute respiratory viral illness. Lancet 1978;1:1132—3.

[73] Vozeh S, Powell JR, Riegelman S, et al. Changes in theophylline clearance in acute illness. J Am Med Assoc 1978;240:1882—4.

[74] Zevin S, Benowitz NL. Drug interactions with tobacco smoking: an update. Clin Pharmacokinet 1999;36:425—38.

[75] Lee BL, Benowitz NL, Jacob P. Cigarette abstinence, nicotine gum and theophylline disposition. Ann Intern Med 1987;106:553—5.

[76] Pesce AJ, Rashkin M, Kotagal U. Standards of laboratory practice: theophylline and caffeine. Clin Chem 1998;44:1124—8.

[77] Natarajan G, Botica ML, Thomas R, Aranda JV. Therapeutic drug monitoring for caffeine in preterm neonates: an unnecessary exercise? Pediatrics 2007;119:936—40.

[78] Hiemke C, Bauman P, Bergemann N, et al. AGNP consensus guidelines for therapeutic drug monitoring in psychiatry: an update 2011. Pharmacopsychiatry 2011;44:195—235.

[79] Roberts JA, Norris R, Paterson DL, Martin JH. Therapeutic drug monitoring of antimicrobials. Br J Clin Pharmacol 2011 August 10 [e-publication ahead of print].

[80] Sedar MA, Sertoglu E, Uyanik M, et al. Determination of 5-fluorouracil and dihydrofluorouracil levels by using a liquid chromatography-tandem mass spectrometry method for evaluation of dihydropyrimidine dehydrogenase enzyme. Cancer Chemother Pharmacol 2011;68:525—9.

[81] Lee NH. Pharmacogenetics of drug metabolizing enzymes and transporters: effects on pharmacokinetics and pharmacodynamics of anticancer agents. Anticancer Agents Med Chem 2010;10:583—92.

[82] Haen E. Therapeutic drug monitoring in pharmacovigilance and pharmacotherapy safety. Pharmacopsychiatry 2011;44:254—8.

Effects of Pre-analytical Variables in Therapeutic Drug Monitoring

Valerie Bush

Bassett Medical Center, Cooperstown, New York, NY

O U T L I N E

INTRODUCTION

Laboratory results are dependent on the quality of the specimen analyzed [1]. The pre-analytical phase accounts for the majority of laboratory errors [2]. It has been estimated that pre-analytical errors account for more than two-thirds of all laboratory errors, while errors in the analytical phase and post-analytical phase account for one-third of all laboratory errors. Carraro and Plebani reported that among 51 746 clinical laboratory analyses performed in a 3-month period in their laboratory (7615 laboratory orders, 17 514 blood collection tubes), clinicians questioned the validity of 393 test results out of which 160 results were confirmed by the authors as being due to laboratory errors. Of the 160 confirmed laboratory errors, 61.9% were determined to be pre-analytical errors, 15% analytical errors and 23.1% post-analytical errors. The pre-analytical phase thus showed the highest percentage of errors, the most frequent problems arising from mistakes in tube-filling with an incorrect blood to anticoagulant ratio for coagulation tests, and empty or inadequately filled tubes. Other common errors in the pre-analytical steps included using the wrong type of blood collection tube, errors in the requested test procedure, wrong patient identification, contradictory demographic data from different information systems, missing tubes, samples diluted with intravenous infusion solution, and other problems. The authors also identified 24 errors in the analytical phase and 37 in the post-analytical stage. The majority of laboratory errors had no impact on patient care (121 errors out of 160), but 1 error caused inappropriate intensive care admission (0.6%), 2 errors caused inappropriate transfusion (1.3%), 9 errors (5.6%) resulted in inappropriate investigation and 27 errors (16.9%) required repeated laboratory tests [3]. By controlling and standardizing practices in the pre-analytical phase, test accuracy can be improved significantly to ultimately benefit patient care and patient safety.

The pre-analytical phase consists of all steps from preparing the patient for collection of the specimen to processing of the specimen prior to the analytical step. Pre-analytical errors can occur *in vivo* or *in vitro*. Many pre-analytical factors can alter test results by producing changes that do not reflect the patient's true physiological or clinical condition. *In vivo* factors are more difficult for laboratory professionals to control, but some pre-analytical errors can be avoided by enforcing specimen-collection and -handling requirements. Certain patient populations (i.e., pediatric, geriatric, dialysis and oncology patients) present additional challenges in obtaining a specimen for therapeutic drug monitoring or other clinical laboratory tests. Some other pre-analytical patient factors include patient identification, time of dose versus collection, hemolysis/lipemia, drug interactions, and degree of protein binding. One of the most common pre-analytical variables associated with therapeutic drug monitoring occurs after the blood has been collected, and is related to the drug's stability in blood collection tubes. *In vitro* drug stability is dependent upon several factors, including the primary tube used, the fill volume in the tube, along with the time and temperature of storage. Another important pre-analytical variable is the collection of hydrophobic antibiotics through intravenous lines. This chapter will focus on pre-analytical variables during collection and processing and their impact on therapeutic drug values, with a brief mention of some *in vivo* factors.

SPECIMEN TYPE

The concentration of a drug in a body fluid depends upon several factors related to the drug's volume of distribution. Each specimen type has advantages and disadvantages, and these are outlined in Table 2.1. Pharmacology is based on the ability to correlate plasma concentration of a drug with observed clinical effects, and it is generally accepted that plasma concentrations correlate with receptor site concentrations. A drug is internalized by cells from extracellular fluid to exert its effect. For this reason, therapeutic drug monitoring is typically performed using serum, plasma or whole blood. These specimen types have been the basis for many methods and therapeutic ranges. Urine is more frequently used for forensics and toxicology testing rather than therapeutic drug monitoring. Urine has also become

TABLE 2.1 Specimen Type Comparison

Specimen type	Advantages	Disadvantages
Blood/plasma/serum	• Correlation to clinical effect • Total and free measurements available • Reference ranges for many therapeutic drugs • Free drug concentration not affected by anticoagulant • Whole blood or plasma can be run without any sample pre-treatment	• Serum/plasma require clotting time prior to centrifugation • Invasive venipuncture required to obtain specimen • Tube components (gel or anticoagulant) may interfere
Urine	• Non-invasive • Ease of collection • Includes metabolites • Estimates a time-averaged concentration • Approximately 3-day window for most abused drugs, therefore commonly used for drugs of abuse testing	• Not commonly used for therapeutic monitoring because urine concentrations may not reflect serum concentration • Assays not widely available for therapeutic drugs except for opioids used for pain management • Influenced by pH of urine • Possibility of adulteration for urine specimen submitted for workplace drug testing.
Saliva	• Non-invasive • Ease of collection • Preferred by children • Results closer to free drug concentration in most cases • Parent drug measured	• Potential for contamination from food particles • Insufficient volume • Needs standardized collecting procedure • Difficulty in pipetting saliva • Metabolites generally absent • Many factors may influence saliva drug concentrations • Lower concentrations require more sensitive methods

a specimen of choice to test opiate compliance in pain management programs [4]. Fritch *et al.* described barbiturate detection in oral fluid, plasma and urine. After a single oral therapeutic dose of butalbital, phenobarbital and secobarbital, these drugs were readily excreted in detectable concentrations in oral fluid over a period of approximately 2 days [5]. Since some parent drugs and their metabolites are excreted in urine, recovery of drugs in urine depends upon renal function, pH of urine and hydration status of the patient, and does not necessarily correlate with plasma concentrations. However, oral fluid (saliva) analysis has provided useful information for monitoring anticonvulsant drugs for many years, particularly in pediatric patients. Urine and saliva have the benefit of non-invasive collections, but validated methods for these samples are not widely available or used. Drug concentrations in saliva are proportional to those in plasma, but this is not true for urine. Drug concentrations in saliva are influenced by many factors, including salivary flow rate, pH, sampling conditions and contamination [6–8]. Serum or plasma still remains the preferred specimen for most therapeutic drug methods.

FACTORS THAT AFFECT THERAPEUTIC DRUG MONITORING RESULTS

Pharmacogenetic, pharmacokinetic and pharmacodynamic factors influence drug efficacy in any given patient. Pharmacogenetics determines how an individual patient's genetic makeup influences drug metabolism and response to therapy [9]. Pharmacokinetics refers to the movement of a drug into, through and out of the body — the time-course of its absorption, bioavailability, distribution, metabolism and excretion. Pharmacokinetics determines the onset, duration and intensity of a drug's effect. Pharmacodynamics defines the pharmacological effect of the drug in the body. This involves receptor binding, postreceptor effects and chemical interactions. Several physiological factors can affect blood levels of therapeutic drugs. Common patient-associated pre-analytical factors include patient compliance, age, diet, body weight changes, exercise, pre-existing diseases, multiple drug administration, time of dose versus time of collection, hemolysis or lipemia, drug interactions, and degree of protein binding. Many of these factors change throughout the lifetime of a patient so periodic monitoring is necessary to ensure current doses are still safe and effective. Assessing patient compliance can be challenging for providers to manage in patients with degenerative mental capacity. Elderly patients frequently forget if they have taken their medication, leading to extra doses or skipping a dose. Some therapies, such as digoxin or warfarin, are lifelong treatments that require long-term monitoring. Additionally, as an individual ages and body habits change, drug dosages should be adjusted accordingly to avoid under- or overdosing the patient.

Recommended times of draw depend on the half-life of the drug of interest, but steady-state trough levels are customarily used. Approximately five half-lives are necessary before equilibrium is reached in serum value after initiation of the drug therapy. Trough levels should be obtained shortly before the next dose. Other sampling schedules may be desired, depending on the properties of the drug and patient needs. For example, measurements of peak and trough concentrations of aminoglycosides and sulfonamides are common in early dosing regimens to achieve proper therapeutic levels and also to avoid toxicity. The time and date of the last dose should be noted, along with the time of collection, to aid in interpretation. Associating the specimen with the correct patient (proper patient identification) by proper labeling is the key to reducing errors and patient mismanagement [10]. A multidisciplinary approach involving the laboratory, pharmacy, nursing staff and providers can help assure that drug concentrations at specified collection times after dosing are meaningful.

Further, drug–food, drug–herb and drug–drug interactions can influence the concentration of some drugs by interfering with the volume of distribution and metabolism of the drug [11–13]. Any of these interactions can either increase or decrease the absorption of a drug, leading to elevated or reduced levels of the drug in the body with subsequent consequences. Patients taking multiple drugs (polypharmacy) for various conditions are at increased risk of these types of interactions. The use of traditional herbal medicines by non-traditional cultures has increased as populations immigrate into Western society. Herbal medicines compete in metabolic pathways and protein binding, and may interfere with the analytical measurement of traditional therapeutic drugs. Certain herbal supplements can interfere with serum digoxin measurement using immunoassays [14, 15]. See Chapter 11 for a detailed discussion on the effect of herbal supplements on digoxin immunoassays.

The use of multiple medications by a patient can impact the physiological effect of a drug. This is most common in elderly patients, but is also found in the general population. Drugs metabolized by common cytochrome P450 (CYP) pathways are known to result in drug–drug interactions. For example, anti-epileptic drugs (e.g. carbamazepine and phenytoin) are known to induce CYP450 enzymes, which can increase the metabolism of other drugs by these enzymes. Naturally occurring compounds may also induce or inhibit CYP activity and influence drug metabolism. A common example is the influence of vitamin K on warfarin therapy. Healthcare professionals at Coumadin® (the trade name of warfarin) clinics are well aware of reduced anticoagulant response from sudden increases in dietary vitamin K [16–18].

Additionally, Digibind is a therapeutic antibody consisting of the Fab fragment of digoxin antibody administered to neutralize digitalis toxicity. At high concentrations, Digibind causes significant interference in many digoxin immunoassays. A blocking agent can be used to reduce interferences from Digibind [19]. Imaging agents have also been reported to interfere with fluorescence polarization immunoassays for vancomycin [20].

The binding of some therapeutic drugs to protein has been shown to be pH dependent. Several investigators have demonstrated that the free fractions of phenytoin, valproic acid and phenobarbital decreased as pH decreased from 8.4 to 7.0, while the free fractions of theophylline and carbamazepine increased [21, 22]. A decrease in blood pH, as may be seen in acid–base imbalances or between serum and plasma, has affected the free fractions of these drugs.

The effect of hemolysis or lipemia on drug analyses is similar to those of other analytes where interferences with the detection method may be observed. Although hemolysis is typically an *in vitro* factor, *in vivo* hemolysis can occur and can be confirmed by serum haptoglobin measurement [23, 24]. Noticeable hemolysis and hyperlipidemia may interfere with antibody–antigen reactions of immunoassays and with some signal detection methods. Depending on the instrument platform used, hemolysis, bilirubin and lipemia can have varying effects. Ryder showed that fewer erroneous results from hemolyzed or lipemic specimens would be expected using EMIT (enzyme multiplied immunoassay technique) and FPIA (fluorescence polarization immunoassay) assays compared to other assays [25]. Most kit manufacturers provide the level of interfering substances for each assay in the package insert. The laboratory can then appropriately set hemolysis or lipemia limits on the instrument or compare the specimen to visual charts for specimen acceptance or rejection.

PROTEIN BINDING ALTERATION: *IN VIVO* AND *IN VITRO*

A brief overview of drug binding with plasma proteins is provided as it relates to pre-analytical error. The reader is referred to reviews of drug binding with plasma proteins for more thorough discussions on the subject [26, 27]. It is well known that drug binding to plasma proteins varies from near zero to over 99% depending upon the drug. The remaining free form of the drug is available to pass through cell membranes and exert its effect. Some drugs are capable of binding to blood cells, but the predominant binding is to serum proteins, primarily albumin. The fraction of free versus bound drug in serum is influenced by endogenous and exogenous compounds that compete with the drug for binding to albumin or other proteins. When the concentration of these proteins is altered through a pathological or physiological condition, the total- to free-drug ratio changes [28]. Because the free fraction is pharmacologically active, measurement of the free fraction is usually desirable. Several factors have been shown to influence protein binding or displacement of therapeutic drugs from proteins. The *in vivo* variables include inflammatory conditions, malignancies, stress, pregnancy, uremia, liver disease, malnutrition, and competition of highly bound drugs with weaker binding drugs. In patients where the total drug level is within the therapeutic range, but the patient presents as either toxic or non-therapeutic, altered protein binding may be responsible. The binding of drugs to proteins in patients with chronic kidney disease is of concern due to decreased albumin-binding capacity. Patients on long-term hemodialysis contain compounds (i.e., 3-carboxy-4-methyl-5-propyl-2-furanpropionate, heparin, etc.) that compete for binding sites on albumin [29]. For these reasons consideration of free drug determination is warranted in uremia, especially for strongly protein-bound classical anticonvulsants such as phenytoin, valproic acid and carbamazepine. *In vitro* factors that may impact the total- to free-drug ratio include the presence of drug-displacement agents in blood collection tubes, heparin, and changes in pH with specimen age and/or exposure to air. Shifts in plasma pH can change the equilibrium of free and bound drug in the specimen. For any drug with a pK_a that is significantly different from the pH of serum (e.g., phenytoin), measurement of free drug levels should be considered. Protein binding of some basic drugs was shown to be inhibited when blood was collected into Vacutainer® tubes in the late 1970s. Cotham and Shand demonstrated spuriously low plasma propranolol concentrations from the redistribution of propranolol between plasma and red blood cells when blood was collected in a specific brand of blood collection tubes [30]. Low plasma drug levels were obtained that were linked to a drug-displacing agent in the Vacutainer tube. This drug-displacing agent was attributed to tris (2-butoxyethyl) phosphate (TBEP) present in the rubber stoppers of the tubes [31]. The displacement interaction was shown to have occurred between TBEP and one or more of the binding proteins (e.g., alpha-1-acid glycoprotein, lipoproteins and albumin). The displacement effect of TBEP with albumin was less likely due to the low concentration of TBEP relative to serum albumin, but the authors noted considerable variability among tubes and between individuals [32]. Drug displacement appeared only to affect highly bound basic drugs (e.g., tricyclic antidepressants). Lidocaine values were also influenced by stopper material yielding spuriously low concentrations in serum or plasma [33]. By 1983 the manufacturer of Vacutainer tubes and catheters had removed the drug-displacing agent, so this is rarely seen today. However, TBEP is a common ingredient in rubber stoppers that may be used in other products in the pre-analytical, analytical or post-analytical steps. Shah *et al.* has outlined a procedure for testing possible interference from TBEP if suspected [34]. Another reported "contaminant" from blood collection tubes, IV lines and IV bags is the phthalate plasticizer (i.e., diethyl-phthalate or di(2-ethylhexlyl) phthalate (DEHP)) that acts as a digoxin-like immunoreactive substance and leads to falsely elevated digoxin concentrations [35, 36].

Anticoagulants, particularly heparin, have also been shown to affect protein binding of drugs as previously mentioned. Heparin in blood collection tubes does not cause changes in pH, as do other anticoagulants, and would not displace protein-bound drugs via this mechanism. Instead, heparin increases the concentration of free fatty acids that, in turn, affects binding of acidic drugs to albumin and basic drugs to alpha-1-acid glycoprotein, thus influencing measurement of the free drug [37, 38]. *In vivo* heparin effects on free fatty acids and disopyramide have been reported in hemodialysis patients. Horiuchi *et al.* found an increase in the free fraction of disopyramide on dialysis days that was associated with elevated free fatty acid levels in the plasma [39]. Others have shown an approximate 24% increase in unbound quinidine in patients during cardiac catheterization, due to the presence of heparin [40].

Not only can heparin interfere with protein binding pre-analytically; it can also interfere analytically if at high enough concentrations. This interference can be method dependent, as demonstrated with aminoglycoside assays. O'Connell *et al.* examined the accuracy of aminoglycoside determinations by three different immunoassays (EMIT, RIA and FPIA) in the presence of heparin [41]. The authors showed the interference was caused by heparin binding to detection enzymes in homogeneous enzyme immunoassays, while no effect was shown with the RIA or FPIA methods. Further, the *in vitro* interference appeared to be dose dependent from 2–1000 USP, depending on the drug assayed. Heparin interferences could occur at concentrations found in blood collection tubes or blood gas syringes, particularly if the tubes are underfilled. Blood collection tubes typically contain 10–30 IU/ml of liquid or dry heparin, while calcium-balanced blood gas syringes contain 40–60 IU/ml dry heparin. Determining the acceptability of blood collection products and enforcing specimen acceptance policies within a laboratory system will minimize errors due to heparin in blood collection tubes.

Several factors have been shown to influence the displacement of therapeutic drugs from proteins, thereby increasing the free fraction of drugs. The type of displacement agent could affect basic drugs differently from acidic drugs.

SPECIMEN COLLECTION SITE

The site of specimen collection can also influence drug levels. It is standard practice that blood should not be collected from the same central line via which drugs or other fluids are infused because such practice may lead to erroneous results due to contamination from the infusion fluid. For example, cyclosporine is a hydrophobic drug. When cyclosporine is administered intravenously, it tends to bind to the hydrophobic surface of some IV catheter tubing. When blood is collected from the indwelling line, cyclosporine concentrations are significantly higher than if collected by direct venipuncture [42]. Conversely, Ptachcinski *et al.* showed the stability of the oral dose form of cyclosporine in plastic syringes [43]. This was confirmed by Shulman *et al.*, who also verified that aminoglycosides and other antibiotics can be collected from central venous lines [44]. The plastic materials used for flexible IV tubing (e.g., polyurethane, polyethylene, polyvinyl, Teflon® or Vialon®) and rigid syringes (e.g., polypropylene polymer) differ, and may be contributing to the differences noted by these two studies. More study is warranted to understand the mechanisms of cyclosporine recovery from flexible IV tubing and plastic syringes. Some variables to consider are the type of plastic or additives used in the manufacture of the device, and the exposed surface area.

A few studies have compared capillary and venous collections on number of analytes tested [45, 46], but little is known about whether drug levels by capillary collection differ from those by venipuncture. In some patient populations (e.g., pediatric, geriatric, oncology) a capillary specimen is preferred because blood volume loss by venipuncture can be limited and venous access may be difficult. However, capillary blood may not necessarily correlate with venous measurements. The major concerns with skin puncture collections are contamination from interstitial fluid, hemolysis and residual contaminates from the surface of the skin. Theoretically, for drugs with a high volume of distribution and a poor puncture necessitating "milking" the finger, drug values could be altered by the presence of tissue fluid in the blood collected. Drugs that are highly protein bound have low volumes of distribution because only a small portion of the drug is free and available to diffuse into extravascular spaces. To verify this concept, the current author and colleagues compared collection methods (fingerstick versus venipuncture) for patients taking phenytoin (90–95% protein bound) and salicylate (~50% protein bound). Serum total phenytoin was measured by EMIT and salicylate by colorimetric technique, and essentially no difference in collection methods for either drug was found (unpublished data). Frazer *et al.* showed a positive bias in capillary specimens for theophylline (~40% protein bound) compared to venous collections [47]. Comparison of capillary blood drug concentrations with venous values deserves further study to determine whether significant differences exist or not.

Some investigators have examined capillary blood drug values of the immunosuppressants cyclosporine and methotrexate. Whole blood measurements of the highly erythrocyte-bound cyclosporine are determined from EDTA (ethylene diamine tetraacetic acid) anticoagulated blood. Several investigators compared fingerstick, ear prick and venipuncture cyclosporine values from organ transplant patients and showed a high degree of correlation among these collection techniques [48, 49]. These investigators also suggested that fingerstick collections were the preferred method to reduce blood loss and preserve venous integrity in this patient population. Ritzmo *et al.* examined capillary and venous methotrexate levels from nine pediatric cancer patients during hospital stays [50]. Venous blood was obtained from a central venous catheter. These authors also showed a high correlation ($r^2 = 0.98$) between fingerstick and venous draws where the venous to capillary plasma concentration ratio was 1.00 for 85% of the data independent of drug concentration. These studies have shown very little difference between capillary collections and venous collections for whole blood measurements of immunosuppressants. Laboratories should understand potential differences that may exist among collection sites and methods. Some national and state accrediting agencies recommend that laboratories verify the use of collection methods and devices used for each method.

VOLUME OF SPECIMEN COLLECTED

All plastic evacuated tubes are composed of polyethylene terephthalate (PET) and contain no additive, an anticoagulant, or a clotting agent. Incorrect filling of the collection tube will cause alterations in the blood to additive ratio. Blood to additive ratios are maintained by allowing the tube to be completely filled with blood. Instrument sampling errors can occur if collection tubes are inadequately filled or if the specimen is not completely clotted and fibrin is aspirated into the sample probe. These issues can be avoided by following the manu-facturer's recommendations for collection and allowing enough time for clotting. If a blood is collected without any anticoagulant, the blood specimen must be allowed to clot for at least 20–30 minutes before centrifugation to separate serum from other blood components. Sampling error by the automated analyzer can be avoided by ensuring that instrument probes are set appropriately, or knowing the maximum depth a liquid-level sensing probe will travel. The effect of specimen volume in gel separator on drug recovery can be signifi-cant, and is discussed later.

GLASS VERSUS PLASTIC TUBES FOR COLLECTION OF BLOOD

Plastic blood collection tubes are lighter than glass, unbreakable, and provide easy disposal. Correlation studies between glass and plastic blood collection tubes for common analytes and some hormones and tumor markers have been published [51, 52]. Many labo-ratories have performed their own evaluations of plastic tubes to document analyte compat-ibility before converting, but haven't always published their findings. Dasgupta *et al.* examined the stability of 13 therapeutic drugs stored in plastic tubes compared to glass tubes, using quality control material [53]. The authors found no significant reduction in concentra-tions of caffeine, primidone, procainamide, NAPA, acetaminophen, salicylate, amikacin, val-proic acid, methotrexate or cyclosporine. When comparing volume of serum in the tube, they observed significant reductions in concentrations of phenytoin, phenobarbital, carbamaze-pine, quinidine and lidocaine after storage of 500 μl of serum versus 1 mL in both glass and plastic gel tubes. The poor recovery of these drugs was attributed to the gel in the tubes, rather than the tube material.

Faynor and Robinson examined the suitability of plastic blood collection tubes for cyclo-sporine measurement [54]. Specimens from renal transplant patients were collected into glass and plastic BD Vacutainer EDTA tubes. Tubes were stored at room temperature and 4°C after collection, and between testing intervals of 0, 1, 4 and 7 days. The drug levels in the plastic tubes were slightly higher than those from the glass tubes at both storage temperatures, and did not appear to be time dependent. All of the differences for individual pairs of samples were within 10%. The authors concluded that cyclosporine levels are stable in plastic tubes over 7 days at room temperature or refrigerated. Boeynaems *et al.* compared Terumo's Venoject® glass tubes with Venosafe® PET tubes with clot activator and heparin for several therapeutic drugs at 2 and 24 hours post-collection [55]. Blood was spiked with the parent drug to low, mid and high therapeutic levels. The authors found no consistent significant differences among the tube types for the panel of drugs tested. These data agree with other comparisons between Venoject II and BD Vacutainer plastic tubes [56].

SERUM VERSUS PLASMA SPECIMEN FOR THERAPEUTIC DRUG MONITORING

Serum and plasma concentrations of analytes and therapeutic drugs are frequently used interchangeably, but they are not necessarily synonymous. Drugs are present in the serum or plasma as free drug or bound to proteins. While some drugs are capable of binding to blood cells — for example, cyclosporine, tacrolimus, sirolimus and everolimus — the prominent and clinically significant binding occurs with serum or plasma proteins. At the time of blood collection into a closed blood collection tube, the drug concentration in the blood is constant and the ratio of free to protein-bound drug does not change. Among the anticoagulants, heparin is frequently preferred because it does not cause shifts in electrolytes and water between plasma and cells. Heparin (*in vitro*) does not cause large changes in pH, as do other anticoagulants, and would not initiate changes in free versus protein-bound drug via this mechanism. For example, no differences in the total or free valproic acid concentrations between samples collected in serum or heparinized plasma have been found [57]. Tricyclic antidepressant (parent and metabolite) concentrations in serum and heparinized plasma are comparable [58, 59]. However, variations in protein binding in the presence of heparin have been shown for other drugs (e.g., carbamazepine, theophylline, and phenobarbital) [60]. This is not a pH effect, but a displacement effect from the release of free fatty acids due to heparin-induced lipolysis. Interference of heparin with aminoglycoside immunoassays is method dependent. The interference is caused by heparin binding to detection enzymes in homogenous enzyme immunoassays (EIA) and radioenzymatic assays. The interference appears to be dose dependent but may occur at concentrations in blood collection tubes, particularly if the tubes are underfilled, with some assays. If anticoagulated blood for amino-glycoside testing is desired, potassium oxalate can be used [61–63].

Measurement of lithium concentrations from blood collected in lithium heparin tubes will yield falsely elevated results that appear toxic. Wills *et al.* examined blood collected into lithium heparin tubes from individuals not taking lithium. Baseline lithium levels were < 0.2 mmol/L. Depending upon the volume of blood collected into the green-top tubes (full draw, 2 ml or 1 ml), the lithium values ranged from 1.0 to 4.2 mmol/L [64].

Many reagent manufacturers claim in their package inserts that serum or plasma can be used for analysis of many therapeutic drugs, although some recommend using only serum specimens for therapeutic drug monitoring. The presence of heparin is not usually a factor with highly automated methods that measure total drug levels. For example, Ortho and Siemens suggest either serum or plasma for their drug assays, although digoxin on the Centaur® is restricted to serum (from respective package inserts). While serum or plasma can be used, plasma values may be 10% higher than serum values by other methods [19]. Amiodarone and desethylamiodarone by HPLC were found to be approximately 11% and 9% higher in serum, respectively [65]. This may necessitate different therapeutic ranges depending upon the sample type and the drug.

Nyberg and Mårtensson conducted an extensive study to test the effects of ten types of blood collection tubes, including two plasma separator tubes, for the stability of the tricyclic antidepressants amitriptyline, imipramine and clomipramine, and their monodemethylated metabolites [66]. The authors found that EDTA-containing (lavender-top) tubes provided the most stable plasma and red-top tubes the most stable serum samples. They also showed that freshly sampled blood from heparin-containing (green-top) tubes could be stored at room temperature for 24 hours without significant losses. Freeze–thaw cycles at −20°C did not influence serum or plasma concentrations.

For cyclosporine, EDTA is preferred over heparin as the anticoagulant of choice. The stability of cyclosporine in EDTA has been demonstrated. The differences in cyclosporine concentrations collected in glass (K$_3$EDTA) and plastic (K$_2$EDTA) tubes is < 10% [54]. The small differences observed could be attributed to dilution effects by the liquid K$_3$EDTA compared to the dry K$_2$EDTA.

Laboratorians should be cognizant of the specimen type recommended and validated for each drug assay on a particular platform. Plasma has the advantage of a faster turnaround time, as the blood does not clot. Serum tends to be a cleaner specimen without potential interferences from particulates when sufficiently clotted, or from anticoagulants. However, for many drugs, values are comparable between plasma and serum [67]. It is important for laboratories to enforce specimen collection and rejection policies to avoid misinterpretation of results due to a pre-analytical error.

SUITABILITY OF SERUM SEPARATOR COLLECTION TUBES FOR SPECIMEN COLLECTION FOR DRUG MONITORING

The use of serum separator tubes in clinical laboratories is common due to the capability of storing serum over time in the primary collection tube. If analysis of the serum is not performed shortly after processing, the laboratory may store the specimen under a variety of conditions. Serum separator tubes provide a closed system that allows for collection, transport, processing, sampling and storage of specimens. Different barrier materials are available among tube manufacturers, but all are thixotropic materials that facilitate separation of serum or plasma from the cells and prevent hemolysis on prolonged storage. The base material in the gel is currently acrylic, silicone or a polyester polymer. The stability of various serum components in gel tubes has been studied and well documented. Errors in drug recovery from specimens collected in gel barrier tubes were first discovered in the early 1980s [68, 69]. Although improvements have been made to the tubes since these early studies, the gel barrier materials have remained relatively unchanged.

An important limitation of gel barrier tubes is the absorption of specific drugs and some steroid hormones into the gel [70, 71]. The stability (or instability) of several drugs in gel tubes has been widely studied, where the instability of drugs in gel serum separator tubes is defined as a loss of recovery of the drug of interest after contact with the gel. This occurs when a drug is absorbed into the gel barrier. The following five factors influence drug stability in gel tubes:

1. The chemical nature of the drug and the gel influence which drugs are absorbed by the gel. While the exact mechanism of this interaction is not well understood, in general the drugs prefer to be associated with the phase where they are most soluble. Thus, if the gel is hydrophobic in nature, then hydrophobic drugs would tend to be absorbed and hydrophilic drugs remain in the aqueous fraction. Those drugs that are susceptible to absorption (instability) are specific and few compared to all drugs that are monitored therapeutically.
2. Sample volume on the barrier, where greater relative absorption is observed with lower sample volumes, has an effect. When blood is collected into a gel tube, the total volume of blood is exposed to a constant surface area of gel. This volume to surface area ratio of whole blood to gel is approximately twice that of the serum on the gel. Drug absorption in

whole blood is typically < 1% of the total concentration, as shown by comparing non-gel tube with gel tube drug levels at an initial time after processing. Additionally, the surface area of the gel centrifuged in a fixed angle centrifuge is greater than that when centrifuged in a swing bucket centrifuge. Higher gel surface area can lead to greater drug absorption into the gel.

3. The length of time the serum is in contact with the gel also influences drug stability for those drugs susceptible to absorption. The longer the serum remains in contact with the gel the more drug is absorbed, until an equilibrium is reached. For those drugs susceptible to absorption, equilibrium is reached at approximately 24 hours.

4. The temperature of storage also influences drug stability. The rate of absorption increases with increasing temperatures until equilibrium is achieved.

Effects of collection of blood in gel separator tubes on therapeutic drug monitoring are summarized in Table 2.2. There have been numerous studies evaluating the stability of various drugs among different types of barrier tubes. Landt *et al.* showed that when blood was processed and analyzed shortly after collection, none of the separator tubes had any effect on seven drugs studied (theophylline, digoxin, phenytoin, phenobarbital, gentamicin, ethanol and cyclosporine). The authors also examined the impact under stressed conditions by partially filling the various barrier tubes of these seven drugs. Only phenytoin, at 1-mL fill volume in a 7-ml polyester separator tube, showed modestly lower recovery (92%). Interestingly, the authors also included cyclosporine because of its known avidity for polymeric materials. It is not surprising that these investigators found no differences in recovery of cyclosporine when using corresponding heparinized versions of each tube type. The majority of the drug itself is protected from interacting with the barrier, as most is bound intracellularly to red blood cells and measurements are performed on whole blood [72].

TABLE 2.2 Effect of Gel Separator Collection Tube on Therapeutic Drug Monitoring

Tube type	Drug affected (Chemical nature)	Comments
Becton-Dickinson SST Tube	Phenytoin (Hydrophobic)	Unstable if stored > 4 h for all drugs listed
	Carbamazepine (Hydrophobic)	
	Lidocaine (Hydrophobic)	
	Quinidine (Hydrophobic)	
Becton-Dickinson SST II tube*	Phenytoin (Hydrophobic)	Unstable if stored > 24 h for both drugs
	Carbamazepine (Hydrophobic)	
Corvac Tube*	Lidocaine (Hydrophobic)	Unstable if stored > 4 h
Greiner Tube Vacuette*	Tricyclic	Unstable if stored > 4 h
	Antidepressant (Hydrophobic)	

*Other therapeutic drugs are stable

The most extensive study on the suitability of gel barrier tubes for therapeutic drug monitoring was published by Karppi *et al.* The authors studied the stability of 41 drugs, including tricyclic antidepressants, benzodiazepines, anti-epileptics, asthma drugs, aminoglycosides, other antibiotics and cardioactive drugs, when specimens were stored in three different gel tubes (BD SST™ tubes, Terumo Autosep and Sarstedt Microvette® gel tubes). After 24 hours' storage time, absorbed drugs ranged from 5% to 20% of the concentration at the initial time for all analyzed drugs. The authors concluded that the studied gel tubes were satisfactory for blood collection for antidepressant drug measurements if the separation step is performed within 3 hours after blood clotting [73].

Bailey *et al.* studied the stability of 11 drugs (amikacin, carbamazepine, digoxin, gentamicin, lithium, methotrexate, phenobarbital, phenytoin, quinidine, theophylline and tobramycin) as well as two heavy metals (copper and zinc) in plasma specimens stored in Corvac® brand gel separation tubes over a week of storage in the refrigerator, and found no significant absorption of any drugs by the barrier gel. The authors used 10 mL serum supplemented with appropriate drugs for their study [74]. Devine also did not observe any decline in drug concentration, either over time or with respect to sample size, when aliquots of heparinized blood (3−9 mL) were supplemented with lidocaine or phenytoin and stored in Corvac® serum separator gel tubes for 24 hours [75]. However, Koch and Platoff demonstrated that both Corvac® and Becton-Dickinson Vacutainer SST serum separator blood collection tubes were unsuitable for storage of specimens containing lidocaine due to a 25−30% decline in concentrations over a 72-hour period. In addition, authors concluded that SST serum separator blood collection tubes were unsuitable for quinidine (storage greater than 24 h), lidocaine (greater than 6 h) and phenytoin. Partially filled tubes caused additional errors [76]. In another report, the authors observed decline in free and total phenytoin concentrations as well as free and total carbamazepine concentrations when specimens were collected in Becton-Dickinson SST serum separator blood collection tubes, but no decline was observed in specimens collected in Terumo Autosep tubes also containing barrier gels [77]. Dasgupta *et al.* studied the stability of several therapeutic drugs in serum following storage in Becton-Dickinson SST serum separator blood collection tubes and Corvac® serum separator blood collection tubes and observed significant reductions in drug concentrations (ranging from 5.9% to 64.5%) for phenytoin, lidocaine, quinidine and carbamazepine. In contrast, concentrations of theophylline and salicylate did not change under identical specimen storage conditions. The reduction in drug concentration was dependent on time of storage (more pronounced effect with storage over 2−6 h) as well as specimen volume, with more significant changes observed in specimens where sample volumes were low. No significant change in the concentration of phenytoin, phenobarbital, carbamazepine, theophylline, quinidine and salicylate was observed when serum was stored in Corvac® serum separator blood collection tubes, while concentration of lidocaine declined (range 31.5% to 72.6%) after storage in these tubes, especially if specimen volume was low (200−500 μL). The decline in drug concentration due to storage of specimens in gel separator tubes was due to slow passive absorption of certain drugs by the gel, as evidenced by recovery of drugs from the gel following chemical extraction with methanol. For phenytoin, the reduction in total drug concentration also resulted in a proportional reduction in free drug concentration and such reduction in the free drug level was also dependent on the extent of protein binding of the drug. As expected, specimens stored in standard red-top Vacutainer tubes without any separator gel showed no reduction in concentration of any drugs [78]. Dasgupta *et al.*, in a later report, investigated the stability of 15 common therapeutic drugs (amikacin, gentamicin, tobramycin, vancomycin, digoxin, quinidine, theophylline, carbamazepine, phenobarbital, phenytoin, valproic acid, tricyclic antidepressants, salicylate, acetaminophen and ethanol) in specimens stored in Greiner Vacuette® blood collection tubes containing serum separator gel, and observed that most drugs did not show any significant decline in concentration except for tricyclic antidepressant and carbamazepine [79].

In order to circumvent the problem of absorption of phenytoin, carbamazepine and phenobarbital by the Becton-Dickinson Vacutainer serum separator SST gels, a new gel tube was formulated and marketed by Becton-Dickinson which was clear gel (SST II tubes) rather than yellow gel. Base on a study, the new gel was superior to the old gel because the concentration of carbamazepine declined by only 10% and the concentration of phenytoin declined by only 4% on prolonged storage. This was a significant improvement over the old gel formulation, and these new tubes are effective for collecting blood for therapeutic drug monitoring if phenytoin and carbamazepine are analyzed within a day of collection [80]. Schouwers *et al.* studied the effect of serum separator gel in Sarstedt S-Monovette® serum tubes on various therapeutic drugs, hormones and proteins by using sera from patients. The authors tested four therapeutic drugs (amikacin, vancomycin, valproic acid and acetaminophen) as well as cortisol, free thyroxine, thyroid stimulating hormone, transferrin, prealbumin and carcinoembryonic antigen. The authors observed no statistically significant difference in values of any analytes on the day of phlebotomy. Although after 1 day statistically significant differences were observed, apart from free T4 the differences were not clinically significant [81].

The data presented by many investigators support the stability of hydrophilic drugs in gel tubes for several days when stored at 4°C. Ambient temperature storage may also be used for many hydrophilic drugs. Some differences may be observed with digoxin due to the magnitude of concentration measured. Some hydrophobic drugs can be underestimated when specimens are stored on the gel over time. The rate of absorption by hydrophobic drugs is temperature and volume dependent. Laboratory policies can allow accurate testing of hydrophobic drugs through monitoring draw volume, time and temperature of storage in gel tubes.

SAMPLE PREPARATION STEPS

Chromatographic techniques for drug analysis usually require sample preparation (liquid or solid phase extraction(s) and derivatization) to isolate the drug and its metabolites from a complex matrix. Sample preparation depends upon the number of analytes in the serum, their concentration, the presence of interfering substances, and the column used for separation. Ineffectual separation can occur from interactions of sample impurities with the stationary phase, increasing the noise level at the detector, interaction of the drug of interest with other matrix components and poor resolution. To minimize these effects, extraction step(s) are employed to isolate the drug(s) of interest from the specimen matrix. There is the potential for components (gel, lubricants and anticoagulants) from the blood collection tube to produce erroneous peaks that could complicate the interpretation of mass spectrometry spectra, particularly at the low molecular weight range [82]. Purification of the sample with high yield of the drug of interest is the goal in sample preparation. By converting the drugs to derivatives, more efficient separation of the components may be achieved. Selecting the proper liquid or solid extraction phase, internal standard, and derivatization agents will enhance the accuracy and resolution of the drugs of interest. The internal standard should behave chemically similarly to the drug of interest so that it reflects losses in sample preparation and inconsistencies in injection volume, as well as chromatographic behavior.

CONCLUSIONS

The quality of test results is dependent on the quality of the specimen analyzed. Several pre-analytical factors have been discussed that could alter test results by producing changes that do not reflect the patient's physiological condition. *In vitro* study designs vary, and may not always represent true practice. Caution should be used in interpreting the outcome of such studies. The materials used in devices for collection, processing and storage may influence plasma or serum drug concentrations. Thorough pre- and post-market medical device evaluations should help minimize many of the pre-analytical errors described herein. Understanding the limitations of blood collection devices and possible mechanisms of interferences allows the laboratory to develop specimen collection and handling policies and procedures to minimize inaccuracies in reporting due to a pre-analytical error. By minimizing errors in the pre-analytical phase, the laboratory can improve the quality of analytical results.

References

[1] Green S. Improving the pre-analytical process. The focus on specimen quality. J Med Biochem 2008;27:343—7.
[2] Lippi G, Guidi GC, Mattiuzzi C, Plebani M. Pre-analytical variability: the dark side of the moon in laboratory testing. Clin Chem Lab Med 2006;44:358—65.
[3] Carraro P, Plebani M. Errors in STAT laboratory; types and frequency 10 years later. Clin Chem 2007;53:1338—42.
[4] Nafziger AN, Bertino JS. Utility and application of urine drug testing in chronic pain management with opioids. Clin J Pain 2009;25:73—9.
[5] Fritch D, Blum K, Nonnemacher S, et al. Barbiturate detection in oral fluid, plasma and urine. Ther Drug Monit 2011;33:1—8.
[6] Lui H, Delgado MR. Therapeutic drug concentration monitoring using saliva samples. Clin Pharmacokinet 1999;36:453—70.
[7] Horning MG, Brown L, Nowlin J, et al. Use of saliva in therapeutic drug monitoring. Clin Chem 1977;23:157—64.
[8] Knott C, Reynolds F. The place of saliva in antiepileptic drug monitoring. Ther Drug Monit 1984;6:35—41.
[9] Daly AK. Pharmacogenetics and human genetic polymorphisms. Biochem J 2010;429:435—49.
[10] Lippi G, Blanckaert N, Bonini P, et al. Causes, consequences, detection and prevention of identification errors in laboratory diagnostics. Clin Chem Lab Med 2009;47:143—53.
[11] Genser D. Food and drug interaction: consequences for the nutrition/health status. Ann Nutr & Metab 2008;52(Suppl. 1):29—32.
[12] Dasgupta A, Bernard DW. Herbal remedies: effects on clinical laboratory tests. Arch Pathol Lab Med 2006;130:521—8.
[13] Lynch T, Price A. The effect of cytochrome P450 metabolism on drug response, interactions and adverse effects. Am Fam Physician 2007;76:391—6.
[14] Dasgupta A, Wu S, Actor J, et al. Effect of Asian and Siberian ginseng on serum digoxin measurement by five digoxin immunoassays. Am J Clin Path 2003;119:298—303.

[15] Datta P, Dasgupta A. Effect of Chinese medicines Chan Su and Danshen in EMIT 2000 and Randox digoxin immunoassays: wide variation in digoxin-like immunoreactivity and magnitude of interference in digoxin measurement by different brands of the same product. Ther Drug Monit 2002;24:637−44.

[16] Lurie Y, Loebstein R, Kurnik D, et al. Warfarin and vitamin K intake in the era of pharmacogenetics. Br J Clin Pharmacol 2010;70:164−70.

[17] Cushman M, Booth SL, Possidente CJ, et al. The association of vitamin K status with warfarin sensitivity at the onset of treatment. Br J Haematol 2001;112:572−7.

[18] Lubetsky A, Dekel-Stern E, Chetrit A, et al. Vitamin K intake and sensitivity to warfarin in patients consuming regular diets. Thromb Haemost 1999;81:396−9.

[19] Datta P. A blocker reagent to reduce Digibind interference in a non-pretreatment digoxin assay [abstract]. Ther Drug Monit 1995;17:407.

[20] Wood FL, Earl JW, Nath C, Coakley JC. Falsely low vancomycin results using the Abbott TDx. Ann Clin Biochem 2000;37:411−3.

[21] Albani F, Riva R, Contin M, Baruzzi A. Valproic acid binding to human serum albumin and human plasma: effects of pH variation and buffer composition in equilibrium dialysis. Ther Drug Monit 1984;6. 31−23.

[22] Ohshima T, Hasegawa T, Johno I, Kitazawa S. Variations in protein binding of drugs in plasma and serum. Clin Chem 1989;35:1722−5.

[23] Carraro P. Hemolyzed specimens: a reason for rejection or a clinical challenge? Clin Chem 2000;46:306−7.

[24] Blank DW, Kroll MH, Ruddel ME, Elin RJ. Hemoglobin interference from *in vivo* hemolysis. Clin Chem 1985;31:343−7.

[25] Ryder KW, Trundle DS, Bode MA, et al. Effects of hemolysis, icterus and lipemia on automated immunoassays. Clin Chem 1991;37:1134−5.

[26] Vallner JJ. Binding of drugs by albumin and plasma proteins. J Pharmaceut Sci 1977;66:447−65.

[27] Koch-Weser J, Sellers EM. Binding of drugs to serum albumin. New Engl J Med 1976;294:311−6, 526−31.

[28] Pike E, Shuterud B, Kiefulf P, et al. Binding and displacement of basic, acidic and neutral drugs in normal and orosomucoid-deficient plasma. Clin Pharmacokinet 1981;6:367.

[29] Henderson SJ, Linup WE. Interaction of 3-carboxy-4-methyl-5-propyl-2-furanpropanoic acid, an inhibitor of plasma protein binding in uraemia, with human albumin. Biochem Pharmacol 1990;40:2543−8.

[30] Cotham RH, Shand D. Spuriously low plasma propranolol concentrations resulting from blood collection methods. Clin Pharmacol Ther 1975;18(5 Pt. 1):535−8.

[31] Misson AW, Dickson SJ. Contamination of blood samples by plasticizer in evacuated tubes. Clin Chem 1974;20:1247.

[32] Borga O, Piafsky KM, Nilsen OG. Plasma protein binding of basic drugs. Clin Pharmacol Ther 1977;22 (5 Pt. 1):539−44.

[33] Stargel WW, Roe CR, Routledge PA, Shand DG. Importance of blood-collection tubes in plasma lidocaine determinations. Clin Chem 1979;25:617−9.

[34] Shah VP, Knapp G, Skelly JP, Cabana BE. Interference with measurements of certain drugs in plasma by a plasticizer in Vacutainer tubes. Clin Chem 1982;28:2327−8.

[35] Malik S, Landicho D, Halverson K, et al. Digoxin like immunoreactivity and plasticizers in hemofiltrate of dialysis patients. Clin Chem 1991;37:931.

[36] Datta P, Hinz V, Klee G. Comparison of four digoxin immunoassays with respect to interference from digoxin-like immunoreactive factors. Clin Biochem 1996;29:541−7.

[37] Daniel R, Thomas JB, Alejandro EDR. Effect of free fatty acids on binding of drugs by bovine serum albumin, by human serum albumin and by rabbit serum. J Pharmacol Exp Ther 1971;176:261−72.

[38] Horiuchi T, Johno I, Kitazawa S, et al. Plasma free fatty acids and protein binding of disopyramide during hemodialysis. Eur J Clin Pharmacol 1987;33:327−9.

[39] Horiuchi T, Johno I, Kitazawa S, et al. Inhibitory effect of free fatty acids on plasma protein binding of disopyramide in haemodialysis patients. Eur J Clin Pharmacol 1989;36:175−80.

[40] Kessler KM, Leech RC, Spann JF. Blood collection techniques, heparin and quinidine protein binding. Clin Pharmacol Ther 1979;25:204.

[41] O'Connell ME, Heim KL, Halstenson CE, Matzke GR. Analytical accuracy of determinations of aminoglycoside concentrations by enzyme multiplied immunoassay, fluorescence polarization immunoassay and radioimmunoassay in the presence of heparin. J Clin Microbiol 1984;20:1080−2.

[42] Blifeld C, Ettenger RB. Measurement of cyclosporine levels in samples obtained from peripheral sites and indwelling lines. New Engl J Med 1987;317:509.

[43] Ptachcinski RJ, Walker S, Burckart GJ, Venkataramanan R. Stability and availability of cyclosporine stored in plastic syringes. Am J Hosp Pharm 1986;43:692—4.

[44] Shulman RJ, Ou C, Reed T, Gardner P. Central venous catheters versus peripheral veins for sampling blood levels of commonly used drugs. J Parenter Enteral Nutr 1998;22:234—7.

[45] Meites S, Levitt MJ. Skin puncture and blood collection techniques in infants. Clin Chem 1979;25:183—9.

[46] Kupke IR, Kather B, Zeugner S. On the composition of capillary and venous blood serum. Clin Chim Acta 1981;112:177—85.

[47] Frazer JF, Stasiowski P, Boyd GK. A clinically useful capillary blood sampling technique for rapid determination of therapeutic levels of theophylline. Ther Drug Monit 1983;5:109—12.

[48] Merton G, Jones K, Lee M, et al. Accuracy of cyclosporine measurements made in capillary blood samples obtained by skin puncture. Ther Drug Monit 2000;22:594—8.

[49] Pettersen MD, Driscoll DJ, Moyer TP, et al. Measurement of blood serum cyclosporine levels using capillary "fingerstick" sampling: a validation study. Transpl Intl 1999;12:429—32.

[50] Ritzmo C, Albertioni F, Cosic K, et al. Therapeutic drug monitoring of methotrexate on the pediatric oncology ward: can blood sampling from central venous accesses substitute for capillary finger punctures? Ther Drug Monit 2007;29:447—51.

[51] Hill BM, Laessig RH, Koch DD, Hassemer DJ. Comparison of plastic vs glass evacuated serum-separator (SST) blood-drawing tubes for common clinical chemistry determinations. Clin Chem 1992;38(8 Pt. 1):1474—8.

[52] Smets EM, Dijkstra—Lagemaat JE, Blankenstein MA. Influence of blood collection in plastic vs glass evacuated serum-separator tubes on hormone and tumour marker levels. Clin Chem Lab Med 2004;42:435—9.

[53] Dasgupta A, Blackwell W, Bard D. Stability of therapeutic drug measurement in specimens collected in VACUTAINER plastic blood-collection tubes. Ther Drug Monit 1996;18:306—9.

[54] Faynor SM, Robinson R. Suitability of plastic collection tubes for cyclosporine measurements. Clin Chem 1998;44:2220—1.

[55] Boeynaems JM, De Leener A, Dessars B, et al. Evaluation of a new generation of plastic evacuated blood collection tubes in clinical chemistry, therapeutic drug monitoring, hormone and trace metal analysis. Clin Chem Lab Med 2004;42:67—71.

[56] Landt M, Wilhite TR, Smith CH. A new plastic evacuated tube with plasma separator. J Clin Lab Anal 1995;9:101—6.

[57] Tarasidis CG, Garnett WR, Kline BJ, Pellock JM. Influence of tube type, storage time and temperature on the total and free concentration of valproic acid. Ther Drug Monit 1986;8:373—876.

[58] Spina E, Ericsson O, Nordin C. Analysis of tricyclic antidepressants in serum and plasma yield similar results. Ther Drug Monit 1985;7:242—3.

[59] Levering SCM, Oostelbos MCJM, Toll PJM, Loonen AJM. Influence of heparin on the assay of amitriptyline, clomipramine and their metabolites. Ther Drug Monit 1996;18:304—5.

[60] Godolphin W, Trepanier J, Farrell K. Serum and plasma for total and free anticonvulsant drug analyses, effects on EMIT assays and ultrafiltration devices. Ther Drug Monit 1983;5:319—23.

[61] Krogstad DJ, Granich GG, Murray PR, et al. Heparin interferes with the radioenzymatic and homogenous enzyme immunoassays for aminoglycosides. Clin Chem 1982;28:1517—21.

[62] Nilsson L, Maller R, Ansehn S. Inhibition of aminoglycoside activity in heparin. Antimicrob Agents Chemother 1981;20:155—8.

[63] Ebert SC, Leroy M, Darcey B. Comparison of aminoglycoside concentrations measured in plasma versus serum. Ther Drug Monit 1989;11:44—6.

[64] Wills BK, Mycyk MB, Mazor S, et al. Factitious lithium toxicity secondary to lithium heparin containing blood tubes. J Med Toxicol 2006;2:61—3.

[65] Siebers RWL, Chen CT, Ferguson FI, Maling TJB. Effect of blood sample tubes on amiodarone and desethylamiodarone concentrations. Ther Drug Monit 1988;10:349—51.

[66] Nyberg G, Mårtensson E. Preparation of serum and plasma samples for determination of tricyclic antidepressants: effects of blood collection tubes and storage. Ther Drug Monit 1986;8:478—82.

[67] Pasciolla P, Ince G, Fay A, et al. An evaluation of selected enzyme immunoassay procedures using serum and plasma. Clin Chem 1980;26:937.

[68] Janknegt R, Lohman JJHM, Hooymans PM, Merkus FWHM. Do evacuated blood collection tubes interfere with therapeutic drug monitoring? Pharm Week Scientific Ed 1983;5:287−90.

[69] Quattrocchi F, Karnes HT, Robinson JD, Hendeles L. Effect of serum separator blood collection tubes on drug concentrations. Ther Drug Monitor 1983;5:359−562.

[70] Bergqvist Y, Eckerbom S, Funding L. Effect of use of gel-barrier sampling tubes on determination of some antiepileptic drugs in serum. Clin Chem 1984;30:465−6.

[71] Smith RL. Effect of serum-separator gels on progesterone assays. Clin Chem 1985;31:1239.

[72] Landt M, Smith CH, Hortin GL. Evaluation of evacuated blood-collection tubes: effects of three types of polymeric separators on therapeutic drug-monitoring specimens. Clin Chem 1993;39:1712−7.

[73] Karppi J, Akerman K, Parviainen M. Suitability of collection tubes with separator gels for collecting and storing blood samples for therapeutic drug monitoring. Clin Chem Lab Med 2000;38:313−20.

[74] Bailey DN, Coffee JJ, Briggs JR. Stability of drug concentrations in plasma stored in serum separator blood collection tubes. Ther. Drug Monit 1988;10:352−4.

[75] Devine JE. Assessment of the Corvac blood collection tube for drug specimen processing. Ther Drug Monit 1986;8:241−3.

[76] Koch T, Platoff G. Suitability of collection tubes with separator gels for therapeutic drug monitoring. Ther Drug Monit 1990;12:277−80.

[77] Mauro L, Mauro V. Effect of serum separator tubes on free and total phenytoin and carbamazepine serum concentrations. Ther Drug Monit 1991;13:240−3.

[78] Dasgupta A, Blackwell W, Bard D. Stability of therapeutic drug measurement in specimens collected in VACUTAINER plastic blood-collection tubes. Ther Drug Monit 1996;18:306−9.

[79] Dasgupta A, Yared MA, Wells A. Time-dependent absorption of therapeutic drugs by the gel of Greiner Vacuette blood collection tubes. Ther Drug Monit 2000;22:427−31.

[80] Bush V, Blennerhasset J, Wells A, Dasgupta A. Stability of therapeutic drugs in serum collected in Vacutainer serum separator tubes containing a new gel (SST II). Ther Drug Monit 2001;23:259−62.

[81] Schouwers S, Brandt I, Willemse J, et al. Influence of separator gel in Sarstedt S-Monovette serum tubes on various therapeutic drugs, hormones and proteins. Clin Chim Acta 2011;412:1428−35.

[82] Luque-Garcia JL, Neubert TA. Sample preparation from serum/plasma profiling and biomarker identification by mass spectrometry. J Chromatogr A 2007;1153:259−76.

CHAPTER

3

Analytical Techniques used in Therapeutic Drug Monitoring

Michael C. Milone

Department of Pathology and Laboratory Medicine, University of Pennsylvania
School of Medicine, Philadelphia, PA

OUTLINE

INTRODUCTION

"All things are poison, and nothing is without poison; only the dose permits something not to be poisonous" said Paracelsus (1493—1541). While Paracelsus astutely recognized the relationship between dose and toxicity five centuries ago, it is evident today that toxicity is also highly dependent upon the concentrations achieved *in vivo* for many drugs and toxins. The absorption, distribution, metabolism and excretion (ADME) characteristics of a compound depend not only upon its chemical properties, but also upon the physiology and environment of the individual exposed to the compound. Differences in physiology and environment lead to wide pharmacokinetic variability for many drugs. Combined with a narrow therapeutic index, knowing the dose of the drug is often not enough to predict the drug response, and potentially lethal consequences can ensue from typically non-lethal doses.

The advent of modern chemical analysis permits a much greater understanding of drug pharmacology through measurement of drugs and their metabolites in blood and bodily fluids. Although the measurement of a drug's concentration is readily accomplished, the precision and accuracy of a measurement depends upon a number of factors, including the analytical platform. Laboratory scientists must balance additional factors beyond precision and accuracy in deciding which analytical platform will best fit the clinical requirements of a particular drug, such as the ease of test performance, the speed with which a test result can be produced, the specimen throughput and, of course, cost. This chapter provides a broad overview of commonly used analytical techniques employed in clinical laboratories today for therapeutic drug monitoring (TDM). Emphasis will be placed upon the general performance characteristics of different methods, and how these characteristics practically affect the application of a method to therapeutic drug monitoring in the clinic. Given the number of methods and variations in each method, it is impossible to cover all aspects of any analytical platform. For a more in-depth discussion of instrumentation and methods of chemical analysis, readers are directed towards textbooks specifically devoted to these subjects.

A GENERAL CLASSIFICATION OF ANALYTICAL METHODS

Analytical methods can be divided into three categories, based upon their precision and accuracy, using a schema original developed by the International Union of Pure and Applied Chemistry (IUPAC) [1]. Those analytical techniques with the highest precision and accuracy are generally referred to as definitive methods. A *definitive method* must have negligible systematic error relative to the application of the measurement. Due to the exacting nature of measurements required for definitive methods, few laboratories have the resources necessary to develop them and they are generally not amenable to routine application in TDM; however, they are typically employed by laboratories such as those of the National Institute of Standards and Technology (NIST, formerly known as the National Bureau of Standards), and are critical for the generation of standardized reference material (SRM) that can be used to aid in method harmonization (discussed further below). In contrast to definitive methods, *reference methods* are those methods possessing "small, estimated inaccuracies relative to the end use requirement". Reference methods are generally complex, but are more amenable to application in clinical laboratories. Methods using liquid chromatography combined with tandem mass spectrometry (LC-MS/MS), with proper validation, often meet the requirements for a reference method. Lastly, *routine methods*, usually immunoassays, generally represent those assays that may have greater uncertainty but have other advantages, such as ease of performance, high throughput and lower cost. Nevertheless, all methods applied in the clinical laboratory should have a degree of uncertainty that is appropriate for the clinical decision that will be based upon the result. Thus, it is important to have a thorough understanding of measurement uncertainty to interpret any test, especially TDM tests.

UNDERSTANDING AND MINIMIZING MEASUREMENT UNCERTAINTY IN THE CLINICAL LABORATORY

Uncertainty is a fundamental part of any measurement. In the case of TDM, the intent is to measure the concentration of a specific drug at a specific time following the administration of a particular dose of the drug. When the measurand (the quantity to be measured) is defined in this way, it should be obvious that uncertainty may exist in all aspects of the TDM sampling and analysis process from the time that the drug is administered to the time that the drug concentration is reported. The complexity of the TDM process and potential for error makes successful TDM a daunting task. Nevertheless, minimizing the uncertainty in the measured concentration of a particular drug in an individual specimen is certainly a major step towards reducing the overall uncertainty in the intended measurement. A thorough understanding of analytical error is therefore essential before one can begin any discussion of analytical techniques in TDM.

The difference between a measured concentration, C_m, and the "true" concentration, C_μ (an idealized quantity that is unknowable) is often termed the total error of the measurement, ε_t, which can be expressed as:

$$C_m - C_\mu = \varepsilon_t \qquad (3.1)$$

The ε_t is commonly viewed as a composite of two types of error, random error ε_R and systematic error ε_S. Random error, as the name implies, varies unpredictably from one measurement to another, arising from the combination of numerous small, immeasurable variations within an analytical system. Factors that might be considered as contributing to random error include small, unpredictable fluctuations in ambient temperature, pressure, power supply and electromagnetic fields around an instrument. While any one of these factors might not be random or normally distributed over time, their combined effects typically lead to error that generally obeys a normal or Gaussian distribution centered on zero. Due to the Gaussian nature of random error, the impact of this error, also known as analytical precision, can generally be accessed through the performance of replicate measurements. In the clinical laboratory, precision is typically assessed by the standard deviation of repeated measurements (σ) expressed as a percentage of the average result (μ) in a quantity termed the coefficient of variation (CV) using the equation:

$$CV = \frac{\sigma}{\mu} * 100 \qquad (3.2)$$

While most laboratories strive for very high precision (%CV less than 10%), this is not always possible. The Federal Drug Administration (FDA) has published a guidance document for validation of bioanalytical drug assays. This document suggests that a CV of < 15% be considered the standard precision goal for bioanalytical drug assays, with an acceptable CV as high as 20% at the lower limit of quantitation (LLOQ) [2]. While precision of this magnitude may be adequate for some TDM applications, some critical-dose drugs may require greater precision. The immunosuppressant tacrolimus is illustrative of the dangers of a "one size fits all" approach. The target range for blood tacrolimus trough concentrations at some transplant centers is 5–8 ng/mL in an effort to reduce the adverse effects of these drugs. At a precision level of 20%, approximately one out of every five individuals with a measured value of 6 ng/mL will have a level below 5 ng/mL, suggesting the need for a dose increase. Given the potentially serious consequences of a subtherapeutic tacrolimus concentration, this error would clearly limit the usefulness of an assay with this precision when using this lower, narrow target range.

In contrast to random error, systematic analytical error represents a consistent, reproducible form of measurement error. Although the distinction between factors that contribute to random and systematic error is often difficult to make, the nature of each error is such that they cannot be dealt with in the same way. Unlike Gaussian-distributed random error, which can generally be handled by repeated measurements of a sample, systematic error, by its nature, cannot be estimated through repeated measurements. A common form of systematic error is method bias, which might arise due to differences between instrument calibration or reagent lots. These differences are generally of sufficient magnitude and consistency to yield a higher or lower average result for one method versus another. While bias between methods can generally be detected at a particular instance in time, their control over time can be quite challenging. Systematic errors within methods can also arise, such as accumulation of debris on a measurement probe that leads to a non-random degradation in the probe's response. Quality control (QC) programs within laboratories often expend great effort to detect and correct systematic errors. Unfortunately, systematic errors may also arise due to incomplete understanding of the measurement procedure resulting in insidious and sometimes challenging problems. The problem of drug interference in immunoassays due to antibody cross-reactivity (discussed further below) is one example of many challenging systematic errors that can be very difficult to predict and detect.

One of the greatest challenges in TDM and clinical chemistry relates to the availability of fully characterized materials for calibration of analytical methods. Under ideal circumstances, a reference material will be available with well-characterized uncertainty for the analyte concentration. This material would provide a way for a laboratory or test kit manufacturer to evaluate a method for systematic error. The NIST currently prepares a number of SRMs for chemical analysis in which the concentrations of the analytes are traceable to the defining units of measurement (e.g., chemical identity, mass and volume for therapeutic drugs). Unfortunately, NIST SRMs exist only for four anti-epileptic drugs (NIST SRM 900, certified in 1979 and currently unavailable) and lithium (NIST SRM 956c). Most laboratories or assay manufacturers therefore must find alternatives to which they can standardize their assays. Practically, this sometimes leads to great difficulty in achieving traceability of results across methods and laboratories. Traceability, or knowledge of the systematic error between methods, therefore remains a critical issue in clinical laboratories, including those that perform testing for TDM. All reputable laboratories participate in external assessments known as proficiency testing. These testing schemes compare results of different laboratories that perform testing on identical samples using either the same or different methods. Laboratories performing tacrolimus testing on the LC-MS/MS platform, considered a reference analytical method due to its specificity and precision, can have an average bias across laboratories of 10% for the same analyte in the same specimens [3]. Differences across platforms can be even higher, highlighting the critical nature of systematic error in measurement. Comparison of sirolimus monitoring by LC-MS/MS compared with the commercial ARCHITECT i2000™ immunoassay from Abbott Diagnostics demonstrates that the immunoassay has an average ~20% positive bias compared with LC-MS/MS methods, most likely due to metabolite interferences ([4] and author's unpublished observations). Clinicians interpreting a TDM result must therefore be cognizant of the laboratory and test platform being used for a particular test, since the combination of random and systematic effects can have a major impact on the uncertainty of the result.

Unfortunately, efforts to harmonize TDM assays have lagged significantly. While there are suggested procedures for harmonization of assays across laboratories, these procedures require collaborative studies across multiple laboratories with standardized test materials and fully validated methods [5]. The increasing number of analytical platforms available as well as the considerable expense required to achieve assay harmonization has led to few tests undergoing harmonization. Unfortunately, the frequent use of multiple laboratories by patients due to third-party payer requirements in the US makes the application of TDM data through personal experience very challenging. Harmonization efforts in TDM assays become increasingly important, and harmonization efforts should be a part of the development for any TDM assay, especially for new drugs in the future.

IMMUNOASSAYS

Antibody-based immunoassays are the workhorses of the modern clinical laboratory. These assays build upon the high affinity (dissociation constant $[K_d]$ of $\sim 10^{-9}$) and specific interaction between an antigen (Ag) and an antibody (Ab). Immunoassays have been applied to measurement of a diverse array of molecules, both small and large. The ability to apply immunoassay methods to a wide array of molecular targets as well as their relative simplicity in operation using automated analyzers makes such assays highly attractive for clinical laboratories. In most cases they do not require expensive equipment, and methods have been developed that can be performed almost anywhere, including directly at the patient's bedside in point of care (POC) applications. Their ready adaptability to high-throughput chemistry analyzers present in most clinical laboratories of moderate to high complexity is also likely to maintain their position as a stable platform in the clinical laboratory over the decades to come.

Immunoassay: Basic Immunochemistry

Immunoassays are classic receptor to ligand binding reactions governed by the fundamental Law of Mass Action:

$$Ag + Ab \underset{K_d}{\overset{K_a}{\rightleftharpoons}} Ag : Ab \tag{3.3}$$

where K_a represents the rate constant for association of free Ag and free Ab and K_d represents the rate constant for dissociation of the Ag:Ab complex. When this binding reaction is carried out to the point of equilibrium, the bound and free Ab are related by:

$$k_{eq} = \frac{[Ag:Ab]}{[Ag] * [Ab]} \qquad (3.4)$$

where k_{eq} represents the constant of equilibrium, [Ag:Ab] represents the concentration of the Ag:Ab complex, [Ab] represents the concentration of free antibody and [Ag] represents the concentration of free antigen. Provided the Ab has high affinity and is present in significant excess of the Ag, measurement of the Ag:Ab complex formed by this reaction becomes a useful endpoint for quantitative immunoassays.

However, antibody molecules are typically divalent rather than monovalent. As a result, complexes composed of multiple Ag and Ab molecules can form as depicted in Fig. 3.1A with reaction kinetics that are more complex than a monovalent receptor to ligand reaction described in equation 3.4. Ag:Ab complexes formed by multivalent Ab may reach sizes that ultimately precipitate from solution, producing the classic precipitin reaction. The formation of these larger Ag:Ab complexes can then be assessed using techniques based upon light scattering, such as turbidimetry and nephelometry, permitting the use of the precipitin reaction for quantitative measurements of the Ag:Ab complex as discussed further below. Importantly, unlike the monovalent binding situation, the precipitin reaction only exhibits increased Ag:Ab complex formation within a low concentration range where antibody exists in excess of antigen. Increasing the concentration of antigen to a point where it exceeds the concentration of antibody (assuming the Ab concentration is held constant) eventually leads to a reduction in Ag:Ab complex formation, producing the typical precipitin curve shown in Fig. 3.1B.

A number of factors influence the kinetics and equilibrium of Ag:Ab complex formation. The ionic strength (i.e., salt concentration) and the ion species of the reaction solution are important since they may alter ionic bonds that contribute to complex formation. This is particular true for basic (i.e., cationic) drugs where cationic salts have been shown to have significant inhibitory effects on antibody binding [6]. Polymers present within the reaction solution can also influence the precipitin reaction, sometimes to the advantage of assay design. This phenomenon, known as the polymer effect, is thought to be a result of steric exclusion of Ab and Ag from solvated polymer. Since the volume of solvent from which Ab and Ag are excluded effectively increases with increasing polymer size and/or concentration, the net result is a decrease in the non-excluded volume available to the Ab and Ag, effectively increasing their local concentration and enhancing their interaction and complex formation [7, 8]. Commonly used polymers include polyethylene glycol (PEG), polypropylene glycol (PPG), dextran, modified cellulose, polyvinyl alcohol (PVA) and polyvinylpyrrolidone (PVP). Temperature certainly affects the kinetics of Ag:Ab complex formation; however, the difference in reaction rate over the thermal range typically afforded by temperature control mechanisms in analytical instruments is rather small. The pH of a solution can profoundly affect the structure and binding of antibodies, particularly at the extremes of pH (i.e., pH < 4.0 or pH > 8.0). Nevertheless, pH changes within the pH 6.0 to pH 8.0 range that are generally attainable with typical buffer systems have also been shown to contribute little to the overall rate and formation of immune complexes [9].

FIGURE 3.1 General scheme of immunoassay: (A) Complexes composed of multiple antigen and antibody; (B) Immune complex formations under various scenarios: antigen excess, equilibrium and antibody excess.

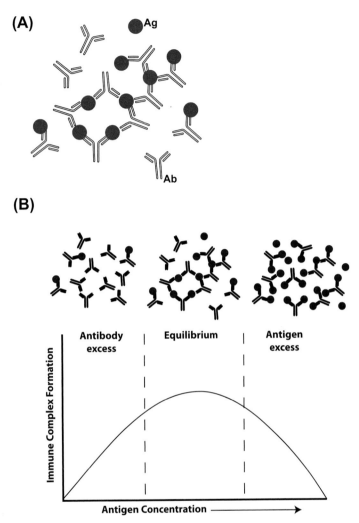

Immunoassay Design Principles

A multitude of immunoassay designs have been developed over the past 50 years since Solomon Berson and Rosalyn Yalow described the radioimmunoassay (RIA) [10]. Broadly, immunoassays can be divided into competitive and non-competitive platforms. In a competitive immunoassay platform, a labeled reagent antigen competes with unlabeled antigen in the specimen for binding to the antibody. The RIA developed for insulin used an insulin polypeptide that was labeled with radioactive iodine (originally ^{131}I, with later assays using ^{125}I). Following mixture of the anti-insulin antibody, labeled insulin and serum containing unlabeled insulin, the resulting immune complexes formed were then separated from unbound antibody, labeled insulin and unlabeled insulin. The greater the concentration of unlabeled insulin in serum, the lower was the radioactivity present in the isolated immune complexes, permitting quantitative measurements of insulin. In addition to being competitive, this reaction format required labor-intensive steps to physically separate the Ag:Ab complex from unbound Ab and Ag prior to measurement − a format often called heterogeneous. Due to the difficulty in controlling the separation, approaches that used direct immobilization of primary antibody onto the walls of a test tube or indirect capture of this primary antibody via Staphylococcal protein A or a secondary antibody directed towards the primary antibody constant domains were developed. Separation is then achieved by washing steps that eliminate unbound Ag and/or Ab. The classic enzyme-linked immunosorbent assay (ELISA) technique is an example of a heterogeneous immunoassay format in common use today [11, 12]. Heterogeneous assay platforms can be performed using both competitive and non-competitive designs.

In addition to the labor associated with the separation steps in heterogeneous immunoassays, the assays also pose challenges to automation, especially on high-throughput analyzers used in clinical laboratories. Soon after the first immunoassay was described, significant effort was devoted to developing homogeneous immunoassay techniques that can be completed in a single step without the need for separation. The first commercial homogenous immunoassay based upon electron spin resonance detection of stable nitroxide radicals, termed the free radical association technique (FRAT), was developed, in part to accommodate the screening of large numbers of specimens for drugs of abuse in Vietnam [13, 14]. Several additional homogenous immunoassay methods have subsequently been developed, and these methods form the majority of immunoassays in common use today for routine TDM, as discussed below.

Immunoassay Methods Commonly used for TDM

There are several immunoassay methods commonly used in clinical laboratories, such as EMIT, CEDIA, FPIA, etc. They are discussed below.

Enzyme Immunoassay (EIA) Platforms

The use of radioactive materials such as ^{125}I poses a number of challenges to widespread application of immunoassays. The health concerns and high costs of waste disposal make them burdensome to use. They are also quite difficult to automate safely and cheaply. Enzyme-based immunoassays overcome the major obstacles associated with RIA, while retaining high analytical sensitivity. Many different EIA methods have been described in the published literature, but only the most commonly employed methods that are frequently used in clinical laboratories will be discussed here.

ENZYME-LINKED IMMUNOSORBENT ASSAY (ELISA)

The enzyme-linked immunosorbent assay (ELISA) was originally developed in the 1970s as a non-radioactive alternative to the earlier described RIA methods [11, 12]. Both techniques are based upon the immobilization of the Ag:Ab complex to a solid support to facilitate separation of bound and unbound reaction components. An enzymatically-labeled antibody is then used to permit detection of the resulting immune complex. A number of configurations for the ELISA technique have been developed, with the common sandwich configuration shown in Fig. 3.2A. These heterogeneous enzymatic immunoassays have proven to be quite sensitive. Assays that can measure target molecules with concentrations in the picomolar range are routinely achieved. The PRO-Trac™ II competitive ELISA (Diasorin, Columbia, MD) for tacrolimus is an example of the application of ELISA technology to therapeutic drug monitoring [15, 16].

The requisite separation step in ELISA techniques represents one of the major barriers to widespread application of these techniques in the modern clinical laboratory. The introduction of automation systems using bench-top robotics has helped to reduce the labor typically associated with these assays. Additional variations on the classic microplate-based ELISA technique using plastic beads or microparticles to facilitate washing of the solid phase support have also been developed and commercialized [17]. The microparticle enzyme immunoassay (MEIA) marketed by Abbott Diagnostics was one of the most widely used heterogeneous immunoassay platforms for the immunosuppressive drug tacrolimus, based upon College of American Pathologist Proficiency Survey Data prior to the discontinuation of this assay platform in 2010.

Although the original ELISA methods were based upon the photometric detection of chromogenic substrates generated by the enzymes used in the assay, additional substrate systems have been developed that can impart increased assay sensitivity. One of the most widely used alternatives is chemiluminescence. In methods that use the enzyme horseradish peroxidase (HRP), the luminol reaction (Fig. 3.3A) is often utilized. A similar reaction using a 1,2-dioxetane compound, adamantyl-1,2-dioxetane aryl phosphate, is available for alkaline phosphatase-conjugated antibodies (Fig. 3.3B). Both reactions produce a photon of light as one of the reaction products, and measurement of the light produced is readily achievable using sensitive detectors such as a photomultiplier tube (PMT). The Immulite® 2000 TDM assays developed by Siemens currently employ the alkaline phosphatase chemiluminescence system. Assay platforms that utilize enzymatically-generated fluorescence are also available, such as the conversion of umbelliferone phosphate to the highly fluorescent umbelliferone by alkaline phosphatase used by the MEIA platform [17]. Both chemiluminescent and fluorescent platforms offer amplification along with the wide dynamic range afforded by fluorescence and photon-counting detectors, which have a number of advantages over colorimetric detection.

ENZYME MULTIPLIED IMMUNOASSAY TECHNIQUE (EMIT)

The EMIT platform represents one of the earliest described homogeneous immunoassay platforms. It is based upon the ability of an antibody to inhibit the activity of an enzyme when bound to an Ag that has been attached the enzyme [18]. When free Ag is present in a sample, the free Ag competes with the Ag-conjugated enzyme for antibody binding with increasing Ag leading to increasing enzymatic activity as depicted in Fig. 3.2B. While the first EMIT assay used bacterial lysozyme and measured the change in turbidity of a killed bacterial cell suspension, this enzyme system was problematic for a number of reasons, including the inability to use serum due to the propensity to agglutinate the bacteria. Alternative enzyme systems were sought and modern EMIT assays typically employ glucose-6-phosphate dehydrogenase (G6PDH). The use of G6PDH makes EMIT assays easily adaptable to large-scale clinical analyzers using the absorbance change at 340 nm between

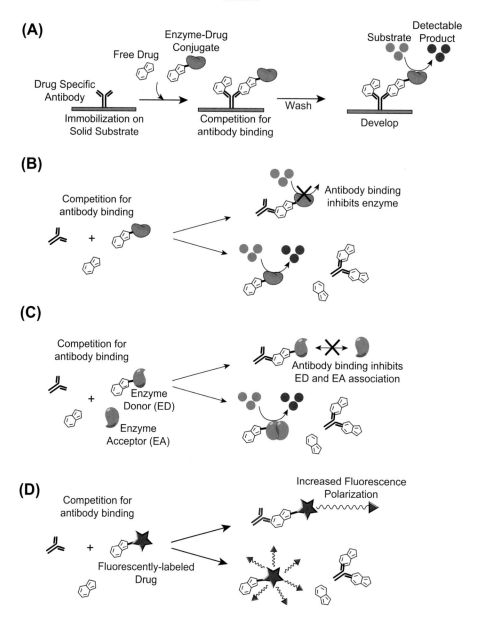

FIGURE 3.2 Immunoassay designs: (A) ELISA (enzyme-linked immunosorbent assay); (B) EMIT (enzyme multiplied immunoassay technique); (C) CEDIA (cloned enzyme donor immunoassay); and (D) FPIA (fluorescence polarization immunoassay).

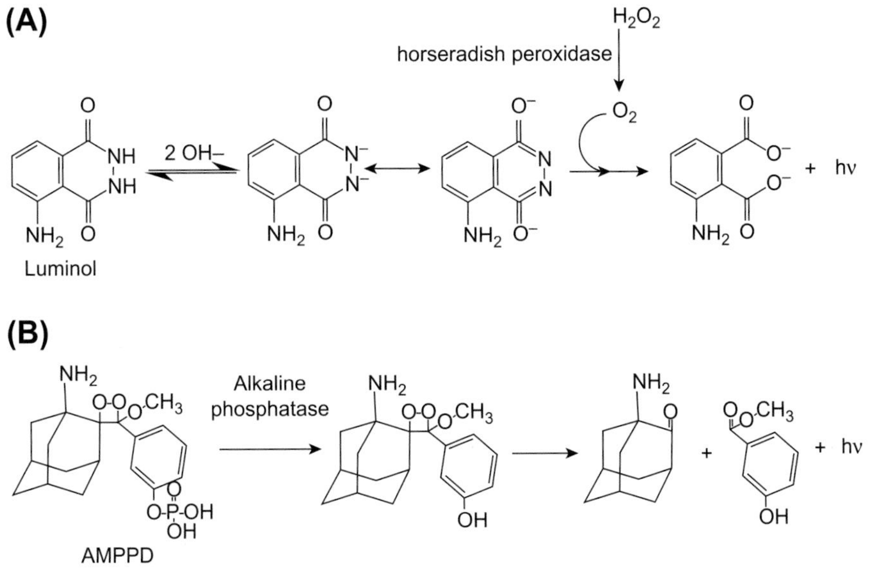

(A)

(B)

FIGURE 3.3 Chemiluminescence reactions: (A) Reaction scheme for production of light from luminol using horseradish peroxidase; (B) Reaction scheme for production of light from 3-(2′-spiroadamantyl)-4-methoxy-4-(3″-phosphoryloxy)-phenyl-1,2-dioxetane (AMPPD) by alkaline phosphatase.

the reaction cofactor NAD+ and its reduced form, NADH. EMIT assays are currently available for most drugs commonly monitored in the clinical laboratory.

CLONED ENZYME DONOR IMMUNOASSAY (CEDIA)

Building upon the earlier success of homogenous assays such as FRAT and EMIT, CEDIA was the first diagnostic assay to use genetic engineering to control enzyme activity of β-galactosidase, an *Escherichia coli* enzyme. This enzyme is involved in the hydrolysis of β-galactosides, and is normally encoded by the Z gene within the Lac operon of this organism. The protein product of the Z gene is enzymatically inactive; however, this gene product spontaneously associates to form a tetrameric complex that displays the β-galactosidase enzymatic activity. Capitalizing upon the requirement for aggregation to form an active enzyme, Henderson *et al.* of Microgenics Corp. determined that active β-galactosidase could be recapitulated using two cloned polypeptide fragments from the enzyme that they termed the enzyme acceptor (EA) and the enzyme donor (ED) [19]. The ED fragment could also be conjugated to small molecules such as a drug without impairing the formation of an active enzyme. Analogous to EMIT, CEDIA is a homogenous immunoassay that is based upon the ability of an antibody to inhibit the spontaneous association between the drug-conjugated ED and the EA required for the formation of an active enzyme complex (Fig. 3.2C). Presence of free drug within a sample can compete for antibody binding, permitting an increase in enzyme activity that can be measured using the chromogenic substrate, chlorophenol red-β-D-glucopyranoside. Several TDM assays are currently available on the CEDIA platform, which can be run on a range of clinical chemistry analyzers using relatively simple photometric detection.

Non-Enzymatic, Fluorescence-Based Immunoassays

While fluorescence can be used in immunoassays by direct labeling with a fluorescent molecule in place of radioactive labeling, these assays, including heterogeneous designs, were initially hampered by background fluorescence due to endogenous components within clinical sample matrices such as bilirubin, hemoglobin, drugs and drug metabolites. Fluorescent labels that are based upon chelates of lanthanide series elements such as europium largely address these interference issues due to extended fluorescence lifetimes of rare earth element chelates compared with the typical endogenous, interfering fluorescent compounds. Combined with time-resolved fluorescence measurements, these labels overcome many of the limitations for fluorescence-based assays using organic fluorophores such as fluorescein isothiocyanate and Rhodamine B. Despite the success of these labeling techniques, they are rarely employed in clinical TDM assays, and there are no FDA-approved or cleared commercial assays currently marketed in the US using this approach. In addition to measuring direct fluorescence label intensity, methods that measure the degree of polarization of emitted fluorescent light (fluorescence polarization immunoassay [FPIA] described below) [20–22] or fluorescence resonant energy transfer (FRET) [23] have also been described. The FPIA platform is currently the only non-enzymatic fluorescence platform in widespread commercial use.

FLUORESCENCE POLARIZATION IMMUNOASSAY (FPIA)

Fluorescence polarization relies on the fact that fluorescent light emitted by a small compound (e.g., a drug) conjugated to a fluorescent molecule exhibits low polarization due to the fast Brownian rotation of the fluorescently-labeled molecule in solution. Upon binding of the fluorescent molecule to a much larger molecule such as an antibody (or other protein), the degree of polarization increases due to the reduced rotation of the bound, fluorescent tracer. Adaptation to a homogeneous immunoassay platform for TDM is therefore relatively simple using a competitive format, where non-conjugated drug present in the sample competes for binding to the antibody, leading to a reduction in polarization (Fig. 3.2D). While these assays are relatively simple to perform with good precision (%CV generally ranges from 1–4%) [24] and good sensitivity [25], they require specialized instrumentation that is not routinely available on commonly used, high-throughput clinical analyzers. In addition, the FPIA tests marketed by Abbott can only be run on Abbott's analyzers (e.g., the TDx or AxSYM analyzer), further restricting the application of this platform, particularly in automated clinical laboratories.

Light-Scattering Based Methods: Turbidimetry and Nephelometry

In turbidimetry, an incident beam of visible light is passed through a sample in a cuvette, and the intensity of the transmitted light is then measured. As Ag:Ab complexes form, light is increasingly scattered away from the incident light path, resulting in a reduction in transmitted light intensity. Provided the antigen and antibody are in an appropriate concentration range for the precipitin reaction, as described earlier, turbidimetric measurements provide a simple and quick way to monitor the formation of Ag:Ab complex formation in a single-step platform. Nephelometry, in contrast to turbidimetry, measures the scattered light rather than transmitted light using photodetectors that are placed at an angle (often 90°) to the incident light path. One of the major advantages of turbidimetry and nephelometry is the ability to perform these measurements using simple photometric systems that are readily incorporated into high-throughput clinical analyzer systems.

In order for light scattering to be used to monitor the formation of immune complexes, the target antigen must exist in a multivalent state. In the case of drugs, this is typically accomplished by the generation of protein (e.g., albumin) [26] or microparticles [27, 28] bearing multiple conjugated molecules. Drug-specific antibody will then lead to the formation of aggregates that scatter light, and free drug in a specimen will then compete for binding to the antibody, leading to a concentration-dependent inhibition of immune complex formation.

While measurement of complex formation at close to the equilibrium state (termed pseudo-equilibrium) can be performed, measurement of the rate of complex formation (either change in intensity over time, or the time to reach a peak rate) can also be used [29–32]. The advantage of rate measurements over pseudo-equilibrium measurements is primarily the benefit of quicker turnaround time. These assays generally have reasonable precision (%CV < 10%) and sensitivity (ng/mL range) for many TDM applications. One of the most important limitations of light-scattering methods, which are based upon the precipitin reaction, is the potential for a pro-zone effect where excess antigen can lead to a reduced signal. The use of competitive inhibition assays typically used for TDM applications avoids this important source of error [27].

Current Challenges for Immunoassay

Immunoassays, like all analytical assays, are subject to both random and systematic measurement error. Some sources of error are platform specific, such as interference produced by endogenous compounds like bilirubin in fluorescence-based immunoassays. The presence of monoclonal proteins such as that found in multiple myeloma can also interfere with some immunoassay platforms [33]. Antibody-based assays are also subject to a particularly insidious error associated with the presence of human antibodies in specimens that may bind to various components within the assay system. The most well recognized form of antibody interference is produced by human antibodies directed towards the constant domains of antibodies produced in other species, such as mice, used in most commercial immunoassay platforms [34]. These antibodies, often termed heterophilic antibodies, can have profound effects on immunoassay results, producing both falsely elevated and falsely reduced concentrations. Although the incidence of clinically significant heterophilic interfering antibodies is likely to be much less than 1%, studies have reported the detectable presence of these antibodies in anywhere from < 1% to 80% of clinical serum/plasma specimens, depending upon the method used for detection. It is often quite difficult for the laboratory to recognize the presence of an interfering heterophilic antibody in routine clinical specimens. Heterophilic antibodies affecting TDM often come to attention only when consumers of TDM data (e.g., physicians and clinical pharmacists) are faced with results that do not make clinical sense [35]. The devastating outcomes that have been reported with heterophilic antibodies illustrate the importance of recognizing this important assay interference, and highlight the benefit of close contact between the laboratory and its clients. Once suspected, a number of techniques are available to confirm their presence [34]. One of the simplest approaches to detecting the presence of an interfering substance affecting an immunoassay is to perform the analysis of a suspected specimen on an alternative assay platform. Heterophilic antibody-induced effects and the effects of other interfering agents may be quite different depending upon the assay platform used. Specimens containing heterophilic antibodies and other interfering substances also often fail to dilute linearly, and dilutional analysis provides another potential method for detecting their presence. Additional tools to specifically demonstrate the presence of a heterophilic antibody include commercial reagents that are specifically designed to neutralize heterophilic antibodies (i.e., antibodies recognizing non-human immunoglobulin) such as the Heterophilic Blocking Reagent (HBR, Scantibodies Laboratories) or Immunoglobulin Inhibiting Reagent (IIR, Bioreclamation), and Protein A/G reagents commonly used for specific adsorption of immunoglobulin. While negative results for any of these tests do not exclude the possibility of an interfering heterophilic antibody or other interfering substance, positive results can confirm their presence. Many manufacturers have also redesigned their immunoassays to make them less sensitive to heterophilic antibody interference.

Beyond analytical interference, immunoassays are also challenged by cross-reactivity between parent drug and metabolite. This problem can be particularly problematic, since drug metabolites may or may not exhibit pharmacologic activity and metabolism may vary considerably from one individual to another. Immunosuppressive drugs (ISDs) illustrate this problem well. The ISDs cyclosporine and tacrolimus each have several metabolites that can achieve concentrations comparable to the parent drug in some individuals [36, 37]. In the case of tacrolimus, the 15-desmethyl and 31-desmethyl metabolites both exhibit significant cross-reactivity with the currently used monoclonal antibodies [38, 39]. While the 31-desmethyl-tacrolimus exhibits ~100% of the activity of tacrolimus, making it potentially useful to measure, the 15-desmethyl metabolite exhibits less than 1% activity. Patients, particularly those with hepatic dysfunction, can also accumulate appreciable concentrations of metabolites that may contribute up to 40% of the immunoreactivity [40]. These forms of interference can sometimes be addressed through improved, more specific antibodies, but they persist for many assays, providing a source of positive bias for immunoassays when compared against more specific methods such as liquid chromatography with mass spectrometry detection (LC-MS).

Digoxin immunoassays are affected by both endogenous and exogenous interfering substances, such as endogenous digoxin-like immunoreactive substances, Digibind (Fab fragment of antidigoxin antibody used in treating acute life-threatening digoxin overdose), spironolactone, potassium canrenoate (not approved by the FDA for use in US but used in other parts of the world), and Chinese medicines like Chan Su, Lu-Shen-Wan and oleander containing herbal products (see Chapter 11 for more detailed discussion on this topic). In fact, digoxin immunoassay is subject to more interferences than any other TDM assay. Immunoassays for tricyclic antidepressants (TC) are also subject to interferences from a variety of compounds structurally related to TCA, including carbamazepine (see Chapter 13 for more detail). Carbamazepine 10, 11-epoxide, an active metabolite of carbamazepine, showed anywhere from 0% to 96% interference with various carbamazepine immunoassays [41].

GAS AND LIQUID CHROMATOGRAPHY

The ability to separate compounds has long been an important part of chemical analysis. The drive to develop improved separation of plant pigments led Russian botanist Michael Tsvet to develop a technique in the early 1900s for their separation using a glass column filled with calcium carbonate through which he passed an extract of plants in a mixture of ether and ethanol. The flow of the plant extract through this column allowed Tsvet to separate many colorful compounds, such as chlorophyll and carotenoids, extracted from the plants, and led him to call this technique chromatography or "color writing". Over the subsequent 100 years since its first description, chromatography has taken a central role in the chemistry laboratory.

All chromatographic methods are based upon the separation of compounds present within a flowing liquid or gas (the mobile phase) by their physical or chemical interaction with an immobile material (the stationary phase), which retards their mobility. Once separated, a variety of techniques can be employed to detect the compounds leaving the chromatographic system, including simple detectors such ultraviolet or visible light spectrophotometry or flame ionization detection (FID), or more complex detectors utilizing mass spectrometry (MS). Fig. 3.4 illustrates a basic schematic for a liquid or gas chromatography system that might be employed in a clinical laboratory.

Time required for analysis is a fundamental parameter in chromatography. In the most simplistic form, the data provided by a chromatography system (the chromatogram, see Fig. 3.5) are the abundance of chemical compounds leaving the system in the mobile phase over time. From these data, several parameters can be derived. The interval between the time of specimen injection and the time of peak elution (i.e., a compound's exit from the chromatography system) is typically referred to as the retention time, t_r (see Fig. 3.5). t_r is often useful to help confirm the identity of a compound of interest; however, more specific techniques such as mass spectrometry are required for robust chemical identification. The chosen mobile and stationary phases are by far the most important factors affecting the t_r for an individual chemical compound. While retention time is important, the primary aim of chromatography is separation. Adequate separation of compound peaks is essential for integration of the area under the peak — the parameter that best correlates with quantity. Thus, resolution (R), which

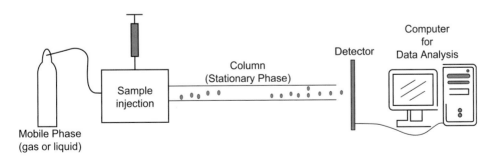

FIGURE 3.4 Scheme for basic chromatography system.

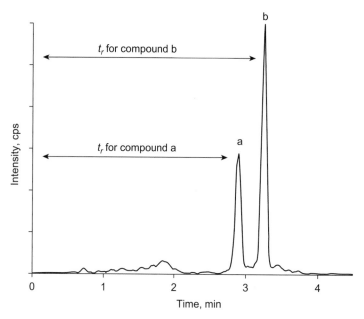

FIGURE 3.5 Basic chromato-graphic analysis showing baseline separation of compounds "a" and "b".

is the ratio of the difference in retention time for two compounds (designated "a" and "b") relative to the average peak width (w) of both compounds, is found as follows:

$$R = \frac{(t_{ra} - t_{rb})}{\frac{1}{2} * (W_a - W_b)} \tag{3.5}$$

R is an important parameter requiring optimization in chromatographic analyses. A discussion of the factors that affect retention time and resolution of chromatographic systems includes, first and foremost, the choice of mobile or stationary phase along with parameters such as the length of the separation column, the nature of the stationary phase (e.g., particle size and packing quality if composed of microparticles), the mobile phase flow rate, the separation column temperature and pressure, to name just a few. A detailed discussion on chromatography is beyond the scope of this chapter, but can be found in any textbook on analytical chemistry.

The choice between gas chromatography (GC) versus liquid chromatography (LC) is generally based upon the compound of interest. GC has high resolution, and can therefore be quite useful in achieving good compound separation. The fact that only ~20% of organic compounds can be separated by GC compared with at least 80% by LC is a major limitation of GC [42]. This is in large part due to the requirement that the compound must be either volatile or able to be made volatile using chemical derivatization. In contrast, LC is capable of separating a wide range of compounds without the need for derivatization. Furthermore, most of the compounds separable by GC are also amenable to LC separation as well, and often with far less sample preparation prior to analysis. Thus, while GC-based methods are still employed for TDM by some laboratories for TDM analytes such as busulfan [43], and have a role for some compounds not amenable to LC, most assays being developed today for therapeutic drugs utilize LC approaches.

LC methods such as high-performance liquid chromatography (HPLC) are widely used in clinical laboratories. A variety of detectors is utilized, from the basic ultraviolet (UV) detector to multi-wavelength photodiode array detectors to mass spectrometry. While HPLC methods using UV absorbance detection (HPLC-UV) are generally quite robust, they are not without their challenges. Most methods require laborious pre-analytical extraction steps. Even with these pre-analytical steps, interfering substances can sometimes pose significant challenges (see Fig. 3.6). The choice of an internal standard that behaves sufficiently similar to the compound of interest during specimen processing and is chromatographically separable from the compound can also be challenging. Despite these limitations, HPLC-UV methods continue to be developed, most likely due to the relatively lower cost of instrumentation compared with LC-MS systems.

Advantages of Liquid Chromatography with Mass Spectrometry Detection

While chromatography alone provides a high degree of specificity in chemical analysis, the potential power of combining LC with highly specific detection provided by MS was recognized very early in the field of analytical chemistry. Unlike GC, where the analyte is already in a vapor phase, LC is faced with the compounds in a liquid. Moving these compounds from the liquid to vapor phase and then introducing them into the vacuum conditions of MS represented a significant technological hurdle. The development of electrospray ionization (ESI) technology by John Fenn in the 1980s proved to be the major advance necessary to make LC-MS approaches possible. Since the development of ESI a number of additional ionization approaches have been developed, such as atmospheric pressure chemical ionization (APCI), particle beam and thermospray. The choice of ionization technique depends greatly upon several factors, especially the compound and the sample matrix.

MASS SPECTROMETRY AND LC-MS/MS APPLICATION TO TDM

A mass spectrometer is an instrument that measures the mass to charge ratio (m/z) of an ion. Several different types of mass spectrometers have been developed over the past century, but all are composed of three basic components. The ion source already discussed above is critical to achieve the charged molecular species in a vapor state amenable to mass analysis. The mass analyzer performs the separation of ions by their m/z. Finally, a sensitive detector is used to detect and quantify the ions successfully passing through the mass analyzer. The detector signals are then used to produce a mass spectrum such as that shown for the drug tacrolimus in Fig. 3.7.

Similar to ion sources, multiple types of mass analyzers have been developed. Each has advantages and disadvantages. In the classic magnetic sector mass analyzer, ions with differing m/z are separated by their different flight paths as they are accelerated through a magnetic and/or electric field. While these analyzers have very high resolution and sensitivity, they are rarely found outside of research environments. Time of flight (TOF)

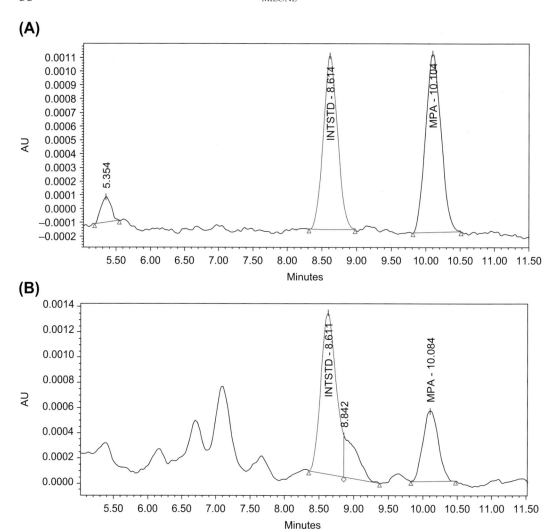

FIGURE 3.6 Chromatograms for mycophenolic acid (MPA) separation by HPLC with UV detection: (A) Chromatogram with good separation of internal standard (IS) and MPA peaks and stable baseline; (B) Chromatogram with good IS and MPA peak separation, but the presence of numerous additional peaks, including one that interferes with the IS.

mass analyzers utilize an electric field to accelerate a pulse of ions toward a detector. The m/z is determined by the time required for the ion to reach the detector. TOF has many attractive qualities − a wide dynamic mass range for analysis, excellent scanning speed and superb efficiency for ion collection. In particular, it is attractive for large molecules like proteins since it theoretically has no upper mass limit. The Fourier transform mass spectrometer (FT-MS) achieves mass analysis by trapping an ion in a cyclotronic motion within a chamber using magnetic and electric fields. As the cycling ions travel past

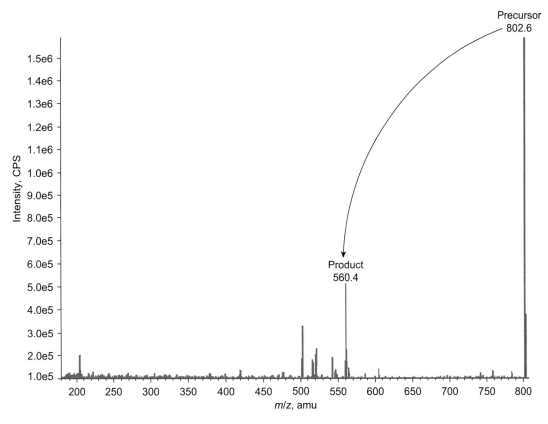

FIGURE 3.7 Mass spectrum of tacrolimus showing precursor and product ions for MRM (multiple reaction monitoring).

spatially fixed detectors, their cycling frequency is transformed to a m/z using Fourier transformation. FT-MS instruments have high resolution, high speed and good resolution. Previously these analyzers were expensive and relegated mostly to research settings for structural elucidation and identification, but have now been incorporated into LC-MS instruments [44]. The quadropole mass analyzer is by far the most common mass analyzer on the market for combined LC and MS systems. This analyzer uses oscillating electric fields to control the flight path of ions through a radiofrequency (RF) electromagnetic field. Thus, this instrument works more as a mass filter where only ions with a certain m/z pass through the system at any particular moment. In order to obtain a full mass spectrum using a quadrupole mass analyzer, the range of m/z must be scanned, reducing the speed at which this instrument can obtain spectra compared with magnetic sector or TOF instruments. Despite this limitation, quadrupole analyzers have gained widespread use, and they are particular suited for use as a mass filter that can be combined with additional quadrupole analyzers in tandem to produce step-wise mass analysis. Variations upon the quadrupole theme have given rise to three-dimensional quadrupole traps that confine the ion to a region in 3D space, rather than along the center of a linear quadrupole. Linear quadrupole ion traps, in which the ion oscillates along the center line of the quadrupole, have also been developed. Ion traps have the advantage of permitting tandem MS analysis beyond two rounds of collision by trapping a particular m/z ion, subjecting it to a round of collision-induced dissociation (CID), trapping a daughter ion and then repeating this process. The interested reader should consult specialized textbooks for a more detailed discussion of LC-MS/MS components and approaches to method selection and validation [45].

The ability to perform tandem MS, whether through the use of several mass analyzers in series or through the use of an ion trap, has significant advantages for bioanalysis of drugs and their metabolites. The specificity of MS is derived from the unique nature of fragmentation that occurs for every molecule. The pattern of fragmentation captured by the mass spectrum often serves as a molecular "fingerprint" that can be used to identify a compound and deduce structure, as commonly used in forensic analysis. Selection of one or a few specific fragment ions is commonly used for detection in LC-MS applications rather than capturing full ion scans to increase the sensitivity of quadrupole analyzers. This process is typically termed selective ion monitoring (SIM). The fragmentation process can be reapplied to a fragment ion derived from an initial ionization process (termed the precursor ion), and the subsequent derived fragments (termed product ions) are also generally unique to an individual compound. Thus, tandem MS allows for monitoring of this very specific serial fragmentation process, frequently termed selective reaction monitoring (SRM) or multiple reaction monitoring (MRM), and it is widely used, accounting for over 90% of LC-MS/MS methods for therapeutic drug analysis.

A particular benefit of the specificity available with MRM is the ability to perform multiplexed LC-MS/MS assays. Fig. 3.8 shows a chromatogram for a single assay that permits simultaneous detection of cyclosporine, $^2H_{12}$-cyclosporine internal standard, tacrolimus and ascomycin (analog standard for tacrolimus). While both drugs as well as their internal standards have very close retention times, each compound is distinguished through the use of unique MRM precursor—production pairs. This approach has been extended to allow simultaneous determination of different immunosuppressive drugs [46], 7 different antidepressants [47, 48], 14 different antimalarial drugs and their metabolites [49] and 30 different antipsychotic drugs [50].

Applying LC-MS/MS to TDM: Current Challenges

While LC-MS/MS has tremendous specificity, it still has its problems. While metabolite interference is not generally a significant problem compared with immunoassay methodologies, LC-MS/MS is still subject to interference. One of the most problematic issues is matrix interference due to ion suppression [51], where components of the matrix and/or co-eluting compounds interfere with the ionization and detection of a molecule of interest, leading to falsely low or high results. This is especially problematic when the analyte and internal standard (IS) are affected very differently, which is more likely to occur with analog IS (e.g., cyclosporine D versus cyclosporine A). Studies have shown ion suppression to be more problematic for ESI compared with APCI, and under some circumstances the "ion suppression" can lead to enhancement of signal [51—54]. Ion suppression and enhancement

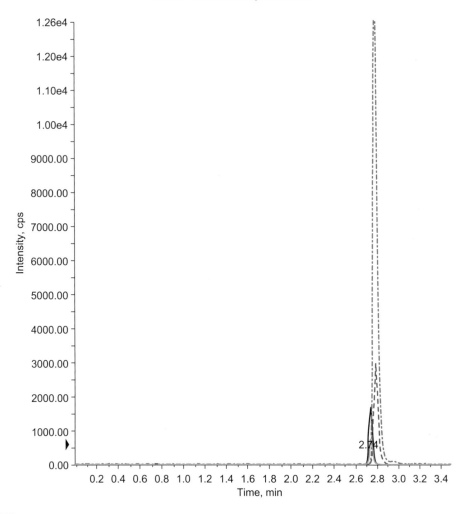

FIGURE 3.8 Distinguishing four different compounds with similar retention time by LC-MS/MS (liquid chromatography/tandem mass spectrometry) through MRM.

effects also occur between stable isotope-labeled internal standard and native analog [55–57]. Although not fully understood from a mechanistic point of view, reduced efficiency of the droplet formation due to the presence of salts or other non-volatile compounds that affect the droplet surface charge in ESI has been proposed as the principle mechanism for ion suppression. Thus, it is imperative that experiments are performed during method validation to evaluate the impact on ion suppression for every analyte, such as those proposed by Thomas Annesley [51]. Additional sources of LC-MS/MS inaccuracy include compound transformations that may occur within the ion source due to molecular disintegration, even with relatively weak ionization. This is particularly problematic for drug analysis where Phase II conjugates, such as glucuronides and sulfates, can be converted into the parent compound if inadequate LC separation occurs, leading to co-elution from the LC into the ion source [58]. Isomers and isobaric compounds (i.e., compounds that share mass but are structurally unrelated) can also contribute to errors even with the high specificity afforded by tandem MS; however, these are certainly more problematic in highly complex metabolomics and proteomic applications compared with TDM applications. Cross-talk between selected SRM precursor—product ion pairs, particularly if mass transitions share a common product ion mass, should also be recognized as a potential source of error [53]. The stability of ionization by APCI has also been shown to vary significantly over time, emphasizing the importance of the internal standard [53].

Finally, one of the greatest challenges in LC-MS/MS remains the lack of standardization. A recent study by Levine *et al.* that evaluated multiple centers using LC-MS/MS compared with immunoassay demonstrated that interlaboratory precision was much lower for LC-MS/MS methods (%CV range 11.4%—18.7%) compared with different labs running the same commercial ARCHITECT tacrolimus procedure (%CV range 3.9%—9.5%) [3]. These results are not entirely surprising, since each LC-MS/MS system is different even when using commercially prepared reagent kits. They illustrate that LC-MS/MS methods are not necessarily superior to immunoassays in the absence of standardization.

Although the versatility of LC-MS/MS permits flexible assay development for drug analysis, there are still a number of barriers that prevent the introduction of LC-MS/MS systems into routine use in most clinical laboratories. First and foremost, a significant amount of technical experience is required to operate these complex systems. Technicians require extensive training extending over weeks to months to gain appropriate competency to operate and maintain these delicate instruments. There are currently no truly "turnkey" systems, but a number of manufacturers of LC-MS/MS systems have made significant strides towards producing much simpler, complete systems for a variety of applications. Costs are also significantly higher than HPLC or immunoassay systems, ranging from ~US$200 000 to US$600 000 for a complete system. Moreover, LC-MS/MS systems have significant space requirements that can add to cost. While the footprint of a basic instrument is not that large, operation requires additional vacuum pumps and a supply of clean nitrogen gas that is often provided by either pressurized tanks or a nitrogen gas generator. These generate abundant heat, and the use of nitrogen generators with an associated air compressor can contribute to substantial noise pollution. Ventilation can also be an issue. With appropriate laboratory design, and perhaps some associated cost, these environmental challenges are generally easily overcome.

Throughput is always an issue, especially in busy clinical laboratories. The use of efficient front-end HPLC systems with short run-times as well as connection of multiple LC systems to a single mass analyzer through a switching valve to maximize usage time of the analyzer have significantly improved operational throughput. The throughput of LC-MS/MS is also superior to that of HPLC or GC-MS due to its greater tolerance for poor separation. Nevertheless, LC-MS/MS throughput is still much lower than that achievable with routine immunoassay platforms, and LC-MS/MS systems do not have the random access capabilities of immunoassay systems. Different drug assays may require significant system change (i.e., change in mobile and/or stationary phase). The development of multiplex assays, as discussed above, partially addresses this challenge.

CONCLUSIONS

Choosing the right analytical platform for a therapeutic drug requires consideration of many variables, including the chemistry of a particular drug, the metabolism, the required precision in relation to the intended clinical use, the specimen volume and throughput, and testing cost. Immunoassays have the benefit of easy performance on automated, high-speed clinical analyzers present in most hospital laboratories with reasonably good precision; however, they are not always available, especially for newer drugs. The LC-MS/MS analytical platform is versatile, and selective assays for almost any drug can be established. While LC-MS/MS holds the potential for greater specificity compared with immunoassays, interference issues are a persistent problem. Failure to recognize interference in any analysis, especially for critical-dose drugs, could lead to serious problems for patients.

References

[1] International Union of Pure and Applied Chemistry. Compendium of Chemical Terminology: Gold Book 2011. Zurich: IUC; 2011.

[2] FDA. Guidance for Industry: Bioanalytical Method Validation. Silver Spring, MD: Center for Drug Evaluation. Available at, http://www.fda.gov/CDER/GUIDANCE/4252fnl.htm; 2001.

[3] Levine DM, Maine GT, Armbruster DA, et al. The need for standardization of tacrolimus assays. Clin Chem 2011;57:1739−47.

[4] Johnson-Davis KL, De S, Jimenez E, et al. Evaluation of the Abbott ARCHITECT i2000 sirolimus assay and comparison with the Abbott IMx sirolimus assay and an established liquid chromatography-tandem mass spectrometry method. Ther Drug Monit 2011;33:453−9.

[5] Greg Miller W, Myers GL, Lou Gantzer M, et al. Roadmap for harmonization of clinical laboratory measurement procedures. Clin Chem 2011;57:1108−17.

[6] Grossberg AL, Chen CC, Rendina L, Pressman D. Specific cation effects with antibody to a hapten with a positive charge. J Immunol 1962;88:600−3.

[7] Laurent TC. The interaction between polysaccharides and other macromolecules. 5. The solubility of proteins in the presence of dextran. Biochem J 1963;89:253−7.

[8] Hellsing K. Immune reactions in polysaccharide media. Investigation on complex-formation between some polysaccharides, albumin and immunoglobulin G. Biochem J 1969;112:483−7.

[9] Tengerdy RP. Reaction kinetic studies of the antigen antibody reactions. J Immunol 1967;99:126−32.

[10] Yalow RS, Berson SA. Immunoassay of endogenous plasma insulin in man. J Clin Invest 1960;39:1157−75.

[11] Van Weemen BK, Schuurs AH. Immunoassay using antigen−enzyme conjugates. FEBS Lett 1971;15:232−6.

[12] Engvall E, Perlmann P. Enzyme-linked immunosorbent assay (ELISA). Quantitative assay of immunoglobulin G. Immunochemistry 1971;8:871−4.

[13] Leute R, Ullman EF, Goldstein A. Spin immunoassay of opiate narcotics in urine and saliva. J Am Med Assoc 1972;221:1231−4.

[14] Leute RK, Ullman EF, Goldstein A, Herzenberg LA. Spin immunoassay technique for determination of morphine. Nat New Biol 1972;236:93−4.

[15] Winkler M, Christians U, Baumann J, Gonschior AK, et al. Evaluation of the Pro-Trac tacrolimus monoclonal whole-blood enzyme-linked immunosorbent assay for monitoring of tacrolimus levels in patients after kidney, heart, and liver transplantation. Ther Drug Monit 1996;18:640−6.

[16] MacFarlane G, Scheller D, Ersfeld T, et al. A simplified whole blood enzyme-linked immunosorbent assay (ProTrac II) for tacrolimus (FK506) using proteolytic extraction in place of organic solvents. Ther Drug Monit 1996;18(6):698−705.

[17] Fiore M, Mitchell J, Doan T, et al. The Abbott IMx automated benchtop immunochemistry analyzer system. Clin Chem 1988;34(9):1726−32.

[18] Rubenstein KE, Schneider RS, Ullman EF. "Homogeneous" enzyme immunoassay. A new immunochemical technique. Biochem Biophys Res Commun 1972;47(4):846—51.

[19] Henderson DR, Friedman SB, Harris JD, et al. CEDIA, a new homogeneous immunoassay system. Clin Chem 1986;32(9):1637—41.

[20] Dandliker WB, Kelly RJ, Dandliker J, et al. Fluorescence polarization immunoassay. Theory and experimental method. Immunochemistry 1973;10(4):219—27.

[21] Jolley ME, Stroupe SD, Wang CH, et al. Fluorescence polarization immunoassay. I. Monitoring aminoglycoside antibiotics in serum and plasma. Clin Chem 1981;27(7):1190—7.

[22] Li TM, Benovic JL, Burd JF. Serum theophylline determination by fluorescence polarization immunoassay utilizing an umbelliferone derivative as a fluorescent label. Anal Biochem 1981;118(1):102—7.

[23] Plebani M, Burlina A. Fluorescence energy transfer immunoassay of digoxin in serum. Clin Chem 1985;31(11):1879—81.

[24] Jolley ME, Stroupe SD, Schwenzer KS, et al. Fluorescence polarization immunoassay. iii. an automated system for therapeutic drug determination. Clin Chem 1981;27(9):1575—9.

[25] Smith DS, Eremin SA. Fluorescence polarization immunoassays and related methods for simple, high-throughput screening of small molecules. Anal Bioanal Chem 2008;391(5):1499—507.

[26] Nishikawa T, Saito M. Competitive nephelometric immunoassay of carbamazepine and its epoxide metabolite in patient blood plasma. J Pharmacobiodyn 1981;4(1):77—83.

[27] Montagne P, Laroche P, Cuilliere ML, et al. Microparticle-enhanced nephelometric immunoassay for human C-reactive protein. J Clin Lab Anal 1992;6(1):24—9.

[28] Montagne P, Laroche P, Cuilliere ML, et al. Polyacrylic microspheres as a solid phase for microparticle enhanced nephelometric immunoassay (NEPHELIA (R)) of transferrin. J Immunoassay 1991;12(2):165—83.

[29] Wieland H, Cremer P, Seidel D. Determination of apolipoprotein B by kinetic (rate) nephelometry. J Lipid Res 1982;23(6):893—902.

[30] Beck OE, Kaiser PE. Rate nephelometry of human IgE in serum. Clin Chem 1982;28(6):1349—51.

[31] Jolliff CR, Cost KM, Stivrins PC, et al. Reference intervals for serum IgG, IgA, IgM, C3, and C4 as determined by rate nephelometry. Clin Chem 1982;28(1):126—8.

[32] Buffone GJ, Savory J, Hermans J. Evaluation of kinetic light scattering as an approach to the measurement of specific proteins with the centrifugal analyzer. II. Theoretical considerations. Clin Chem 1975;21(12):1735—46.

[33] Alexander NM, Gattra R, Nishimoto M. Myeloma immunoglobulin interferes with serum thyroxine analysis by homogeneous enzyme immunoassay. Clin Chim Acta 1980;100(3):301—5.

[34] Kricka LJ. Human anti-animal antibody interferences in immunological assays. Clin Chem 1999;45(7):942—56.

[35] Altinier S, Varagnolo M, Zaninotto M, et al. Heterophilic antibody interference in a non-endogenous molecule assay: an apparent elevation in the tacrolimus concentration. Clin Chim Acta 2009;402(1-2):193—5.

[36] Alak AM. Measurement of tacrolimus (FK506) and its metabolites: a review of assay development and application in therapeutic drug monitoring and pharmacokinetic studies. Ther Drug Monit 1997;19(3):338—51.

[37] Ozbay A, Karamperis N, Jorgensen KA. A review of the immunosuppressive activity of cyclosporine metabolites: new insights into an old issue. Curr Clin Pharmacol 2007;2(3):244—8.

[38] Alak AM, Moy S. Biological activity of tacrolimus (FK506) and its metabolites from whole blood of kidney transplant patients. Transplant Proc 1997;29(5):2487—90.

[39] Murthy JN, Davis DL, Yatscoff RW, Soldin SJ. Tacrolimus metabolite cross-reactivity in different tacrolimus assays. Clin Biochem 1998;31(8):613—7.

[40] Gonschior AK, Christians U, Winkler M, et al. Tacrolimus (FK506) metabolite patterns in blood from liver and kidney transplant patients. Clin Chem 1996;42(9):1426—32.

[41] McMillin GA, Juenke JM, Tso G, Dasgupta A. Estimation of carbamazepine and carbamazepine 10, 11—epoxide concentrations in plasma using mathematical equations generated with two carbamazepine immunoassays. Am J Clin Pathol 2010;133:728—36.

[42] Snyder LR, Kirkland JJ, Dolan JW. Introduction to modern liquid chromatography. 3rd ed. New York, NY: Wiley; 2009.

[43] Lai WK, Pang CP, Law LK, et al. Routine analysis of plasma busulfan by gas chromatography-mass frag-mentography. Clin Chem 1998;44(12):2506—10.

[44] Sanders M, Shipkova PA, Zhang H, Warrack BM. Utility of the hybrid LTQ-FTMS for drug metabolism applications. Curr Drug Metab 2006;7(5):547−55.

[45] Willoughby RC, Sheehan E, Mitrovich S. A global view of LC/MS: how to solve your most challenging analytical problems. 2nd ed. Pittsburgh, PA.: Global View Publ.; 2002.

[46] Koster RA, Dijkers EC, Uges DR. Robust, high-throughput LC-MS/MS method for therapeutic drug monitoring of cyclosporine, tacrolimus, everolimus, and sirolimus in whole blood. Ther Drug Monit 2009;31(1):116−25.

[47] Kollroser M, Schober C. Simultaneous determination of seven tricyclic antidepressant drugs in human plasma by direct-injection HPLC-APCI-MS-MS with an ion trap detector. Ther Drug Monit 2002;24(4):537−44.

[48] de Castro A, Ramirez Fernandez Mdel M, Laloup M, et al. High-throughput on-line solid phase extraction-liquid chromatography-tandem mass spectrometry method for the simultaneous analysis of 14 antidepressants and their metabolites in plasma. J Chromatogr A 2007;1160(1−2):3−12.

[49] Hodel EM, Zanolari B, Mercier T, et al. A single LC-tandem mass spectrometry method for the simultaneous determination of 14 antimalarial drugs and their metabolites in human plasma. J Chromatogr B Analyt Technol Biomed Life Sci 2009;877(10):867−86.

[50] Saar E, Gerostamoulos D, Drummer OH, Beyer J. Identification and quantification of 30 antipsychotics in blood using LC-MS/MS. J Mass Spectrom 2010;45(8). p. 915−295.

[51] Annesley TM. Ion suppression in mass spectrometry. Clin Chem 2003;49(7):1041−4.

[52] Van Eeckhaut A, Lanckmans K, Sarre S, et al. Validation of bioanalytical LC-MS/MS assays: evaluation of matrix effects. J Chromatogr B Analyt Technol Biomed Life Sci 2009;877(23):2198−207.

[53] Vogeser M, Seger C. Pitfalls associated with the use of liquid chromatography-tandem mass spectrometry in the clinical laboratory. Clin Chem 2010;56(8):1234−44.

[54] Taylor PJ. Matrix effects: the Achilles heel of quantitative high-performance liquid chromatography-electrospray-tandem mass spectrometry. Clin Biochem 2005;38(4):328−34.

[55] Remane D, Wissenbach DK, Meyer MR, Maurer HH. Systematic investigation of ion suppression and enhancement effects of fourteen stable-isotope-labeled internal standards by their native analogues using atmospheric-pressure chemical ionization and electrospray ionization and the relevance for multi-analyte liquid chromatographic/mass spectrometric procedures. Rapid Commun Mass Spectrom 2010;24(7):859−67.

[56] Wang S, Cyronak M, Yang E. Does a stable isotopically labeled internal standard always correct analyte response? A matrix effect study on a LC/MS/MS method for the determination of carvedilol enantiomers in human plasma. J Pharm Biomed Anal 2007;43(2):701−7.

[57] Lindegardh N, Annerberg A, White NJ, Day NP. Development and validation of a liquid chromatographic-tandem mass spectrometric method for determination of piperaquine in plasma stable isotope labeled internal standard does not always compensate for matrix effects. J Chromatogr B Analyt Technol Biomed Life Sci 2008;862(1−2):227−36.

[58] Yan Z, Caldwell GW, Jones WJ, Masucci JA. Cone voltage induced in-source dissociation of glucuronides in electrospray and implications in biological analyses. Rapid Commun Mass Spectrom 2003;17(13):1433−42.

Clinical Utility of Free Drug Monitoring

Florin Marcel Musteata

Department of Pharmaceutical Sciences, Albany College of Pharmacy and Health Sciences, Albany, NY

OUTLINE

Therapeutic Drug Monitoring: Newer Drugs and Biomarkers
DOI: 10.1016/B978-0-12-385467-4.00004-V

INTRODUCTION

Therapeutic drug monitoring is highly dependent on the ability to measure drug concentrations in the body fluid, most commonly serum, plasma or whole blood. Since biological samples are complicated mixtures containing lipids and proteins that can bind the compound, only some of the drug molecules will be dissolved directly in the serum. The free concentration of a drug represents the freely diffusible drug fraction that is immediately available to distribute in the body, pass through biological membranes, and bind to receptors (Fig. 4.1). Accordingly, the free drug concentration correlates to clinical efficacy and drug toxicity better than total concentration. However, the great majority of decisions in clinical pharmacokinetics and research continue to be made based on the sum of free plus bound molecules, which is the conventionally monitored total drug concentration [1, 2]. Some authors claim that free concentrations do not need to be measured when there is a constant free drug fraction within and between individuals. However, this is rarely the case: while the free fraction is fairly constant when drug concentrations are much lower than protein concentrations, the free fraction always depends on the concentration of binding protein, which is seldom the same between individuals. Furthermore, the binding characteristics of proteins can change dramatically in genetic or metabolic diseases, as well as in patients who suffer from burns or malnutrition. In all these cases, total drug concentration is not necessarily proportional to pharmacodynamic activity and the free drug concentration should be monitored instead for better patient management.

Drug distribution throughout the body is mostly influenced by the flow of blood, which contains two main drug-binding proteins: albumin (human serum albumin; HSA, with a normal concentration of 662 μM) and alpha-1-acid glycoprotein (AGP, with a normal concentration of 24 μM). If the free drug concentration cannot be measured, the concentration of these binding proteins should be determined in addition to total drug

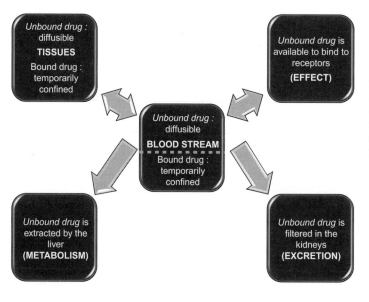

FIGURE 4.1 Drug molecules that are freely diffusible in the body and can pass through biological membranes are the driving force for distribution, elimination and effect. Movement of drug between central compartment (blood stream), tissue compartment and effect compartment is reversible. Elimination by metabolism and excretion is irreversible.

concentration. Subsequently, the normalized drug concentration or the free drug concentration can be calculated from total drug concentration and the concentration of the binding protein.

FREE CONCENTRATIONS VERSUS TOTAL CONCENTRATIONS

The process of therapeutic drug monitoring usually includes measurement of drug concentration in the body as a parameter that can guide the therapeutic regimen and confirm attainment of suitable drug levels. Drug concentration is most often measured in blood (using serum, plasma or whole blood), since this is the main connective tissue that equilibrates with all the other tissues of the body. However, most drug targets are located outside the blood compartment, and total drug concentration in the blood is not equal to total drug concentration in the body. Therefore, drug concentration in the blood is simply used as a surrogate for drug concentration at the intended target. Since drug molecules must diffuse from the central circulatory system into tissues in order to reach their targets, a better surrogate for drug concentration at its target is the freely diffusible drug concentration in blood — the free drug. There are mathematical models to calculate the free drug fraction based on total drug concentration and plasma protein concentration. In order to calculate the free drug fraction (f_u) and the plasma protein binding (PPB), most models are based on the assumption that plasma contains a binding protein P (representing the active binding sites on all proteins) with the concentration C_p and the binding constant K between drug (D) and protein. The binding equilibrium can then be described as:

$$P + D \rightarrow \rightleftarrows P[D]$$

$$K = \frac{[PD]}{[D] \cdot [P]} = \frac{C_{total} - C_{free}}{C_{free} \cdot (C_P - C_{total} + C_{free})} \tag{4.1}$$

where C_{total} is the total drug concentration and C_{free} is the free drug concentration.

When the concentration of the drug is much lower than the concentration of proteins, the bound drug concentration ($C_{total} - C_{free}$) is negligible with respect to C_p and equation 4.1 becomes:

$$K = \frac{C_{total} - C_{free}}{C_{free} \cdot C_P} = \frac{C_{total}/C_{free} - 1}{C_P} \tag{4.2}$$

Since most drugs are active at low µM concentrations, this assumption is certainly applicable in the case of binding to albumin, which is present in plasma at a concentration of 600−750 µM. Furthermore, some studies suggest that the binding sites are not limited even at drug concentrations higher than 2000 µM [3]. The values of the unbound fraction and that of PPB% can easily be derived from equation 4.2:

$$f_u = 1 - \frac{PPB}{100} = \frac{C_{free}}{C_{total}} = \frac{1}{1 + C_p \cdot K} => PPB = \frac{100}{1 + 1/(C_p \cdot K)} \tag{4.3}$$

PHARMACOKINETIC CONSEQUENCES OF DRUG–PROTEIN BINDING

Drugs with high plasma protein binding tend to be confined mostly in the central compartment, have a low volume of distribution, and are mostly eliminated by metabolism. In order for these drugs to be active, they must achieve total blood concentrations significantly higher than those required for receptor activation in tissues. Such drugs, with low free concentration and high total concentration in blood, require routine free concentration monitoring – for example, phenytoin, valproic acid and to some extent carbamazepine. Drugs that have similar plasma and tissue binding distribute relatively homogeneously throughout the body, and for these drugs plasma concentration is a good indicator of target site concentration. Lastly, drugs that have limited binding to plasma proteins but distribute to a large extent in tissues tend to produce low total plasma concentrations that are an underestimation of tissue levels. In all these cases, the most convenient indicator of target site concentration would be the free drug concentration in plasma, since receptor occupancy is directly proportional to the unbound fraction of drug in plasma [4]. Onset of drug action depends on achieving a minimum effective concentration, as well as the rate at which the free drug reaches the receptor. More drug molecules are available to cross cell membranes when protein binding decreases and the free drug fraction increases, resulting in a more intense pharmacological effect. Sometimes this increased effect is only temporary, since an increased free fraction can result in higher clearance from the body. However, the concentration of plasma proteins tends to decrease at the same time as liver and kidney function decrease, in which case a regular dosage regimen results in sustained increased free drug levels.

In practice, the free drug concentration is usually used to calculate the percentage of binding to plasma proteins (PPB as %):

$$PPB = \frac{C_{total} - C_{free}}{C_{total}} \cdot 100 \qquad (4.4)$$

Representation of drug binding as a percentage of bound fraction leads to substantial compression of the free concentration range in the case of strongly bound drugs, and to broadening of values for weakly bound drugs. This can easily be observed by rearranging equation 4.4 and expressing the change in free concentration (ΔC_{free}) as a function of the change in protein binding (ΔPPB) and the drug's normal protein binding (PPB):

$$\frac{\Delta C_{free}}{C_{free}} = \frac{-\Delta PPB}{100 - PPB} \qquad (4.5)$$

Equation 4.5 can be used to generate graphs that illustrate the change in free concentration as a function of the change in protein binding, as shown in Fig. 4.2. For drugs that are less than 70% bound to proteins, the change in free concentration is relatively small and may not be clinically significant. However, for drugs more than 90% bound to proteins, the free concentration can increase significantly with clinical consequences when protein binding changes.

The clinical consequences of decreased plasma protein binding are sometimes unclear and controversial. In the case of anti-epileptic drugs, decreased binding to albumin is correlated

FIGURE 4.2 Dependence of free concentration changes on variations in protein binding and normal protein binding.

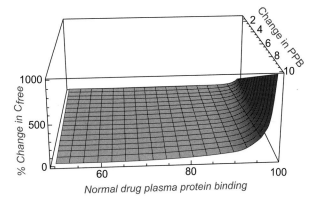

with an increased risk of toxicity, and lower doses are recommended. On the other hand, in the case of antibiotics, hypoalbuminemia usually results in higher drug clearance and suboptimal treatment, with higher doses being recommended. Obviously, significantly more research is needed in this area, and this can only be accomplished if suitable analytical methods become available. The utility of free concentration monitoring has been investigated for numerous classes of drugs, among which anti-epileptics, antibiotics, immunosuppressants, and anesthetics are most studied.

MONITORING FREE CONCENTRATIONS OF CLASSICAL ANTI-EPILEPTICS

Some of the most commonly monitored free drug concentrations in clinical practice are several classical anti-epileptics. Of these, phenytoin and valproic acid are well-known drugs for which clinical utility of free fraction monitoring has been extensively studied in clinical practice. Free carbamazepine concentration is monitored less often compared to monitoring free phenytoin and free valproic acid concentration. Free phenobarbital concentration is not monitored, due to modest protein binding of the drug. In general, free phenytoin and free valproic acid concentrations should be monitored in all patients with renal insufficiency, hepatic dysfunction, hypoalbuminemia, critically ill patients, pregnant women, the elderly and patients suffering from AIDS. In addition, drug–drug interactions may cause elevated concentration of free phenytoin, free valproic acid and, to a lesser extent, free carbamazepine concentration [5].

Iwamoto *et al.* evaluated the relationship between free phenytoin concentrations and clinical responses, as well as the factors influencing protein binding of phenytoin, in 119 plasma samples from 70 patients treated orally with phenytoin. Their results show that the free phenytoin concentration is more useful than the total concentration for monitoring anti-epileptic effects in patients receiving phenytoin monotherapy. The authors also found that the free phenytoin fraction was significantly influenced by aging, creatinine clearance and serum albumin levels [6]. Similar results were obtained by Banh *et al.*, who investigated the relationship between total and free serum concentrations of phenytoin in 48 hospitalized patients. The authors found significant intra-individual variation in the free fraction of phenytoin, of up to 94%, rendering corrections for albumin concentrations useless [7]. Other researchers used the same monitoring approach to validate a new equation for calculating normalized phenytoin levels for patients with abnormal serum albumin levels [8]. A team from the Miyazaki Medical College Hospital has published several papers regarding the free concentration of phenytoin in pediatric patients. Binding parameters of phenytoin to pediatric serum proteins were compared with *in vivo* and *in vitro* binding parameters in adult subjects reported by other investigators. Their results suggest that although the number of binding sites is the same, there are some differences in binding constants between pediatric and adult subjects, with adult albumin having an affinity approximately 1.2 times higher [9]. Monitoring free phenytoin, free valproic acid and, to some extent, free carbamazepine concentration is essential in uremic patients and patients with hepatic dysfunction due to a disproportionately high amount of free phenytoin compared to total phenytoin concentration. Therefore, if dosage adjustment is made based on total phenytoin or total valproic acid concentration, a patient may experience severe drug toxicity.

It has been speculated that many uremic toxins are responsible for displacement of strongly bound classical anticonvulsants from protein binding sites causing elevated concentrations of free drugs. Hippuric acid and indoxyl sulfate, the two compounds that are present in elevated concentrations in uremia, can cause displacement of strongly protein-bound drugs [10]. Takamura identified 3-carboxy-4-methyl-5-propyl-2-furanpropionate (CMPF) as the major uremic toxin that causes impaired protein binding of furosemide [11]. Hepatic disease alters the pharmacokinetic parameters of valproic acid, as Klotz *et al.* reported that alcoholic cirrhosis and viral hepatitis decreased valproic acid protein binding from an average of 88.7% to 70.3% and 78.1%, respectively, with a significant increase in volume of distribution. Elimination half-life was also prolonged [12]. An increase in unbound concentration of carbamazepine has been also reported in patients with hepatic disease [13]. Critically ill patients also exhibit elevated concentrations of free anticonvulsants. Kemper *et al.* reported severe phenytoin intoxication in two patients with hypoalbuminemia: one 35-year-old woman and one 60-year-old man developed severe phenytoin toxicity, but both patients showed total phenytoin concentrations within the recommended therapeutic range. However, the free phenytoin level was 4 μg/mL in the first patient and 8 μg/mL in the second, explaining the severe phenytoin toxicity experienced by these two patients. The authors concluded that despite total phenytoin concentrations within the therapeutic range, free phenytoin levels were disproportionately elevated in both patients due to severe hypoalbuminemia (albumin below 2.5 mg/dL) in both patients. Although the first patient (the 35-year-old woman) survived after discontinuation of phenytoin, the second patient died from phenytoin overdose [14]. In one report the authors investigated free phenytoin fractions in 60 critically ill pediatric patients, and concluded that total phenytoin concentrations did not accurately reflect free phenytoin concentrations in these patients. The authors reported that 10% of their patients demonstrated toxic concentrations of free phenytoin (over 2 μg/mL) despite total phenytoin concentrations being within the recommended therapeutic range of less than 20 μg/mL. Although the mean free phenytoin fraction was 13%, the free fraction varied widely, from 6% to 42%. The free phenytoin concentrations were particularly elevated in patients with severe hypoalbuminemia (albumin < 2.5 gm/dL) [15].

Zielmann *et al.* studied protein binding of phenytoin in 39 critically ill patients, and observed that in 76% of these patients free phenytoin fractions were increased (by over 10% up to 24%) due to hypoalbuminemia, hepatic failure or renal failure. The authors concluded that free phenytoin monitoring is essential in critically ill patients [16]. Valproic acid is extensively bound to serum proteins, mainly albumin. Other than uremia and liver disease, hypoalbuminemia is a major cause of a disproportionate increase in free valproic acid concentration. Gidal *et al.* reported a case where markedly elevated plasma free valproic acid in a hypoalbuminemic patient contributed to neurotoxicity. The total valproic acid concentration was 103 μg/mL, but the free valproic acid concentration was 26.8 μg/mL. This unexpected elevation was due to a low albumin level (3.3 gm/dL) of the patient [17].

Mamiya *et al.* investigated drug–drug interactions between phenytoin and valproic acid in patients with severe motor and intellectual disabilities with epilepsy, and found that hypo-albuminemia and valproate coadministration with phenytoin increased the free fraction. Patients with these double risk factors have a higher danger of exceeding the therapeutic range of serum free phenytoin concentration even when their total phenytoin concentration is within therapeutic range [18]. Strongly protein-bound drugs that are known to cause displacement of phenytoin, valproic acid and carbamazepine include non-steroidal anti-inflammatory drugs such as salicylate, ibuprofen, tolmetin, naproxen, mefenamic acid and fenoprofen, and antibiotics such as ceftriaxone, nafcillin, oxacillin, dicloxacillin and sulfame-thoxazole [5].

Although valproic acid is a widely prescribed anticonvulsant and mood stabilizer, the therapeutic range of free valproic acid has not been established properly, while for free phenytoin the well-accepted therapeutic range is 1–2 μg/mL. Most investigators used a protein-free ultrafiltration method with commercially available filters (one common example is Amicon Centrifree Micropartion System with a filter cut-off of 30 000 Da marketed by Millipore Corporation, Billerica, MA) for determination of free anticonvulsant concentrations. The free drug level in the protein-free ultrafiltrate can be determined by a commercially available immunoassay or an appropriate chromatographic method. Recently, Alvarez *et al.* commented that measurement of free fractions is complicated, and developed an equation for predicting free valproic acid concentration as a function of total concentration and albumin concentration. The new equation was validated against experimental data obtained by ultrafiltration. Their study showed that there are significant differences between calculated and measured free valproate concentrations, which further confirms the need to measure or predict the free fraction [19]. Ueshima *et al.* investigated the relationship between free valproic acid concentrations and clinical efficacy of valproate in intractable epileptic children. This is particularly significant, since the dose of valproic acid required for intractable seizures is higher than that used in standard therapy, exposing the patients to greater risk of adverse reactions. An increased unbound serum concentration of valproic acid observed in such high-dose therapy is the likely cause of frequent toxicity, but the unbound concentration is rarely monitored in therapeutic drug monitoring activity and the total valproic acid concentration is commonly determined instead. The authors showed that the unbound concentration non-linearly increased as the total concentration increased, and that unbound valproic acid concentrations in infants are generally higher and vary more widely than those in adult patients. The authors concluded that unbound concentrations in neonates and infants should be closely monitored, and should be used to individualize dosage regimens of valproic acid in intractable epileptic children [20]. The free concentration of valproic acid can also vary unexpectedly following rapid intravenous administration. Important research on this topic characterized valproate protein binding in patients with epilepsy who achieve transient high (> 150 mg/L) total plasma concentrations following rapid infusion at very high doses. This was done by measuring both total and unbound valproic acid concentrations. One- and two-binding site models were explored in a non-linear mixed effects population analysis framework. The relative importance of weight, age, sex, race and enzyme-inducing co-medications on the binding site association constant was examined using the likelihood ratio test. Because of the rapid administration of high doses, the authors found unbound valproate concentrations much higher than in previous studies, further highlighting the importance of monitoring free concentrations [21]. Sproule *et al.* also acknowledge that interpreting total valproate concentrations can be challenging. In addition to its variable protein binding properties, valproate is a low hepatic extraction drug and its clearance has been shown to be concentration dependent. These complex changes in total valproate concentration do not accurately reflect active drug concentration. The authors recommend monitoring unbound valproate concentrations in order to simplify interpretation of drug levels, particularly with dosage changes at higher concentrations and in elderly patients, even if albumin concentrations are within the normal range [22].

MONITORING FREE CONCENTRATIONS OF ANTIBIOTICS, ANTIMALARIALS AND ANTIRETROVIRALS

The results of antibiotic therapy are highly dependent on achieving suitable concentrations of unbound drug at the target site of infection. Many antibiotics exhibit a high degree of binding to plasma proteins, which results in pharmacokinetic and pharmacodynamic differences between patients, especially in the case of elderly and critically ill patients. Ulldemolins *et al.* reported that the incidence of hypoalbuminemia in the intensive care units can be as high as 50%, resulting in markedly increased clearance and volume of distribution of many antibiotics in these patients, which ultimately translates to lower antibacterial exposures that can compromise the achievement of suitable therapeutic targets, especially for time-dependent antibiotics. For example, the volume of distribution and clearance for ceftriaxone (85–95% protein binding) in hypoalbuminemic critically ill patients were increased two-fold. A similar phenomenon was reported with teicoplanin, aztreonam, fusidic acid, daptomycin and ertapenem (85–95% protein binding), which led to failure to attain the desired the desired pharmacodynamic effect. Measurement of free antibiotic concentrations is particularly important since many new antibacterials under development exhibit a high level of protein binding, while hypoalbuminemia is rarely considered in clinical trials in critically ill patients [23].

A thorough investigation of the binding of antimalarial drugs to serum proteins was performed by Zsila *et al.* [24]. The investigators used multiple techniques, such as induced circular dichroism and affinity chromatography, to study specific interactions between six antimalarial agents of quinoline and acridine types, and AGP. Association constant values of about $10^5–10^6 M^{-1}$ could be determined. HSA association constants estimated from affinity chromatography ($10^3-10^5\,M^{-1}$) were found to lag behind those for AGP. The authors also discussed the pharmacological and clinical aspects of the results in great detail [24].

Antiviral activity is also well known to be dependent on unbound concentrations. Fayet *et al.* developed a modified ultrafiltration method enabling the accurate measurement of unbound concentrations of ten antiretroviral drugs by liquid chromatography-tandem mass spectroscopy, which circumvents the problem of loss by adsorption in the early ultra-filtration fractions. The method was applied to assess the variability of free fractions of anti-retroviral drugs during routine therapeutic drug monitoring in 144 patients with HIV. Free fraction values obtained with this modified ultrafiltration method revealed substantial inter-individual variability, suggesting that monitoring unbound antiretroviral drug concentrations can increase the clinical usefulness of antiretroviral therapy, especially for lopinavir, saquinavir and efavirenz [25]. A thorough study of free atazanavir pharmacokinetics was performed by Barrail-Tran *et al.* Their results indicated that atazanavir pharmacokinetics is moderately influenced by its protein binding, especially to AGP. This binding has only minor clinical consequences when the concentration of proteins is normal, since atazanavir is less than 90% bound to plasma proteins [26]. However, the therapeutic regimen should be adjusted based on free atazanavir concentration when AGP levels are significantly above normal.

MONITORING FREE CONCENTRATIONS OF IMMUNOSUPPRESSANTS

Most immunosuppressants currently in use have a narrow therapeutic window and exhibit a high degree of protein binding (> 90%), and would therefore be good candidates for free concentration monitoring. Furthermore, organ transplant procedures are lengthy, intricate, and often involve changes in the concentration of plasma proteins. However, cyclo-sporine, tacrolimus, sirolimus and everolimus are preferentially monitored in whole blood, mostly because they tend to have a higher concentration in the blood cells. Accordingly, although the free concentration of these drugs is important, only their total whole blood concentration is currently monitored [27].

The main immunosuppressant whose free concentration is currently investigated is myco-phenolic acid. The drug is successfully used to prevent rejection in cases of renal and liver transplant. Since the pharmacokinetics of mycophenolic acid is highly variable from patient to patient, therapeutic drug monitoring is vital for dose individualization. However, consid-eration of total mycophenolic acid can be misleading in clinical situations in which protein binding may be altered, as changes in total concentration of the drug may not be associated with parallel changes in free concentration. The plasma protein binding of mycophenolic acid increases as a function of time after liver transplant, and protein binding may increase from 92% to 98%, which may cause intraindividual variation in active free fraction of myco-phenolic acid [28]. Atcheson *et al.* reported that mycophenolic acid free fraction varied eleven-fold, from 1.6% to 18.3%, while the metabolite glucuronide fraction varied three-fold, from 17.4% to 54.1%, in transplant recipients. There were positive correlations between blood urea nitrogen and creatinine concentrations and free mycophenolic acid concentra-tions, while there was a negative correlation between albumin concentration and free mycophenolic acid concentration. The authors further reported that in average free mycophenolic acid the free fraction was 70% higher in patients with albumin concentrations below 3.1 g/dL than in patients with normal albumin concentrations. Patients with marked renal impairment showed higher free concentrations of mycophenolic acid. The exposure to unbound mycophenolic acid was significantly related to infections and hematological toxicity, but neither free nor total mycophenolic acid concentration was related to rejection episodes [29]. High unbound mycophenolic acid concentration was also encountered in a hematopoietic cell transplant patient with sepsis and renal and hepatic dysfunction [30]. Concentrations of free mycophenolic acid can be measured in protein free ultrafiltrate after solid phase extraction using C-18 cartridges and liquid chromatography combined with tandem mass spectrometry [31]. Shen *et al.* also described a liquid chromatography combined with tandem mass spectrometric method for determination of total, free and saliva mycophenolic acid concentrations in healthy volunteers and renal transplant recipients [32]. In the most recent study, Benichou *et al.* found that the apparent clearance (CL/F) of mycophenolic acid correlated significantly with the free drug fraction. Enhanced CL/F in relation with an increase in the free fraction of mycophenolic acid results in a low AUC (area under the concentration curve) of total drug during the first postoperative month, but on average the exposure to free mycophenolate is not altered. The authors conclude that total drug AUC should not be used to adjust dosing during this period, and free concentration should be used instead [33].

MONITORING FREE CONCENTRATIONS OF OTHER DRUGS

Several other classes of drugs, such as anesthetics, antineoplastics and anticoagulants, have high inter-individual pharmacokinetic variability that is partly caused by changes in plasma protein binding. Anesthetics are a class of drugs that have to be particularly well monitored, given the high risk of toxicity from these drugs. Since numerous investigations showed that their effect is better associated with free concentrations, several researchers are investigating drug–drug interactions by measuring the binding constants between anesthetics and HSA. For example, propofol and halothane are clinically used general anesthetics which are transported primarily by HSA in the blood. Researchers from the University of Pennsylvania Medical Center characterized anesthetic–HSA interactions in solution using elution chromatography, isothermal titration calorimetry, hydrogen-exchange experiments, and geometric analyses of high-resolution structures. They found that propofol has a much higher binding affinity for HSA than halothane. The binding stoichiometry of the two drugs was also considerably different, with propofol binding to albumin in a 2 : 1 ratio as compared with 7 : 1 for halothane. Hydrogen-exchange studies in isolated recombinant domains of HSA showed that propofol-binding sites are primarily found in domain III, whereas halothane sites are more widely distributed. In addition to pharmacokinetic implications of propofol displacing halothane from some HSA sites, their data suggest that HSA might be a suitable platform for further characterization of the general anesthetic structure–activity relationship [34]. More recently, the group has published lack of competition between bilirubin and propofol for binding sites on HSA, based on the fact that binding of these two compounds occurs at different sites [35].

Gefitinib, an inhibitor of epidermal growth factor receptor-tyrosine kinase, exhibits wide inter-subject pharmacokinetic variability which may contribute to differences in treatment outcome. Since unbound drug concentrations are more relevant to pharmacological and toxicological responses, gefitinib binding in plasma and factors affecting this process were studied both *in vitro* and in cancer patients. An equilibrium dialysis method using 96-well microdialysis plates was optimized and validated for determining the unbound fraction of gefitinib in plasma. It was found that gefitinib was extensively bound in human, rat, mouse and dog plasma. Accordingly, the variable plasma protein concentrations observed in cancer patients will affect gefitinib unbound fraction with implications for inter-subject variation in drug toxicity and response, warranting the need to monitor the levels of free drug [36]. Similar investigations were performed for anticoagulants such as warfarin and phenprocoumon [37, 38].

APPLICATIONS AND METHODS FOR MONITORING FREE DRUG CONCENTRATIONS

Several methods have been applied for measuring free drug concentrations, most of which involve the physical separation of the free from the bound fractions followed by a conventional analysis step (Table 4.1). Examples of methods based on separation of the free fraction include equilibrium dialysis, ultrafiltration, gel filtration, ultracentrifugation, liquid chromatography and capillary electrophoresis. These approaches are usually time-consuming, can suffer loss of analyte if the analyte binds non-specifically to membranes, and can shift the binding equilibrium between drug and protein during separation. Chromatographic techniques usually employ a mobile phase that is very different from physiological conditions, which can further disturb binding. The same is true for methods based on electrospray ionization mass spectrometry (ESI-MS), which work only when particular buffer solutions are used and when the combination ratio between protein and drug is 1:1.

While chromatographic methods used for the assay of free concentrations and binding constants assume a very fast equilibrium (less than a few seconds) between the drug and the binding proteins, ultrafiltration and ultracentrifugation techniques assume a slow equilibrium (more than 30 minutes), so the free fraction can pass through a membrane without shifting the equilibrium in the other compartment. Electrophoretic methods are very flexible and have been applied for both 1 : 1 and 1 : n combination ratios between protein and drug, but they are restricted to certain buffer solutions and do not allow for precise control of the temperature.

One of the most recent sample preparation methods that have found applications for the assay of free concentrations is solid phase microextraction (SPME) [3, 39, 40]. The main strength of SPME is the small size of the extractive phase and the partial extraction approach, which allows for simultaneous investigation of the analyte and the matrix. Compared to other methods, SPME offers several advantages, including small sample size, short analysis time, possibility to automate, and ability to directly study complex samples (e.g., whole blood). While ESI-MS, CE and chromatographic methods are only effective when the samples are dissolved in certain buffer solutions, SPME methods can be used for extraction from any media, and at any concentration range, if a suitable extraction phase is selected.

TABLE 4.1 Selected Applications Based on Monitoring of Free Drug Concentrations

Drug(s)	Protein or biological fluid	Application	Separation and detection	Reference(s)
18 serotonin and dopamine transporter inhibitors	Rat brain	Relationship between free concentrations and brain receptor occupancy	Rapid equilibrium dialysis and LC-MS/MS	[57, 58]
Amodiaquine, primaquine, tafenoquine, quinacrine, chloroquine	Alpha-1-acid glycoprotein and human serum albumin (isolated)	Binding constants, number of binding sites	Affinity chromatography and induced circular dichroism	[24]
Atazanavir	Alpha-1-acid glycoprotein and human serum albumin (isolated and in human plasma)	Influence of protein concentrations on drug pharmacokinetics	Ultrafiltration and LC-MS/MS	[26]
Bilirubin	Cell culture containing human serum albumin	Cytotoxicity of free versus total bilirubin	Horseradish peroxidase assay	[64]
Carbamazepine	Alpha-1-acid glycoprotein (immobilized on column)	Binding constant	Affinity chromatography (frontal analysis)	[41]
Chlorpromazine, chloroquine, propranolol and a proprietary compound	Human whole blood	New analytical approaches, prediction of non-linear pharmacokinetics	Rapid equilibrium dialysis and LC-MS/MS	[56]
Clarithromycin, levofloxacin, amiodarone, metoclopramide, gabapentin, meloxicam	Mouse plasma and adipose tissue	Free concentration in plasma versus adipose tissue	Equilibrium dialysis and LC-MS/MS	[68]
Diazepam, nordiazepam, warfarin, verapamil, loperamide	Human plasma	Plasma protein binding	Solid phase microextraction and LC-MS/MS	[69]
Gefitinib	Alpha-1-acid glycoprotein and human serum albumin (isolated), as well as plasma from four species: human, rat, mouse, and dog	Free fraction, binding constants	Equilibrium dialysis and LC-MS/MS	[36]

Drug	Matrix	Topic	Method	Reference
Ibuprofen, warfarin, verapamil, propranolol, caffeine	Human plasma	Plasma protein binding	Solid phase microextraction and LC-MS/MS	[3]
Lidocaine	Alpha-1-acid glycoprotein and human serum albumin (immobilized on column)	Binding constants	Affinity chromatography (frontal analysis, zonal elution, and competitive binding)	[42]
Mycophenolic acid	Human serum albumin (isolated) and human plasma	Factors influencing the free fraction	(a) Equilibrium dialysis and scintillation counter (b) Ultrafiltration and scintillation counter	[55]
Naproxen	Human plasma	Fraction unbound, number of binding sites	Ultrafiltration and LC-MS	[48, 49]
Octylphenol	Human serum albumin, bovine serum albumin	Free concentration, exploration of matrix effects	Solid phase microextraction and LC-MS/MS	[46]
Phenytoin	Human serum	Calculation of normalized concentrations in special populations	Ultrafiltration and fluorescence polarization immunoassay	[8]
	Human plasma	Free fraction, factors influencing protein binding	Ultrafiltration and fluorescence polarization immunoassay	[6]
	Human serum (pediatric)	*In vivo* binding in pediatric patients	Ultrafiltration and fluorescence polarization immunoassay	[9]
	Human serum (pediatric)	Influence of temperature on protein binding	Ultrafiltration and fluorescence polarization immunoassay	[47]
	Human serum albumin (immobilized on column)	Study of phenytoin binding to serum albumin	Affinity chromatography (frontal analysis and competitive binding zonal elution)	[43]
Phenytoin and valproic acid	Human serum	Free fraction, drug interactions	Ultrafiltration and fluorescence polarization immunoassay	[18]
Propofol and halothane	Human serum albumin (isolated)	Binding constants, comparative binding	Affinity chromatography (zonal elution), isothermal titration calorimetry, hydrogen-tritium exchange, and geometric analyses of high-resolution structures	[33, 34]

Continued

TABLE 4.1 Selected Applications Based on Monitoring of Free Drug Concentrations—cont'd

Drug(s)	Protein or biological fluid	Application	Separation and detection	Reference(s)
Propofol, fatty acids, indomethacin and lidocaine	Human serum albumin (isolated) and human plasma	Relationship between free fraction and drug concentration	Ultrafiltration and GC-MS or LC-UV	[52, 53]
Quinine, quinidine, naproxen, ciprofloxacin, haloperidol, paclitaxel, nortriptyline	Human serum albumin (isolated)	Protein binding study	Solid phase microextraction and LC-UV/LC-FL	[45]
Roscovitine	Alpha-1-acid glycoprotein, human serum albumin, blood, and plasma	Bound fraction, binding protein	(a) Equilibrium dialysis and LC-MS/MS (b) Ultrafiltration and LC-MS/MS	[54]
Testosterone	Human serum	Free concentration, prediction based on equations	Isotope dilution equilibrium dialysis and scintillation counter	[59]
Valproic acid	Human plasma (children)	Individualized dosing based on free concentration	Ultrafiltration and fluorescence polarization immunoassay	[20]
	Human plasma	Influence of serum albumin on free fraction	Ultrafiltration and fluorescence polarization immunoassay	[19]
	Human plasma	Protein binding at transient high doses	Ultrafiltration and immunoassay	[21]
	Human serum	Usefulness of monitoring free concentrations	Ultrafiltration and fluorescence polarization immunoassay	[22]
Vitamin D binding protein	Human serum	Association with lipoproteins	Gel permeation, ultracentrifugation, and immunonephelometry	[63]
Warfarin and phenprocoumon	Human serum albumin (isolated) and serum samples	Binding constants, influence of fatty acids	Equilibrium dialysis and spectrophotometry	[37, 38]

Methods that can measure free drug concentrations without separating the drug from the binding protein include surface plasmon resonance, calorimetry, and spectroscopy. These methods demonstrate least interference with the binding equilibrium, but are not suitable for complex biological samples such as serum, plasma and whole blood. All applications have direct or indirect clinical significance and were selected based on sample type, analytical approach and investigated drug(s).

Methods Suitable for Isolated Protein Samples

Investigation of the interaction of drugs with proteins is an important initial step in drug discovery, whether it is focused on the determination of plasma protein binding or the interaction between drugs and receptors. While the value of plasma protein binding is an important parameter in clinical practice, the drug—protein binding constants are much more important in research. In order to obtain accurate results, the binding constants are usually determined with purified proteins attached to a solid support or dissolved in buffers that mimic biological conditions. In order to carry out a thorough study of biological responses to molecular stimuli, the strength of binding of a ligand to its receptor must be investigated. Drug binding to purified proteins should also be investigated in clinical practice when it is suspected that a patient may have atypical receptors or binding proteins. Also, identification of the drug-binding proteins and measurement of the binding constants allows prediction of drug pharmacokinetics in cases of changing pathophysiology.

Affinity Chromatography

Most tests regarding binding of drugs to specific serum proteins are based on affinity chromatography with the protein immobilized on the column. With this approach, the investigated drug is injected as a small volume (zonal elution) or very large volume (frontal analysis) onto a column containing the protein, and the profile of the eluate is monitored. Once an affinity chromatography column is prepared, it can be used numerous times for many compounds, greatly reducing the per-sample cost of analysis. The greatest challenges for this approach are to minimize non-specific binding to the support and to prepare reproducible columns without altering the binding affinity and native configuration of the protein.

The free concentration of carbamazepine in the presence of alpha-1-acid glycoprotein (AGP) was investigated using an immobilized AGP column under controlled temperature. The authors found low-affinity interactions with the chromatographic support, and high-affinity ones with the protein. Competition studies showed that these interactions were occurring at the same site that binds propranolol on AGP. Their results provided a much more complete picture of how carbamazepine binds to AGP in human serum [41]. In another report, the same research group studied binding of lidocaine to two serum proteins, HSA and AGP. It was shown that lidocaine has strong binding to AGP and weak to moderate binding to HSA [42]. A very carefully conducted study regarding the binding of phenytoin to immobilized HSA demonstrated that the drug can interact with the protein at the warfarin-azapropazone, indole-benzodiazepine, tamoxifen and digitoxin sites. The authors concluded that this rather complex binding system indicates the importance of identifying the binding regions on HSA for specific drugs as a means of understanding their transport in blood and characterizing their potential for drug—drug interactions [43].

Solid Phase Microextraction

SPME is a rapid sample preparation technique in which a small amount of extracting phase is put in contact with a sample for a controlled period of time. Because of the partial extraction approach, the method can be used to determine free drug concentrations in either negligible or non-negligible mode [44]. However, the partial extraction mode also makes the outcome of the method more susceptible to variations in temperature, time and contaminants. Also, the extraction phase must be carefully selected so that it does not adsorb the binding protein. Nevertheless, although method development must be carefully addressed, solid phase microextraction allows for significant flexibility in the choice of extraction phase and analytical method as demonstrated by published reports. SPME was applied to study the binding of seven drugs to human serum albumin. The preferred extraction mode was "negligible depletion", where the concentration of drug in the sample remains almost the same after extraction. The author found experimental results to be in agreement with literature data and ultrafiltration experiments performed in parallel, indicating the feasibility of SPME for such bioanalytical purposes [45]. Since matrix effects are crucial when measuring free concentrations, Heringa *et al.* investigated the influence of proteins on the kinetics of microextraction. It was found that although there is a large effect of protein presence on the kinetics of drug uptake, the apparent affinity constant for proteins can still be measured [46].

Methods Suitable for Complex Biological Samples Including Blood

Measurement of free drug concentrations in complex biological samples is performed either to determine the extent of overall serum protein binding (without necessarily identifying a specific binding protein) or to assure therapeutic efficiency for drugs with a low therapeutic window and high binding to plasma proteins. Determining the overall amount of drug binding to serum proteins is an essential step in both drug discovery and the clinical phases of drug development. The largest contribution to serum protein binding of drugs is given by HSA and AGP. Usually, HSA shows higher binding affinity for acidic and neutral compounds while AGP preferentially binds basic drugs. AGP is a protein synthesized in the liver, and is often associated with acute-phase reactions. Accordingly, its influence on drug pharmacokinetics is often missed when drugs are tested on healthy volunteers. Many pathological conditions are associated with increased levels of AGP. Among these, chronic inflammation, myocardial infarction and advanced cancer are the most notable, since drug distribution can be significantly altered and the risk for adverse reactions is increased. Furthermore, most drugs that bind to AGP also bind to HSA; even if the binding constant to HSA is lower than that to AGP, the influence of albumin can still be significant given its much higher concentration in plasma. Although the main drug-binding proteins are HAS and AGP, serum contains many other proteins; consequently, there is a high probability that many drug molecules will exhibit some levels of binding which should be checked in biological samples.

Ultrafiltration

Perhaps the most popular separation method for determination of free drug concentrations in complex biological samples is ultrafiltration. Ultrafiltration is the method of choice, especially in clinical laboratories, due to its ease of use and rapidity. The serum or plasma is usually centrifuged in tubes with semipermeable membranes, and the free drug is measured in the ultrafiltrate.

Two of the most problematic aspects when using ultrafiltration in clinical practice are the temperature at which the process is carried out, and the specificity and sensitivity of the analytical method. Although it is now well known that changes in temperature significantly affect the extent of drug-binding to proteins, most clinical laboratories continue to measure free concentrations by ultrafiltration at room temperature (25°C). In a comprehensive study, Kodama et al. measured the free phenytoin concentration by ultrafiltration at body temperature and room temperature and discovered a difference of 44% in binding affinity, which clearly shows the importance of controlling the temperature for such measurements [47].

Another issue is the fact that many clinical assays are based on antibodies that have cross-reactivity to drug metabolites and sometimes even to endogenous compounds. While this may still be a problem when total drug concentrations are measured, it can definitely lead to more problems when the metabolite is less bound to serum proteins than the parent drug and the metabolite cross-reacts with the immunoassay used for the drug measurement. In this case, the ratio of drug to metabolite concentration in the ultrafiltrate can increase in an unpredictable manner, as a function of the metabolic rate and time of sample collection. Depending on the extent of metabolite cross-reactivity, errors can be as high as 100%. In such cases, analytical methods based on chromatography should be used. Unfortunately, because of speed and convenience, immunoassays continue to be the analytical method of choice in many clinical laboratories. In addition, some ultrafiltration-based assays suffer from non-specific binding of drugs to the ultrafiltration device. Finally, there is a lot of variability between studies regarding the molecular mass cutoff of the membrane used for ultrafiltration, ranging from 3 kDa to 50 kDa.

Several publications challenge the current knowledge regarding the validity of calculation of free drug concentration [48–51]. These research papers show that the unbound drug fraction is concentration dependent, which should be taken into account in the interpretation of drug pharmacokinetics as well as in modeling. Dawidowicz et al. recently published two papers about the anomalous relationship between the free fraction of a drug and its total concentration in drug–protein systems. Their reports are surprising, indicating that the free fraction of some drugs increases with the decrease in total drug concentration. They used both isolated albumin and human plasma to study the binding of propofol, fatty acids, indomethacin and lidocaine to proteins. Free drug molecules were separated by ultrafiltration through a 10-kDa molecular mass cutoff membrane and measured by liquid chromatography. The experiments carried out in this study show that ligand hydrophobicity affects the dependence between the free ligand fraction and its total concentration, and that similar anomalous changes of the free drug fraction are observed not only for drugs interacting with different binding sites on HSA, but also for basic local anesthetics that bind to AGP [52, 53]. The importance of these findings in clinical practice is currently unclear, and further research is needed.

Equilibrium Dialysis

While ultrafiltration is the most popular method, especially in clinical settings, equilibrium dialysis is still considered the gold standard for monitoring free drug concentrations and continues to be used in many research settings. The method is based on drug diffusion across a semipermeable membrane that separates the sample to be investigated from a buffer solution. The membrane should be permeable to the drug and not to the protein. The device is incubated until equilibrium is reached, and the free drug is measured in the buffer solution. The main challenges with this method are long equilibration times (up to 2 days), difficulties for compounds with low solubility in water, volume shifts due to differences in osmotic pressure, artifacts created by electrically charged drugs or proteins, and non-specific adsorption to the device. Although rapid equilibrium dialysis devices have been introduced, the equilibration time is still long, at up to 6 hours. Furthermore, this quick equilibration approach requires stirring and mixing, which may result in sample loss and/or leakage through the membrane. Since equilibrium dialysis is mostly used in research settings, analysis of the free fraction is usually done by chromatography combined with mass spectrometry, and not immunoassays as is the case for ultrafiltration.

Several publications used both equilibrium dialysis and ultrafiltration to determine free drug concentrations. For example, Vita *et al.* used both methods to investigate plasma protein binding of roscovitine and observed that although binding of roscovitine to HSA was constant (about 90%) within the concentration range studied, binding to AGP decreased with increasing drug concentration, indicating that albumin is more important in binding protein in clinical settings [54]. Nowak *et al.* used equilibrium dialysis to validate results for free mycophenolic acid measurements obtained by ultrafiltration. HSA, high concentrations of the primary glucuronide metabolite, and sodium salicylate were found to significantly affect mycophenolic acid binding to proteins. The conclusion of the study was that the pharmacological activity of the drug is a function of unbound concentration [55]. A very practical method for measuring free drug concentrations in whole blood using rapid equilibrium dialysis was developed by Chen *et al.* Their experimental results can be used to explain non-linear pharmacokinetic profiles and to predict effect and doses across species [56]. Using a similar method, Liu *et al.* showed that drug activity in the brain is much more accurately determined by the unbound brain drug concentration [57, 58].

Significant challenges in measuring free concentrations are encountered for compounds with high binding that are active in low concentrations. Furthermore, some compounds have significantly different binding depending on patient gender, age and disease state. For these complicated cases, the gold standard method for measuring free concentrations is isotope dilution equilibrium dialysis. This approach was used by Hackbarth *et al.* to investigate the accuracy of calculated free testosterone levels. Although total testosterone is generally believed to be sufficient for diagnosing significant androgen excess or deficiency, the free (bioactive) testosterone is of superior diagnostic value, especially under circumstances of altered sex-hormone binding globulin serum concentrations or binding affinity. Such cases are encountered in hyper- or hypothyroidism, liver cirrhosis, obesity, or exogenous sex hormone use – especially estrogen treatments. Serum concentrations of the globulin also increase with age, often affecting free testosterone levels disproportionately to total testosterone concentrations. The authors concluded that application of equations for calculating free testosterone concentrations to wider populations will frequently yield results that differ substantially from isotope dilution equilibrium dialysis [59]. Obviously, the best approach in this case would be to always measure the free testosterone concentration.

Methods Suitable for *In Vivo* Analysis

All approaches discussed so far in this chapter are based on a defined sample that is collected from a human (or in a few cases an animal) and analyzed at a later time. An important direction in recent years has been the push to analyze target compounds *in vivo*, without removing a portion of the investigated system. This can be done either with non-invasive spectroscopic methods or by *in vivo* microextraction. The methods that are currently applicable in clinical practice are ultrafiltration and microdialysis. SPME is also increasingly being used in animal models, and will most likely become available for clinical testing in the near future [60, 61].

Ultrafiltration is a filtrate selection method with a wide range of biomedical and clinical applications. Ultrafiltration probes for pharmacokinetic studies are small, flexible tubes with a surface area of a few square millimeters that can be implanted into living animals or humans. Once installed, fluid can be painlessly removed from the extracellular space of the surrounding tissue by exerting negative pressure and thus drawing the interstitial cell fluid out through a semipermeable membrane with a molecular weight cut-off between 20 kDa and 50 kDa. The probe should be implanted in tissues with a high fluid turnover that can tolerate some loss of fluid [62]. The technique has proved particularly useful for monitoring the tissue pharmacokinetics of antineoplastic drugs and for probing tumor secretions.

Microdialysis can be used to measure drugs in the extracellular fluid by means of a small probe that is equipped with a semipermeable membrane. The equipment needed for microdialysis usually consists of a pump, an implantable catheter (probe), and a vial where the sample is collected. Sampling is accomplished by implanting the probe into the target biological fluid or tissue, followed by slowly pumping a suitable perfusate through the catheter. Microdialysis probes are manufactured to have a specific molecular weight cutoff (usually from 10 to 50 kDa) and can differ in their form and material, depending on the tissue to be investigated. While the perfusate passes through the probe, some molecules diffuse from the sample into the probe based on their concentration gradient, generating a dialysate that is collected for analysis. Microdialysis has basically been used for sampling drugs in human and animal tissue, from blood to hard bone. Both ultrafiltration and microdialysis can measure the free drug concentration if the semipermeable membrane allows passage of drug molecules and prevents removal of binding proteins. One of the methods that is increasingly being used for free concentration assays in research settings is SPME. The ability of SPME to measure protein binding for drugs with very high affinity is particularly important, since this is difficult to perform with popular methods such as equilibrium dialysis and ultrafiltration. In order to investigate such drugs, extraction phases with high affinity for the investigated compound should be selected.

Other Methods

Many other methods have been developed to measure free drug concentrations, but their applicability is currently rather limited. The best non-invasive methods that can be used to measure drug concentrations are positron emission tomography and magnetic resonance spectroscopy. These approaches could in the future become the ideal therapeutic drug monitoring methods, but currently they are very expensive and cannot measure free concentrations. Positron emission tomography has good spatial resolution, but requires potentially hazardous radioactive tracers and cannot distinguish between the drug and its metabolites. Magnetic resonance spectroscopy is more specific and avoids the use of radioactivity, but has poor spatial resolution when it comes to drug analysis.

A very interesting study that extends the concept of free concentrations to larger molecules such as proteins was conducted by Speeckaert *et al.* in order to investigate the potential association of vitamin D binding protein with lipoproteins. The presence of vitamin-D binding protein in lipoprotein fractions was examined using precipitation, gel permeation chromatography and ultracentrifugation. The study revealed that the lipid-bound vitamin-D binding protein fraction is of greater clinical importance than initially thought [63]. Similarly, Calligaris *et al.* measured free bilirubin using the diluted peroxidase method to show that bilirubin-induced cytotoxicity in a given cell line can be accurately predicted by free bilirubin irrespective of the source and concentration of albumin, or total bilirubin level [64].

Perhaps the ideal devices for continuously monitoring free drug concentrations in clinical practice would be based on biosensors. These sensors are usually small and portable, and allow for selective quantitation of chemical and biochemical analytes. Chemical recognition is generally accomplished by exploiting the natural selectivity of biochemical species such as enzymes, antibodies, receptors and nucleic acids. Due to their selectivity, small size and equilibrium approach, and the fact that they don't remove any analyte from the investigated system, sensors naturally measure the free drug concentration in the sample. Regrettably, biosensors continue to be difficult to produce, may not be suitable for complex biological samples, and are mostly found in research laboratories.

Choosing an Appropriate Technique

When deciding on a method for measuring free drug concentrations, the sample type should be considered first, followed by the desired throughput. Two general types of samples are usually monitored for free drug concentrations: isolated proteins, and biological samples including blood (Fig. 4.3). When the binding of drugs to isolated proteins is investigated, more convenient methods can be built if the protein can be immobilized on a solid surface. In this case, affinity chromatography and surface plasmon resonance can be used. When the protein is preferred to be free in solution, the free concentrations can be monitored by capillary electrophoresis or parallel artificial membrane assay. Methods for complex biological samples can be divided into those that are mostly used in research laboratories and those with clinical applicability. Ultrafiltration is by far the preferred method in clinical settings, due to speed and simplicity, but may suffer from non-specific binding and lack of temperature control (it is still used at room temperature in clinical laboratories). SPME is a new potential candidate in this area; it is a fast and simple approach, but method development can be lengthy.

Currently, there are many disadvantages related to the available methods for measuring the free fraction of drugs. Although free concentrations are well recognized as being more useful for therapeutic decisions and research than total concentrations, they will not be regularly monitored in hospitals unless the following issues are addressed by clinical chemists:

- Cost: free concentration assays are costlier and more difficult to perform than total concentration assays
- Accuracy and precision: current methods for free concentrations are less accurate and more variable than those for total concentrations

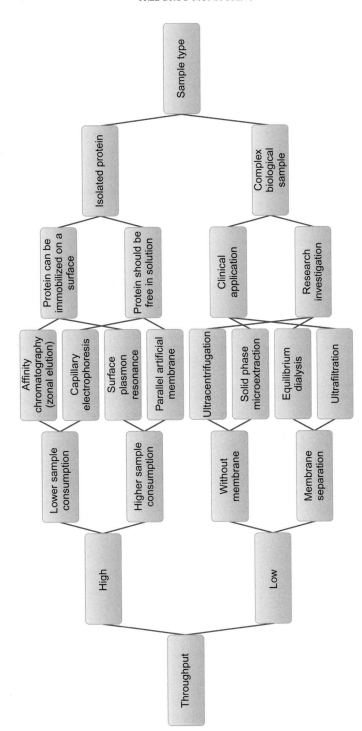

FIGURE 4.3 Selection of the most appropriate method for measuring free drug concentrations.

- Reference methods: while equilibrium dialysis is regarded as the reference method, the long time for analysis is unsuitable in a clinical setting when a result within few hours is needed
- Reliability: practitioners continue to complain about a high proportion of physical failures of the ultrafiltration and equilibrium dialysis devices
- Establishment of standardized test conditions: plasma (or serum) characteristics change after removal from the body, potentially changing the free concentration; all biological samples should be processed at a similar temperature, pH, and CO_2 partial pressure.

ALTERNATIVE METHODS

Given the many technical difficulties in measuring free concentrations in samples derived from blood, researchers have found several alternatives, such as using other samples or calculating either the free concentration or normalized concentration.

Alternative Samples

When free concentrations cannot be measured in blood, other body fluids that naturally contain fewer proteins can be used as substitute samples. Saliva and tears are largely secreted from the plasma water, and therefore contain most of the small molecules that are found in blood, including drugs. While the concentration of drugs in these secretions is usually not exactly the same as the free concentration in serum, the values are generally proportional. Therefore, once the proportionality constant is determined, saliva and tears can be used as substitutes for determining free concentrations in serum.

Calculated Values

When the free concentration cannot be measured due to technical difficulties or financial constraints, it may be possible to calculate it instead. In order to perform the calculations, the protein concentration and the drug–protein binding constants need to be known. Since many researchers and clinicians are not comfortable with using free concentrations, a "normalized concentration" is often calculated for some drugs. The normalized drug concentration is the drug level that would produce the same free concentration in plasma samples with a normal concentration of binding proteins. The calculations are usually based on the observed total drug concentration and serum albumin concentration.

Several equations for calculating normalized phenytoin levels are listed in the scientific literature, leading to different results. Regrettably, all the equations in the current literature are based on an outdated drug binding model to human serum albumin and are based on the fraction of unbound drug, which is known to depend on both protein and drug concentration. To address this problem, a general method for calculating normalized drug levels in the presence of altered plasma protein binding was recently proposed [65]. Regardless of the binding model, the normalized drug concentration (C_{norm}) may be expressed as:

$$C_{norm} = C_{obs} \cdot R - C_f \cdot (R - 1) \qquad (4.6)$$

TABLE 4.2 Examples of Drugs for which the Normalized Concentration can be Calculated

Drug & ref.	Range of reported fu %	Binding to HSA (L/mole)	Binding to AGP (L/mole)	V_D (L/kg)	$t_{1/2}$ (hr)	Therapeutic range
Carbamazepine [31]	20–30	$K_1 = 1.0 \cdot 10^3$	$K_2 = 1.0 \cdot 10^5$	1.3 ± 0.7	14 ± 2	15–50 µM
Lidocaine [35]	20–40	$K_1 = 4.7 \cdot 10^4$	$K_2 = 1.1 \cdot 10^5$	1.6 ± 0.5	1.7 ± 0.3	4–16 µM
Paclitaxel [55]	2–12	Stoichiometric $k_1 = 2.4 \cdot 10^6$ $k_2 = 1.0 \cdot 10^5$	n/a	2.0 ± 1.2	3 ± 1	0.5–1 µM (dose of 135 –250 mg/m^2)
Valproic acid [12]	6–8	Site oriented $b_1 = 1.98$ $K_1 = 15.5 \cdot 10^3$	n/a	0.22 ± 0.07	14 ± 3	350–1000 µM
Phenytoin [41]	1–34	Site-oriented $K_1 = 1.04 \cdot 10^4$ $K_2 = 6.50 \cdot 10^3$	n/a	0.64 ± 0.04	15 ± 9	40–80 µM

where C_{obs} is the observed drug concentration, R is the ratio between the normal protein concentration and observed protein concentration, and C_f is the calculated free drug concentration derived from the binding model. This method is applicable for any drug–protein pair, as long as the corresponding binding constants are known. Examples of drugs for which the normalized concentration can easily be calculated based on literature data are listed in Table 4.2.

As a direct clinical application, equation 4.6 can be used for calculating normalized phenytoin and paclitaxel levels (Fig. 4.4) in patients with altered albumin concentration,

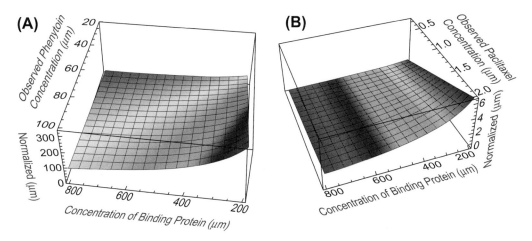

FIGURE 4.4 Variation of normalized drug concentration as a function of observed drug concentration and binding protein concentration: (A) phenytoin; (B) paclitaxel.

such as the elderly, trauma patients and pediatric patients. However, it should be noted that the equations are never as good as actually measuring the free drug concentrations [66, 67].

CONCLUSIONS

Free drug concentrations correlate to therapeutic effects better than total drug concentrations, for both small and large molecules. Unfortunately, current technical difficulties in accurately measuring free concentrations prevent full clinical application, and further research in this field is needed. Nevertheless, in clinical laboratories ultrafiltration followed by measurement of the drug in the protein-free ultrafiltrate using a commercially available immunoassay or a chromatographic method is routinely used for free drug monitoring of phenytoin, valproic acid, carbamazepine and mycophenolic acid. Such routine monitoring of free drug concentrations certainly has demonstrated clinical usefulness. As bioanalytical methods become more sensitive, accurate and precise we will certainly witness an increase in monitoring of free drug concentrations, which represent the "active" fraction of the drug.

As an alternative, when free drug concentrations are too complicated to monitor or the procedure is too costly, the total drug concentration can be normalized by using equation 4.6, or specific equations such as those proposed for phenytoin [1, 8] or testosterone [54]. However, direct measurement of free drug is certainly superior to indirect estimation of free drug using a mathematical equation.

An important trend in the next decade will be the development of new analytical methods based on *in vivo* microextraction and biosensors. These new approaches will naturally determine free drug concentrations, and will also allow investigation of pharmacokinetics in target tissues, further expanding the utility of free drug monitoring.

References

[1] Lee M. Basic Skills in Interpreting Laboratory Data. Bethesda, MD: American Society of Health-System Pharmacists; 2009.
[2] Bauer LA. Applied Clinical Pharmacokinetics. New York, NY: McGraw-Hill Medical; 2008.
[3] Musteata FM, Pawliszyn J, Qian MG, et al. Determination of drug plasma protein binding by solid phase microextraction. J Pharm Sci 2006;95:1712—22.
[4] Trainor GL. The importance of plasma protein binding in drug discovery. Expert Opin Drug Discov 2007;2:51—64.
[5] Dasgupta A. Usefulness of monitoring free (unbound) concentrations of therapeutic drugs in patient management [Review]. Clin Chim Acta 2007;377:1—13.
[6] Iwamoto T, Kagawa Y, Naito Y, et al. Clinical evaluation of plasma free phenytoin measurement and factors influencing its protein binding. Biopharm Drug Dispos 2006;27:77—84.
[7] Banh HL, Burton ME, Sperling MR. Interpatient and intrapatient variability in phenytoin protein binding. Ther Drug Monit 2002;24:379—85.
[8] Anderson GD, Pak C, Doane KW, et al. Revised Winter-Tozer equation for normalized phenytoin concentrations in trauma and elderly patients with hypoalbuminemia. Ann Pharmacother 1997;31:279—84.
[9] Kodama H, Kodama Y, Shinozawa S, et al. *In vivo* binding characteristics of phenytoin to serum proteins in monotherapy pediatric patients with epilepsy. Intl J Clin Pharmacol Ther 2008;38:25—9.
[10] Gulyassy PF, Jarrard E, Stanfel L. Roles of hippurate and indoxyl sulfate in the impaired ligand binding by azotemic plasma. Adv Exp Med Biol 1987;223:55—8.

[11] Takamura N, Maruyama T, Otagiri M. Effects of uremic toxins and fatty acids on serum protein binding of furosemide: possible mechanism of the binding defect in uremia. Clin Chem 1997;43:2274–80.

[12] Klotz U, Rapp T, Muller WA. Disposition of VPA in patients with liver disease. Eur J Clin Pharmacol 1978;13:55–60.

[13] Hooper W, Dubetz D, Bochner F, et al. Plasma protein binding of carbamazepine. Clin Pharmacol Ther 1975;17:433–40.

[14] Kemper EM, van Khan HJ, Speelman P, et al. Severe phenytoin intoxication in patients with hypoalbuminemia. Ned Tjdschr Geneeskd 2007;151:138–41 [in Dutch].

[15] Wolf GK, McClain CD, Zurakoski D, et al. Total phenytoin concentrations do not accurately predict free phenytoin concentrations in critically ill children. Pediatr Crit Care Med 2006;7:434–9.

[16] Zielmann S, Mielck F, Kahl R, et al. A rational basis for the measurement of free phenytoin concentration in critically ill trauma patients. Ther Drug Monit 1994;16:139–44.

[17] Gidal BE, Collins DM, Beinlich BR. Apparent valproic acid neurotoxicity in a hypoalbuminemic patient. Ann Pharmacother 1993;27:32–5.

[18] Mamiya K, Yukawa E, Matsumoto T, et al. Synergistic effect of valproate coadministration and hypoalbuminemia on the serum-free phenytoin concentration in patients with severe motor and intellectual disabilities. Clin Neuropharmacol 2002;25:230–3.

[19] Alvarez MTR, Valino LE, Gabriel EF, et al. Relation between total and unbound valproate concentration and serum albumin. Pharm World Sci 2010;32:289.

[20] Ueshima S, Aiba T, Sato T, et al. Individualized dosage adjustment of valproic acid based on unbound serum concentration in intractable epileptic children. Yakugaku Zasshi-J Pharm Soc Jpn 2008;128:92.

[21] Dutta S, Faught E, Limdi NA. Valproate protein binding following rapid intravenous administration of high doses of valproic acid in patients with epilepsy. J Clin Pharm Ther 2007;32:365–71.

[22] Sproule B, Nava-Ocampo AA, Kapur B. Measuring unbound versus total valproate concentrations for therapeutic drug monitoring. Ther Drug Monit 2006;28:714–5.

[23] Ulldemolins M, Roberts JA, Rello J, et al. The effects of hypoalbuminaemia on optimizing antibacterial dosing in critically ill patients. Clin Pharmacokinet 2011;50:99–110.

[24] Zsila F, Visy J, Mady G, Fitos I. Selective plasma protein binding of antimalarial drugs to alpha(1)-acid glycoprotein. Bioorg Med Chem 2008;16:3759–72.

[25] Fayet A, Beguin A, de Tejada BM, et al. Determination of unbound antiretroviral drug concentrations by a modified ultrafiltration method reveals high variability in the free fraction. Ther Drug Monit 2008;30:511–22.

[26] Barrail-Tran A, Mentre F, Cosson C, Piketty C. Influence of alpha-1 glycoprotein acid concentrations and variants on atazanavir pharmacokinetics in HIV-infected patients included in the ANRS 107 Trial. Antimicrob Agents Chemother 2009;54:614–9.

[27] Dasgupta A. Monitoring free drug concentrations. In: Dasgupta A, editor. Handbook of Drug Monitoring Methods: Therapeutics and Drugs of Abuse. Totawa, NJ: Humana Press; 2007, p. 41–65.

[28] Pisupati J, Jain A, Burckart G, et al. Intraindividual and interindividual variation in the pharmacokinetics of mycophenolic acid in liver transplant patients. J Clin Pharmacol 2005;45:34–41.

[29] Atcheson BA, Taylor PJ, Mudge DW, et al. Mycophenolic acid pharmacokinetics and related outcomes early after renal transplant. Br J Clin Pharmacol 2005;59:271–80.

[30] Jacobson P, Long J, Rogosheske J, et al. High unbound mycophenolic acid concentrations in a hematopoietic cell transplantation patient with sepsis and renal and hepatic dysfunction [Letter]. Biol Blood Marrow Transplant 2005;11:977–8.

[31] Patel CG, Mendonza AE, Akhlaghi F, et al. Determination of total mycophenolic acid and its glucuronide metabolite using liquid chromatography with ultraviolet detection and unbound mycophenolic acid using tandem mass spectrometry. J Chromatogr B Analyt Technol Biomed Life Sci 2004;813(1–2):287–94.

[32] Shen B, Li S, Zhang Y, Yuan X, et al. Determination of total, free and saliva mycophenolic acid with LC-MS/MS method: application to pharmacokinetic study in healthy volunteers and renal transplant patients. J Pharm Biomed Anal 2009;50:515–21.

[33] Benichou AS, Blanchet B, Conti F, et al. Variability in free mycophenolic acid exposure in adult liver transplant recipients during the early posttransplantation period. J Clin Pharmacol 2010;50:1202–10.

[34] Liu RY, Meng QC, Xi J, et al. Comparative binding character of two general anaesthetics for sites on human serum albumin. Biochem J 2004;380:147–52.

[35] Zhou R, Liu R. Does bilirubin change the free concentration of propofol? Acta Anaesthesiol Scand 2010;54:653−4.

[36] Li J, Brahmer J, Messersmith W, et al. Binding of gefitinib, an inhibitor of epidermal growth factor receptor-tyrosine kinase, to plasma proteins and blood cells: *in vitro* and in cancer patients. Invest New Drugs 2006;24:291−7.

[37] Vorum H, Honore B. Influence of fatty acids on the binding of warfarin and phenprocoumon to human serum albumin with relation to anticoagulant therapy. J Pharm Pharmacol 1996;48:870−5.

[38] Vorum H, Jorgensen HRI, Brodersen R. Variation in the binding affinity of warfarin and phenprocoumon to human serum albumin in relation to surgery. Eur J Clin Pharmacol 1993;44:157−62.

[39] Vuckovic D, Cudjoe E, Musteata FM, Pawliszyn J. Automated solid phase microextraction and thin-film microextraction for high-throughput analysis of biological fluids and ligand−receptor binding studies. Nat Protocols 2010;5:140−61.

[40] Musteata ML, Musteata FM. Analytical methods used in conjunction with SPME: a review of recent bio-analytical applications. Bioanalysis 2009;1:1081−102.

[41] Xuan H, Joseph KS, Wa CL, Hage DS. Biointeraction analysis of carbamazepine binding to alpha(1)-acid glycoprotein by high-performance affinity chromatography. J Sep Sci 2010;33:2294−301.

[42] Soman S, Yoo MJ, Jang YJ, Hage DS. Analysis of lidocaine interactions with serum proteins using high-performance affinity chromatography. J Chromatogr B 2010;878:705−8.

[43] Chen JZ, Ohnmacht C, Hage DS. Studies of phenytoin binding to human serum albumin by high-performance affinity chromatography. J Chromatogr B 2004;809:137−45.

[44] Musteata FM, Pawliszyn J. Study of ligand−receptor binding using SPME: investigation of receptor, free, and total ligand concentrations. J Proteome Res 2005;4:789−800.

[45] Theodoridis G. Application of solid phase microextraction in the investigation of protein binding of pharmaceuticals. J Chromatogr B 2006;830:238−44.

[46] Heringa MB, Hogevonder C, Busser F, Hermens JLM. Measurement of the free concentration of octylphenol in biological samples with negligible depletion-solid phase microextraction (nd-SPME): analysis of matrix effects. J Chromatogr B 2006;834:35−41.

[47] Kodama H, Kodama Y, Itokazu N, et al. Effect of temperature on serum protein binding characteristics of phenytoin in monotherapy paediatric patients with epilepsy. J Clin Pharm Ther 2001;26:175−9.

[48] Berezhkovskiy LM. On the calculation of the concentration dependence of drug binding to plasma proteins with multiple binding sites of different affinities: determination of the possible variation of the unbound drug fraction and calculation of the number of binding sites of the protein. J Pharm Sci 2007;96:249−57.

[49] Berezhkovskiy LM. Consideration of the linear concentration increase of the unbound drug fraction in plasma. J Pharm Sci 2009;98:383−93.

[50] Berezhkovskiy LM. Some features of the kinetics and equilibrium of drug binding to plasma proteins. Expert Opin Drug Metab Toxicol 2008;4:1479−98.

[51] Berezhkovskiy LM. On the possibility of self-induction of drug protein binding. J Pharm Sci 2010;99:4400−5.

[52] Dawidowicz AL, Kobielski M, Pieniadz J. Anomalous relationship between free drug fraction and its total concentration in drug−protein systems − II. Binding of different ligands to plasma proteins. Eur J Pharm Sci 2008;35:136−41.

[53] Dawidowicz AL, Kobielski M, Pieniadz J. Anomalous relationship between free drug fraction and its total concentration in drug−protein systems − I. Investigation of propofol binding in model HSA solution. Eur J Pharm Sci 2008;34:30−6.

[54] Vita M, Abdel-Rehim M, Nilsson C, et al. Stability, pK_a and plasma protein binding of roscovitine. J Chromatogr B 2005;821:75−80.

[55] Nowak I, Shaw LM. Mycophenolic acid binding to human serum albumin − characterization and relation to pharmacodynamics. Clin Chem 1995;41:1011−7.

[56] Chen S, Zhang J, Huang TN, et al. A practical method for measuring free drug concentration in whole blood using rapid equilibrium dialysis (RED) device. Drug Metab Rev 2007;39:290.

[57] Liu XR. Unbound brain concentration determines brain receptor occupancy. Drug Metab Rev 2009;41:27.

[58] Liu XR, Vilenski O, Kwan J, et al. Unbound brain concentration determines receptor occupancy: a correlation of drug concentration and brain serotonin and dopamine reuptake transporter occupancy for eighteen compounds in rats. Drug Metab Dispos 2009;1548−56.

[59] Hackbarth JS, Hoyne JB, Grebe SK, Singh RJ. Accuracy of calculated free testosterone differs between equations and depends on gender and SHBG concentration. Steroids 2011;76:48−55.

[60] Musteata FM, de Lannoy I, Gien B, Pawliszyn J. Blood sampling without blood draws for *in vivo* pharmacokinetic studies in rats. J Pharm Biomed Anal 2008;47:907−12.

[61] Musteata FM. Pharmacokinetic applications of microdevices and microsampling techniques. Bioanalysis 2009;1:171−85.

[62] Leegsma-Vogt G, Janle E, Ash SR, et al. Utilization of *in vivo* ultrafiltration in biomedical research and clinical applications. Life Sci. 2003;73:2005−18.

[63] Speeckaert MM, Taes YE, De Buyzere ML, et al. Investigation of the potential association of vitamin D binding protein with lipoproteins. Ann Clin Biochem 2010;47:143−50.

[64] Calligaris SD, Bellarosa C, Giraudi P, et al. Cytotoxicity is predicted by unbound and not total billrubin concentration. Pediatr Res 2007;62:576−80.

[65] Musteata FM. Interpretation of plasma concentrations in the case of drugs with high protein binding. In: AAPS Northeast Regional Discussion Group. Rocky Hill, CT: AAPS; 2011, p. 42−3.

[66] Mauro LS, Mauro VF, Bachmann KA, Higgins JT. Accuracy of two equations in determining normalized phenytoin concentrations. Dalian Inst Chem Phys 1989;23:64−8.

[67] Tandon M, Pandhi R, Garg SK, Prabhakar SK. Serum albumin-adjusted phenytoin levels: an approach for predicting drug efficacy in patients with epilepsy, suitable for developing countries. Intl J Clin Pharmacol Ther 2004;42:550−5.

[68] Hsueh MM, Wang MM, Sleckza B, et al. Theory vs reality: is free drug concentration in adipose equal to free concentration in plasma? Drug Metab Rev 2009;41:130.

[69] Musteata ML, Musteata FM, Pawliszyn J. Biocompatible solid phase microextraction coatings based on polyacrylonitrile and SPE phases. Anal Chem 2007;79:6903−11.

Current Practice of Therapeutic Drug Monitoring
Dose Adjustment of Drugs using Pharmacokinetic Models

Franck Saint-Marcoux

Department of Pharmacology and Toxicology, Limoges University Hospital, Limoges France

INTRODUCTION

Dose adjustment in therapeutic drug monitoring (TDM) is based on estimating relevant pharmacokinetic parameters with the aim of first determining the exposure to the drug and, secondly, modifying the dosing to achieve a desired level of exposure. The starting point of this chapter is to define whether a dose adjustment based on modeling will have any added value. Consequently, by focusing on a particular drug, the emerging questions would be: Are the exposure indices defined? If such indices are well defined, then next question should be: Are these parameters easily accessible in the routine clinical setting or not? When establishing TDM for a drug, single blood concentration levels have been traditionally, and almost systematically, proposed; most of the time, trough concentrations or maximum concentrations (C_{max}). A trough level can be pertinent when the concentration—effect relationship suggests that efficacy (or toxicity) of a drug is linked to the maintenance of blood concentrations above a predefined targeted concentration (glycopeptides, antiviral or antiretroviral drugs, for instance). Accordingly, a C_{max} has to be measured when high enough concentrations are needed to increase the efficacy (aminoglycosides, for example). However, the use of a single blood concentration is questionable when effects are linked to the global exposure over the entire dosing interval. In such cases, area under the concentration—time curve (AUC), reflecting the evolution of concentrations over the dosing interval, is logically considered as a more relevant exposure index. At this stage, the logical question is to ask whether a single blood concentration is a good representative of the AUC or not. If not, a switch to tools that will allow the determination of the AUC is unavoidable. This is typically the case for different immunosuppressive compounds, such as cyclosporine, tacrolimus or, more recently, mycophenolate mofetil, for which reports of consensus conferences have promoted the use of the AUC to improve TDM efficacy [1—3]. Precisely, for these drugs traditional trough levels have been shown to be either poor representatives of the global exposure or/and not predictive of patients' behavior, even if largely employed.

The further question, then, is to know how to reach the AUC or, more precisely, for practical, ethical and economic reasons, how to limit the number of concentration measurements while maintaining accuracy. Different processes of determining at which times samples should be taken to produce the most accurate estimation using as few samples as possible have been proposed. The simplest method of estimating AUC is multiple regression analysis (MRA). Basically, in MRA a large number of drug concentration measurements are made within a dosing interval in a population of patients. From this database, a reference AUC is determined by the trapezoidal method and a statistics program is run to perform the multiple regressions of all combinations of time points that produce the combination with the best correlation between the estimated and the reference AUC. The resulting equation is in the form of $AUC = A + B_1 \times Ct_1 + B_2 \times Ct_2...$; where A is a constant corresponding to the intercept on the y-axis, Ct_i are the blood concentrations measured at time t_i, and B_i are the associated coefficients determined by MRA. Due to its simplicity, MRA has been largely employed. However, MRA has major drawbacks: it can only be applied in an exact copy of the dosing schedule used to develop the regression equation; errors in timing lead to errors in estimation; and extrapolations can only be used with any accuracy in the population in which they have been developed [3]. Even if sometimes helpful when rigorously validated and appropriately used, such tools are not pharmacokinetic tools, as they do not refer to any kind of individualized estimation of pharmacokinetic parameters.

Even then, if the added value of a pharmacokinetic-based (PK-based) dose adjustment strategy is accepted, the question remains regarding which program. This is obviously the hardest step to get through: Should I develop my own models? If so, will I be able to develop them? Or should I buy a licence for a ready-to-use program which should provide reliable results for my patients? A huge number of PK or PK/PD (PD, pharmacodynamics) programs exist [4], but not all of them have been developed with the aim of being usable by everyone, from the experienced pharmacometrician to inexperienced personnel. The question should not be whether one program or another is the most suitable for a routine activity, but rather an evaluation of whether a black box system which proposes new dosages based on individual information is preferable, or a system that can be upgraded and customized.

This chapter reports the experience of a so-called "pharmacometrician" whose activity is dedicated to the development of models and Bayesian estimators for the dose adjustment of drugs in a clinical routine activity. Its objectives are to describe some methodologies that can be employed to develop such models and Bayesian estimators (MAP-Bes), although none can be recognized as a gold standard.

BAYESIAN ESTIMATION

Bayesian estimation methods have been frequently used to estimate patients' pharmacokinetic parameters, and have been extensively applied in TDM. The definition for a Bayesian estimator proposed by Jelliffe *et al.* [5] is as follows: Bayesian estimation is a method that aims to provide "a patient-specific model of drug behavior in an individual patient, based on dosage, serum concentration, and other relevant clinical descriptors".

Principles

The fundamental behind Bayesian statistics have been accurately defined in some books [6–8] and published papers [9, 10]. Nevertheless, a reasonable view could be that:

1. A Bayesian estimator combines population parameter values (and their standard deviations) and individual data, including measured concentrations.
2. If the covariance matrix of the parameters is diagonal (i.e., the simplest case where no correlation between parameters is considered), the Bayesian posterior parameter values are estimated by minimizing the so-called "Bayesian objective function":

$$\sum_{j=1}^{p} \left(\frac{P_{j(pop)} - P_{j(pat)}}{SD\ P_{j(pop)}} \right)^2 + \sum_{i=1}^{n} \left(\frac{C_{i(obs)} - C_{i(pat)}}{SD\ C_{i(obs)}} \right)^2$$

where $P_{(pop)}$ are the parameter values of the population pharmacokinetic model, $P_{(pat)}$ the patient's individualized model, $C_{(obs)}$ the measured concentrations in the patient, $C_{(pat)}$ the estimates of these concentrations obtained when applying the patient's individualized PK model, and $SDP_{(pop)}$ the standard deviations of population parameter values. The last component, $SDC_{(obs)}$, is the standard deviation of the observed concentrations. More precisely, Bayesian estimation takes into account the pharmacokinetic characteristics of a typical population in the form of mean values and SDs of the pharmacokinetic parameters that represent all the patients included beforehand in a given study. Then, to estimate individual pharmacokinetic parameter values, the Bayesian estimator combines the prior knowledge of the probability density function of the population parameters and the fractional individual patient data — for example, one or two blood concentrations measured after drug administration and, possibly, physiological parameters such as body weight, age, gender, etc. This leads to initial parameters corresponding to the results obtained by substituting the patient's observable features values into the expressions for the kinetic parameters. In the next step, "guesses" are made to slightly alter the initial parameters to explain the observed data. Consequently, by minimizing the above expression, a parameter becomes different from its initial value only to the extent that this difference is compensated by a reduction in the "concentration deviation" (i.e., the difference between observed and estimated concentrations).

Therefore, intuitively, before any drug levels are measured, a patient is regarded as a typical member of the population of all similar patients with respect to PK parameter values, but once drug levels have been measured this patient is regarded as a unique individual whose PK parameters are distinct from the others, and the point of view is gradually shifted from the population to the patient by accumulating information about that individual.

At this point, looking at the previous equation, remaining questions might be: Where do the parameter values of the population PK model ($P_{(pop)}$) come from? What is the importance of the standard deviation of the observed concentrations?

Impact of the Assay Employed to Measure Concentration of the Drug

When looking at the above expression, it can be seen that the standard deviation (SD) of the assay (so-called "assay error") in measuring drug level most commonly serum, plasma or whole blood, is thus a key point of the objective function in the Bayesian fitting procedure. Thus the assay error has to be carefully quantified before any calculation, as the credibility of each measured concentration is directly linked to the reciprocal of its variance. To compute this probable variance, and so the probable SD with which a blood concentration is measured, it is necessary to build an analytical error model that expresses the relationship between SD and concentration. For that, it is recommended to make replicates of several representative samples (e.g., blank, low, intermediate, high and very high concentrations) and to calculate the mean and SD of each. Then, the data can be fitted with a polynomial (most of the time a second order) that is further used to calculate the SD with which any concentration is measured. An example is depicted in Fig. 5.1. Obviously, each analytical

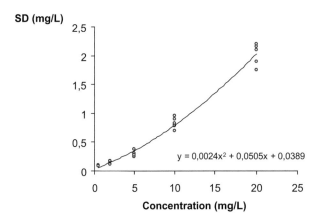

FIGURE 5.1 Typical example of an analytical error model. Data were obtained from five replicates performed at five different levels of concentration with an immunoassay dedicated to the measurement of mycophenolic acid in plasma (author's own data).

SD (mg/L)

$y = 0{,}0024x^2 + 0{,}0505x + 0{,}0389$

Concentration (mg/L)

technique exhibits its own analytical error model. Consequently, a MAP-BE developed using concentrations measured with a particular assay might not be suited to concentrations measured with a different assay. In a study where 45 full PK profiles of tacrolimus were measured with three different techniques (EMIT, Siemens Healthcare Diagnostics Inc., Newark, DE, USA; CMIA, Abbott Diagnostics, Abbott Park, IL, USA; and liquid chromatography-tandem mass spectrometry, LC-MS/MS), it was demonstrated that when using an MAP-BE developed from LC-MS/MS concentrations in patients monitored by CMIA or EMIT the imprecision in the AUC estimation was greater than 20% in about a third of the cases, whereas this proportion was much lower when using MAP-BEs with analytical error models corresponding to the assay actually employed [11]. This implies that a specific concentration database is required to develop a MAP-BE for each existing assay. However, taking into account the large number of immunoassays proposed for a single drug and their different versions (for instance for different analytical platforms), this is hardly feasible. As an example, for tacrolimus, when looking at the International Tacrolimus Proficiency Testing Scheme records [12], at least five different brands of immunoassays are currently employed to measure this drug, in addition to LC-MS/MS, notwithstanding the platforms on which they are run. However, databases corresponding to different analytical techniques are not easily available. As a solution, the feasibility of developing MAP-BE without having any specific database for an analytical technique was proposed. Briefly, taking into account the correlation between concentrations measured with either immunoassays or a reference LC-MS technique, as well as the analytical error model of the techniques, new databases were simulated and 2 MAP-BEs dedicated to the immunoassays were developed from full PK profiles of tacrolimus [11]. The performances of these MAP-BEs were found to be similar to those of the respective MAP-BEs developed using the actual immunoassay concentration results.

Method for Obtaining Population PK Parameters

As mentioned above, what is needed to run a Bayesian estimator is a prior distribution of PK parameters in the form of a population PK model. Therefore, first, a database of observational or experimental data is required. Briefly, this database will consist of patient records containing patient-specific data (the so-called covariates) such as age, body weight, plasma creatinine level and, obviously, concentration–time points of the drug.

At this stage, some information concerning the pharmacokinetics of the targeted drug of interest should already be available in order to anticipate whether a simple (or basic) model or something more sophisticated will be built. This is a key point to decide the structure of the database required for further PK developments − i.e., start with the end in mind. In fact, it is possible to fail in developing and validating a precise and valuable PK tool just because the needs in terms of data were not anticipated. For instance, if working with a drug with a high interpatient variability in absorption, the trial has to take into account that multiple samples will have to be collected in the first hours after administration. Such a case is depicted in Fig. 5.2.

Keeping in mind that the final objective will be to have a PK tool dedicated to the dose adjustment of a drug, several methods of population modeling can be considered. Briefly, population modeling methods can be divided into parametric and non-parametric methods.

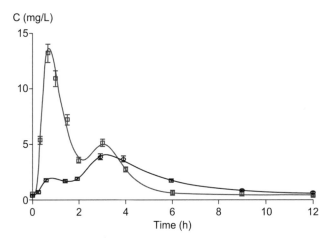

C (mg/L)

Time (h)

FIGURE 5.2 Typical pharmacokinetic profile of mycophenolic acid observed in two different kidney recipients. According to the complexity of the PK profiles, it is necessary to collect blood samples within the whole dose interval, especially by multiplying them during the absorption phase (author's own data).

Parametric methods work under the assumption that each population PK parameter has a specific inter-individual distribution, this distribution being normal or lognormal. Non-parametric methods do not need to make such an assumption.

For the development of PK tools dedicated to TDM, four methods are usually used: the standard two-stage (STS) approach, the iterative approaches (IT2S, IT2B), the non-linear mixed-effect modeling (NONMEM) approach, and the non-parametric expectation maximization (NPEM) approach. Each one is described in detail elsewhere [12–17], but the following paragraph provides the salient features of each of these methods.

The *STS approach* is a well known and widely used procedure [18–21]. It is available, for example, in the ADAPT program [22]. It consists of estimating individual parameters in the first stage by separately fitting each subject's data, then, in the second stage, parameters across individuals are pooled to get a mean and a variance that are considered as the population parameter estimates. With the STS approach, estimates of individual parameters are combined as if this set of estimates were a true sample from a multivariate distribution. Consequently, this approach can be recommended when dealing with individual estimates of PK parameters derived from experimental PK studies with "clean" and homogeneous data coming from full-PK profiles. Nevertheless, STS tends to overestimate parameter dispersion, which can limit further use as prior information for Bayesian estimation [17].

The *ITS methods* rely on repeated fittings of individual data. They are implemented, for instance, with the USC-PACK collection of programs [23]. To run such a method, an approximate *a priori* knowledge about parameter values and variability is required (a previous analysis through STS can be helpful to start out). Based on this information, in a first stage the population model is used as a set of prior distributions for Bayesian estimation of the individual parameters for each patient. This estimation is irrespective of the number of samples provided by each patient, and ITS can be theoretically applied to rich, sparse or mixture data. However, full-PK profiles with samples collected over the dosing interval are preferable [24]. In the second stage, the population parameters are re-obtained from the new individual parameters and used as a new set of prior distributions. These two stages are performed iteratively until the difference between the new and the previous prior distribution becomes null. This is the so-called convergence. Numerous applications in the field of TDM have been published using this approach [25–28].

The first attempt at using the *non-linear mixed-effects approach* model was made by Sheiner *et al.* in the early 1970s [29] and was then rendered available through the well-known NON-MEM program [30]. This approach is a pillar of population pharmacokinetics, and has created a paradigm shift in the role of pharmacokinetics in drug development. However, it has also been extensively applied to develop PK tools for the dose adjustment of drugs [31–35]. Briefly, the non-linear mixed-effects approach aims at estimating the pharmacokinetic parameters and the sources of their variability in the population. Contrary to the previous approaches, in this one the population parameters are calculated by studying all the patients simultaneously, and the patient's individual data are further obtained using MAP-BE based on these parameters' values. The non-linear mixed-effects modeling methods estimate the parameter by the maximum likely approach, and the probability of the data obtained by the model is considered as a function of the model parameters — these parameters' estimates being chosen to maximize this probability. In other words, the idea is to look for parameter estimates that render the observed concentrations more probable than they would be using other parameter estimates.

Moreover, this approach refers to something being "mixed". It is because such models consist of two components: a structural or base model that describes the mean response in the studied population, and another describing how much the value of the parameters varies from one individual to another. This last variability makes the parameter a random effect, as opposed to a fixed effect that has no variability. Keep in mind that if projecting to obtain individual empirical Bayes estimates, the random effects still have to be properly determined, even if the goal is not actually to quantify and explain the variability of the parameters among subjects. Technically, because of the non-linear dependence of the observed data on the random variabilities, it is difficult to reach the maximum likelihood of the data. Therefore, different approximate methods that represent the probability distribution of inter-individual random effects have been proposed. Among the different methods available in the NON-MEM program, the FOCE (first-order conditional estimate) is the most employed — this estimation method being also available in S-Plus as the NMLE function.

The *non-parametric approach* provides an estimate of the whole probability distribution of the pharmacokinetic parameters without any assumption that they exhibit a specific inter-individual distribution [37]. It relies on maximization of the likelihood of the observed data of all individuals to estimate the distribution of the parameters. Conceptually, the individual parameters are assumed to be independent events of a given random variable that has a discrete probability distribution. This probability involves so-called "locations" whose frequencies are determined using a specific algorithm called expectation-maximization. The non-parametric maximum likelihood (NPML) of Mentre and Mallet and the expectation-maximization (NPEM) of Schumitzky share this algorithm. As in NONMEM, this method allows the inclusion of patient-specific covariates, covariates being regarded here as additional parameters and the algorithm providing an estimate of the joint distribution of parameters and covariates. Non-parametric modeling is sometimes considered as being an approach that better describes population PK parameters than parametric methods, especially when distributions are obviously non-Gaussian. However, Bayesian estimation needs parametric population parameters as priors. Discrete non-parametric distributions, as proposed in the multiple model of the software package USC-PACK [38], offer this possibility and can give reliable results if the number of patients is large enough [39].

Determine the Best Limited Sampling Strategy

At this stage, a model is considered to have been built, enabling an accurate estimation of PK parameters. The remaining question is to evaluate whether this prior information will ensure good predictive performances to a MAP-BE using a limited sampling strategy. This approach unfortunately leads to several other questions: To which reference values will the Bayesian estimates be confronted? How can optimal sampling times be determined? Which indicators of predictive performances will be used? How can the developed tools be validated?

Reference Value

In the case of AUC, most of the time the reference value is the AUC determined using the trapezoidal rule that calculates the AUC between every consecutive two measured concentrations and adds all the trapezoidal areas. For other exposure indices, such as C_{max}, the reference values can be those obtained by Bayesian estimation using all available samples.

The so-called "Monte-Carlo simulation" is another suitable technique. Briefly, in the Monte Carlo simulation, simulated patients are created by randomly drawing PK parameters from the distribution of the developed PK model. Provided a sufficient number are created, these "virtual" patients are considered as representatives of the entire distribution of the population, and consequently their PK parameters or concentration–time curves can be used as reference values. This approach has been widely and successfully used [40–41].

Determination of the Limited Sampling Strategy

An intuitive method of determining optimal sampling times could be to perform a comparison of predictive performance of all relevant (possible) combinations of sampling times. Obviously, this cannot be considered as actually optimal, because the possible combinations are limited by the sampling times of the study design. For instance, if sampling is performed hourly in the study design, the limited sampling strategy will automatically be a combination of one or more of these sampling times.

The optimal sampling theory with the determination of D-optimality criterion is a more robust method [42]. D-optimality can be determined in ADAPT, for instance [22]. Briefly, it assumes that there are sampling times providing more information about PK parameters than others. The D-optimality criterion relies on the concept of Fisher information. Fisher information is a method of measuring the amount of predictive information a variable carries about a parameter, and, in the specific case of optimal sampling, the Fisher information represents the available amount of information about the PK parameters at each sampling time. This approach also has some limitations, mainly because the optimal time points are actually optimal for the value of the mean population PK parameters, and because D-optimality reflects a sort of compromise for the simultaneous determination of all PK parameters (even if only one is of interest). However, in a review reporting published Bayesian estimators in the field of TDM, van der Meer *et al.* observed that the D-optimality criterion was used in almost a third of the cases when looking for the best limited sampling strategy [43].

Indicators of Predictive Performance

In the literature, there are multiple indicators of predictive performance. The coefficient of determination (r^2) and the coefficient of correlation (r, or Pearson's correlation coefficient) have been extensively used to express whether the data provided by a PK tool are somehow "well correlated" to the actual data observed in the patients or not. Mean prediction error (MPE) as a measure of bias or mean absolute error (MAE) and root mean squared error (RMSE) as a measure of precision, have been also used. What constitutes a good r^2 or r value is still debatable, and many cautionary notes have been written on their misuse [44] emphasizing that they do not provide quantitative information about predictive performance. For the author, a bias value (MPE) should always be provided with specifications about its spread or magnitude, and ideally with the proportion of patients being "badly" estimated (for instance, the proportion of patients for whom the bias in the estimation of the AUC is greater than 15 or 20%).

As previously mentioned, predictive performance of a PK tool using a limited number of concentrations is most of the time judged by the results of comparisons between estimated AUCs and the actual AUCs (or any estimated exposure index versus its actual value). However, considering that the main objective of the PK tool will be to propose adjustments, the dose proposals coming from the developed PK tool should always be compared to those that would have been proposed using "non-PK" approaches. For instance, knowing the targeted AUC, it seems pertinent to address to what extent a MAP-BE is able to propose a similar dose to that proposed using the trapezoidal rule, and to express the proportion of patients having been proposed the "good" dose.

Validation of a Limited Sampling Strategy

At this stage, *a priori* information coming from a PK model has been obtained, and a MAP-BE has been built, enabling the determination of PK parameters or exposure indices using a limited sampling strategy. The next compulsory step of the development is validation. Instinctively, it might be expected that validation is performed in an independent group of patients, these patients being similar to the clinical target population of the tested tool (the so-called "validation group"). If D-optimality has been used to determine the optimal sampling times, the corresponding samples are taken in the test group and Bayesian estimation is applied. Based on the same reference values as for the determination of optimal sampling times, predictive performances are consequently obtained. However, the use of a "validation group" implies that a significant part of the available information is not used for the development, and thus reduces the precision: It remains a matter of debate whether or not the "intuitive" advantage of independent validation counterbalances the better precision of a procedure using all the available information. Nevertheless, numerous variations of resampling strategies have been proposed. Briefly, the concept is still to split the dataset into a "building group" (i.e., the one used to develop) and a "validation group", but to resample the patients a number of times to ensure that each of them belongs consecutively to both the building and the validation group. Such strategies are the well-known "Jack-knife" method, bootstrapping and cross-validation. Here, as previously mentioned, Monte Carlo simulation can also be a viable alternative, especially when limited patient data are available, but the applied PK distribution has to be as close as possible to the true population distribution. Readers can obtain exhaustive information on this topic from a paper by J. H. Proost that compared the predictive performance of PK tools validated either with a building group or by a cross-validation [45].

EXAMPLES OF CLINICAL TRANSFERABILITY

For the most part, during the development process of a drug excellent PK or PK/PD or PK/PD/PG (PG, pharmacogenetics) analyses are performed and robust models are developed and applied, but not with the aim of being used in clinical settings where actual individual dose adjustment has to be done. In literature, it is also not unusual to find very elegant models with perfect descriptions of the behavior of a drug, excellent predictive performance and a full explanation of interpatient variability, but requiring multiple covariates, which are obviously difficult to obtain in a routine setting. In reality, these models built during a drug's development are by definition not meant for disclosure; instead, sophisticated models from academic research teams are the single best candidates for publication. As a consequence, pharmacometricians are often regarded as scientists living in an ivory tower, and effective application of pharmacometrics, even if practiced in many centres, is not well known.

In the following paragraphs, examples of effective connexions of PK tools at the clinical interface are presented.

Aminoglycosides

Aminoglycosides represent a typical candidate to discuss the feasibility and utility, not to mention the obligation, of using PK/PD modeling for individual dose adjustments based on PK/PD modeling. First, the so-called "targets of concentrations" are defined. Thus, according to findings about aminoglycosides' PK—PD relationships, and despite controversial results of meta-analyses which have been designed to compare efficacy of the "traditional" and "once-daily" regimens, it is consensually recognized that administration should aim to obtain (1) the highest peaks to maximize concentration-dependent killing and post-antibiotic effect, and to prevent adaptive resistances; and (2) the "drug free" periods within the administration interval to avoid drug accumulation linked to the well-known nephrotoxicity and ototoxicity.

Relying on common sense, a TDM strategy might be systematically introduced where, after reaching a presumed steady state, a patient given gentamicin or amikacin should be sampled at the end of an infusion and just before the next one. However, there are major limitations with such an approach: (1) the lack of intervention in the choice of the starting dose; (2) the loss of time waiting for the presumed steady-state; (3) the necessity of respecting strict sampling times to interpret concentrations; and (4) that it will result in nothing more than vague recommendations for a decrease or increase in the dose or in the administration interval. In this context, strategies where aminoglycoside dosing is preceded and immediately followed by individualized pharmacokinetic monitoring are more powerful. They can ensure that both the C_{max}/MIC targets are achieved early in therapy and that the "safe" trough concentrations are kept after several infusions.

However, even though the added value of a PK-based dose adjustment strategy might be obvious, numerous questions remain concerning the organization of such a service.

First, which programs are required to run the models? Numerous PK or PK/PD software applications are available and have been used (see references in the preceding paragraphs), but not all of them have been developed with the aim of being easily used for a routine activity. Among others, MW/PHARM [46] or extensions of the USC*PACK clinical PC programs [23] belong to the category of the ready-to-use tools especially dedicated to clinical use to guide and adjust therapy: they allow estimation of pharmacokinetic parameters on the basis of medication history, can take into account a varying status of the patient with respect, for instance, to body weight and kidney function, optionally using a Bayesian procedure, and include curve-fitting facilities. Using such programs, desired target goals (C_{max}, C_{min}, length of infusion, etc.) can be defined. The option to run such a program off the shelf may be sufficient to start the activity, but, using structural models of the program, it is also possible to enter and store parameter values derived from particular populations. Ideally, a local study should be designed where a few patients are extensively sampled. Based on this database, tests have to be performed to evaluate the performances of the program. If the results are not satisfactory, then mean clearance, volume of distribution and the covariates influencing them have to be calculated and implemented into the program. Such a strategy will satisfy the key question: Will the models of the program adequately describe and forecast the concentrations of my patients?

Aminoglycosides represent the most favorable case to start out with, to build experience in developing PK models and MAP-BEs. Indeed, we are talking about drugs usually described by the simplest models, with CL/F and/or V_c/F variability that can be explained by simple covariates such as body weight or serum creatinine. The following example illustrates the strategy employed at the Limoges University centre to propose dose adjustments of amikacin in elderly patients.

Sixty geriatric-medicine patients (aged 59–95 years) were enrolled in a pharmacokinetic study with the aim of obtaining population pharmacokinetic parameters of amikacin. The population was separated into a building group of 40 patients, the remaining patients being kept for validation. The PK analysis was performed by the NPEM-2 algorithm, using a two-compartment model. In this study, the fitted parameters were renal clearance, expressed as a fraction of creatinine clearance; and volume of the central compartment, expressed as a fraction of body weight. Non-renal clearance of amikacin and transfer constants between the two compartments (k_{12} and k_{21}) being held constant, the distribution of each pharmacokinetic parameter was characterized by the median and the 50% dispersion factor (DF50). The parameters were found to be: CL = 0.91 ± 0.45 and $V_d = 0.29 \pm 0.10$ L $\times$ kg^{-1}. In this population the inter-individual variability was high, and although the median value of CL was close to unity (i.e., indicating that for most patients the elimination of amikacin followed that of creatinine), there was a non-negligible probability of observing much higher values of CL (up to 5). This indicated that for some of these aged patients the elimination of amikacin was less altered than that of creatinine, and consequently that a dose adjustment of this drug could not be systematically performed on the basis of a simple calculation of the creatinine clearance. Concomitantly, the analytical error model of the technique used to measure amikacin blood concentrations had to be defined. From replicates of several representative samples (blank, low, intermediate, high and very high concentrations) analyzed using a fluorescence polarization immunoassay (Abbott, TDx), it was demonstrated that the inter-assay standard deviation (SD) was linearly related to measured concentration (C) with the equation: $SD = 0.3 + 0.028\,C$ (mg/L). This equation was used to compute, for each measured concentration, a weight inversely proportional to the variance (SD^2). In the second step, the population parameters were used as reference population values to estimate the pharmacokinetics of amikacin in a second group of 20 patients by Bayesian estimation, with two blood samples per patient; one at the end of the infusion and another within 8–24 hours after. In this validation group where concentrations ranged from 0.2 to 70.9 mg/L, the bias between observed and estimated concentrations (mean prediction error) was 0.8 mg/L (CI 95%: −0.4, 2.1) and precision (root mean squared error) was 3.5 mg/L. These results illustrated the ability of the MAP-BE to predict the plasma concentrations of amikacin in this specific population and its clinical transferability.

A lack of indubitable clinical-based evidence is often put forward as an argument when not confident in applying any kind of "PK dose adjustment". When focusing on antibiotic therapy, the objective endpoints that have to be explored to evaluate the added value of a "PK dose adjustment" strategy are decreased durations of treatment, shortened lengths of hospitalization, or reduced institutional expenditure. Despite the fact that numerous confounding factors appear in any antibiotic therapy, some interesting results showing higher antibiotic efficacy, shorter hospitalization, and reduced incidence of nephrotoxicity when practicing a so-called PK dose adjustment have been reported [47–50]. For example, a well-designed prospective concentration-controlled study was performed in 232 inpatients from four different hospitals [49]. In this study, a PK dose adjustment at the start of treatment with subsequent Bayesian adaptive control was applied to 105 patients whose outcome was compared to that of 127 "not adjusted" patients followed up as controls. Among other results, the study reported significantly higher peak concentrations in "PK-adjusted patients" (10.6 ± 2.9 mg/L versus 7.6 ± 2.2 mg/L; $P < 0.01$) and significantly lower trough levels ($P < 0.01$). From a clinical point of view, there was a significantly lower mortality for patients with an infection on admission (1/48 patients versus 9/62; $P = 0.023$), a reduced length of hospital stay (12.6 ± 0.8 days versus 18.0 ± 1.4; $P < 0.001$), a lower incidence of nephrotoxicity (2.9% versus 13.4%; $P < 0.01$), and finally a mean reduction of 24.3% of the total costs ($P < 0.01$).

To evaluate the impact on the dose adjustments of aminoglycosides when performed using Bayesian estimators, a local study was performed at the Limoges University Hospital (France). This query was roughly aimed at answering the following questions: When using MAP-BEs, do we propose any change in the dosage when a dose adjustment is requested? Do the clinicians respect our proposals? What are the predictive performances of the employed MAP-BEs? For this, a retrospective study over 1 year of activity was performed in patients given gentamicin and for which multiple dose adjustments were done by the pharmacokinetic unit. A summary of the observed results is presented in Table 5.1. Briefly, in 134 hospitalized patients, when performing a first dose adjustment, an increase in the dose was proposed in about half, although more than two-thirds had been prescribed a dose around the consensually recommended 3 mg/kg. At the next visit, the prescribed doses remained those previously recommended by the PK unit in more than three-quarters of the patients, which illustrated a good adherence by the clinicians. To estimate the predictive performance of the Bayesian estimation, patients with no significant change in their renal function (i.e., creatinine clearance remaining stable) who came for a second dose adjustment and had been prescribed the dose proposed on their first visit were analyzed. Predictive performance

TABLE 5.1   Results of a Retrospective Study Performed in 134 Patients given Gentamicin and for whom Multiple Dose Adjustments were Performed using Bayesian Estimators*

		n	%
DO WE CHANGE THE DOSE?			
MRE between the prescribed dose and that proposed after PK modeling	> 20%	12	9%
	0 ± 20 %	56	42%
	< −20%	66	49%
DO THE CLINICIANS RESPECT THE DOSE PROPOSALS?			
MRE between the prescribed dose and that previously recommended	> 5%	8	6%
	0 ± 5%	103	77%
	< −5%	23	17%
WHAT ARE THE PREDICTIVE PERFORMANCES OF THE BAYESIAN ESTIMATION?			
MRE between the dose proposed on visit $n + 1$ and that proposed on visit n	> 15%	14	10%
	0 ± 15 %	109	79%
	< −15%	15	11%

*Author's own data.
MRE: Mean Relative Error.

of the MAP-BE was considered good if the dose did not need to be changed again, which was the situation in almost 80% of the cases. Looking at the practice in the Limoges Hospital: Bayesian forecasting is usually based on a peak level after the first dose is administered, followed by a second level 6−12 hours later. This service is available 6 days/week, and gives the pharmacologists access to all patient data (by electronic patient files) in addition to measured levels. In this 2000-bed hospital, about 1500 dose adjustments of aminoglycosides are performed per year (giving a written advised dosing strategy in the EPF) by an expert system combining in-house, NPEM and NONMEM programs (https://pharmaco.chu-limoges.fr).

Tacrolimus in Transplantation

Tacrolimus is a calcineurin inhibitor widely used for the long-term prevention of allograft rejection in solid organ transplantation. This drug is available as a "classical" tacrolimus formulation, requiring twice-daily administration (b.i.d.), and a once-daily formulation. Since its commercialization, TDM of tacrolimus has been performed on the basis of trough-level measurement. However, in 2009 a consensus report noted the lack of concentration-controlled trials to study formally the relationship between tacrolimus concentration and clinical outcome, and from which tacrolimus target blood concentrations could be derived, and consequently, that it was impossible to conclude whether one particular TDM strategy is more effective than others [2]. Interestingly, in this consensus report AUC was described as the best marker of drug exposure. As the measurement of the AUC is generally considered to be financially or practically unfeasible, its calculation based on a limited number of blood samples using maximum *a posteriori* Bayesian estimation (MAP-BE) has been proposed. These tools have been helpful to monitor kidney transplant patients given tacrolimus (either the immediate-release formulation, which requires twice-daily administration (b.i.d.) or the once-daily formulation) and to define consensual tacrolimus AUC_{0-12h} targets [26, 51–54]. The following illustrates the strategy that has been employed at the Limoges University centre to develop one of its Bayesian estimators for the dose adjustment of tacrolimus in renal transplant patients.

Thirty-two patients (145 full PK profiles with 10–12 samples in the first 4 hours) given tacrolimus b.i.d. and 41 patients (41 PK profiles collected at $>$ M12 post-transplantation) given tacrolimus once daily and enrolled in two different PK studies were used to develop a PK model and a Bayesian estimator allowing the estimation of AUC using three blood samples. As said, the structure of the database in terms of time of sampling was crucial. There, patients were sampled eight times in the first 4-hour period after drug intake (at pre-dose and 0.33, 0.66, 1, 1.5, 2, 3 and 4 hours post-dose) according to the high interpatient variability in the absorption phase. The distribution of population parameters was studied by a non-linear mixed-effect approach (NONMEM version VI) using the first-order conditional estimation (FOCE) method. A two-compartment open model with an Erlang distribution (which is a particular case of the gamma distribution) to describe the absorption was used [55]. Such a model is obviously more complicated than a classical model with a zero-order rate constant, but was characterized by an excellent goodness-of-fit (the coefficient of determination between individual predicted concentrations and observed concentrations was greater than 0.98). This opportunity to accurately describe each profile in a population is of great interest when the objective is to then apply the model to Bayesian forecasting. Thus, considering that Bayesian estimation uses the distribution of the PK parameters determined in a population and some individual information to estimate the most likely PK parameters in a given subject, this approach requires the development beforehand of an accurate PK model able to calculate unbiased and precise estimates of the individual and population PK parameters. Then, the screening and selection of covariates was performed as part of population pharmacokinetic analysis following a classic stepwise approach [56]. The covariates that finally remained significant in the final model were the hematocrit and CYP3A5 status on CL/F. At this stage, a kind of validation was needed. In this context, the whole population was split into two parts: 49 patients were used as a "building group" and the remaining 24 patients for further validation. First, it was confirmed that (1) the population pharmacokinetic parameters obtained in the new building group were similar to the parameters obtained in the entire database ; and (2) the same significant covariates as previously identified in the whole dataset remained significant in this group. Secondly, the best limited sampling strategy among the combinations of a maximum of three sampling times was selected in the building group based on the D-optimality criterion (Adapt Software) [22]. As previously mentioned, D-optimality has the drawback of producing results that render optimal the estimation of all PK parameters (i.e., a kind of compromise), and so it was decided that the study of optimal sampling design would only focus on CL/F (the inverse of AUC/dose). The optimal limited-sampling schedules were 0, 1.2 and 3 hours post-dose, the closest available sampling times of these optimal times being 0, 1 and 3 hours. In the remaining 24 independent patients, this LSS was characterized by accurate estimation of AUC_{0-12h} (RMSE $= 8.5\%$) and AUC_{0-24h} (RMSE $= 8.2\%$), with only 1 out of the 58 estimated AUC having a bias which was outside the $\pm20\%$ interval. Finally, to illustrate the feasibility of actual clinical transfer after PK developments, this tool has been implemented (with others) on an expert system for immunosuppressants Bayesian dose adjustment to render it accessible to transplantation centres worldwide through a free and secured website (https://pharmaco.chu-limoges.fr). This service has been offering tacrolimus dose adjustment since 2007, by providing: the AUC estimated using MAP-BEs on the basis of three blood samples collected in the first three hours following drug intake; the modelled concentration-time curve; and one or a range of recommended dose(s) to reach the AUC target. By spring 2012, about 30 transplantation centres regularly used this service and had sent more than 3500 requests for adult renal transplant patients given tacrolimus.

CONCLUSION

Whichever drug is concerned, even if the need for an individual dose adjustment is obvious, it is always a hard task to convince clinicians that a model could improve the quality of their drug prescription, prevent their patients from under-dosing or drug intoxication, reduce the number of concentration measurements or shorten the duration of hospitalization.

However, a PK-based dose adjustment service can usually be offered on a consultation basis. From our experience, we think that such an activity can become an active and viable part of patient care with a probable positive impact. When such a service is available 6 days a week, most of the staff become rapidly acquainted with it. When handling a dose adjustment request, one is required to contact the patient care areas to obtain information which significantly increases the visibility to the physicians, resulting in better interdepartmental communication. This also increases the interest and knowledge of younger colleagues in the overall care of the patient, and prevents them focusing only on the theoretical aspects of pharmacology and pharmacokinetics. Such considerations, if not accountable in a financial plan, obviously increase motivation to provide optimal patient care and improve job satisfaction.

References

[1] Oellerich M, Armstrong VW, Schütz E, Shaw LM. Therapeutic drug monitoring of cyclosporine and tacrolimus. Update on Lake Louise Consensus Conference on cyclosporin and tacrolimus. Clin Biochem 1998; 31:309—16.
[2] Wallemacq P, Armstrong VW, Brunet M, et al. Opportunities to optimize tacrolimus therapy in solid organ transplantation: report of the European consensus conference. Ther Drug Monit 2009;31(2):139—52.
[3] Kuypers DR, Le Meur Y, Cantarovich M, et al. Transplantation Society (TTS) Consensus Group on TDM of MPA. Consensus report on therapeutic drug monitoring of mycophenolic acid in solid organ transplantation. Clin J Am Soc Nephrol 2010;5(2):341—58.
[4] Pharmacokinetic software site. Available at http://www.boomer.org/pkin/soft.html (accessed November 2011).
[5] Jelliffe RW, Schumitzky A, Van Guilder M, et al. Individualizing drug dosage regimens: roles of population pharmacokinetic and dynamic models, Bayesian fitting, and adaptive control. Ther Drug Monit 1993;15(5): 380—93.
[6] Gelman A, Carlin JB, Stern HS, et al. Bayesian Data Analysis. 2nd ed. Boca Raton, FL: Chapman & Hall/CRC; 2004.

[7] Gilks WR, Richardson S, Spiegelhalter DJ. Markov Chain Monte Carlo in Practice. London: Chapman & Hall/CRC; 1996.

[8] Migon HS, Gamerman D. Statistical Inference: An Integrated Approach. London: Arnold; 1999.

[9] Best NG, Tan KK, Gilks WR, Spiegelhalter DJ. Estimation of population pharmacokinetics using the Gibbs sampler. J Pharmacokinet Biopharm 1995;23(4):407−35.

[10] Lunn DJ, Best N, Thomas A, et al. Bayesian analysis of population PK/PD models: general concepts and software. J Pharmacokinet Pharmacodyn 2002;29(3):271−307.

[11] Saint-Marcoux F, Debord J, Parant F, et al. Development and evaluation of a simulation procedure to take into account various assays for the Bayesian dose adjustment of tacrolimus. Ther Drug Monit 2011;33(2):171−7.

[12] Analytical Services International website. Available at www.bioanalytics.co.uk (accessed November 2011).

[13] Ette EI, Williams PJ. Pharmacometrics. The Science of Quantitative Pharmacology. John Wiley & Sons; 2006.

[14] Bustad A, Terziivanov D, Leary R, et al. Parametric and nonparametric population methods: their comparative performance in analysing a clinical dataset and two Monte Carlo simulation studies. Clin Pharmacokinet 2006;45(4):365−83.

[15] Ette EI, Williams PJ. Population pharmacokinetics II: estimation methods. Ann Pharmacother 2004 Nov;38(11):1907−15.

[16] Jelliffe RW, Schumitzky A, Bayard D, et al. Model-based, goal-oriented, individualised drug therapy. Linkage of population modeling, new "multiple model" dosage design, Bayesian feedback and individualised target goals. Clin Pharmacokinet 1998 Jan;34(1):57−77.

[17] Steimer JL, Mallet A, Golmard JL, Boisvieux JF. Alternative approaches to estimation of population pharmacokinetic parameters: comparison with the nonlinear mixed-effect model. Drug Metab Rev 1984;15(1−2):265−92.

[18] Leger F, Debord J, Le Meur Y, et al. Maximum *a posteriori* Bayesian estimation of oral cyclosporine pharmacokinetics in patients with stable renal transplants. Clin Pharmacokinet 2002;41(1):71−80.

[19] Doz F, Urien S, Chatelut E, et al. Limited-sampling method for evaluation of the area under the curve of ultrafiltrable carboplatin in children. Cancer Chemother Pharmacol 1998;42(3):250−4.

[20] Overholser BR, Brophy DF, Sowinski KM. Development of an efficient sampling strategy to predict enoxaparin pharmacokinetics in stage 5 chronic kidney disease. Ther Drug Monit 2006;28(6):807−12.

[21] Bullock JM, Smith PF, Booker BM, et al. Development of a pharmacokinetic and Bayesian optimal sampling model for individualization of oral busulfan in hematopoietic stem cell transplantation. Ther Drug Monit 2006;28(1):62−6.

[22] D'Argenio DZ, Schumitzky A, Wang X. ADAPT 5 User's Guide: Pharmacokinetic/Pharmacodynamic Systems Analysis Software. Los Angeles, CA: Biomedical Simulations Resource; 2009.

[23] USC*PACK PC Pharmacokinetic Programs. Available at: http://www.lapk.org (accessed November 2011).

[24] Proost JH, Eleveld DJ. Performance of an iterative two-stage Bayesian technique for population pharmacokinetic analysis of rich data sets. Pharm Res 2006;23(12):2748−59.

[25] Saint-Marcoux F, Royer B, Debord J, et al. Pharmacokinetic modeling and development of Bayesian estimators for therapeutic drug monitoring of mycophenolate mofetil in reduced-intensity haematopoietic stem cell transplantation. Clin Pharmacokinet 2009;48(10):667−75.

[26] Scholten EM, Cremers SC, Schoemaker RC, et al. AUC-guided dosing of tacrolimus prevents progressive systemic overexposure in renal transplant recipients. Kidney Intl 2005;67(6):2440−7.

[27] Prémaud A, Le Meur Y, Debord J, et al. Maximum *a posteriori* Bayesian estimation of mycophenolic acid pharmacokinetics in renal transplant recipients at different postgrafting periods. Ther Drug Monit 2005;27(3):354−61.

[28] Langers P, Cremers SC, den Hartigh J, et al. Easy-to-use, accurate and flexible individualized Bayesian limited sampling method without fixed time points for ciclosporin monitoring after liver transplantation. Aliment Pharmacol Ther 2005;21(5):549−57.

[29] Sheiner LB, Rosenberg B, Melmon KL. Modeling of individual pharmacokinetics for computer-aided drug dosage. Comp Biomed Res 1972;5:441−59.

[30] Sheiner LB, Beal SL. Bayesian individualization of pharmacokinetics: simple implementation and comparison with non-Bayesian methods. J Pharm Sci 1982;71:13344−8.

[31] Delattre IK, Musuamba FT, Nyberg J, et al. Population pharmacokinetic modeling and optimal sampling strategy for Bayesian estimation of amikacin exposure in critically ill septic patients. Ther Drug Monit 2010;32(6):749−56.

[32] Salinger DH, Vicini P, Blough DK, et al. Development of a population pharmacokinetics-based sampling schedule to target daily intravenous busulfan for outpatient clinic administration. J Clin Pharmacol 2010;50(11):1292−300.

[33] Benkali K, Rostaing L, Premaud A, et al. Population pharmacokinetics and Bayesian estimation of tacrolimus exposure in renal transplant recipients on a new once-daily formulation. Clin Pharmacokinet 2010; 49(10):683−92.

[34] Plard C, Bressolle F, Fakhoury M, et al. A limited sampling strategy to estimate individual pharmacokinetic parameters of methotrexate in children with acute lymphoblastic leukemia. Cancer Chemother Pharmacol 2007;60(4):609−20.

[35] Irtan S, Saint-Marcoux F, Rousseau A, et al. Population pharmacokinetics and Bayesian estimator of cyclosporine in pediatric renal transplant patients. Ther Drug Monit 2007;29(1):96−102.

[36] S-Plus™. Seattle, WA: Insightful Corporation; 2002.

[37] Mallet A. A maximum likelihood estimation method for random coefficient regression models. Biometrika 1986;73:645−56.

[38] Jelliffe R, Bayard D, Milman M, et al. Achieving target goals most precisely using nonparametric compartmental models and "multiple model" design of dosage regimens. Ther Drug Monit 2000;22(3):346−53.

[39] Rousseau A, Sabot C, Delepine N, et al. Bayesian estimation of methotrexate pharmacokinetic parameters and area under the curve in children and young adults with localised osteosarcoma. Clin Pharmacokinet 2002;41(13):1095−104.

[40] Bonate PL. A brief introduction to Monte Carlo simulation. Clin Pharmacokinet 2001;40(1):15−22.

[41] Schoemaker NE, Mathôt RA, Schöffski P, et al. Development of an optimal pharmacokinetic sampling schedule for rubitecan administered orally in a daily times five schedule. Cancer Chemother Pharmacol 2002;50:514−7.

[42] D'Argenio DZ. Optimal sampling times for pharmacokinetic experiments. J Pharmacokinet Biopharm 1981;9:739−56.

[43] van der Meer AF, Marcus MAE, Touw DJ, et al. Optimal sampling strategy development methodology using maximum *a posteriori* Bayesian estimation. Ther Drug Monit 2011;33(2):133−46.

[44] Bonate PL. Pharmacokinetic−Pharmcodynamic Modeling and Simulation. New York, NY: Springer Science+Business Media; 2006.

[45] Proost JH. Validation of limited sampling models (LSM) for estimating AUC in therapeutic drug monitoring − is a separate validation group required? Intl J Clin Pharmacol 2007;45(7):402−9.

[46] Proost JH, Meijer DK. MW/Pharm, an integrated software package for drug dosage regimen calculation and therapeutic drug monitoring. Comput Biol Med 1992;22(3):155−63.

[47] Destache CJ, Meyer SK, Rowley KM. Does accepting pharmacokinetic recommendations impact hospitalization? A cost−benefit analysis. Ther Drug Monit 1990;12(5):427−33.

[48] Burton ME, Ash CL, Hill Jr DP, et al. A controlled trial of the cost benefit of computerized Bayesian aminoglycoside administration. Clin Pharmacol Ther 1991;49(6):685−94.

[49] van Lent-Evers NA, Mathôt RA, Geus WP, et al. Impact of goal-oriented and model-based clinical pharmacokinetic dosing of aminoglycosides on clinical outcome: a cost-effectiveness analysis. Ther Drug Monit 1999;21(1):63−73.

[50] Bartal C, Danon A, Schlaeffer F, et al. Pharmacokinetic dosing of aminoglycosides: a controlled trial. Am J Med 2003;114(3):194−8.

[51] Woillard JB, de Winter BC, Kamar N, et al. Population pharmacokinetic model and Bayesian estimator for two tacrolimus formulations − twice daily Prograf and once daily Advagraf. Br J Clin Pharmacol 2011; 71(3):391−402.

[52] Benkali K, Rostaing L, Premaud A, et al. Population pharmacokinetics and Bayesian estimation of tacrolimus exposure in renal transplant recipients on a new once-daily formulation. Clin Pharmacokinet 2010; 49(10):683−92.

[53] Saint-Marcoux F, Debord J, Undre N, et al. Pharmacokinetic modeling and development of Bayesian estimators in kidney transplant patients receiving the tacrolimus once-daily formulation. Ther Drug Monit 2010; 32(2):129−35.

[54] Benkali K, Prémaud A, Picard N, et al. Tacrolimus population pharmacokinetic−pharmacogenetic analysis and Bayesian estimation in renal transplant recipients. Clin Pharmacokinet 2009;48(12):805−16.

[55] Rousseau A, Léger F, Le Meur Y, et al. Population pharmacokinetic modeling of oral cyclosporin using NONMEM: comparison of absorption pharmacokinetic models and design of a Bayesian estimator. Ther Drug Monit 2004;26(1):23−30.

[56] Wählby U, Jonsson EN, Karlsson MO. Comparison of stepwise covariate model building strategies in population pharmacokinetic−pharmacodynamic analysis. AAPS PharmSci 2002;4(4):E27.

CHAPTER

6

An Introduction to Personalized Medicine

Annjanette Stone[1], Joshua Bornhorst[2]

[1]Central Arkansas Veterans Healthcare System (Pathology and Laboratory Medicine, Research Service) Little Rock, AR

[2]Department of Pathology, University of Arkansas for Medical Sciences, School of Medicine, Little Rock, AR

OUTLINE

Therapeutic Drug Monitoring: Newer Drugs and Biomarkers
DOI: 10.1016/B978-0-12-385467-4.00006-3

2012, Published by Elsevier Inc.

INTRODUCTION

The chemical blueprint for DNA was elucidated six decades ago, providing a biochemical mechanism for genetic inheritance observed originally by Mendel in 1866 [1]. These discoveries provided the basis for the "central dogma of molecular biology", which involved transfer of genetic information from DNA to RNA to protein expression (phenotype). It has now been a decade since the Human Genome Project supplied a blueprint of the human genetic material, and scientists are beginning to realize the implications of this enormous amount of information [2, 3]. The knowledge gained from the Human Genome Project serves as the foundation for new therapeutic treatments and diagnostic tests based upon an individual's genetic variation, broadly termed as personalized medicine [4, 5].

Pharmacogenomics is the study of how genetic information (or genotype) encoded by genes can be used to predict pharmacological responses to exogenous compounds. In principle, this information can be used to guide drug selection and dosing. The metabolism of exogenous compounds has been classified into Phase I oxidative reactions and Phase II conjugation reactions (Fig. 6.1) [6]. The term "pharmacogenomics (PGo) testing" is used to denote the study of sources of genetic variation in metabolism, representative of multiple genes and/or a genomic profile, while pharmacogenetic testing is sometimes used to denote testing of response alteration based on an individual gene [7]. However, in practice the terms are often used interchangeably, with both pharmacogenomics and pharmacogenetic testing denoted as PGx. In addition to PGx methodologies that obtain genetic information directly from the DNA, phenotyping or characterization of the metabolic activity of a gene product can be used to classify potential drug response.

Several phenotyping approaches are employed in the practice of medicine, and traditional therapeutic drug monitoring is also a phenotyping approach. For example, determination of pseudocholinesterase enzyme activity for susceptibility testing of extended paralysis after administration of succinylcholine, or the activity of Phase II enzyme thiopurine methyltransferase (TPMT) for the detection of variation in potential toxicity of azathioprine administration represent phenotyping approaches [8–10]. Isoelectric focusing to visualize differences in alpha-1-antitrypsin protein variants in the course of investigation of potential alpha-1-antitrypsin deficiency can also be considered phenotype-based testing [11]. In some cases, phenotypic tests are utilized in concert with more traditional direct genetic testing approaches [12]. In general, phenotyping provides information regarding the "state" of enzyme activity.

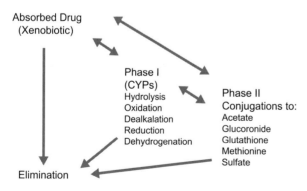

FIGURE 6.1 Metabolic pathways of xenobiotics. Phase I reactions predominately denote oxidizations catalyzed by the P450(CYP) isozymes. Phase II reactions involve conjugation of xenobiotic compounds. Phase I and Phase II reactions generally increase water solubility of compounds and promote excretion.

Although the phenotypic state is strongly influenced by the underlying genetic "traits", factors such as differential expression or induction of enzymes often play a role in pharmacokinetic processes [6].

PGx-related genetic testing uses the information provided by an individual's unique genetic makeup to predict both pharmacokinetic profiles and pharmacodynamic responses. Xenobiotics are typically metabolized by Phase I and Phase II reactions; both processes can be greatly influenced by genetic variation [6]. Thus, PGx testing may be used to guide drug selection and dosing protocols for increased efficacy and minimizing toxicity. Approximately 100 000 fatal adverse drug reactions occur each year in the United States [13]. Several dosing guidelines relying on PGx testing information have been proposed [14, 15]. However, in some cases, dosing alterations based on PGx testing have met with limited clinical success, emphasizing the need for further study to fully realize the potential of personalized medicine [16].

OVERVIEW OF CLASSICAL SEQUENCE VARIATION PROFILING TECHNIQUES

DNA polymorphisms exhibit significant variation between individuals, typically at frequencies of greater than 1%. Human DNA sequence variants include single nucleotide polymorphisms (SNPs) or single nucleotide variants (SNVs), and insertions/deletions (indels). Other polymorphisms include short tandem repeat polymorphisms (STRPs) and variable number of tandem repeats (VNTRs) — highly polymorphic markers used in human linkage mapping, forensics, and paternity testing. If two or more polymorphisms are located near each other (i.e., a few thousand bases apart) they may be studied jointly as a haplotype, since the recombination rate between these two markers is usually low. All SNP genotyping methods share two common steps: sample preparation for investigating a SNP, followed by measurement of the allele-specific product using a variety of physical methods.

Prior to the availability of direct sequencing technologies, a number of advances in methodology for the identification of genetic variation had been developed. Paul Berg's use of restriction enzymes to cut specific DNA sequences, as well as Cohen and Boyer's work with plasmid cloning vectors, provided a foundation for the development of new molecular techniques [17, 18]. Edward Southern described his use of restriction endonucleases to probe the variation in sequence of DNA fragments, a process known as "Southern Blotting" [19]. This technique involved hybridization of probes to DNA sequences separated by size and charge during electrophoresis. Southern Blotting was the basis for one of the first DNA profiling techniques used in molecular biology, Restriction Fragment Length Polymorphism analysis (RFLP), a time-consuming, low-throughput yet inexpensive technology. RFLP is based on PCR (polymerase chain reaction) amplification of DNA using primer pairs and DNA polymerase. The PCR product is then digested using restriction-site enzymes specifically chosen for the base change at the SNP position; the fragments are visualized using gel electrophoresis.

Another DNA profiling technique, known as "DNA fingerprinting", was developed as a variation on the principle of hybridization of labeled DNA probes to immobilized DNA. The fingerprinting method has many diverse applications, and relies on examining probes against regions of genomic DNA which contain variable numbers of tandem repeats (VNTRs) that differ considerably between individuals [20]. These relatively inexpensive techniques were utilized extensively for molecular biology applications to analyze sequence variation, some of which involved PGx applications. For example, RFLPs were used to analyze polymorphisms of drug metabolizing enzymes [21].

A number of other methods have been developed which rely on detecting conformational changes in DNA based on changes in electrophoretic migrations. These methods include denaturing gel electrophoresis, single strand conformation, and heteroduplex analysis. Other methods rely on the ability of enzymes or chemicals to recognize sequence mismatches, such as ribonuclease A cleavage or chemical/enzymatic mismatch cleavage [22]. However, these methods and the probing methods described above are not readily adaptable for high-throughput analysis, which limits their utility in modern applications.

Polymerase chain reaction (PCR), a scientific technique where DNA sequences are exponentially amplified, was developed by Kary Mullis in 1983 [23]. This advancement in molecular biology provided the foundation for modern techniques including the Sanger method for direct sequencing of DNA [24]. Sanger sequencing can be combined with PCR to amplify specific DNA sequences from a labeled probe. The incorporation of different dideoxynucleotides into the PCR reaction resulted in the occasional termination of growing radiolabeled PCR fragments at each base. These terminations could be visualized by electrophoresis and assembled into sequence with high accuracy. Later variations of direct sequencing incorporated fluorescence-based labeling in combination with capillary electrophoresis for automated sequencing [25].

Genotype sequencing technology has advanced rapidly in the past three decades, resulting in reduced costs, enhanced accuracy and genetic coverage, improved simplicity of operation, and increased throughput rates [26, 27]. Automated Sanger method sequencing, as well as major advances in computing technology that enabled the assembly of overlapping sequence fragments into a continuous sequence, spurred the initiation of human genome sequencing projects. Two methodologies were instrumental in sequencing the human genome: direct sequencing of vectors containing large amounts of DNA, or reassembly of overlapping DNA sequences from small fragments of the genome [2, 3]. These efforts produced a human genome sequence comprised of ~3 billion base pairs [28]. This achievement did not produce a complete or accurate map of the human genome. Some regions of the genome (i.e., areas near telomeres) are resistant to sequencing.

RECENT MOLECULAR PROFILING TECHNOLOGIES

A technological revolution in molecular profiling from expensive, single-locus methodologies to more cost-effective, genome-wide analysis formats is in progress [29]. Technologies employed within the past decade include new variations in DNA sequencing, real-time PCR techniques, mass spectrometry-based analysis, and oligonucleotide microarrays. Additionally, advances in molecular profiling technologies within the fields of research known as "-omics" (i.e., genomics, transcriptomics, proteomics, metabolomics and pharmacogenomics) are essential for new approaches to diagnosis, drug development and personalized treatments, as well as the identification of new therapeutic targets. A partial list of highly specialized molecular technologies, and applications specific to each system, is provided in Table 6.1.

TABLE 6.1 Overview of Molecular Technologies

Tools	Throughput	Applications
Real-time quantitation	Moderate	• SNP genotyping and copy number analysis • microRNA analysis • Gene expression analysis • Protein expression analysis
Mass spectrometry	Moderate	• SNP genotyping • DNA methylation • Molecular typing • Somatic mutation profiling • Quantitative gene expression
BeadXpress system with VeraCode technology	Moderate	• Custom low- to mid-plex genotyping • Custom low- to mid-plex methylation analysis • Gene expression analysis • Protein screening • Epigenetic analysis (microRNA) • ADME core panel
Microarray systems	High	• Custom and whole-genome genotyping, and copy number analysis • Cytogenetic analysis • Linkage analysis • Whole-genome methylation analysis • Transcriptome analysis • FFPE sample analyses • Whole-genome gene expression analysis
Next-generation sequencing	High	• DNA sequencing • Gene regulation analysis • Transcriptome analysis • SNP discovery and structural variation analysis • Cytogenetic analysis • DNA–protein interaction analysis (ChIP-Seq) • Sequencing-based methylation analysis • Small RNA discovery and analysis
Third-generation sequencing	High	• Direct detection of haplotypes and whole chromosome phasing • Rare variant detection • Single molecule real-time sequencing • Observe and capture kinetic information • Real-time DNA sequencing using fluorescence resonance energy transfer (FRET)

Real-Time PCR

In real-time PCR, fluorescent reporter molecules are used in conjunction with rapid cycle times to generate information on the quantity and sequence composition of nucleic acid samples [30]. This technique detects product formation as it amplifies and can be readily utilized to genotype specific SNPs based on melting analysis of PCR probes and DNA target sequencing at the end of the PCR cycling process [31, 32]. Although there are many examples of available quantitative real-time PCR genotyping platforms, one is Applied Biosystem's 7900 Sequencing Detection System (i.e., TaqMan®) [33]. The TaqMan assay is based on rapid cycling and hybridization of complementary oligonucleotide probes to a small target DNA sequence containing the SNP of interest, and can monitor the amount of fluorescently-labeled amplified product. Real-time PCR systems such as the TaqMan can process thousands of samples per day and are widely used to investigate multiple SNPs of clinical interest, although they have somewhat limited multiplexing capacity [34, 35].

Next-Generation Sequencing

The traditional Sanger sequencing methodology is now referred to as "first-generation technology". Newer DNA sequencing methods are collectively referred to as next-generation sequencing, and have been comprehensively reviewed [36]. Next-generation analyzers started to become available in 2005 [37]. A number of commercial platforms have been developed, such as the Illumina/Solexa genome analyzer [38]. One novel method of genotyping is by Pyrosequencing™ (www.pyrosequencing.com), or "sequencing by synthesis". This method sequences short single strands of DNA and their complementary strands by enzymatically adding one base pair at a time, and ultimately releasing pyrophosphate which drives a chemiluminescent reaction that is measured by the sequencer. At present, 454 Life Sciences have purchased the pyrosequencing technology license and developed a large-scale genome sequencing platform, known as the GS FLX, capable of genotyping 400 million nucleotides in a single day's run. Next-generation sequencing technologies allow for repeat sequencing of the same template for more accurate sequence generation than conventional Sanger sequencing methods [29].

Some investigators have already begun to term next-generation sequencing as "second generation sequencing", in an attempt to distinguish it from "third-generation sequencing". Third-generation sequencing refers to sequencing methods which sequence single DNA molecules without wash steps [37]. Platforms such as the Helicos genetic analysis platform have achieved single molecule sequencing. Further improvements in read accuracy, read length, genome coverage and cost of sequencing are expected. Using next-generation and third-generation sequencing technologies, the achievement of a personal genome sequence for US$1000 or even US$100 is now plausible, although the quality and timetable are still uncertain [37, 39, 40]. These technologies are certain to exert wide-ranging effects on the study of the molecular pathophysiology of various diseases [41, 42].

Mass Spectroscopy

Matrix-assisted, laser-desorption/ionization, time-of-flight mass spectrometry (i.e., MALDI-TOF) uses a soft ionization technique that is capable of multiplex SNP genotyping. More specifically, an ultraviolet (UV) laser beam triggers the ionization of a biomolecule (often a PCR amplification product) embedded in a matrix. The ionization products can be used to generate spectra with high resolution and, therefore, accurate allele calling. This technique has been used to effectively detect SNPs [43–45]. New applications of related techniques are currently being explored in rapid microbial identification [46]. Some disadvantages of mass spectrometry-based techniques are (1) expense of purchasing and maintaining mass spectrometers, (2) requirement for high purity samples, and (3) technical expertise needed for operation.

Microarrays

Another important conceptual development was the idea of generating DNA arrays [47]. In this model, short DNA oligonucleotides of varying sequence from tissue-specific sources are attached to solid supports [48]. "Microarrays" or "DNA chips" were developed to enable large numbers of DNA sequences or expressed sequence tags (ESTs) to bond covalently to solid surfaces at known locations. The FDA-approved Roche Amplichip™ CYP450, for example, can genotype 27 polymorphisms in CYP2D6 [49]. These personalized data can be used to alter drug therapy [50].

Increasing numbers of specific microarrays are available, many of them targeted toward specific disease states; however, there are barriers to widespread adoption in clinical practice [49, 51]. Two top competitors in the field of array-based technologies are the companies Illumina, Inc. and Affymetrix, Inc. Affymetrix arrays are tiling arrays, where DNA is hybridized to probes attached to solid surfaces. Affymetrix arrays include traditional gene expression chips, methylation chips, array-based comparative genomic hybridization chips, copy number variation and genotyping arrays (www.affymetrix.com). Illumina's Omni family of arrays, next-generation genotyping arrays, is designed to capture human variations down to 1% minor allele frequency (MAF; see www.illumina.com). By the end of 2011, Illumina's Infinium genotyping array will be able to investigate more than 5 million polymorphisms per DNA specimen. Illumina's Infinium chemistry involves an enzymatic labeling step using single-base extension, followed by DNA hybridization to the oligo array. After washing and fluorescent staining, the beadchip is scanned with a confocal laser reader for final genotype identification. See Chapter 7 for more in-depth discussion on this subject.

Genomics

Genomics is the study of nucleotide sequences (including structural genes, regulatory sequences and non-coding segments) in the chromosomes of individuals, and incorporates a wide range of scientific subdisciplines such as toxicogenomics, bioinformatics, and network and systems biology [52]. This section will include an overview of "omics" technologies used to discover novel pharmacogenetic effects, and discuss molecular profiling systems used to advance pharmacogenomics research and diagnostics. Two of these technologies, microarray-based genomics and next-generation sequencing, are rapidly changing the landscape of PGx testing.

Identification of genes associated with disease or responsiveness to drug therapy can be accomplished by candidate gene, whole-genome linkage or whole-genome association (WGA) studies. In whole-genome linkage studies, large family-based sets of DNAs are tested for meiotic linkage to disease using a panel of polymorphisms spread over comparatively large chromosomal regions [53]. Then, a candidate gene study is conducted on the region of interest found in the whole-genome linkage study using microarray or other molecular approaches. In contrast, genome-wide association studies (GWAS) use dense microarray panels with more than 1 million polymorphisms and copy number variant markers run on unrelated individuals from case—control studies of complex diseases. GWAS can detect small effects for trait loci but only over small distances, whereas linkage studies have limited capacity to detect small effects from rare variants. A summary table of selected genome-wide association studies in pharmacogenomics conducted since 1998 is presented (Table 6.2); only those attempting to assay at

TABLE 6.2   Selected Whole-Genome Association Studies in Pharmacogenomics

Journal	Pharmacological response	Platform [# of SNPs passing QC]
J. Natl Cancer Inst. (2011) **103**(10), 817—825	Response to platinum-based chemotherapy in non-small-cell lung cancer	Illumina [307 260]
N. Engl. J. Med. (2011) **364**(12), 1134—1143	Adverse response to carbamazepine	Illumina [~1.2 million] (imputed)
Pharmacogenet. Genomics (2011) **21**(5), 280—288	Response to cerivastatin	Illumina [292 461]
Nat. Genet. (2011) **43**(2), 117—120	Response to metformin	Affymetrix [705 125]
Toxicol. Sci. (2011) **120**(1), 33—41.	Response to acetaminophen (hepatotoxicity)	Affymetrix & Illumina [1 348 864]
Hum. Mol. Genet. (2010) **19**(23), 4735—4744; Epub 10 Sep 2010	Warfarin maintenance dose	Illumina [485 227]
Am. J. Psychiatry (2010) **167**(5), 555—564	Response to antidepressants	Illumina [539 391]
Pharmacogenet. Genomics (2009) **19**(9), 666—674	Response to antidepressant treatment	Illumina [100 864]
PLoS One (2010) **5**(3), e9763	Response to statin therapy	Illumina [~2.5 million](imputed)
J. Am. Med. Assoc. (2009) **302**(8), 849—857	Response to clopidogrel therapy	Affymetrix [400 230]
Am. J. Psychiatry (2009) **166**(6), 718—725	Response to lithium treatment in bipolar disorder	Affymetrix [~1.4 million] (imputed)
Circ. Cardiovasc. Genet. (2009) **2**(2), 173—181; Epub 12 Feb 2009	Response to statin therapy	Perlegen [291 998]
PLoS Genet. (2009) **5**(3), e1000433; Epub 20 Mar 2009	Warfarin maintenance dose	Illumina [325 997]
N. Engl. J. Med. (2008) **359**(8), 789—799	Response to statin therapy	Illumina [316 184]
Blood (2008) **112**(4), 1022—1027	Warfarin maintenance dose	Illumina [538 629]

Data extracted from the NHGRI Office of Population Genomics Catalog (www.genome.gov/gwastudies, May 2011). Only selected whole-genome association studies conducted on at least 100 000 polymorphisms in the initial stage are listed. The number of SNPs passing quality control metrics if multiple platforms are used without imputation, or the total number of imputed SNPs in each study, is shown in brackets.

least 100 000 single nucleotide polymorphisms are included (data extracted from the NHGRI Office of Population Genomics Catalog: www.genome.gov/gwastudies).

One current effort that has evolved from the Human Genome Project and the availability of more advance sequencing platforms is the international research consortium known as the 1000 Genomes Project, sponsored by the National Human Genome Research Institute (NHGRI), the Wellcome Trust and the Beijing Genome Institute (www.1000genomes.org) [54]. The 1000 Genomes Project is producing a catalog of genetic variation of the human population by using next-generation sequencing technologies (i.e., Illumina's Solexa platforms and Applied Biosystems' SOLiD™) to sequence 1000 genomes from various ethnic groups. Data from the 1000 Genomes Project is publicly accessible to the worldwide research community on a web-based Ensemble browser (www.1000genomes.org). The success of large-scale sequencing projects like the 1000 Genomes Project is due to "next-generation" or "massively parallel" sequencing platforms capable of processing millions of sequencing reads in parallel, both rapidly and inexpensively [55, 56]. These data will be used to characterize functional variants with complex traits, and will deepen our understanding of how genetic information relates to an individual's susceptibility to treatment for disease and response to treatment for disease [57, 58].

Another major genomics initiative sponsored by the NHGRI in collaboration with the National Cancer Institute is The Cancer Genome Atlas (TCGA) [59]. TCGA is scanning large groups of ovarian, lung and glioblastoma multiform biospecimens for DNA methylation and copy number variations, as well as gene mutations associated with oncogenesis. Techniques used by TCGA program include SNP genotyping, whole-genome gene expression profiling, genome-wide methylation, exon sequencing, microRNA and copy number variation profiling.

Copy number variants (CNV) are large DNA sequences (> 1000 nucleotides in length) that are duplicated, deleted, inserted or inverted a variable number of times as copies of a genome relative to a reference genome. CNVs have been associated with drug efficacy, toxicity, and disease prevalence, and may be used as diagnostic tools in the clinical setting [60, 61]. For example, CYP2D6, a highly polymorphic drug-metabolizing gene expressed in the human liver, metabolizes over 25% of drugs used clinically today [62]. CYP2D6 is an isoenzyme in the cytochrome P450 mixed function oxides family of enzymes responsible for metabolism of a majority of drugs and endogenous hormones. Some CNVs of CYP2D6 result in nonfunctional or reduced activity CYP2D6 alleles which alter the activity of the CYP2D6 enzyme. Individuals with impaired metabolism of CYP2D6 substrates are known as poor metabolizers (PMs). Individuals who inherit more than two copies of CYP2D6 normal alleles are known as ultrarapid metabolizers (UMs) because these individuals are capable of rapidly metabolizing drugs that are substrates for CYP2D6, compared to normal subjects [63]. Efficacy of several drug classes, including antidepressants, estrogen receptor modulators and β-adrenergic antagonists are affected by CYP2D6 activities. In addition, duplications of the functional CYP2D6 gene have been associated with drug toxicity from central nervous system sedatives like codeine because codeine is more rapidly metabolized to morphine, which is mostly responsible for the analgesic effect of codeine [61, 64–67].

Conventional methods for detection of copy number variants include long-distance and multiplex PCR followed by gel electrophoresis or TaqMan® real-time quantification. New methodologies for CNV detection are based on microarray hybridization technology. For example, de Smith *et al.* used a two-stage array comparative genomic hybridization (aCGH) method to identify 1284 new CNV polymorphisms in a Caucasian population [68]. This genome-wide screening technique uses high resolution arrays with oligonucleotides spaced on average 500 bp apart, spanning 2475 regions of the genome. Resolution is better than chromosome-based CGH [69], and CNVs of 5–10 kb of DNA sequence can be detected. Another array-based hybridization method known as the Roche AmpliChip CYP450 system is the first FDA approved pharmacogenetics test for clinical use. It detects gene variations, including deletions and duplications of the CYP2D6 and CYP2C19 genes. Illumina, Inc. offers genome-wide association high-density SNP microarrays with millions of probes for detection of copy number variants and loss of heterozygosity in addition to SNPs. One advantage of some SNP microarrays is the ability to detect copy neutral loss of heterozygosity (CN-LOH). CN-LOH, also known as uniparental disomy (UPD), cannot be detected by traditional clinical techniques such as karyotyping, fluorescence *in-situ* hybridization (FISH), or aCGH [70]. An increasing number of commercial tools are available. Both Affymetrix, Inc. and Illumina, Inc. offer unique tools for pharmacogenomics research that feature "core" markers, including copy number variants, in essential drug metabolizing genes selected by the PharmADME working group. CNVs belonging to CYP2D6, CYP2A6, UGT2B17 (genes that encode the uridine diphosphate glucuronosyltransferase enzyme, UDP-glucuronosyltransferase), GSTM1 and GSTT1 (genes that encode glutathione S-transferase enzyme) are covered by these panels [68, 71]. The Illumina ADME panel uses digitally inscribed microbeads in a microplate format, and allele-specific fluorescence detection is achieved by Illumina's BeadXpress™ reader [72]. The Affymetrix DMET™ Plus panel also includes polymorphisms in drug transporters, in addition to genes encoding Phase I and Phase II enzymes [71].

Transcriptomics

Next-generation sequencing and microarray systems can analyze entire "transcriptomes" from large numbers of tissues simultaneously, and find the causal genetic variants that influence gene expression [73]. Genome-wide expression profiling, using high-quality RNA extracted from human tissue, is providing new functional information about complex traits and diseases [74]. Recently, the field of transcriptomics has been transformed by RNA sequencing of alternate splice variants [75], novel transcripts from gene fusion events, and new classes of non-coding RNAs (ncRNAs) using next-generation sequencing [73, 76, 77].

Metabolomics

Current advances in metabolomics, the study of small-molecule metabolite profiles which are the end products of cellular processes, offer unique opportunities to discover new biomarkers [78]. New approaches in bioinformatics approaches and the development of computational tools to integrate the data obtained from metabolomics and other "omics" can discover potential biomarkers. For example, FDA's National Center for Toxicological Research (Jefferson, AR) Center for Excellence on Metabolomics and Division of Systems Toxicology uses mass spectrometry, nuclear magnetic resonance (NMR) and a software tool known as Scaled-to-Maximum, Aligned, and Reduced Trajectories (SMART) analysis to analyze endogenous materials found in biological fluids (www.fda.gov/nctr) [79].

Proteomics

Proteomics is the large-scale study of proteins, their structures and their functions. High-throughput proteomic approaches, including protein microarray platforms, isotope-coded affinity tags and next-generation sequencing, are emerging as powerful tools for the analysis of proteins. Next-generation sequencing identifies and quantifies proteins on a genome-wide scale by parallel processing of clonally amplified molecules; massive numbers of analytes as well as samples are processed simultaneously [80, 81]. Other platforms for proteomics include matrix-assisted laser desorption/ionization time-of-flight, and liquid chromatography-tandem mass spectrometry. These technologies have fast scanning capabilities, in addition to high resolution and mass accuracy, and have been used "to profile small protein molecules, biomarkers, and whole organism proteomes" [82]. One practical application of proteomics is the identification of potential disease biomarkers (novel fusion proteins or alternate splice isoforms). The high-throughput platforms mentioned previously can help mine the proteome in a rapid, comprehensive manner.

Epigenetics

Epigenetics is the study of epigenetic changes (DNA methylation, post-translational histone modifications, and regulation) on a genome scale, contributing to the fundamental biological knowledge of development, differentiation and disease. Epigenetic changes are inherited patterns of DNA and RNA activity unrelated to the naked nucleotide sequence; they change the phenotype of a cell or organism without affecting the genotype. Aberrant epigenetic mechanisms are implicated in the development of many diseases, including cancer, type II diabetes, autoimmune disease, and cardiovascular and neuropsychiatric disorders [83–86].

Next-generation sequencing platforms used to study DNA methylation and histone modifications include the Solexa (Illumina), SOLiD (Applied Biosystems) and 454 (Roche) platforms [87]. These platforms depend upon massive parallel sequencing of the entire genome following bisulfite pre-treatment of DNA specimens – a technique used to distinguish methylated CpG (Cytosine-phosphate-Guanine) sites from unmethylated ones. Another whole-genome DNA methylation profiling technology is Illumina's HumanMethylation 450 BeadChip™ array, which contains probes for more than 480 000 CpGs. An accompanying methylation analysis software module allows the integration of gene expression and methylation data for a side-by-side comparison of gene transcript levels and methylation profiles from the same samples. Another exciting development in high-throughput methylation technology is a single-molecule, real-time (SMRT) DNA sequencing system (Pacific Biosciences) that directly detects DNA methylation without bisulfite conversion or other treatments [88].

Histone modifications, including acetylation, phosphorylation, methylation and ubiquitination, affect the gene-regulatory function of proteins. Chromatin immunoprecipitation sequencing (ChIP-seq) is a next-generation sequencing technology for the investigation of genome-wide DNA–protein interactions [77, 89]. More than 800 microRNAs (miRNAs) have been discovered in humans, and they control cellular proliferation, differentiation and apoptosis [90]. MicroRNAs, a class of non-coding RNAs transcribed by RNA polymerase II, regulate epigenetic modification by directly targeting histone deacetylases and DNA methyltransferases [91]. The development of microarray and sequencing technologies for whole-genome miRNA profiling has advanced the fields of cancer genomics and diagnostics, as well as discovery of novel microRNA biomarkers [92, 93]. Dr. Carlo M. Croce and colleagues have performed whole-genome miRNA expression analysis on more than 10 000 human cancer specimens [94]. Applied Biosystems has developed the TaqMan Array Human MicroRNA Panel, a tool for microRNA discovery [95]. In 2008, Asuragen introduced the first validated microRNA diagnostic assay for differentiation of chronic pancreatitis from pancreatic cancer [96], and Rosetta Genomics introduced the first microRNA diagnostic test for squamous-cell lung cancer [97].

To summarize, the pace of pharmacogenomics research is changing due to the rapid development of high-throughput genomic technology, including microarray-based tools, next-generation sequencing and mass spectrometry. New data management tools will be needed to handle the extraordinary amount of genomic information generated; this includes storage and retrieval databases, bioinformatics algorithms for analysis, and electronic medical records.

SELECT BIOMARKERS IN PHARMACOGENOMICS

Biomarkers in pharmacogenomics are already playing an important role in guiding pharmacotherapy of certain drugs. In this section, brief information regarding the application of pharmacogenomics techniques in selected drugs is presented.

Warfarin

Individual genetic variations contribute to the efficacy and toxicity of warfarin, the most widely prescribed oral anticoagulant in North America and Europe [98]. Warfarin is used to reduce the risk of stroke, thrombosis, pulmonary embolism and coronary failure. Pharmacogenetic studies have identified warfarin candidate genes belonging to the drug-metabolizing and vitamin K pathways, vitamin K-dependent clotting factors, and other minor pathways. Genetic variants in cytochrome p450 2C9 (CYP2C9) and vitamin K epoxide reductase complex 1 (VKORC1) genes contribute to 40% of warfarin dosing variance in Caucasians [99, 100], while non-genetic factors account for another 15% [101]. A retrospective genome-wide association study (GWAS) used the Illumina HumanHap 550K v3 Beadchip (> 550 000 markers) to search for common genetic variation in genes correlated with warfarin dosing [99]. A number of GWASs have been utilized to search for common genetic variation in genes correlated with warfarin dosing, and these studies further indicate that CYP2C9 and VKORC1 polymorphisms are the main genetic determinants of a stabilized warfarin dose [98, 99]. The inclusion of genotype information into warfarin dosing algorithms can improve effective warfarin dose predictability and reduce hospitalization rates [102–104]. In 2007 the FDA updated the warfarin label to encourage the use of pharmacogenomics data in guiding dosing, and further revision in 2010 provided genotype specific dose ranges [105, 106]. See Chapter 8 for more in-depth discussion on this subject.

Statins

Statins, one of the most prescribed drugs in the world, lower total and plasma LDL-C (low density lipoprotein-cholesterol) by inhibition of the rate control enzyme of the cholesterol biosynthetic pathway [107]. Statins are well tolerated, but adverse effects associated with dose include liver and muscle toxicity. The Study of the Effectiveness of Additional Reductions in Cholesterol and Homocysteine (SEARCH) conducted a genome-wide association study on a subset of cardiovascular patients in whom myopathy developed while taking simvastatin daily [108]. A non-coding SNP located within intron 11 of *SLCO1B1* (rs4363657) was strongly associated with myopathy. A candidate gene approach and haplotype analysis identified additional SNPs within *SLCO1B1* linked to statin metabolism. A larger cohort from the Treating to New Targets (TNT) study comprising 1984 individuals with cardiovascular disease was genotyped for ~300 000 SNPs [109]. Associations were found in apoE and PCSK9 SNPs for response of LDL-C. Additional SNPs, one located within the CLMN gene (rs8014194) and one located in APOC1 near APOE (rs4420638), also demonstrated associations with statin-mediated lipid response [110].

Clopidogrel

Clopidogrel, a prodrug used to decrease the morbidity and mortality of some cardiovascular diseases, is extensively metabolized by CYP1A2, CYP2B6, CYP2C9, CYP2C19 and CYP3A4/5 in the liver to the active thiol metabolite which inhibits ADP (adenosine diphosphate)-stimulated platelet activation [106, 111]. Several drugs such as atorvastatin, omeprazole, etc. interact with clopidogrel and decrease the concentration of the active metabolite [112]. It is known that polymorphisms in the CYP2C19 and ABCB1 genes (which determine the activity of P-glycoprotein, also known as multiple drug resistance protein) affect the responsiveness of clopidogrel [113]. The common CYP2C19*2 variant of the gene encoding the enzyme produces an enzyme with very little activity. Therefore, as expected individuals with CYP2C19*2 allele suffered from associated decreased antiplatelet effect after therapy with clopidogrel and an increased likelihood of a cardiovascular event [106]. A meta-analysis of nine genotyping studies on clopidogrel involving patients with acute coronary syndrome found associations between CYP2C19 polymorphisms and increased risk of death from cardiovascular diseases. In response, the FDA added a boxed warning regarding CYP219 in 2010; also, the American College of Cardiology endorsed CYP219 genotyping for some patients treated with clopidogrel [114].

Irinotecan

Specific drugs have significant potential for unexpected toxicity due to genetic variation. One example is irinotecan, an anticancer drug approved by the Food and Drug Administration (FDA) for treatment of colorectal cancer. The FDA recommends but does not require pharmacogenetic testing before irinotecan is prescribed [115]. Toxic effects associated with irinotecan include diarrhea and myelosuppression; adverse side effects are increased in patients with seven TA dinucleotide repeats rather than the common six repeats found in the promoter of UGT1A1 (the gene that determines activity of UDP-glucuronosyltransferase,

UGT, responsible for metabolism of irinotecan). The $(TA)_7$ repeat (or UGT1A1*28) is associated with low UGT enzymatic activity [116], Gilbert and Crigler-Najjar syndromes [117] and neutropenia in patients treated with irinotecan [118]. The current FDA-approved UGT1A1 assay for clinical applications (Invader™ molecular assay) tests the *28 polymorphism and does not include other UGT1A1 polymorphisms that affect enzymatic activity. Additional genes are also involved in the irinotecan pathway, so a more comprehensive genome-wide approach for irinotecan metabolism may be required to optimize therapeutic dosage. Life Technologies' Personal Genome Machine™ (PGM), a third-generation sequencer, may provide a solution that is cost- and time-effective. The PGM uses ion torrent sequencing technology, a massively parallel array of semiconductor sensors for direct real-time measurement with ion semiconductor chips [119]. See Chapter 14 for more in-depth discussion on pharmacogenomics of anticancer agents.

TRANSLATIONAL APPROACHES ASSOCIATED WITH PHARMACOGENOMICS AND PERSONALIZED MEDICINE

A number of new initiatives have emerged to expand the use of new technologies. The following examples, along with many other existing and emerging genomic medicine initiatives, will allow for further advances in personalized medicine.

Health Information Technology in Pharmacogenetics

The American Recovery and Reinvestment Act of 2009 (Stimulus or Recovery Act) came into law in February 2009 as an economic stimulus package intended to promote consumer spending and create jobs; it included US$23 billion in appropriations for improvements in health information technology (HIT) and its infrastructure over a 5-year period [120]. More than US$19 billion in incentives is offered to physicians who invest in electronic medical records (EMRs) in 2011 and 2012; however, they face cuts in their Medicare fee schedule if they do not implement EMRs by 2015 [121]. The Patient Protection and Affordable Care Act of 2010 provides additional incentives for physicians who implement EMRs by 2015.

Electronic Medical Records and BioBanks

Electronic medical records (EMRs) allow storage, retrieval and modification of medical records using digital media instead of paper-based records systems. EMRs include databases of patient demographic data, clinical laboratory results, radiology images and pharmaceutical records, as well as patient diagnosis, treatment, disease progression and survival data. The potential of personalized medicine will be realized when genomic data, environmental exposures and family medical history are added to these databases. Since genome-wide approaches using high-throughput technology are replacing conventional methodologies in "omics", entire genomic sequences will soon be linked via EMRs to clinical and demographic data [40, 122]. To reach this objective, several health organizations have constructed large data and specimen bio-repositories [123, 124]. The PopGen Biobank (University Hospital of Kiel, Germany) is one example of a successful European bio-repository involving more than 100 scientific and 50 medical partners [125]. This biobank holds specimens from 45 000 participants in an effort to investigate genetic risk factors associated with complex diseases, and, like other biobanks, could potentially be used for pharmacogenetic research [123].

The United States Veterans Administration (VA) Healthcare System has a nationally-connected EMR system accessed through the Veterans Health Information Systems and Technology Architecture (VistA) by VA-authorized employees [126]. In 2006, the US Department of Veterans Affairs launched a Genomic Medicine program to examine the potential of emerging genomic technologies, optimize medical care for veterans, and enhance the development of tests and treatments for relevant diseases.

Natural Language Processing Algorithms

Natural Language Processing (NLP) algorithms are used to find unstructured clinical data embedded in free-text notes. NLP algorithms have been used successfully in pharmacogenetic studies to extract medication history from clinical narratives [127]. The NIH-funded i2b2 initiative (Informatics for Integrating Biology and the Bedside) uses NLP software to extract clinical data from existing datasets, which are then combined with genomic data for the purpose of designing personalized medicine for patients with genetic diseases [128]. NLP-based extraction of pharmacogenomics data from biobanks linked to EMRs is an ongoing effort within the National Institutes of Health-funded Pharmacogenomics Research Network (PGRN) to quantify breast cancer treatments in patients exposed to tamoxifen (http://www.PharmGKB.org) [129]. PGRN is a nationwide research consortium with a central repository — the PharmGKB database of genetic, genomic, molecular and cellular phenotype data, as well as clinical data from participants of pharmacogenomics research studies. A similar study using EMRs to investigate adverse drug response to tamoxifen is under way at the NIH-funded eMERGE network of biobanks (https://www.mc.vanderbilt.edu/victr/dcc/projects/acc/index.php/Main_Page).

Implementation of PGx Testing

Although it has been clearly demonstrated that PGx testing provides clinically relevant data for many gene–drug combinations, there are several challenges for implementation of PGx testing in routine clinical practice. Such challenges include ethical issues, costs of pharmacogenomics testing, proper utilization of test results by clinicians, and regulatory concerns. Due at least in part to these concerns, the implementation of PGx testing has in some cases lagged behind evidence indicating that testing should be adopted [130, 131]. In some cases, the lack of PGx testing on a well-characterized CYP2D6 has resulted in a fatality that could potentially be avoided [132]. However, in other cases the evidence for testing may be less clear, and further efforts need to be made to clarify the benefits of testing versus questions regarding efficacy and cost [130, 133]. In some areas, such as antidepressant drug dosing, there is enormous potential benefit for implementation of pharmacogenomics [133].

Some of the major ethical issues in pursuing PGx-related clinical studies, and clinical testing, are safeguarding patient consent and confidentiality. Although consent is sought from research participants who contribute specimens for specific genetic studies or permanent banks of genetic specimens and/or related medical information, the question often remains as to whether the consent is sufficient to allow for these specimens and data to be used in any future studies that are currently technically infeasible or unanticipated [131]. Furthermore, there is debate as to whether there is an obligation to disclose the results of research studies to participants even though in some cases the results of such studies may not be completely understood [134]. Electronic medical records, which are becoming progressively more available, could be used to help readily integrate genetic information from PGx testing into clinical practice, yet increase the risk and ease of inappropriate sharing and release of PGx testing results [135, 136].

The increase in availability of PGx testing and resulting information could have several potential deleterious consequences for patients, and federal legislation in the United States has been passed in an attempt to address some of these concerns. The Genetic Information and Non-discrimination Act (GINA) of 2008 has several important provisions. Broadly, these include prohibiting genetic information from being used in setting health insurance premiums or being used by employers for employment or job assignment decisions. Furthermore, this law prohibits insurers or employers from requiring genetic testing to be performed. However, it does not prohibit the use of genetic testing for determination of eligibility for cost of life, disability, or long-term care insurance. Additionally, many members of the military are exempt from some of the genetic information safeguards present in GINA [131, 137].

Regulation of PGx testing is also evolving rapidly. The Clinical Laboratory Improvement Act of 1988 (CLIA) regulates which laboratories can offer PGx testing. Currently, there is little external validation of the clinical efficacy of laboratory-developed testing outside of the FDA purview. Recently, the FDA has signaled its intention to perform further assessment of laboratory developed tests [131]. The increasing availability of direct-to-consumer PGx testing in the absence of healthcare provider involvement has also raised concerns [138, 139]. Another hotly debated issue is the validity and applicability of patents of genetic information. Currently, as much as 20% of the human genome is patented in the United States. The outcome of this debate may have a lasting effect on PGx testing practices [131, 140, 141].

CONCLUSIONS

Personalizing drug therapy for maximizing the efficacy of a drug and minimizing the risk is the goal of pharmacogenomics. The major goal of personalized medicine is to take the practice of medicine into a new level of highly improved patient safety and effectiveness of a drug therapy. At this time, at least 77 drug labels contain PGx information for improving pharmacotherapy using these agents, but in many cases fail to fully elucidate testing or dosing guidance for physicians [131]. Table 6.3 lists some of these drugs where pharmacogenomics testing could be useful. Despite calls for additional training in pharmacogenomics, physicians' knowledge in this area has been reported to be "suboptimal" [130, 142, 143]. Finally, reimbursement for PGx testing has not been standardized and is inconsistent. There is little to suggest that current reimbursement of PGx testing is reflective of cost-effectiveness analysis of that testing [144–146]. Efforts are underway to provide evidence-based guidelines for the evaluation of the benefit and proper use of PGx testing. It is hoped that these efforts will stimulate wider use of beneficial PGx testing [130].

TABLE 6.3 Selected FDA Labeling Events Involving PGx

Drug*	Enzyme	Goal	Year
6-Marcaptourea	TPMT	Safety	2003
Azathioprine	TRMT	Safety	2003
Atomoxetine	CYP2D6	Safety	2003
Irinotecan	UGT1A1	Safety	2004
Warfarin	CYP2C9, VKORC1	Safety/efficacy	2007
Abacavir	HLA-B85701	Safety	2007
Carbamazepine	HLA-B*1502	Safety	2007
Phenytoin/Fosphenytoin	HLA-B*1502	Safety	2008
Clopidogrel	CYP2C19	Efficacy	2010

*Selected drug labels introduced by the FDA containing PGx-related genetic information. See also Drugs@FDA at www.accessdata.fda.gov/cder/drugsatfda.
TPMT, thiopurine methyltransferase; VKORC1, vitamin K epoxide reductase complex 1.
Table adapted from a presentation of Professor Steven H.Y. Wong of Wake Forrest University, with author's permission.

References

[1] Watson JD, Crick FH. Molecular structure of nucleic acids; a structure for deoxyribose nucleic acid. Nature 1953;171:737–8.
[2] Lander ES, Linton LM, Birren B, et al. Initial sequencing and analysis of the human genome. Nature 2001;409(6822):860–921.
[3] Venter JC, Adams MD, Myers EW, et al. The sequence of the human genome. Science 2001;291(5507):1304–51.
[4] Lander ES, Weinberg RA. Genomics: journey to the center of biology. Science 2000;287(5459):1777–82.
[5] McLeod HL, Evans WE. Pharmacogenomics: unlocking the human genome for better drug therapy. Annu Rev Pharmacol Toxicol. 2001;41:101–21.
[6] McMillin GA, Linder MW, Bukaveckas BL. Pharmacogenetics. In: Burtis CA, Ashwood ER, Bruns DE, editors. Tietz Textbook of Clinical Chemistry and Molecular Diagnostics. St Louis, MO: Elsevier; 2006. p. 1393–406.
[7] Linder MW, Valdes RJ. Fundamentals of pharmacogenetics. In: Wong S, Linder MW, Valdes RJ, editors. Pharmacogenomics and Pharmacogenetics. Washington, DC: AACC Press; 2006.
[8] McQueen MJ. Clinical and analytical considerations in the utilization of cholinesterase measurements. Clin Chim Acta 1995;237(1–2):91–105.
[9] Eichelbaum M, Ingelman-Sundberg M, Evans WE. Pharmacogenomics and individualized drug therapy. Annu Rev Med 2006;57:119–37.
[10] Evans WE. Pharmacogenetics of thiopurine S-methyltransferase and thiopurine therapy. Ther Drug Monit 2004;26(2):186–91.
[11] Crystal RG. Alpha 1-antitrypsin deficiency, emphysema, and liver disease. Genetic basis and strategies for therapy. J Clin Invest 1990;85(5):1343–52.
[12] Snyder MR, Katzmann JA, Butz ML, et al. Diagnosis of alpha-1-antitrypsin deficiency: an algorithm of quantification, genotyping, and phenotyping. Clin Chem 2006;52(12):2236–42.
[13] Lazarou J, Pomeranz BH, Corey PN. Incidence of adverse drug reactions in hospitalized patients: a meta-analysis of prospective studies. J Am Med Assoc 1998;279(15):1200–5.
[14] Klein TE, Altman RB, Eriksson N, et al. Estimation of the warfarin dose with clinical and pharmacogenetic data. N Engl J Med 2009;360(8):753–64.
[15] Johnson JA, Gong L, Whirl-Carrillo M, et al. Clinical Pharmacogenetics Implementation Consortium Guidelines for CYP2C9 and VKORC1 Genotypes and Warfarin Dosing. Clin Pharmacol Ther 2011;90(4):625–9.

[16] Grossman I, Sullivan PF, Walley N, et al. Genetic determinants of variable metabolism have little impact on the clinical use of leading antipsychotics in the CATIE study. Genet Med 2008;10(10):720—9.

[17] Jackson DA, Symons RH, Berg P. Biochemical method for inserting new genetic information into DNA of Simian Virus 40: circular SV40 DNA molecules containing lambda phage genes and the galactose operon of *Escherichia coli*. Proc Natl Acad Sci USA 1972;69(10):2904—9.

[18] Cohen SN, Chang AC, Boyer HW, et al. Construction of biologically functional bacterial plasmids *in vitro*. Proc Natl Acad Sci USA 1973;70:3240—4.

[19] Southern EM. Detection of specific sequences among DNA fragments separated by gel electrophoresis. J Mol Biol 1975;98(3):503—17.

[20] Jeffreys AJ, Turner M, Debenham P. The efficiency of multilocus DNA fingerprint probes for individualization and establishment of family relationships, determined from extensive casework. Am J Hum Genet 1991;48(5):824—40.

[21] Gaikovitch EA, Cascorbi I, Mrozikiewicz PM, et al. Polymorphisms of drug-metabolizing enzymes CYP2C9, CYP2C19, CYP2D6, CYP1A1, NAT2 and of P-glycoprotein in a Russian population. Eur J Clin Pharmacol 2003;59(4):303—12.

[22] Weber WW. Techniques for analyzing pharmacogenetic variation. In: Wong S, Linder MW, Valdes RJ, editors. Pharmacogenomics and Proteomics. Enabling the Practice of Personalized Medicine. Washington, DC: AACC Press; 2006.

[23] Mullis KB, Faloona FA. Specific synthesis of DNA *in vitro* via a polymerase-catalyzed chain reaction. Methods Enzymol 1987;155:335—50.

[24] Sanger F, Nicklen S, Coulson AR. DNA sequencing with chain-terminating inhibitors. Proc Natl Acad Sci USA 1977;74(12):5463—7.

[25] Hutchison III CA. DNA sequencing: bench to bedside and beyond. Nucleic Acids Res 2007;35(18):6227—37.

[26] Kwok PY. Methods for genotyping single nucleotide polymorphisms. Annu Rev Genomics Hum Genet 2001;2:235—58.

[27] Davey JW, Hohenlohe PA, Etter PD, et al. Genome-wide genetic marker discovery and genotyping using next-generation sequencing. Nat Rev Genet 12(7):499—510.

[28] International Human Genome Sequencing Consortium. Finishing the euchromatic sequence of the human genome. Nature 2004;431(7011):931—45.

[29] Nielsen R, Paul JS, Albrechtsen A, et al. Genotype and SNP calling from next-generation sequencing data. Nat Rev Genet 2011;12(6):443—51.

[30] Wittwer CT, Kusukawa N. Nucleic acid techniques. In: Burtis CA, Ashwood ER, Bruns DE, editors. Tietz Textbook of Clinical Chemistry and Molecular Diagnostics. St Louis, MO: Elsevier; 2006.

[31] Millward H, Samowitz W, Wittwer CT, et al. Homogeneous amplification and mutation scanning of the p53 gene using fluorescent melting curves. Clin Chem 2002;48(8):1321—8.

[32] Bernard PS, Ajioka RS, Kushner JP, et al. Homogeneous multiplex genotyping of hemochromatosis mutations with fluorescent hybridization probes. Am J Pathol 1998;153(4):1055—61.

[33] Livak KJ, Flood SJ, Marmaro J, et al. Oligonucleotides with fluorescent dyes at opposite ends provide a quenched probe system useful for detecting PCR product and nucleic acid hybridization. PCR Methods Appl 1995;4(6):357—62.

[34] Stamer UM, Bayerer B, Wolf S, et al. Rapid and reliable method for cytochrome P450 2D6 genotyping. Clin Chem 2002;48(9):1412—7.

[35] Ranade K, Chang MS, Ting CT, et al. High-throughput genotyping with single nucleotide polymorphisms. Genome Res 2001;11(7):1262—8.

[36] Metzker ML. Sequencing technologies — the next generation. Nat Rev Genet 2010;11(1):31—46.

[37] Schadt EE, Turner S, Kasarskis A. A window into third-generation sequencing. Hum Mol Genet 2010;19(R2):R227—240.

[38] Bentley DR, Balasubramanian S, Swedlow HP, et al. Accurate whole human genome sequencing using reversible terminator chemistry. Nature 2008;456(7218):53—9.

[39] Bennett ST, Barnes C, Cox A, et al. Toward the 1,000 dollars human genome. Pharmacogenomics 2005;6(4):373—82.

[40] Lifton RP. Individual genomes on the horizon. N Engl J Med 2010;362(13):1235—6.

[41] Mardis ER, Ding L, Dooling DJ, et al. Recurring mutations found by sequencing an acute myeloid leukemia genome. N Engl J Med 2009;361(11):1058—66.

[42] Sastre L. New DNA sequencing technologies open a promising era for cancer research and treatment. Clin Transl Oncol 2011;13(5):301—6.

[43] Harksen A, Ueland PM, Refsum H, et al. Four common mutations of the cystathionine beta-synthase gene detected by multiplex PCR and matrix-assisted laser desorption/ionization time-of-flight mass spectrometry. Clin Chem 1999;45(8 Pt 1):1157—61.

[44] Millis MP. Medium-throughput SNP genotyping using mass spectrometry: multiplex SNP genotyping using the iPLEX® Gold assay. Methods Mol Biol 2011;700:61—76.

[45] Blievernicht JK, Schaeffeler E, Klein K, et al. MALDI-TOF mass spectrometry for multiplex genotyping of CYP2B6 single-nucleotide polymorphisms. Clin Chem 2007;53(1):24—33.

[46] Emonet S, Shah HN, Cherkaoui A, et al. Application and use of various mass spectrometry methods in clinical microbiology. Clin Microbiol Infect 2010;16(11):1604—13.

[47] Schena M, Shalon D, Davis RW, et al. Quantitative monitoring of gene expression patterns with a complementary DNA microarray. Science 1995;270(5235):467—70.

[48] Kricka LJ, Fortina. Microarray technology and applications: an all-language literature survey including books and patents. Clin Chem 2001;47(8):1479—82.

[49] de Leon J, Susce MT, Murray-Carmichael E. The AmpliChip CYP450 genotyping test: integrating a new clinical tool. Mol Diagn Ther 2006;10(3):135—51.

[50] Lorizio W, Rugo H, Beattie MS, et al. Pharmacogenetic testing affects choice of therapy among women considering tamoxifen treatment. Genome Med 2011;3(10):64.

[51] Savage MS, Mourad MJ, Wapner RJ. Evolving applications of microarray analysis in prenatal diagnosis. Curr Opin Obstet Gynecol 2011;23(2):103—8.

[52] Choudhuri S. Looking back to the future: from the development of the gene concept to toxicogenomics. Toxicol Mech Methods 2009;19(4):263—77.

[53] Penny MA, McHale D. Pharmacogenomics and the drug discovery pipeline: when should it be implemented? Am J Pharmacogenomics 2005;5(1):53—62.

[54] 1000 Genomes Project Consortium. A map of human genome variation from population-scale sequencing. Nature 2010;467(7319):1061—73.

[55] Ansorge WJ. Next-generation DNA sequencing techniques. N Biotechnol 2009;25(4):195—203.

[56] Mardis ER. Next-generation DNA sequencing methods. Annu Rev Genomics Hum Genet 2008;9: 387—402.

[57] Stranger BE, Stahl EA, Raj T. Progress and promise of genome-wide association studies for human complex trait genetics. Genetics 187(2):367-383.

[58] Zhang W, Dolan ME. Impact of the 1000 Genomes Project on the next wave of pharmacogenomic discovery. Pharmacogenomics 2010;11(2):249—56.

[59] The Cancer Genome Atlas Research Network. Comprehensive genomic characterization defines human glioblastoma genes and core pathways. Nature 2008;455(7216):1061—8.

[60] Johansson I, Ingelman-Sundberg M. CNVs of human genes and their implication in pharmacogenetics. Cytogenet Genome Res 2008;123(1—4):195—204.

[61] He Y, Hoskins JM, McLeod HL. Copy number variants in pharmacogenetic genes. Trends Mol Med 2011;17(5):244—51.

[62] Zhou SF. Polymorphism of human cytochrome P450 2D6 and its clinical significance: Part I. Clin Pharmacokinet 2009;48(11):689—723.

[63] Ingelman-Sundberg M. Genetic polymorphisms of cytochrome P450 2D6 (CYP2D6): clinical consequences, evolutionary aspects and functional diversity. Pharmacogenomics J 2005;5(1):6—13.

[64] Dalen P, Dahl ML, Bernal Ruiz ML, et al. 10-Hydroxylation of nortriptyline in white persons with 0, 1, 2, 3, and 13 functional CYP2D6 genes. Clin Pharmacol Ther 1998;63(4):444—52.

[65] Wood CE, Kaplan JR, Fontenot MB, et al. Endometrial profile of tamoxifen and low-dose estradiol combination therapy. Clin Cancer Res 2010;16(3):946—56.

[66] Fux R, Morike K, Prohmer AM, et al. Impact of CYP2D6 genotype on adverse effects during treatment with metoprolol: a prospective clinical study. Clin Pharmacol Ther 2005;78(4):378—87.

[67] Kirchheiner J, Schmidt H, Tzvetkov M, et al. Pharmacokinetics of codeine and its metabolite morphine in ultra-rapid metabolizers due to CYP2D6 duplication. Pharmacogenomics J 2007;7(4): 257—65.

[68] de Smith AJ, Tsalenko A, Sampas N, et al. Array CGH analysis of copy number variation identifies 1284 new genes variant in healthy white males: implications for association studies of complex diseases. Hum Mol Genet 2007;16(23):2783—94.

[69] Pinkel D, Segraves R, Sudar D, et al. High resolution analysis of DNA copy number variation using comparative genomic hybridization to microarrays. Nat Genet 1998;20(2):207—11.

[70] O'Keefe C, McDevitt MA, Maciejewski JP. Copy neutral loss of heterozygosity: a novel chromosomal lesion in myeloid malignancies. Blood 2010;115(14):2731—9.

[71] Burmester JK, Sedova M, Shapero MH, et al. DMET microarray technology for pharmacogenomics-based personalized medicine. Methods Mol Biol 2010;632:99—124.

[72] Lin B, Strickland SJ, Wang J, et al. Meeting report: the 2009 Westlake International Conference on Personalized Medicine. OMICS 2009;13(4):285—9.

[73] Maher CA, Kumar-Sinha C, Cao X, et al. Transcriptome sequencing to detect gene fusions in cancer. Nature 2009;458(7234):97—101.

[74] Montgomery SB, Dermitzakis ET. From expression QTLs to personalized transcriptomics. Nat Rev Genet 2011;12(4):277—82.

[75] Mortazavi A, Williams BA, McCue K, et al. Mapping and quantifying mammalian transcriptomes by RNA-Seq Nat Methods 2008;5(7):621—8.

[76] Guttman M, Amit I, Garber M, et al. Chromatin signature reveals over a thousand highly conserved large non-coding RNAs in mammals. Nature 2009;458(7235):223—7.

[77] Hawkins RD, Hon GC, Ren B. Next-generation genomics: an integrative approach. Nat Rev Genet 2010;11(7):476—86.

[78] Jordan KW, Nordenstam J, Lauwers GY, et al. Metabolomic characterization of human rectal adenocarcinoma with intact tissue magnetic resonance spectroscopy. Dis Colon Rectum 2009;52(3):520—5.

[79] Mendrick DL, Schnackenberg L. Genomic and metabolomic advances in the identification of disease and adverse event biomarkers. Biomark Med 2009;3(5):605—15.

[80] Meyer JM, Ginsburg GS. The path to personalized medicine. Curr Opin Chem Biol 2002;6(4):434—8.

[81] Turner DJ, Tuytten R, Janssen KP, et al. Toward clinical proteomics on a next-generation sequencing platform. Anal Chem 2011;83(3):666—70.

[82] Renuse S, Chaerkady R, Pandey A. Proteogenomics. Proteomics 2011;11(4):620—30.

[83] Feinberg AP, Irizarry RA, Fradin D, et al. Personalized epigenomic signatures that are stable over time and covary with body mass index. Sci Transl Med 2010;2(49):49—67.

[84] Satterlee JS, Schubeler D, Ng HH. Tackling the epigenome: challenges and opportunities for collaboration. Nat Biotechnol 2010;28(10):1039—44.

[85] Young M. Epigenetics — Expanding on Genomic Foundations. NEB Expressions 2010:3—5.

[86] Portela A, Esteller M. Epigenetic modifications and human disease. Nat Biotechnol 2010;28(10):1057—68.

[87] Esteller M. Epigenetic changes in cancer. In: Faculty of 1000 Ltd, F1000 Biology Reports 3 May. Available at, http://f1000.com/reports/b/3/9/; 2011 (open access).

[88] Flusberg BA, Webster DR, Lee JH, et al. Direct detection of DNA methylation during single-molecule, real-time sequencing. Nat Methods 2010;7(6):461—5.

[89] Huss M. Introduction into the analysis of high-throughput-sequencing based epigenome data. Brief Bioinform 2010;11(5):512—23.

[90] Pietrzykowski AZ. The role of microRNAs in drug addiction: a big lesson from tiny molecules. Intl Rev Neurobiol 2010;91:1—24.

[91] Rivera RM, Bennett LB. Epigenetics in humans: an overview. Curr Opin Endocrinol Diabetes Obes 2010;17(6):493—9.

[92] Ahmed FE. Role of miRNA in carcinogenesis and biomarker selection: a methodological view. Expert Rev Mol Diagn 2007;7(5):569—603.

[93] Calin GA, Sevignani C, Dumitru CD, et al. Human microRNA genes are frequently located at fragile sites and genomic regions involved in cancers. Proc Natl Acad Sci USA 2004;101(9):2999—3004.

[94] Croce CM. Causes and consequences of microRNA dysregulation in cancer. Nat Rev Genet 2009;10(10):704—14.

[95] Zanette DL, Rivadavia F, Molfetta GA, et al. miRNA expression profiles in chronic lymphocytic and acute lymphocytic leukemia. Braz J Med Biol Res 2007;40(11):1435—40.

[96] Szafranska AE, Doleshal M, Edmunds HS, et al. Analysis of microRNAs in pancreatic fine-needle aspirates can classify benign and malignant tissues. Clin Chem 2008;54(10):1716–24.

[97] Lebanony D, Benjamin H, Gilad S, et al. Diagnostic assay based on hsa-miR-205 expression distinguishes squamous from nonsquamous non-small-cell lung carcinoma. J Clin Oncol 2009;27(12):2030–7.

[98] Takeuchi F, McGinnis R, Bourgeois S, et al. A genome-wide association study confirms VKORC1, CYP2C9, and CYP4F2 as principal genetic determinants of warfarin dose. PLoS Genet 2009;5(3):e1000433.

[99] Cooper GM, Johnson JA, Langaee TY, et al. A genome-wide scan for common genetic variants with a large influence on warfarin maintenance dose. Blood 2008;112(4):1022–7.

[100] Crawford DC, Ritchie MD, Rieder MJ. Identifying the genotype behind the phenotype: a role model found in VKORC1 and its association with warfarin dosing. Pharmacogenomics 2007;8(5):487–96.

[101] Wadelius M, Chen LY, Lindh JD, et al. The largest prospective warfarin-treated cohort supports genetic forecasting. Blood 2009;113(4):784–92.

[102] Epstein RS, Moyer TP, Aubert RE, et al. Warfarin genotyping reduces hospitalization rates: results from the MM-WES (Medco-Mayo Warfarin Effectiveness study). J Am Coll Cardiol 2010;55(25):2804–12.

[103] Linder MW, Looney S, Adams III JE, et al. Warfarin dose adjustments based on CYP2C9 genetic polymorphisms. J Thromb Thrombolysis 2002;14(3):227–32.

[104] Schwab M, Schaeffeler E. Warfarin pharmacogenetics meets clinical use. Blood 2011;118(11):2938–9.

[105] Gage BF, Lesko LJ. Pharmacogenetics of warfarin: regulatory, scientific, and clinical issues. J Thromb Thrombolysis 2008;25(1):45–51.

[106] Wang L, McLeod HL, Weinshilboum RM. Genomics and drug response. N Engl J Med 2011;364(12):1144–53.

[107] Giorgi MA, Caroli C, Arazi HC, et al. Pharmacogenomics and adverse drug reactions: the case of statins. Expert Opin Pharmacother 2011;12(10):1499–509.

[108] Link E, Parish S, Armitage J, et al. SLCO1B1 variants and statin-induced myopathy — a genome-wide study. N Engl J Med 2008;359(8):789–99.

[109] Thompson JF, Hyde CL, Wood LS, et al. Comprehensive whole-genome and candidate gene analysis for response to statin therapy in the Treating to New Targets (TNT) cohort. Circ Cardiovasc Genet 2009;2(2):173–81.

[110] Barber MJ, Mangravite LM, Hyde CL, et al. Genome-wide association of lipid-lowering response to statins in combined study populations. PLoS One 2010;5(3):e9763.

[111] Sangkuhl K, Klein TE, Altman RB. Clopidogrel pathway. Pharmacogenet Genomics 2010;20(7):463–5.

[112] Lau WC, Waskell LA, Watkins PB, et al. Atorvastatin reduces the ability of clopidogrel to inhibit platelet aggregation: a new drug–drug interaction. Circulation 2003;107(1):32–7.

[113] Momary KM, Dorsch MP, Bates ER. Genetic causes of clopidogrel nonresponsiveness: which ones really count? Pharmacotherapy 2010;30(3):265–74.

[114] Holmes Jr DR, Dehmer GJ, Kaul S, et al. ACCF/AHA clopidogrel clinical alert: approaches to the FDA "boxed warning": a report of the American College of Cardiology Foundation Task Force on clinical expert consensus documents and the American Heart Association endorsed by the Society for Cardiovascular Angiography and Interventions and the Society of Thoracic Surgeons. J Am Coll Cardiol 2010;56(4):321–41.

[115] Ikediobi ON. Personalized medicine: are we there yet? Pharmacogenomics J 2009;9(2):85.

[116] Beutler E, Gelbart T, Demina A. Racial variability in the UDP-glucuronosyltransferase 1 (UGT1A1) promoter: a balanced polymorphism for regulation of bilirubin metabolism? Proc Natl Acad Sci USA 1998;95(14):8170–4.

[117] Strassburg CP. Pharmacogenetics of Gilbert's syndrome. Pharmacogenomics 2008;9(6):703–15.

[118] Innocenti F, Undevia SD, Iyer L, et al. Genetic variants in the UDP-glucuronosyltransferase 1A1 gene predict the risk of severe neutropenia of irinotecan. J Clin Oncol 2004;22(8):1382–8.

[119] Glenn TC. Field guide to next-generation DNA sequencers. Mol Ecol Resour 2011;11(5):759–69.

[120] Lee JC, Lau DT. Health information technology and the American Recovery and Reinvestment Act: some of the challenges ahead. Clin Ther 2009;31(6):1276–8.

[121] D'Avolio LW. Electronic medical records at a crossroads: impetus for change or missed opportunity? J Am Med Assoc 2009;302(10):1109–11.

[122] Ashley EA, Butte AJ, Wheeler MT, et al. Clinical assessment incorporating a personal genome. Lancet 2010;375(9725):1525–35.

[123] McCarty CA, Wilke RA. Biobanking and pharmacogenomics. Pharmacogenomics 2010;11(5):637–41.

[124] Zika E, Schulte In den Baumen T, Kaye J, et al. Sample, data use and protection in biobanking in Europe: legal issues. Pharmacogenomics 2008;9(6):773–81.

[125] Vijverberg S, Daly AK, Maitland-van der Zee AH. Conference scene: initiatives on future biobanking in pharmacogenomics. Pharmacogenomics 2009;10(7):1135–8.

[126] D'Avolio LW, Farwell WR, Fiore LD. Comparative effectiveness research and medical informatics. Am J Med 2010;123(12 Suppl. 1):e32–37.

[127] Jagannathan V, Mullett CJ, Arbogast JG, et al. Assessment of commercial NLP engines for medication information extraction from dictated clinical notes. Intl J Med Inform 2009;78(4):284–91.

[128] Chhieng D, Day T, Gordon G, et al. Use of natural language programming to extract medication from unstructured electronic medical records. AMIA Annual Symposium Proceedings 2007:908.

[129] Wilke RA, Dolan ME. Genetics and variable drug response. Jama 2011;306(3):306–7.

[130] Mrazek DA, Lerman C. Facilitating clinical implementation of pharmacogenomics. Jama 2011;306(3):304–5.

[131] Hudson KL. Genomics, health care, and society. N Engl J Med 2011;365(11):1033–41.

[132] Sallee FR, DeVane CL, Ferrell RE. Fluoxetine-related death in a child with cytochrome P450 2D6 genetic deficiency. J Child Adolesc Psychopharmacol 2000;10(1):27–34.

[133] Porcelli S, Drago A, Fabbri C, et al. Pharmacogenetics of antidepressant response. J Psychiatry Neurosci 2011;36(2):87–113.

[134] Greely HT. The uneasy ethical and legal underpinnings of large-scale genomic biobanks. Annu Rev Genomics Hum Genet 2007;8:343–864.

[135] Scheuner MT, de Vries H, Kim B, et al. Are electronic health records ready for genomic medicine? Genet Med 2009;11(7):510–7.

[136] McGuire AL, Fisher R, Cusenza P, et al. Confidentiality, privacy, and security of genetic and genomic test information in electronic health records: points to consider. Genet Med 2008;10(7):495–9.

[137] Baruch S, Hudson K. Civilian and military genetics: nondiscrimination policy in a post-GINA world. Am J Hum Genet 2008;83(4):435–44.

[138] Li C. Personalized medicine – the promised land: are we there yet? Clin Genet 2011;79(5):403–12.

[139] Bates BR, Poirot K, Harris TM, et al. Evaluating direct-to-consumer marketing of race-based pharmacogenomics: a focus group study of public understandings of applied genomic medication. J Health Commun 2004;9(6):541–59.

[140] Gold ER, Carbone J. Myriad genetics: in the eye of the policy storm. Genet Med 2010;12(4 Suppl):S39–70.

[141] Huys I, Berthels N, Matthijs G, et al. Legal uncertainty in the area of genetic diagnostic testing. Nat Biotechnol 2009;27(10):903–9.

[142] Shields AE, Lerman C. Anticipating clinical integration of pharmacogenetic treatment strategies for addiction: are primary care physicians ready? Clin Pharmacol Ther 2008;83(4):635–9.

[143] Winner JG, Goebert D, Matsu C, et al. Training in psychiatric genomics during residency: a new challenge. Acad Psychiatry 2010;34(2):115–8.

[144] Ramsey SD, Veenstra DL, Garrison Jr LP, et al. Toward evidence-based assessment for coverage and reimbursement of laboratory-based diagnostic and genetic tests. Am J Manag Care 2006;12(4):197–202.

[145] Garrison Jr LP, Carlson RJ, Carlson JJ, et al. A review of public policy issues in promoting the development and commercialization of pharmacogenomic applications: challenges and implications. Drug Metab Rev 2008;40(2):377–401.

[146] Meckley LM, Neumann PJ. Personalized medicine: factors influencing reimbursement. Health Policy 2010;94(2):91–100.

Application of Ultra-High Throughput Sequencing and Microarray Technologies in Pharmacogenomics Testing

Gary Hardiman

Department of Medicine, and BIOGEM, School of Medicine, University of California, San Diego, CA; Computational Science Research Center and Biomedical Informatics Research Center, San Diego State University, San Diego, CA

OUTLINE

DOI: 10.1016/B978-0-12-385467-4.00007-5

INTRODUCTION

The sequencing of the human genome over a decade ago was a critical scientific milestone. The draft human genome sequence has revolutionized the pharmaceutical industry, providing a framework for the identification of novel drug targets, and elucidation of the genetic factors that affect drug metabolism and toxicity and of those that contribute to the wide variability in pharmacological treatment responses. The emergence and wide acceptance of genomic technologies, including microarray and deep sequencing technologies, has allowed geneticists, biologists and pharmacologists to bridge the gap between gene sequence and function on a scale that was not possible previously. These newer technological approaches have been integrated into multiple aspects of the drug discovery process, including target validation, pharmacokinetics and toxicology, and clinical pharmacogenomics [1].

The adoption of a novel technology is met by a paradigm shift in how biological assays are designed and executed. Throughput is increased by at least an order of magnitude and accompanied by an exponential cost reduction compared to older traditional approaches. The economic benefit and efficacy of nascent technologies is often realized by process-miniaturization combined with the multiplexing of millions of reactions. A classic example of this scheme is the DNA microarray which was developed in the early 1990s [2, 3]. DNA arrays or (bio)chips evolved steadily over time from archetypal in-house boutique efforts to robust commercial arrays. This progression was accompanied by the availability of higher density chips with increased content, lower per-sample costs, and concomitant increases in sensitivity, accuracy and precision [3–7]. Frequently, an appreciation of the benefits and long-term impact of nascent technologies is not immediate, as their initial use is restricted to developers, beta-testers and early adopters. The impact of a given technology and its long-term value is not realized until its wider acceptance by the scientific community.

In the past five years, ultra-high throughput or deep sequencing of DNA has transitioned from development to widespread use, with several well-established academic and commercial efforts in place [8–10]. Deep sequencing has reduced the cost per base of DNA sequencing by several orders of magnitude, and has effectively introduced genome sequencing center capability into every laboratory [8]. Incorporation of next-generation sequencing approaches into drug discovery programs has become an important issue for many biotechnology and pharmaceutical companies. As the technology is in a state of flux with constant improvements and upgrades, and with new players being added to this space almost monthly, this creates complexity as to the choice of the most appropriate platform.

Many changes can be expected in the next few years, mirroring the early days in the development of microarray technology, where early adopters were forced to build on their initial investment and commit additional resources in the form of equipment upgrades or hardware replacement to remain current with the technology. Cost, ease of use, versatility, peer review in the form of published data, platform stability and the quality of long-term technical support will continue to guide the technology selection process. Data management also poses challenges, with the need for high-speed fiber-optic networks, and ample storage capacity for long-term data storage, annotation, query and retrieval. The microarray comparison is again appropriate when one considers the current state of analytical tools for next-generation sequencing analysis. Better analytical tools will emerge over time, likely from open source efforts, permitting additional analyses and enhanced information mining from raw data sets compared to the tool kits provided with the instruments themselves.

DNA MICROARRAY

A DNA microarray (commonly referred to as gene or genome chip, cDNA array, DNA chip or biochip) is a collection of DNA features attached to a solid support – commonly silanized glass, plastic, film or silicon. The array features or "spots" contain individual DNA probes which are used to interrogate mRNAs (expression) or polymorphisms (genotype). Most of the arrays in use today contain hundreds to thousands of probes. The utility of this technology is that it permits highly parallel measurements from an individual sample or patient specimen.

In the case of gene expression profiling, the substantial number of data points obtained from a single experiment provides an insight into the state of a transcriptome in, for example, healthy and diseased cells, or cells before and after exposure to a therapeutic. The knowledge obtained from such comparisons permits the identification of gene families and pathways pertinent to a malady or drug treatment, in addition to those that remain unaffected. Similar expression profiles may infer that genes are co-regulated; enabling the formulation of hypotheses about genes with hitherto unknown functions by comparison of their expression patterns to well-characterized genes [11–15]. This approach permits the discovery of DNA biomarkers and facilitates the development of diagnostic and prognostic tests.

The applicability of microarrays in genomics research has expanded with the evolution and maturation of the technology. Biochips have found utility in exon-based gene expression analyses, genotyping and re-sequencing applications, comparative genomic hybridization studies and genome-wide (epigenetic) localization. Biochips are being widely applied to improve the processes of disease diagnosis, pharmacogenomics, and toxicogenomics [12–15].

PHARMACOGENETIC TESTING AND HEALTHCARE

Heterogeneity is observed in the manner in which individuals respond to medications. Clinical observations of inherited differences in drug effects were first noted in the 1950s. By the 1990s, it was well established that inherited differences in drug metabolism and disposition, and genetic polymorphisms in the targets of drug therapy, could have a profound effect on the efficacy and toxicity of medications [16, 17]. Pharmacogenetics is concerned with the relationship between a patient's inherited genetic makeup and his or her response to pharmaceutical drugs. Pharmacogenetic testing aims at determining the underlying genotypic and phenotypic differences in the pharmacodynamics and pharmacokinetics of drug metabolism. Whereas pharmacogenetics refers to genetic differences (variation) in drug metabolism and response, pharmacogenomics refers to the study of the multiplicity of genes that ultimately determine drug behavior. Pharmacogenomics is in essence a whole-genome application of pharmacogenetics, correlating gene expression or single nucleotide polymorphisms (SNPs) with drug efficacy and toxicity. Genetic variability in drug response occurs as a result of molecular alterations in the enzymes involved in the metabolism of a particular drug, in addition to the drug receptors and transport proteins [18].

The grand promise of pharmacogenomics is the development of therapeutics targeted for specific patient subgroups. The vision has been the application of high-throughput molecular diagnostics approaches, DNA microarrays and next-generation sequencing technologies as sensitive screening tools for genetic predisposition to the adverse effects of therapeutics. These approaches would facilitate patient stratification and robust selection of medications and dosages tailored to address inter-individual variability [19, 20]. An advance and fundamental shift in healthcare has been the emergence of personalized medicine [21]. This model emphasizes the customization of healthcare, with all decisions and practices being tailored to individual patients. This approach makes use of genetic and/or other information about individual patients to select or optimize their preventative and therapeutic care.

Drug—drug interactions (DDIs) can have serious consequences such as adverse drug reactions (ADRs), and extreme outcomes including death. A drug interaction occurs when a substance affects the activity of a drug, either increasing or decreasing its efficacy, or, alternatively, a new effect is observed that is not observed with just the drug alone [22—24]. DDIs have become a serious issue, particularly in the care of elderly patients, who are often prescribed a wide variety of medications [25]. ADRs are presently the fourth leading cause of death in US. The economics of drug-related morbidity and mortality has become a pressing issue, with current costs exceeding US$177 billion annually in the USA alone [23].

Pharmacogenetic approaches are being used more widely for therapeutic monitoring and health management of patients, with patient genotyping and stratification performed well in advance of drug treatments, thereby eliminating completely or greatly reducing adverse effects. The testing itself can generally be performed in a non-invasive manner using DNA obtained from saliva, hair root or buccal swab samples, and can provide predictive values for many drugs rather than a single drug [18].

DNA MICROARRAY PLATFORMS

The platforms most widely utilized in the past decade for expression profiling include those developed commercially by Affymetrix, Agilent, Nimblegen, Applied Microarrays CodeLink, and Illumina. Affymetrix (Santa Clara, CA) pioneered this crowded field by developing a GeneChip™ comprising short 25-mer oligonucleotide probes that were fabricated *in situ* using a combination of photolithographic techniques (borrowed from the silicon chip industry) and solid phase DNA synthesis [5, 6]. Agilent (Palo Alto, CA) coupled inkjet printing (developed by Hewlett Packard) with standard phosphoramidite chemistry [7, 8] to synthesize 60-mer probes. Nimblegen (Madison, WI) coupled photolithography and solid phase DNA synthesis but, unlike the related Affymetrix technology, Nimblegen disposed of solid chromium mask photolithography in favor of digital micro-mirrors (DMDs or DLPs). DMDs flip mirrors on and off, thereby providing the highly specific light patterns required for photo-activation and DNA chain extension components of DNA chip synthesis [26]. Nimblegen designed isothermal probes to mini-mize hybridization artifacts and bias, with probe lengths ranging from 45 to 85 mers, depending on the particular application. Applied Microarrays (Tempe, AZ) utilized a non-contact, piezoelectric dispensing method optimized by Motorola to deposit 30-mer oligonucleotides on a three-dimensional polyacrylamide gel (CodeLink™) matrix [27]. A bead-based microarray technology was developed by Illumina (San Diego, CA) permitting multiplexing of up to 96 samples. These substrates contain thousands of tiny etched wells, into which thousands to hundreds of thousands of 3-micron beads are randomly self-assembled. Gene-specific probes (50 mers) concatenated with "address or zip-code" sequences are immobilized on the bead surface. Once bead assembly has occurred the array is "decoded", to uncover which bead type containing a particular sequence is present in each well of the substrate [28–30].

The net result of a microarray experiment is a list of significant probe sets or genes that are differentially expressed across given experimental conditions. The standard experimental design utilizes biological replicates, permitting an estimate of the statistical relevance of a given fold-change between a control and treated condition. The subsequent steps in inter-pretation of this data are appending biological knowledge to this list. This process has matured considerably over the past decade, and relied on the expansion of public databases such as Entrez Gene, Unigene, UniProt, Gene Ontology (GO) and KEGG pathways in addi-tion to commercial proprietary efforts.

In an effort to minimize the need to replicate microarray experiments, and to provide exact descriptions for experimenters wishing to utilize public datasets, gene expression data is today stored in public repositories such as Gene Expression Omnibus (GEO) and EBI Array Express, which have become the major portals for deposition and retrieval of genomics data. The "Minimum Information about a Microarray Experiment (MIAME)" standard today requires experimenters to report in detail their experimental design, sample description, labeling and hybridization protocol, data-imaging conditions and data analysis using a pre-determined set of criteria. In order to publish microarray data in the majority of peer-reviewed journals today, mandatory submission of the dataset to one of the databases precedes publication.

In order to assess the performance and reliability of different microarray platforms, a comprehensive study known as the MicroArray Quality Control (MAQC) project was undertaken. This global effort had FDA (Federal Drug Administration of the United Sates Government) oversight and brought together academic and industrial scientists. The outcome was a detailed assessment of the strengths and weaknesses of the major platforms in terms of their performance and reliability, and better strategies for integrating data from different platforms.

Array comparative genomic hybridization (a-CGH) has today superseded traditional chromosome-based methods for detection of genomic copy number variations. It permits higher resolution levels than chromosome-based methods, facilitating identification of chro-mosomal changes such as micro-deletions and duplications. The Agilent Human Genome CGH Microarray is one such high-resolution platform that has been widely applied for profiling genome-wide DNA variation without genome amplification or complexity reduc-tion approaches. The output of a CGH experiment is a series of copy number variations

(CNV), namely DNA segments which range in size from under 1 kilobase to several megabases of DNA.

MICROARRAYS AND GENOTYPE

Single nucleotide polymorphisms (SNPs) are highly abundant, with over 10 million present in the human genome. SNPs serve as valuable markers of genome-wide variation. A chromosome region may contain many SNPs, but just a few "tag" SNPs is all that is required to provide information on the pattern of genetic variation. The high costs associated with most SNP detection strategies have until recently made genome-wide approaches impractical. The relatively low-cost and high-throughput capabilities of Illumina bead-based technology made genome-wide approaches a reality. Genome-wide genotyping of defined sets of up to 1 million SNPs can be performed using the Infinium assay, developed by Illumina. A whole-genome amplification step is initially employed to enrich the target DNA up to 1000-fold. Once amplified, the DNA is subsequently fragmented and mobilized by hybridization to SNP-specific primers present on the array. An oligonucleotide primer is hybridized adjacent to the SNP site and is extended with a single labeled dideoxynucleotide terminator corresponding to the minor or major allele. Genotyping calls can then be made, based on the dye-labeled terminator that is incorporated [29–30].

Since their development in 2005, the Illumina whole-genome genotyping (WGGT) arrays have become an important tool for discovering variants that contribute to human diseases and phenotypes. Illumina arrays permit two different types of study: genome-wide association studies (GWAS) and copy-number variant (CNV) analyses. The genome-wide association study (GWA study or GWAS) is an unbiased examination of the entire genome of different individuals to see if any variant is associated with a phenotypic (disease) trait. Single nucleotide polymorphisms (SNPs) are investigated. These studies typically compare the DNA of two groups of participants: people with the disease (cases), and age- and sex-matched people without (controls). If genetic (SNP) variations are more frequent in people with the disease, the variations are "associated" with the disease. The associated genetic variations provide pointers to the genomic region responsible for the disease.

Structural variation (SV) is defined as the variation that exists in the structure of an organism's chromosomes. Many types of variation exist, encompassing alterations such as deletions, duplications, copy-number variants, insertions, inversions and translocations. SVs comprise millions of nucleotides of heterogeneity within every genome. Consequently SVs contribute to human diversity, disease susceptibility and pharmacogenomic responses. Copy-number variants (CNVs) are important SVs, and are alterations of the DNA of a genome that results in a cell having an abnormal number of copies of one or more sections of the DNA. This variation accounts for roughly 12% of human genomic DNA, and ranges from about 1 kilobase to several megabases in size [31].

The most recent iteration of Infinium WGGT products is the Omni family of microarrays. This platform provides up to 5 million markers per sample. The content has been designed from next-generation sequencing data from international projects such as the 1000 Genomes

Project. The HumanOmni5-Quad4 and HumanOmni1-Quad4 provide approximately 4.3 and 1.1 million markers, respectively.

MICROARRAYS IN CLINICAL DIAGNOSIS

Microarrays are today being applied in the clinical diagnostics arena. Their successful utilization and survival in the clinic will depend on the ability of the technology to meet the rigorous requirements applied to human diagnostics in a cost-effective manner. A greater degree of robustness is needed in the clinical environment compared to the research laboratory. Arrays in the clinic must provide binary answers, and the assay itself must be simple and versatile and be scalable to the higher-throughput needs of the clinical laboratory. In terms of robustness, the same sample should give the same result and be independent of variables associated with different operators. Assays should provide straightforward "YES" or "NO" binary-style answers.

Two clinical scenarios can be envisaged: a Case A trial where potential responders need to be assayed based on the mRNA levels of a specific gene expressed in a given target tissue, and Case B, where the assay is based on a specific polymorphic variant on the receptor for the particular compound being tested. In Case A the binary answer is more difficult to achieve, as high variability may be associated with the isolation of target tissue. Important issues include the purity of the sample, the timing of the sample collection and the inherent variability associated with complex organisms. It is well known that genetic complexity exists amongst populations, but this is further confounded by the time of day sampling occurs and the status of each patient. In Case B, the binary answer is easier to implement and independent of variables associated with sample collection. The presence or absence of the polymorphic variant in patients' alleles remained a fixed value. The Case B scenario will always be *a priori* the more successful and easier to implement in a clinical setting. Case A may benefit from clustering (examination of the mRNA levels of subsets of genes) rather than selecting a single marker. The clinical setting demands simplicity and versatility, capable of performing in various settings. Protocols must reduce the variables associated with sample collection and processing.

One obstacle to immediate acceptance of newer genomics technology is the reluctance of the pharmaceutical industry and healthcare providers to introduce new techniques lying outside their current expertise. Careful and convincing cost–benefit studies must be carried out to justify the costs associated with the introduction of the technology and the hiring of an expert workforce.

The first pharmacogenetic microarray-based test approved for clinical use is the AmpliChip CYP450™ from Roche Diagnostics (Basel), which measures genetic variation, both deletions and duplications, for the CYP2D6 and CYP2C19 genes. The test was approved by the FDA in December 2004, and is unique in that it is the first FDA-approved pharmacogenetic test. The AmpliChip is a marriage of expertise in polymerase chain reaction (Roche) and microarray (Affymetrix) technologies. The test determines the associated predictive phenotype (poor, intermediate, extensive or ultra metabolizer) and can aid physicians in individualizing patient treatment and dosing for drugs metabolized through these P450 genes. It detects up to 33 CYP2D6 alleles and 3 CYP2C19 alleles.

Once patient genomic DNA has been extracted, the test involves a series of five steps, and the analysis time from start to finish is approximately 8 hours. A minimum of 25 ng of input genomic DNA is required for the assay and the preferred tissue source is blood, although buccal swab-derived DNA would also suffice. First, PCR amplification is carried out to amplify the genes of interest using gene-specific primers. This is followed by fragmentation and biotin labeling of the amplicons at their 3' termini with Terminal Transferase (TdT). The biotin labeled target is subsequently hybridized to the AmpliChip DNA microarray. Following washing and staining via a streptavidin–phycoerythrin conjugate, the chip is scanned on an Affymetrix GeneChip® Scanner, the data features are extracted and analyzed, and genotyping calls are made. As CYP2D6 substrates are primarily psychiatric drugs, including antidepressant and antipsychotics, this test has been extensively used in psychiatry.

The INFINITI™ Analyzer is an automated, continuous flow, microarray platform for clinical applications that has been developed by Autogenomics (Carlsbad, CA) [32]. The underlying component of the Autogenomics technology is the BioFilm™, which consists of multiple layers of porous hydrogel matrices 8- to 10-μm thick on a polyester solid base. This provides an aqueous microenvironment that is highly compatible with biological materials and permits analyses of both nucleic acid and proteins [33]. It can be tailored to clinical genetic testing for custom polymorphisms of interest.

The INFINITI™ integrates all the discrete processes of sample handling, reagent management, hybridization and detection. A confocal microscope has been integrated into the analyzer with two lasers (red and green). In addition, a thermal stringency station and a thermal cycler for denaturing nucleic acids for primer extension studies or hybridization reactions in solution have been incorporated. A series of *in vitro* diagnostic assays have been developed and commercialized on this platform. They include the INFINITI™ CYP2C19 Assay, which has been developed for use as an aid to clinicians in determining therapeutic strategy for therapeutics that are metabolized by the CYP450 2C19 gene product, specifically *2, *3, *17; the INFINITI™ Warfarin Assay, indicated for use to identify individuals at risk for sensitivity to Warfarin; the INFINITI™ System Assay for Factor II, indicated for use as an aid to diagnosis in the evaluation of patients with suspected thrombophilia (genetic variants in Factor II − Prothrombin); and the INFINITI™ Factor V Leiden Assay, indicated for use as an aid to diagnosis in the evaluation of patients with suspected thrombophilia (genetic variants in Factor V Leiden).

SEQUENCING TECHNOLOGIES − THE FIRST GENERATION

Since its development the most widely used DNA sequencing approach has been the "chain-termination" method, developed by Sanger and colleagues, which utilizes dideoxynucleoside triphosphates (ddNTPs) as DNA chain terminators [34]. This methodology advanced the throughput of genome sequencing, culminating with a draft of the human genome over a decade ago. An inherent disadvantage with the Sanger method is the need for fragmentation of large DNA polynucleotides into smaller pieces, followed by their individual amplification and sequencing. This process is very costly, highly laborious and incredibly time consuming.

The time line for the development of Sanger sequencing is as follows. In 1975, Sanger and Coulson published the seminal "plus-minus method" of DNA sequencing which primes DNA synthesis using DNA polymerase [35], and sequenced the 5375-nucleotide genome of bacteriophage phi [36]. Two years later, an alternate DNA sequencing method was described by Maxam and Gilbert which was based on the chemical modification of DNA and subsequent cleavage at specific bases [37]. Although both represented ground-breaking advances, the "chemical modification" and "plus-minus" methods lacked the efficiency of the "chain-termination" method, subsequently developed by Sanger and coworkers. This approach utilized dideoxynucleoside triphosphates (ddNTPs) as DNA chain terminators [34].

Technological and instrument improvements have advanced the throughput of genome sequencing to routine projects lasting just a few months. However, the costs associated with sequencing a single human genome using traditional Sanger sequencing remain elevated, and are estimated in the region of US$10 to US$25 million [38].

SEQUENCING TECHNOLOGIES — NEXT GENERATION

Traditional sequencing approaches require the fragmentation of large DNA polymers into smaller pieces, followed by the amplification and sequencing of the individual fragments, data quality control and, finally, the assembly of contiguous sequences. One of the primary objectives of the next-generation sequencing technologies has been circumvention of the cumbersome library construction and DNA cloning steps. Massively parallel signature sequencing (MPSS) approaches have replaced the Sanger capillary-based electrophoresis method for high-throughput sequencing projects. These shotgun methods have been termed "next-generation" or "second-generation" technologies.

Margulies *et al.* described an early 454 Life Sciences instrument, capable of sequencing 25 million bases in a 4-hour period — an advance 100 times more rapid than Sanger-based capillary-based electrophoresis [39]. In this methodology, the DNA was amplified via a "clonal" approach and sequenced yielding sequencing tags 100 bp in length. Adaptors were ligated to sheared genomic DNA fragments, 300 bp in length, permitting their capture on tiny beads (28 mm in diameter), and reaction conditions were optimized to promote the attachment of just one fragment per bead. Subsequently, oil droplets containing all the requisite reactants for DNA amplification were allowed to encase the beads, forming an emulsion which maintains each bead distinct from another bead. This emulsion or e-PCR ensured uncontaminated amplification of approximately 10 million copies of the initial fragment. The beads were then dispensed into the open wells of a fiber-optic slide and pyrosequenced (via luciferase-based real-time monitoring of pyrophosphate release) [40, 41]. Shotgun sequencing and *de novo* assembly of the *Mycoplasma genitalium* genome was carried out as a test case to validate the approach. In just one 4-hour run using this system, 96% genome coverage with 99.96% accuracy was obtained.

Another approach for ultra-high throughput DNA sequencing was reported by Shendure *et al.* [42]. This method of sequencing by synthesis on a solid support is similar in principle to that described by Margulies *et al.* [39]. This approach differed, however, with regard to the method utilized for library construction, the sequencing chemistry and signal detection (a modified epifluorescence microscope). The method relied on polonies (polymerase colonies), discrete clonal amplifications of a single DNA molecule, grown on a solid phase surface. A "polony" protocol was employed to generate a DNA library containing approximately 1.6 million fragments, each 135 bp in length with 100 bp in common, in addition to two "mate-pairs" sequence tags 17 and 18 bp in length, respectively, which derived from the genome being sequenced. The tags representing random sequences were located approximately 1 kb apart on the genome. Each fragment was attached to a separate bead (1 μm in size), amplified using emulsion PCR, and immobilized in a poly-acrylamide gel. Parallel sequencing was carried out using a four-dye ligation protocol to identify each base. For each fragment, a 26-bp sequence (13 bp from each tag) was determined. An *Escherichia coli* strain, MG1655, engineered for deficiencies in tryptophan biosynthesis was re-sequenced using this approach, with an error rate estimated at 1 per million consensus bases.

The first commercial next-generation sequencing platform was introduced in 2005 by 454 Life Sciences (Branford, CT). The current Genome Sequencer™ FLX from 454 Life Sciences has improved error rates and reads lengths of 250 bp on average. Other commercial efforts include technologies from Illumina (San Diego, CA), Applied Biosystems (Foster City, CA) and Helicos BioSciences (Cambridge, MA).

The Illumina HiSeq™ platform is based on the massively parallel sequencing of millions of fragments using a proprietary clonal single molecule array technology coupled to a novel reversible terminator-based sequencing chemistry. For short sequence reads (up to 125 bp), the approach has been determined to be highly robust and accurate. Applications in whole-genome association studies, expression analysis, and sequencing in addition to genome-wide location studies have been described [43, 44]. The short individual read lengths have led to primary applications in re-sequencing where an established reference genome exists, rather than *de novo* sequencing.

The Applied Biosystems (Foster City, CA) "supported oligo ligation detection" (SOLiD) DNA sequencing system developed by Agencourt Personal Genomics utilizes a related clonal amplification approach on beads, employing four fluorescent tags with a two-base readout system. Each ligation step interrogates a pair of adjacent nucleotides, with each base interrogated twice for higher accuracy. Applications include detection of sequence variation, including SNPs (single nucleotide polymorphisms), gene copy-number variations, and single base duplications, inversions, insertions and deletions.

Ion Semiconductor Sequencing (Ion Torrent Systems Inc.) is a recent addition to DNA sequencing, and is based on the detection of hydrogen ions that are released during DNA polymerization. A microwell containing a template DNA strand is inundated with a single deoxyribonucleotide (dNTP) species. If the introduced dNTP is complementary to the leading template nucleotide it is incorporated into the growing complementary strand, releasing a hydrogen ion, and ultimately triggers an ion sensor. This technology is unique in that it is fluorescence-free, and no modified nucleotides or optics are used. Ion torrent sequencing represents pH-mediated sequencing, and is a true post-light sequencing technology.

The majority of sequencing by synthesis approaches requires nucleic acid amplification steps, so that an adequate signal level can be achieved. In contrast, single-molecule or third-generation approaches circumvent amplification and involve direct sequencing of single DNA molecules. One popular single-molecule approach gaining momentum is nanopore sequencing. As DNA passes through a 1.5-nm nanopore (a small pore in an electrically insulating membrane) different base pairs obstruct the pore to varying degrees, causing measurable variations in the electrical conductance of the pore, which can then be used to infer the DNA sequence [45].

Pacific Biosciences has developed Single Molecule Real Time (SMRT™) DNA sequencing technology, permitting observation of natural DNA synthesis by a DNA polymerase as it occurs. The approach is based on eavesdropping on a single DNA polymerase molecule which works in a continuous, processive manner. One of the advantages of SMRT™ sequencing is its long reads. There are three sequencing modes possible with the Pacific Biosciences technology: standard sequencing, circular consensus sequencing and strobe sequencing. Standard SMRT™ sequencing generates single-pass long reads from 2-kb DNA templates. Continuous polymerase synthesis occurs along a single DNA strand. Circular consensus sequencing uses a circular DNA template to enable multiple reads across a single molecule. This approach provides both forward and reverse reads with a double stranded template, and increases the accuracy of the sequence data. Strobe sequencing is applicable to long inserts > 6 kb. Physical coverage of the DNA is increased by "strobing" the laser illumination on and off, and the polymerase works its way across the DNA molecule. Read lengths are extended by minimizing the enzymatic damage that results from the continuous laser illumination. Data are then collected at user-defined illumination intervals. When the illumination is set to off, the sequencing continues at a predictable rate. The net result of this approach is the generation of multiple sub-reads with varying lengths from a single molecule.

EXON CAPTURE AND OLIGONUCLEOTIDE-BASED GENOMIC SELECTION

In order to fully leverage the power of this technology, obstacles in template preparation need to be overcome. PCR, which has been the dominant enrichment technology for conventional sequencing, is rate limiting with newer technologies, as it requires the synthesis of large numbers of oligonucleotides and performing large numbers of individual PCR reactions. Furthermore, PCR does not multiplex efficiently. Complex eukaryotic genomes are at this time simply too large to explore without the use of complexity-reduction methods. Exome sequencing or targeted exome capture has proven a robust approach to selectively sequence the coding regions present in the genome that contains the majority of disease-causing mutations. The exome constitutes approximately 1% of the genome spanning all the exons or the transcribed component of the human genome. Exons are derived from genomic regions that are translated into protein and the flanking untranslated regions (UTRs).

A new utility for DNA microarrays has been described recently in the context of exome capture. High-density oligonucleotide microarrays can be repurposed as hybrid-selection matrices to capture defined genomic fragments as substrates for sequencing. This represents a paradigm shift from conventional array-based approaches, where DNA hybridization to a cognate probe generates a coordinate signal and the intensity is translated into biological information.

Microarray-based genomic selection (MGS) permits enrichment of pre-defined sequences (for example, exomes) from complex eukaryotic genomes. Although several related techniques have been described, MGS essentially consists of shearing genomic DNA into smaller fragments which are ligated with unique adaptors, and subsequently hybridized to high-density oligonucleotide microarrays or oligonucleotides in solution derived from microarrays. The bound fragments are eluted and amplified with PCR, using the adaptor primers, and sequenced.

Okou et al. reported MGS capable of enriching targeted sequences from complex eukaryotic genomes without the repeat blocking steps necessary for bacterial artificial chromosome (BAC)-based genomic selection [46]. Custom oligonucleotide microarrays from NimbleGen Systems, Inc. (Madison, WI) containing 385 000 capture probes 50–93 bp in length were designed to achieve optimal isothermal hybridization across the microarray. Re-sequencing was carried out using a custom Nimblegen microarray.

Hodges et al. [47] focused on coding exons and their adjacent splice sites, a sequence range representing roughly 1% of the human genome. Nimblegen arrays with overlapping 60- to 90-nt probes were designed to tile approximately 6 Mb of exonic sequence. The enriched material was sequenced using an Illumina instrument. Analysis of the captured fragments revealed that 55–85% derived from the targeted regions and up to 98% of the intended exons were recovered. Albert et al. coupled high-density Nimblegen microarrays with 454 Life Sciences FLX sequencing to perform MGS [48]. A total of 6726 base "exon" segments approximately 500 bp in size, and "locus-specific" regions 200 kb to 5 Mb in size were enriched and sequenced. The majority of the sequence reads represented selection targets.

Porreca et al. [49] described an interesting variation of MGS which utilized a modification of the molecular inversion probe methodology to enrich sequences for Illumina 1G Analyzer sequencing. In this approach, 100-mer oligos are synthesized and released from a programmable microarray (Agilent Technologies, Santa Clara, CA), amplified using PCR, and restriction digested to release a single-stranded 70-mer "capture probe" mixture. Each individual mature probe contains a universal 30-nt motif, flanked by unique targeting arms each 20 nt in length. The arms facilitate hybridization immediately upstream and downstream of a specific genomic target, which is copied by polymerase-driven extension from the 3' end of the capture probe. Ligation to the 5' end completes a circle which is enriched and amplified. Advantages of this approach include compatibility with extensive multiplexing (facilitating capture of up to 10 000 targets in an individual reaction), high specificity with 98% of amplicons corresponding to targets, and the precise specification of target boundaries.

MICROARRAY TECHNOLOGY VERSUS DEEP SEQUENCING

The commercial microarray platforms in use today have been applied very successfully to a wide range of biomedical studies. They have established efficiencies with regard to signal dynamic range, the ability to discriminate related mRNA species and the reproducibility of the data (i.e., raw data, fold-change and expression levels). However, these arrays are not without their limitations. Expression or cDNA microarrays facilitate the analysis of the relative levels of mRNA species in one tissue sample compared to another. Although a measure of transcript abundance is achieved with each sample assayed, the arrays do not enable absolute quantification of specific mRNA species. A further limitation is that the analog data obtained merely determines whether a given messenger RNA is above the threshold level of detection for the particular array platform. If the signal is significantly above the background intensity, one can say with confidence that the transcript is expressed in that tissue. However, the absence of signal does not indicate lack of expression for a particular mRNA; it merely indicates that it is below the detection capability of the platform and it remains a possibility that the mRNA is expressed, albeit at low levels, and this basal expression may have biological relevance to the disease under study.

Analysis of gene expression using DNA microarrays provides a measure of the transcriptome, and mRNA can be ranked on the basis of abundance. However, cellular mRNA abundance often correlates poorly with the amount of protein synthesized. Translation regulation controls the levels of protein synthesized from a specific mRNA. It involves specific RNA secondary structures on the mRNA and ribosomal recruitment on the initiation codons, and modulation of the elongation or termination stages of protein synthesis. Important regulation is in place at the levels of translation and enzymatic activities. The only effect of a signal transduction pathway that is observed via a gene expression experiment is the end point, the downstream effects. DNA microarrays currently have little utility in determining these post-translational modifications, which influence the diversity, affinity, function, cellular abundance and transport of proteins.

One argument for the use of next-generation sequencing approaches for the analysis of gene expression (RNA sequencing or RNAseq) is that the genome is in flux from the viewpoint of its annotation. Updates to the human genome consensus sequence are frequent. This means that a given microarray build is frozen in time from the viewpoint of probe content, as it is dependent on the genome build which guided its probe design and fabrication. Arrays contain probes that, over time, may become irrelevant. Furthermore, arrays may lack probes for newly discovered or annotated genes. Transcriptome sequencing does not have this limitation, as it is not dependent on the selection of probes at a given time point. The output from a transcriptome-sequencing experiment is a collection of short sequence tags or reads. As the annotation of the human genome and transcriptomes becomes more refined, older sequencing data still have relevance as they can be mapped to the newest genome build, permitting additional analysis of the particular experiment. This luxury is not afforded by microarrays. Additionally, microarrays rely on the energy kinetics of probe binding, meaning that a low copy number transcript can be swamped by non-specific hybridization events and therefore remain undetected. DNA sequencing, on the other hand, can produce a very small number of true hits. A summary of the salient features of DNA microarray and massively parallel sequencing technology is presented in Table 7.1.

SEQUENCING AND IMPLICATIONS FOR PHARMACOGENOMICS TESTING

In the past, the methods employed for genetic testing have been both labor-intensive and complex. Today, genetic testing laboratories demand the simultaneous analysis of multiple nucleic acid markers per patient sample. Microarray technology has proven a practical approach to obtain multiplexed analysis permitting rapid biomarker interrogation in large

TABLE 7.1   Salient Features of Massively Parallel Sequencing and DNA Microarrays

Massively parallel sequencing	DNA microarrays
a priori knowledge of sequences not required	Prior knowledge of sequences required
High precision and high sensitivity	Less precision and sensitivity
Expensive and labor-intensive	Cost effective; streamlined catalog arrays available
Complex data storage and manipulation	Modest data storage and manipulation
Digital data (sequence tags and counts)	Analog data (intensity information)
Ordered Poisson-based process, high sensitivity, limited noise	Hybridization based technology, limited sensitivity, background noise
Genome-wide analysis	Genome-wide analysis, but not truly genome wide as dependent on probes

patient cohorts. The transition from the research laboratory to the clinical setting has been steady but slow. Continued success of microarrays in the clinical laboratory will depend on their ability to perform in the more rigorous clinical environment and deliver high quality, reproducible and robust results.

The clinical environment poses a different set of challenges for array technology, as performance criteria are measured differently to the research laboratory. An important consideration from an economic standpoint is that the cost per reportable result holds greater significance than the cost per data point. Other key factors are the requirements for automation from sample processing to end result, precision and accuracy of the results, and the need to process multiple tests in parallel under strict regulatory guidelines and compliances.

The emergence and rapidly diminishing cost of high-throughput sequencing technologies will have consequences for the future use of microarrays in both research and clinical settings. The full-genome arrays widely utilized at present will eventually be replaced with low-cost sequencing approaches which are immune from the problems that plague current microarray experiments, namely cross-hybridization of related species, poor hybridization kinetics, interference from DNA secondary structure, noise from DNA repetitive elements, poor sensitivity in relation to low-abundance transcripts, and the inability to distinguish between genes of interest and pseudogenes. A severe limitation of most of the microarray platforms in use today is the inability to discriminate between mRNA splice-variants, an obstacle that is easily addressed via high-throughput sequencing approaches.

Ultra-high throughput technologies have found considerable use in re-sequencing human genomes, epigenetic studies using sodium bisulfite sequencing expanded to whole-genome analysis, novel discovery efforts such as uncovering small RNAs and microRNAs relevant to disease, and the characterization of microbial communities in diseased tissues permitting pathogen identification and the potential of tailored therapy. *In vitro* and *in situ* expression profiling during the development of an organism from fertilized egg to maturity will become a routine exercise in the future. The sequence information obtained will provide discrete digital tags, facilitating a direct count of transcript copy number in healthy and diseased cells.

These biomarkers will provide novel targets for early diagnosis and therapeutic intervention for many human diseases.

Individual genome sequencing is finding its niche in personalized and preventative medicine approaches. Diminishing costs have reduced human genome sequencing to under US$10 000 at the time of writing, and with continued technology advances and improvements the US$100 genome should be a reality within the next decade. Presently the costs remain prohibitive to support routine re-sequencing of individual human genomes at sufficient depth of coverage to accurately call single nucleotide polymorphisms, insertions and deletions with a high degree of confidence. In the short term, the focus will therefore be on characterizing defined genomic regions that encompass disease-causing genes. This strategy involves selection of disease-related target sequences using capture or target enrichment approaches — processes which are not without selection bias.

"Retail genomics" has emerged in the past few years, with clinical diagnostic and prognostic testing routinely available for common and rare inherited disease conditions, risk assessment and prevention, and *a priori* stratification for pharmacogenetic contraindications using microarray-based approaches. As this evolves from genotyping to complete genome sequencing, ethical issues currently under consideration will become even more pertinent. A scenario where a patient opts to remain ignorant of a predisposition to a late-onset disease — particularly one that cannot be treated, prevented or ameliorated — is understandable. That public disclosure of such information could influence health insurability and employment prospects is a frightening possibility. Greater pressure to live healthy lives, predictive diagnoses, and treatment long before any physical evidence of disease manifests will exploit the use of personalized genome sequencing methods. Appropriate retraining of medical personnel in genomic medicine will be an *a priori* requirement so that they are better equipped to counsel and treat patients presenting with the awareness of possessing genetic aberrations.

CONCLUSIONS

Many of the traditional methods that have been employed for genetic testing are labor-intensive and complex. Microarray technology has provided a practical approach to multiplex genetic analysis, allowing high-throughput measurements of gene expression. Although widely accepted as a research tool for over a decade, acceptance of microarray technology in the clinical environment has been slow. The long-term success of microarrays in the clinical laboratory will depend on their ability to adapt to this more rigorous environment and provide high quality, cost-effective, reproducible and robust results. In the clinical setting, automation from sample processing to end result is mandatory. Furthermore, strict regulatory guidelines must be carefully adhered to.

Next-generation sequencing technology is redefining clinical diagnostics and ultimately will make current microarray approaches obsolete. The challenge moving forward will be for healthcare providers to assimilate the vast genomic information relating to all variations in an individual and prescribe effective and customized modes of treatment. How to correlate this information with patient phenotype, particularly in the context of disease predisposition and pharmacogenomics, will be the topic of much study in the coming years.

References

[1] Marton MJ, DeRisi JL, Bennett HA, et al. Drug target validation and identification of secondary drug target effects using DNA microarrays. Nature Med 1998;4:1293—301.

[2] Brown PO, Botstein D. Exploring the new world of the genome with DNA microarrays. Nat Genet 1999;21:33—7.

[3] Hardiman G, Carmen A. DNA biochips — past, present and future; an overview. In: Carmen A, Hardiman G, editors. Biochips as Pathways to Discovery. New York, NY: Taylor & Francis; 2006. p. 1—13.

[4] Hardiman G. Microarray platforms — comparisons and contrasts. Pharmacogenomics 2004;5:487—502.

[5] Chee M, Yang R, Hubbell E, et al. Accessing genetic information with high-density DNA arrays. Science 1996;274:610—4.

[6] Lipshutz RJ, Fodor SPA, Gingeras TR, Lockhart DJ. High density synthetic oligonucleotide arrays. Nat Gen Suppl 1999;21:20—4.

[7] Hughes TR, Mao M, Jones AR, et al. Expression profiling using microarrays fabricated by an ink-jet oligonucleotide synthesizer. Nat Biotechnol 2001;19:342—7.

[8] Mardis ER. The impact of next-generation sequencing technology on genetics. Trends Genet 2008;24:133—41.

[9] Margulies M, Egholm M, Altman WE, et al. Genome sequencing in microfabricated high-density picolitre reactors. Nature 2005;437:376—80.

[10] Shendure J, Mitra RD, Varma C, Church GM. Advanced sequencing technologies: methods and goals. Nat Rev Genet 2004;5:335—44.

[11] Vilo J, Kivinen K. Regulatory sequence analysis: application to the interpretation of gene expression. Eur Neuropsychopharmacol 2001;11:399—411.

[12] Waring JF, Ciurlionis R, Jolly RA, et al. Microarray analysis of hepatotoxins *in vitro* reveals a correlation between gene expression profiles and mechanisms of toxicity. Toxicol Lett 2001;120:359—68.

[13] Hamadeh HK, Amin RP, Paules RS, Afshari CA. An overview of toxicogenomics. Curr Issues Mol Biol 2002;4:45—56.

[14] Johnson JA. Drug target pharmacogenomics: an overview. Am J Pharmacogenomics 2001;1:271—81.

[15] Kruglyak L, Nickerson DA. Variation is the spice of life. Nat Genet 2001;27:234—6.

[16] Evans WE, Relling MV. Pharmacogenomics: translating functional genomics into rational therapeutics. Science 1999;286:487—91.

[17] Bhasker CR, Hardiman G. Advances in pharmacogenomics technologies. Pharmacogenomics 2010;11:481—5.

[18] Ensom MH, Chang TK, Patel P. Pharmacogenetics: the therapeutic drug monitoring of the future? Clin Pharmacokinet 2001;40:783—802.

[19] Collins FS. Medical and societal consequences of the Human Genome Project. N Engl J Med 1999;341:28.

[20] Kleyn PW, Vesell ES. Genetic variation as a guide to drug development. Science 1998;281:1820.

[21] PricewaterhouseCoopers' Health Research Institute. The new science of personalized medicine. Available at, http://www.pwc.com/personalizedmedicine; 2009.

[22] Hardiman G. Applications of microarrays and biochips in pharmacogenomics. Methods Mol Biol 2008;448:21—30.

[23] Lundkvist J, Jönsson B. Pharmacoeconomics of adverse drug reactions. Fund Clin Pharmacol 2004;18:275—80.

[24] Amur S, Zineh I, Abernethy DR, et al. Pharmacogenomics and adverse drug reactions. Personal Med 2010;7:633—42.

[25] Routledge PA, O'Mahony MS, Woodhouse KW. Adverse drug reactions in elderly patients. Br J Clin Pharmacol 2004;57:121—6.

[26] Nuwaysir EF, Huang W, Albert TJ, et al. Gene expression analysis using oligonucleotide arrays produced by maskless photolithography. Genome Res 2002;12:1749—55.

[27] Ramakrishnan R, Dorris D, Lublinsky A, et al. An assessment of Motorola CodeLink™ microarray performance for gene expression profiling applications. Nucleic Acids Res 2002;30:e30.

[28] Gunderson KL, Kuhn KM, Steemers FJ, et al. Whole-genome genotyping of haplotype tag single nucleotide polymorphisms. Pharmacogenomics 2006;7:641—8.

[29] Steemers FJ, Chang W, Lee G, et al. Whole-genome genotyping with the single-base extension assay. Nat Methods 2006;3:31—3.

[30] The International HapMap Consortium. A second generation human haplotype map of over 3.1 million SNPs. Nature 2007;449:851—62.

[31] Stankiewicz P, Lupski JR. Structural variation in the human genome and its role in disease. Annu Rev Med 2010;61:437—55.

[32] Mahant V, Kureshy F, Vairavan R, Hardiman G. The INFINITI system — an automated multiplexing microarray platform. In: Hardiman G, editor. Microarray Methods and Applications. Eagleville, PA: DNA Press Inc.; 2003. p. 325—8.

[33] Kim P, Fu YKK, Mahant V, et al. The next generation of automated microarray platform for a multiplexed CYP2D6 assay. In: Carmen A, Hardiman G, editors. Biochips as Pathways to Discovery. New York, NY: Taylor & Francis; 2006. p. 97—108.

[34] Sanger F, Nicklen S, Coulson AR. DNA sequencing with chain-terminating inhibitors. Proc Natl Acad Sci USA 1977;74:5463—7.

[35] Sanger F, Coulson AR. A rapid method for determining sequences in DNA by primed synthesis with DNA polymerase. J Mol Biol 1975;94:441—8.

[36] Sanger F, Air GM, Barrell BG, et al. Nucleotide sequence of bacteriophage phi X174 DNA. Nature 1977;265:687—95.

[37] Maxam AM, Gilbert W. A new method for sequencing DNA. Proc Natl Acad Sci USA 1977;74:560—4.

[38] Rogers YH, Venter JC. Genomics: massively parallel sequencing. Nature 2005;437:326—7.

[39] Margulies M, Egholm M, Altman WE, et al. Genome sequencing in microfabricated high-density picolitre reactors. Nature 2005;437:376—80.

[40] Wheeler DA, Srinivasan M, Egholm M, et al. The complete genome of an individual by massively parallel DNA sequencing. Nature 2008;452:872—6.

[41] Korbel JO, Urban AE, Affourtit JP, et al. Paired-end mapping reveals extensive structural variation in the human genome. Science 2007;318:420—6.

[42] Shendure J, Mitra RD, Varma C, Church GM. Advanced sequencing technologies: methods and goals. Nat Rev Genet 2004;5:335—44.

[43] Johnson DS, Mortazavi A, Myers RM, Wold B. Genome-wide mapping of *in vivo* protein—DNA interactions. Science 2007;316:1497—502.

[44] Barski A, Cuddapah S, Cui K, et al. High-resolution profiling of histone methylations in the human genome. Cell 2007;129:823—37.

[45] Winters-Hilt S, Vercoutere W, DeGuzman VS, et al. Highly accurate classification of Watson—Crick basepairs on termini of single DNA molecules. Biophys J 2003;84:967—76.

[46] Okou DT, Steinberg KM, Middle C, et al. Microarray-based genomic selection for high-throughput resequencing. Nat Methods 2007;11:907—9.

[47] Hodges E, Xuan Z, Balija V, et al. Genome-wide *in situ* exon capture for selective resequencing. Nat Genet 2007;39:1522—7.

[48] Albert TJ, Molla MN, Muzny DM, et al. Direct selection of human genomic loci by microarray hybridization. Nat Methods 2007;11:903—5.

[49] Porreca GJ, Zhang K, Li JB, et al. Multiplex amplification of large sets of human exons. Nat Methods 2007;11:931—6.

CHAPTER

8

Pharmacogenomics and Warfarin Therapy

Jennifer Martin[1], Andrew Somogyi[2]

[1]School of Medicine, University of Queensland, Princess Alexandra Hospital, Brisbane, Australia
[2]Discipline of Pharmacology, University of Adelaide, Adelaide, Australia

INTRODUCTION

Warfarin is the most commonly prescribed anticoagulant drug for the prophylaxis and treatment of venous and arterial thromboembolic disorders, with more than 20 million scripts each year in United States alone. This volume of use persists despite newer anticoagulation medications now entering the market, predominantly because warfarin has a wealth of efficacy data around its use, is relatively cheap and is routinely used by many patients with atrial fibrillation. However, warfarin has a narrow therapeutic index, multiple clinically-important drug—drug interactions and an erratic safety profile — conditions which would impede its market approval if developed today. In reality though, its use has been well managed by clinicians by using the international normalized ratio (INR) measurements and adjustment of dose to reduce the risk of bleeding. Time in INR therapeutic range has been shown to directly correlate with efficacy and bleeding [1]. However, with current management, patients remain on average within their target INR range for only 70% of the time [1] and bleeding events do occur. The 10-fold variability around dose, target INR and side effects has therefore led to interest in whether testing for genetic variations in warfarin metabolism and target site could be useful for predicting the optimum dose, reducing bleeding risk and reducing the time to achieve a therapeutic prothrombin time, expressed as the INR.

THE POTENTIAL OF PHARMACOGENETICS FOR WARFARIN

Warfarin is a potential candidate for pharmacogenetic testing as it is a commonly used medication, has a narrow therapeutic window and displays highly variable pharmacokinetics and responses between individuals such that achieving and maintaining INRs within the therapeutic range that reduces adverse drug events can be difficult and time consuming. Further, warfarin has a mechanism of action and elimination pathways that involve enzymes that are polymorphic; variations that account for 30—50% of the variability in dosing. Thus there has been much interest in whether testing for these variants improves warfarin safety and efficacy.

There have been a number of retrospective studies examining the relationship between pharmacogenetics, clinical variations and outcomes. However, the effect sizes are variable and clinical outcomes often not measured; thus there has been discussion as to the actual clinical relevance of these genetic tests. Whilst there remains some uncertainty, it is agreed both that the analytical validity of these tests has been met and that there is strong evidence to support association between these genetic variants and the therapeutic dose of warfarin [2]. The FDA (Federal Drug Administration of the United States) updated warfarin's label in 2007 to reflect the influence of genetic polymorphisms, with recommendations to consider lower initiation doses for warfarin-naïve patients with genetic variations. At that stage it was recommended that prospective clinical trials were needed to inform the degree of benefit or disadvantage before recommending routine genetic testing in warfarin-naïve patients. In 2010 the FDA recommended that prescribers now refer to a table showing stable maintenance doses and dosing ranges observed in multiple patients having different combinations of genetic variants [3]. This information actually resulted from examination of a pharmacogenetic dose algorithm derived from a study of an over 4000-patient dataset [4]. This study showed that dosage recommendations that were based on the combined pharmacogenetic-clinical algorithm were significantly better than those that were based on an algorithm that used only clinical variables or those that were based on a fixed-dose strategy. The combined algorithm in this study included variables of age, height, weight, amiodarone use, race and presence of enzyme inducer, as well as the genetic polymorphisms in the C1 sub-unit of the vitamin K 2, 3 epoxide reductase complex (VKORC1) and CYP2C9 (an isoenzyme in the

Cytochrome P450 family of enzymes responsible for metabolism of majority of drugs), and is available at www.warfarindosing.org.

PHARMACOLOGY

Warfarin is an equal mixture of the enantiomers S-warfarin and R-warfarin, with S-warfarin being approximately three to five times more potent than R-warfarin (Fig. 8.1). It is generally considered that S-warfarin is the pharmacologically active enantiomer and that R-warfarin plays only a small role. Metabolism of S-warfarin occurs through the cytochrome P450 2C9 enzyme to the 6- and 7-hydroxy metabolites, while metabolism of the less potent R-warfarin occurs through CYP2C19 (8-hydroxy), CYP1A2 (6-hydroxy), CYP3A4 (10-hydroxy) and carbonyl reductase of the side chain ketone to form the alcohols 1 and 2 [5] (Fig. 8.2).

CYP2C9 Status

People who metabolize warfarin "normally" are homozygous for the usual (wild-type) allele CYP2C9*1. Two clinically relevant single nucleotide polymorphisms have been identified in CYP2C9 (*2[C430T] and *3[A1075C]). These result in reduced enzymatic activity (*2 has about 12% S-warfarin metabolic activity and *3 has <5% activity compared to the wild-type) and therefore reduced S-warfarin metabolism. The *2/*2 homozygous genotype leads to a 12% reduction in CYP2C9 activity, and the *3/*3 homozygous genotype has less than 5% of wild-type CYP2C9 activity. These single nucleotide polymorphisms are relatively common in Caucasians. Approximately 1% of the population is homozygous for CYP2C9*2 and 20% are heterozygous carriers of this allele. The corresponding figures for CYP2C9*3 are 0.4% and 8%. Another 1.4% of people are compound heterozygotes (CYP2C9*2/*3). However, there are wide inter-ethnic differences in the frequencies of the *2 allele (practically absent in Asian and Indian populations, and very low in Africans and African-Americans) and *3 (high incidence in Indians and low in Africans and African-Americans) (Table 8.1).

Patients requiring a low dose of warfarin (1.5 mg daily or less) have a high likelihood of having a CYP2C9 variant allele (*2 or *3) and an increased risk of major bleeding complications [6]. A number of studies have shown that knowing the patient's genotype helps in achieving the target INR more quickly [7—9]. However, if this does not result in a reduction of hospital bed stay, reduction of bleeding or other clinical endpoint, the relevance of

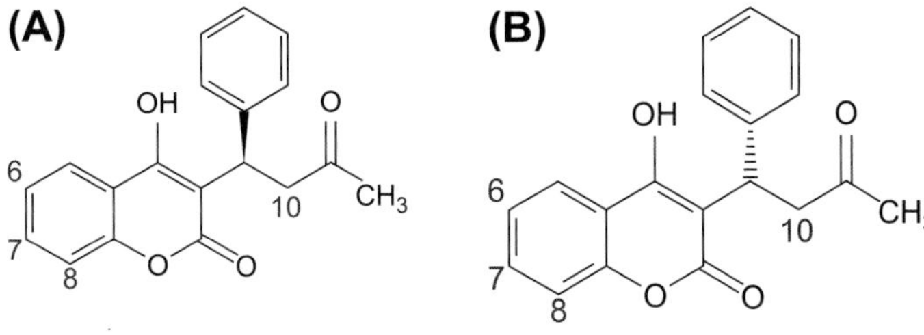

FIGURE 8.1 Structures of (A) R-warfarin and (B) S-warfarin. Numbers are the sites of metabolism.

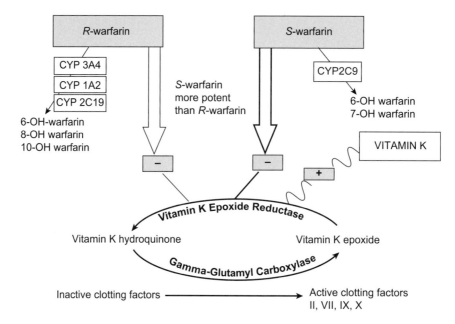

FIGURE 8.2   Summary of metabolism of warfarin.

reducing time to target INR by a small amount many not provide any meaningful benefit. Specifically, using this knowledge to predict dose may not necessarily even reduce bleeding events, as CYP2C9 genotype *per se* predicts only 10–15% of dose variability [9]. Even after adjusting the warfarin dose for the variability in CYP2C9 status, there is still a considerable amount of dosing variability in patients who have similar CYP2C9 alleles. This variability appears to be partly attributable to genetic polymorphisms in the C1 subunit of the vitamin K 2, 3 epoxide reductase complex (VKORC1). The VKORC1 complex is the rate-limiting step in the vitamin K-dependent gamma carboxylation system which activates clotting factors. Warfarin exerts its anticoagulant effect by inhibiting VKORC1 (Fig. 8.3).

TABLE 8.1   Frequencies (%) of the Two Major CYP2C9
Variant Alleles in Various Populations

Population	*2	*3
Caucasian	15	7
Asian (Han Chinese, Korean, Japanese)	0	3
Indian	0	18
African	0	1
African-American	0	1
Hispanic	7	6

FIGURE 8.3 Vitamin K-dependent gamma carboxylation system. Warfarin reduces the regeneration of vitamin K by inhibiting vitamin K epoxide reductase. This reduces the gamma-carboxylation of coagulation factors, reducing their functionality.

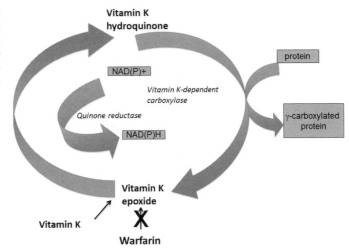

VKORC1 Status

A number of common polymorphisms in non-coding sequences have been identified in VKORC1; seven were found to be significantly associated with warfarin maintenance dosage and five were in strong linkage disequilibrium [10]. As such, low-dose (A) (2.7 ± 0.2 mg/day) and high-dose (B) (6.2 ± 0.3 mg/day) haplotypes were identified, and again these haplotypes showed substantial inter-ethnic differences with Caucasians and Indians having 40–45% A and 45–55% B, Chinese almost 90% A, and Africans 15% A and 50% B and a sizable missing haplotype (Table 8.2). Polymorphisms of this receptor are associated with a need for lower doses of warfarin [10]. The *VKORC1* genotype alone may explain up to 35% of the variability in warfarin dosage [11].

TABLE 8.2 Frequencies (%) of the Two Major *VKORC1* Haplotypes in Various Populations

Population	A (Low dose)[1]	B (High dose)[2]
Caucasian	40	45
Asian (Han Chinese, Korean, Japanese)	90	10
Indian	45	45
African	15	50
African-American	10	50
Hispanic	44	40

[1]includes −1639G > A (rs9923231), 1173C > T(rs9934438); 2.7 ± 0.2 mg/day [9].
[2]3730G > A (rs7294); 6.2 ± 0.3 mg/day [9].

Other Genetic Mutations

It is likely that point mutations in the genes other than those for CYP2C9 or VKORC1 add to the variability in warfarin requirements. Evidence for this comes from at least two models which have demonstrated that the CYP2C9 and VKORC1 genotypes, together with known factors such as age and body size, only explain half to two-thirds of the inter-individual variability in warfarin requirements [9, 12]. Although this is an improvement on current non-pharmacogenetic algorithms, at least one-third of the variability is still unaccounted for. There are at least 30 other genes involved in the pharmacodynamics of warfarin which may explain this variability, including polymorphisms in apolipoprotein E, multidrug resistance 1 (MDR1), genes encoding vitamin K-dependent clotting factors and possibly genes encoding additional components of the vitamin K epoxide reductase complex. Evidence for these is lacking. However, recently polymorphisms in CYP4F2, an enzyme involved in vitamin K oxidation, have been associated with altered warfarin dosage requirements, although the contribution is minor at less than 3% in Caucasians but up to 10% in some Asian populations [13].

The first genome-wide association study (GWAS) was recently conducted in over 1000 Swedish subjects and investigated about 326 000 markers, confirming the major role of VKORC1 followed by CYP2C9, and the minor role of CYP4F2 [14].

NON-GENETIC FACTORS AFFECTING WARFARIN DOSING

One of the difficulties with focusing solely on the effect of polymorphisms in the metabolizing pathways of S-warfarin and vitamin K epoxide reductase is that there are a number of important non-genetic factors that affect the INR and warfarin dosing requirements (Tables 8.3–8.5). Age, racial group and sex are well known, but increasingly recognized yet understudied is the effect of dietary and gut-derived vitamin K.

Vitamin K

Vitamin K is an essential cofactor for the normal production of clotting factors II, VII, IX and X. By inhibiting VKORC1, warfarin reduces the regeneration of vitamin K and thereby inhibits the activation of vitamin K-dependent clotting factors. It is known that a patient's vitamin K status when starting warfarin affects the time to reach a therapeutic INR. In addition, a daily dietary intake of more than 250 μg reduces warfarin sensitivity. Interesting from a therapeutic

TABLE 8.3 Non-genetic Factors Associated with Variation in Warfarin Requirements

Dietary vitamin K (average plus daily intake)	Altering vitamin K intake alters warfarin requirements
Variation in concomitant medications or CYP-interacting foods	Includes alteration in dose of drugs such as amiodarone or thyroxine, plus short courses of antibiotics, intermittent ingestion of foods such as grapefruit juice or St John's wort
Diarrhoea	Reduces vitamin K recycling in gut wall

TABLE 8.4 Factors Associated with Lower Warfarin Requirements

VKORC1;−1639 AA	This genotype affects warfarin requirement less than GA or GG genotypes
CYP2C9 *2 or *3 CYP2C9 *2 and *3	Both heterozygotes of *2 or *3 or homozygotes of *2 and *3 result in a reduced warfarin requirement
Factor X insertion genotype	Mildly lower reduction
Factor VII deletion genotype	Mildly lower reduction
Reduced vitamin K intake	For example, if starving or in institutional care
Some racial groups	May be independent or secondary to known racially divergent CYP2C9 or VKORC1 mutations, different diet or additional factor
Gender	Gender did not make any significant contribution to the regression models but it is likely that the differences in warfarin requirements noted clinically are attributable to body size, with females in general smaller than males
Age	Reduced requirements for age may be secondary to altered distribution, altered receptor sensitivity or reduced clearance
Advanced malignancy	Reduced requirements may be due to liver metastases, lower body weight and drug interactions
Malabsorption syndromes	Affects vitamin K production and absorption in gut
Liver disease	Affects synthetic functions of liver, including production of clotting factors and warfarin metabolism
Heart disease	Causes hepatic congestion, resulting in abnormal liver function and reduced clotting factor synthesis
Pyrexia	Increases warfarin sensitivity by enhancing the rate of degradation of vitamin K-dependent clotting factors

TABLE 8.5 Factors Associated with Higher Warfarin Requirements

Increased body weight	Higher total and lean body weight increase warfarin requirements, possibly through their effect on increasing body surface area
Smoking	Increased metabolism, particular of the R-enantiomer
CYP2C9 inducers	Induces metabolism of the more potent S-enantiomer

perspective is the finding that giving patients with an unstable INR daily doses of vitamin K of 150 µg decreases the variability of INR and increases the time in the target range [15].

Diet

Until recently it had been assumed that all dietary effects on warfarin were due to vitamin K content. However, the role of other chemicals and vitamins in food may also have an effect on warfarin carboxylation or activity, perhaps by changing gut flora (and gut-derived vitamin K), pharmacodynamic effects on other blood coagulation pathways — for example, as seen with dong quai, garlic, papaya and St John's wort (serotonin effect) — or competing reductase systems [16]. However, this effect has not been as rigorously studied, and instead most of the studied dietary effects are due to intake of vitamin K in foods such as green tea, turnips, avocados and green leafy vegetables (e.g., Brussels sprouts, broccoli, lettuce and cabbage) [17]. Similarly, certain beverages can increase the effect of warfarin on bleeding outcomes, such as cranberry juice and alcohol intake. The latter may also contribute to a higher risk of bleeding due to increased likelihood and severity of falls and gastritis.

Age

The use of warfarin is expanding among the population over 70 years of age in part because of the increasing prevalence of atrial fibrillation but also because of increased longevity and quality of life. However, there is still limited availability of dose data for this population, although dosing regimens in most medical centers opt for a 5 mg or lower dosage of warfarin per day as the starting dose in people over 70. The lower requirement for the induction and maintenance dose is likely to be due to a number of factors, including drug interactions (owing to a higher likelihood of co-morbidity and polypharmacy in this age group); reduced dietary vitamin K intake (especially in residential/nursing home subjects or recipients of "meals on wheels"); and reduced absorption of vitamin K due to changes in bowel flora (also likely to be related to dietary changes). Reduced volume of distribution may be an issue if lower total body fat or low serum albumin occurs, but there is uncertainty in the literature as to whether clearance changes with age. For example, there are some studies, including a population pharmacokinetic model, showing that warfarin clearance is inversely related to age [18, 19], especially the clearance of R-warfarin; however there are many others not showing any significant difference of clearance with age, albeit in studies with small numbers of elderly subjects [20, 21]. Measuring free as opposed to total warfarin clearance may be relevant to this debate, as it has recently been demonstrated that the unbound clearance of R- and S-warfarin decreases by approximately 0.5% per year [22]. There is also known to be an up to 30% decline in hepatic drug metabolism and cytochrome P450 content with age; the clinical effect of this on INR has not been clearly reported. However, there is a large amount of literature on the effect of weight and body size on clearance, and thus it is possible that the effect of age on warfarin is a surrogate of the factors above such as diet and reduction in body weight or change in body composition with age.

A recent prospective study of 4616 patients, including 2359 patients over 80 years of age, has shown that the warfarin dose is not only inversely related to age but also strongly associated with gender. The weekly warfarin dose declined by 0.4 mg/y (95% confidence interval [CI], 0.37–0.44; $P < 0.001$) [23]. Among patients who were > 70 years of age, an initiation dose of 5 mg daily would have been excessive for 82% of women and 65% of men.

Gender

It has been well established that women in general need a lower maintenance dose of warfarin that men. For example, in the large study conducted above, females required 4.5 mg less warfarin per week than males (95% CI, 3.8–5.3; $P < 0.001$). The effects of age were clear (and additive) to gender; however, the effects of differences in lean versus fat body mass on this gender difference were not reported.

Anthropometric Variables

There is a large literature examining the effect of body size variables on warfarin dosage requirements. By themselves, body surface area and body weight have significant correlations with warfarin dose; however, they do not appear to make a significant contribution to the regression model for dose once genotype and other factors are added [24]. In a later model, age, height and CYP2C9 genotype were shown to significantly contribute to the more potent S-warfarin and total warfarin clearance, whereas only age and body size significantly contributed to R-warfarin clearance. The multivariate regression model including the variables of age, CYP2C9 and VKORC1 genotype, and height produced the best model for estimating warfarin dose ($r^2 = 55\%$) [12].

CLINICAL RELEVANCE

Pharmacogenetic testing for warfarin therapy is not yet a routine practice because alone it does not predict all the variability in a patient's response to warfarin. However, it has far greater clinical effect than the non-genetic factors, especially when pharmacogenetics is combined with the clinical factors. Furthermore, clinicians require easily available information that can help them to predict an individual's warfarin requirements with close to 100% accuracy in both the induction and maintenance phases of therapy. This is especially relevant when starting treatment, as this is when the risk of bleeding due to over-anticoagulation is high. The induction regimens in current use are only moderately successful in achieving the target INR, especially in older people [25]. It also takes up to 14 days to reach a therapeutic INR for some people. Additionally, once treatment is started using induction doses tailored for elderly patients, the contribution of VKORC1 and CYP2C9 genotypes in dose refinement appears to be negligible compared with two INR values measured during the first week of treatment [26]. Nevertheless, patients with either *VKORC1 A/A* haplotype or *CYP2C9 *2* or **3* genotype had a significantly reduced time to first INR being in the therapeutic range and to the first INR of more than 4; however, this was not a significant predictor of the time to the first INR within the therapeutic range. Both the genotypes had a significant influence on the required warfarin dose after the first 2 weeks of therapy [27].

Interestingly, the initiation regimen and long-term rules that have specifically been developed and included in a computerized dosage program improve quality of anticoagulation in elderly inpatients [28]. In non-elderly patients, even knowing the patient's CYP2C9 and VKORC1 status predicts less than half of the variation in the response to warfarin. Better predictions are achieved by incorporating pharmacogenetics into a dosing algorithm such as that based on the regression model of Sconce [12]. In this model, the variables age, height, and CYP2C9 and VKORC1 genotypes were the best predictors for estimating the starting dose of warfarin. This algorithm also confirmed that the mean warfarin daily dose requirement is significantly lower with some genotypes.

This model is a marked improvement on current algorithms, although it still only explains about half of the variability in dose requirements. However, it has been shown that, despite the shortcomings, a pharmacogenetics algorithm is clinically helpful to predict appropriate initial doses of warfarin in high-risk patients. In a recent study in almost 900 patients, providing CYP2C9 and VKORC1 genotype information to the prescribers resulted in a 28% reduction in hospitalizations due to hemorrhage over 6 months [12].

There are other algorithms for warfarin dosing that take into account genetic and non-genetic factors, some of which are web-based (www.warfarindosing.org). In addition, the FDA has now made specific dosing recommendations for warfarin based on genotype and non-genetic factors [3], and has made strong suggestions that genotype be considered when warfarin is to be initiated. In addition, a recent analysis of 13 warfarin algorithms concluded that most performed well in the intermediate-dose range (21−49 mg/week) compared to the low- (< 21 mg/week) and high- (> 49 mg/week) dose ranges and that admixed population algorithms were in general better performers than race-specific algorithms [29].

COST-EFFECTIVENESS OF PHARMACOGENOMICS TESTING IN WARFARIN THERAPY

As with all new technologies, it is important to evaluate the incremental cost-effectiveness of pharmacogenetic testing versus standard clinical practice. Pharmacogenetic testing for warfarin is relatively cheap compared to other anti-clotting medications such as new clotting factor inhibitors, or new health technologies such as nuclear medicine/magnetic resonance imaging fusion techniques. The extra costs of this warfarin service would have to include both the diagnostics of genotyping and clinical interpretative support. Analyzing CYP2C9 and VKORC1 genes, with the costs of clinical interpretation, is estimated at 100 Australian dollars (AUD) per person, with a clinically realistic turnaround time (within 1 day). As multiple platforms are now available, the costs are rapidly declining.

For the cost-effectiveness analysis, the efficacy of pharmacogenetic tests is measured as the reduction in the number of expensive adverse effects, the time in hospital, and the improvement in quality of life due to less frequent INR monitoring. None of this has been accurately quantified in a prospective study, yet it is clear that a reduction in hospital stay by even 1 day would provide a sizeable cost saving. However, while testing seems relatively good value for money, there are additional issues to consider − for example, the cost of screening all potential warfarin users, and the cost of pharmacist or clinical pharmacologist time. It would also be an additional cost to current therapy, with INR testing still required, albeit possibly less often. Additionally, although the prevalence of heterozygotes is relatively high (approximately 30% for CYP2C9, depending on the ethnic group studied), patients with a null genotype (those likely to get life-threatening and expensive adverse effects) are rare (less than 1%). The detection rate for a genotype associated with serious adverse events is therefore low. Lastly, clinical outcomes such as bleeding are rare in patients followed in anticoagulation clinics because warfarin therapy is closely monitored and individualized. Thus, the benefit is likely to be much smaller in tertiary centers and much larger for the small numbers of patients that live in rural or remote settings away from easily available medical care. Further, the INR is a well-validated and inexpensive surrogate marker for warfarin effects which is already used widely in clinical practice. However, it is not helpful for predicting which dose of warfarin to use for starting anticoagulation, which is where pharmacogenetics testing could make a difference, especially in high-risk groups.

Comparative-effectiveness research is a developing field. Its relationship with individualized medicine to combine pharmacogenetic and clinical markers of warfarin use and response is of interest for its ability to accurately estimate and quantify comparative efficacy and toxicity with other medicines [30]. Decision tree analyses have also been developed to evaluate the potential clinical and economic outcomes of using genotype data to guide the management of warfarin therapy. In a recent study, a decision tree was designed to simulate the clinical and economic outcomes of patients newly started on warfarin with either no genotyping or CYP2C9 genotyping prior to initiation of warfarin therapy. The total number of events and the direct medical cost per 100 patient-years in the genotyped and non-genotyped groups were US\$9.58 and US\$155,700, and US\$10.48 and US\$150,500, respectively. The marginal cost per additional major bleeding averted in the genotyped group was US\$5778. The model was sensitive to the variation of the cost and reduction of bleeding rate in the intensified anticoagulation service, and concluded that incorporating pharmacogenetic management into warfarin therapy is potentially more effective in preventing bleeding with a marginal cost, depending on the relative local costs and local effectiveness, which would alter depending on patient-specific factors [31]. Additional local clinical and epidemiological studies, including studying benefits in different racial groups, are needed to assess the association between genotype and the absolute risk of adverse effects before a cost-effectiveness analysis can be completed for warfarin pharmacogenetic testing [32].

NEW MEDICATIONS TO REPLACE WARFARIN

As well as warfarin, other traditional anticoagulant drugs, including unfractionated heparin (UFH) and low-molecular-weight heparins (LMWH), have therapeutic issues such as slow onset of action, narrow therapeutic index, requirement for monitoring, and multiple food and drug interactions that make use expensive, slightly unpredictable and time-consuming.

New anticoagulants have been developed that target a single coagulation factor and have more predictable dose–response relationships than warfarin. These include direct thrombin inhibitors (DTIs) and Factor Xa inhibitors. However, despite being more pharmacologically "pure", in order to replace warfarin use they need to have all, or most of, the following: equivalent or superior efficacy, an easily available antidote, predictable toxicities with no unexpected toxicities, and a reasonable cost. So far, data are emerging for some of these newer anticoagulants on both efficacy and safety grounds. Dabigatran is a direct thrombin inhibitor, and is a new medication used in anticoagulation therapy. Oldgren et al. compared risk for stroke, bleeding and death in patients with atrial fibrillation receiving either warfarin or dabigatran, and observed that rates of stroke or systematic embolism in patients with dabigatran 150 mg twice daily and/or intracranial bleeding with dabigatran 150 mg b.i.d. or 110 mg b.i.d. were lower than those in patients receiving warfarin [33].

Selective inhibitors of specific coagulation factors represent a potentially exciting development in antithrombosis therapy, and may in time replace warfarin use. As compared to conventional drugs such as warfarin, they have the potential to be as effective, and safer and easier to use. However, clinical evidence so far has not yet shown superiority to older anticoagulants in all spheres, although data are promising. In particular, studies examining the potential for warfarin replacement in people with atrial fibrillation are encouraging.

CONCLUSIONS

The variability in warfarin dosage requirements is multifactorial, although genetic polymorphisms play a part. Current warfarin dosing algorithms fail to take into account genetics and other individual patient factors. Theoretically, including these factors could help in predicting an individual's loading and maintenance doses for safer anticoagulation. However, linear regression analysis, taking into account genetic polymorphisms of CYP2C9 and VKORC1 (additive effect), body weight, body surface area and height, has so far been able to capture only approximately half of the large inter- and intra-patient variation in dose requirements. Vitamin K status and alcohol intake, together with additional genetic factors, are likely to account for some of the remaining difference in warfarin requirements, but still need to be studied in a regression analysis. For now, incorporation of age, body surface area, and CYP2C9 and VKORC1 genotypes allow the best estimate of warfarin induction and maintenance dose. In addition, CYP2C9 and VKORC1 genotypes explain more of the dose variability than the other clinical variables, and several large prospective clinical trials are underway [28]. Pharmacogenomics *per se*, apart from a few examples such as homozygosity for the *CYP2C9*3* alleles, although attractive, seems to be unable to explain enough of the variation to ensure it is a helpful tool to predict dosing for all-comers currently. It is clear, however, that in certain situations CYP2C9 and VKORC1 testing may be useful, and warranted, in determining the cause of unusual therapeutic responses to warfarin therapy or in high-risk patients.

References

[1] Wieloch M, Sjalander A, Frykman V, et al. Anticoagulation control in Sweden: reports of time in therapeutic range, major bleeding, and thrombo-embolic complications from the national quality registry AuriculA. Eur Heart J 2011;32:2282.

[2] Flockhart DA, O'Kane D, Williams MS, et al. Pharmacogenetic testing of CYP2C9 and VKORC1 alleles for warfarin. Genet Med 2008;10:139–50.

[3] FDA. Drug advice for Coumadin® tablets (Warfarin Sodium Tablets, USP) and Crystalline Coumadin® for injection (Warfarin Sodium for Injection, USP). Available at, http://www.accessdata.fda.gov/drugsatfda_docs/label/2010/009218s108lbl.pdf; 2010. pp. 26–27.

[4] International Warfarin Pharmacogenetics Consortium. Estimation of the warfarin dose with clinical and pharmacogenetic data. N Engl J Med 2009;360:753–64.

[5] Kaminsky LS, Zhang ZY. Human P450 metabolism of warfarin. Pharmacol Ther 1997;73:67–74.

[6] Aithal GP, Day CP, Kesteven PJ, Daly AK. Association of polymorphisms in the cytochrome P450 CYP2C9 with warfarin dose requirement and risk of bleeding complications. Lancet 1999;353:717–9.

[7] Wilke RA, Berg RL, Vidaillet HJ, et al. Impact of age, CYP2C9 genotype and concomitant medication on the rate of rise for prothrombin time during the first 30 days of warfarin therapy. Clin Med Res 2005;3:207–13.

[8] Taube J, Halsall D, Baglin T. Influence of cytochrome P-450 CYP2C9 polymorphisms on warfarin sensitivity and risk of over-anticoagulation in patients on long-term treatment. Blood 2000;96:1816—9.

[9] Caldwell MD, Berg RL, Zhang KQ, et al. Evaluation of genetic factors for warfarin dose prediction. Clin Med Res 2007;5:8016.

[10] Rieder MJ, Reiner AP, Gage BF, et al. Effect of VKORC1 haplotypes on transcriptional regulation and warfarin dose. N Engl J Med 2005;352:2285—93.

[11] Bodin L, Verstuyft C, Tregouet DA, et al. Cytochrome P450 2C9 (CYP2C9) and vitamin K epoxide reductase (VKORC1) genotypes as determinants of acenocoumarol sensitivity. Blood 2005;106:135—40.

[12] Sconce EA, Khan TI, Wynne HA, et al. The impact of CYP2C9 and VKORC1 genetic polymorphism and patient characteristics upon warfarin dose requirements: proposal for a new dosing regimen. Blood 2005;106:2329—33.

[13] Caldwell MD, Awad T, Johnson JA, et al. CYP4F2 genetic variant alters required warfarin dose. Blood 2008;111:4106—12.

[14] Takeuchi F, McGinnis R, Bourgeois S, et al. A genome-wide association study confirms VKORC1, CYP2C9, and CYP4F2 as principal genetic determinants of warfarin dose. PLoS Genet 2009;5:e1000433.

[15] Sconce E, Avery P, Wynne H, Kamali F. Vitamin K supplementation can improve stability of anticoagulation for patients with unexplained variability in response to warfarin. Blood 2007;109:2419—23.

[16] Campbell P, Roberts G, Eaton V, et al. Managing warfarin therapy in the community. Aust Prescr 2001;24:86—9.

[17] Pittet D, Zingg W, Pfister R, et al. Secular trends in antibiotic use among neonates 2001—2008. Ped Infect Dis J 2011;30:365—70.

[18] Mungall DR, Ludden TM, Marshall J, et al. Population pharmacokinetics of racemic warfarin in adult patients. J Pharmacokinet Biopharm 1985;13:213—27.

[19] James AH, Britt RP, Raskino CL, Thompson SG. Factors affecting the maintenance dose of warfarin. J Clin Pathol 1992;45:704—6.

[20] Chan E, McLachlan AJ, Pegg M, et al. Disposition of warfarin enantiomers and metabolites in patients during multiple dosing with rac-warfarin. Br J Clin Pharmacol 1994;37:563—9.

[21] Routledge PA, Chapman PH, Davies DM, Rawlins MD. Factors affecting warfarin requirements. A prospective population study. Eur J Clin Pharmacol 1979;15:319—22.

[22] Jensen B, Chin P, Roberts RR, et al. Total and free clearance of R- and S-warfarin in elderly people. Basic Clin Pharmacol Toxicol 2010;107:354—5.

[23] Garcia D, Regan S, Crowther M, et al. Warfarin maintenance dosing patterns in clinical practice: implications for safer anticoagulation in the elderly population. Chest 2005;127:2049—56.

[24] Kamali F, Khan TI, King BP, et al. Contribution of age, body size, and CYP2C9 genotype to anticoagulant response to warfarin. Clin Pharmacol Ther 2004;75:204—12.

[25] Oates AJ, Jackson PR, Austin CA, Channer KS. A new regimen for starting warfarin therapy in out-patients. Br J Clin Pharmacol 1998;46:157—61.

[26] Moreau C, Pautas E, Gouin-Thibault I, et al. Predicting the warfarin maintenance dose in elderly inpatients at treatment initiation: accuracy of dosing algorithms incorporating or not VKORC1/CYP2C9 genotypes. J Thromb Haemost 2011;9:711—8.

[27] Schwarz UI, Ritchie MD, Bradford Y, et al. Genetic determinants of response to warfarin during initial anti-coagulation. N Engl J Med 2008;358:999—1008.

[28] Gouin-Thibault I, Levy C, Pautas E, et al. Improving anticoagulation control in hospitalized elderly patients on warfarin. J Am Geriatr Soc 2010;58:242—7.

[29] Shin J, Cao D. Comparison of warfarin pharmacogenetics dosing algorithms in a racially diverse large cohort. Pharmacogenomics 2011;12:125—34.

[30] Epstein RS, Teagarden JR. Comparative effectiveness research and personalized medicine: catalyzing or colliding? Pharmacoeconomics 2010;28:905—13.

[31] You JH, Chan FW, Wong RS, Cheng G. The potential clinical and economic outcomes of pharmacogenetics-oriented management of warfarin therapy — a decision analysis. Thromb Haemost 2004;92:590—7.

[32] Garber AM, Phelps CE. Economic foundations of cost-effectiveness analysis. J Health Econ 1997;16:1—31.

[33] Oldgren J, Allins M, Darius H, et al. Risks for stroke, bleeding and death in patients with atrial fibrillation receiving dabigatran or warfarin in relation to the CHADS2 score: a subgroup analysis of the RE-LY trial. Ann Intern Med 2011;155:660—7.

CHAPTER

9

Applications of Pharmacokinetic and Pharmacodynamic Principles to Optimize Drug Dosage Selection
Example of Antibiotic Therapy Management

Jill Butterfield, Thomas P. Lodise Jr., Manjunath P. Pai

Albany College of Pharmacy and Health Sciences, Albany, NY

OUTLINE

INTRODUCTION

The probability for a lead new molecular entity (NME) to enter the clinical domain is currently very low. The reasons for this high rate of failure are multifactorial, but a key determinant is often the result of serious adverse events or insufficient therapeutic response

Therapeutic Drug Monitoring: Newer Drugs and Biomarkers
DOI: 10.1016/B978-0-12-385467-4.00009-9

175

during Phase III clinical trials [1]. This failure during Phase III trials adds significant expense to the pharmaceutical industry, and ultimately the "shelving away" of compounds that are potentially active [1, 2]. Often, this failure can be linked to the evaluation of the "wrong" dosage regimen in Phase III trials. Hence, informed drug dose design can improve the probability of success for a NME within the current clinical drug development model. However, this probability of success hinges on an astute understanding of the specific exposure—response relationships.

Over the past 50 years, newer study designs and mathematical approaches have emerged to aid our understanding of exposure—response relationships [1]. Regulatory agencies have also outlined definite guidance to advocate for the integrated evaluation of exposure—response relationships into all phases of clinical drug development [3, 4]. Notably, sophisticated mathematical techniques are used to develop structural models with key covariates that accurately predict exposure—response relationships in the intended patient population [3]. This approach, known as pharmacokinetic—pharmacodynamic systems analyses, seeks to maximize the exposure—response information obtained from clinical trials [5]. The models developed from these analyses can then be used to extrapolate doses into more heterogeneous populations than were initially studied [5]. In addition, improvements in our measurements of therapeutic and toxicologic effects of a drug using novel biomarkers can also be used to refine drug dose design for currently marketed drugs [6]. This goal of optimizing drug dosing is particularly applicable to special patient populations. Regulatory bodies currently recognize pregnancy, gender, geriatric and pediatric patients, and patients with kidney and liver dysfunction as special populations where additional pharmacokinetic and pharmacodynamic studies are needed to ensure optimal dosing [7]. However, as can be expected, other special populations such as the obese, patients with HIV and patients that receive various modalities of chronic renal replacement therapy exist. Specific dosing guidance in these populations that are not as yet recognized to be "special" by regulatory bodies is often lacking. This is concerning because these special populations comprise a large and emerging segment of the global population. As examples, 1 in 3 Americans are obese, 1 million Americans will require hemodialysis by the year 2015, and 33 million people are living with HIV worldwide [8—10]. Optimizing drug dosing and treatment strategies in special populations will improve health outcomes and reduce overall healthcare costs.

The current chapter outlines the key approaches to pharmacokinetic and pharmacodynamic systems analyses as tools for optimal drug dose design. Specific examples are provided from an antimicrobial perspective to demonstrate the applicability of this science to optimize dose selection. We advocate the use of these principles to improve extant drug dosing regimens as well as the probability of success of NME in clinical drug development.

PHARMACOKINETICS AND PHARMACODYNAMICS

Evaluation of the drug exposure—response relationship is a fundamental necessity for optimal dose selection [4]. Drug exposure evaluation includes evaluation of the time-course relationship of drug absorption, distribution, metabolism and elimination by an organism, a science known as pharmacokinetics [5]. The relationship of pharmacologic or toxicologic response in an organism as a function of the drug concentration time-course is the science known as pharmacodynamics [5]. Pharmacodynamic relationships are therefore dependent on pharmacokinetics, and so these branches of pharmacology are commonly referred to in the same breath as pharmacokinetic/pharmacodynamic or PK/PD systems analyses. Over the past 50 years, studies have demonstrated that the response of an organism to a drug can be more clearly explained using PK/PD relationships. This is important because utilization of single concentration measurements to independently predict drug response often fails due to the phenomenon of system hysteresis [11]. Sophisticated mathematical modeling approaches have been developed to maximize the prediction of response from limited subject-specific information to overcome the aforementioned limitation [12]. The following sections seek to clarify the current approaches to PK/PD modeling that lead to optimal dose selection.

Pharmacokinetic Modeling

Several approaches currently exist to accurately model the drug concentration–time profile in subjects receiving the drug [13–15]. The development of an "optimal" model requires varying degrees of technical expertise, and is dependent on the amount of information that is available from each individual subject [16]. In simple terms, a more homogenous subject population with multiple concentration–time points can be explained using a simple model. In contrast, a more heterogeneous subject population with sparse concentration–time data requires more complex hierarchical and covariate dependent models to accurately define the concentration–time profile. The key pharmacokinetic modeling approaches that are currently utilized in drug development are explained as follows.

Non-Compartmental Analysis

Non-compartmental analysis (NCA) represents the simplest approach to PK analysis. This approach is reliant on theories that support statistical moment analysis. The reader is directed to the excellent work by Cobelli and Toffolo [13] for additional details regarding the assumptions and theory that support NCA. This modality of PK analysis is sufficient in key clinical settings. The initial clinical Phase I study, for example, often includes a relatively homogeneous sample of 10–30 subjects who receive a single dose of a NME. The goal of this initial study includes descriptive characterization of the maximum drug concentration (C_{max}), minimum drug concentration (C_{min}), and time of maximum concentration (T_{max}). Quantitative assessments are also performed to determine the elimination rate constant (K_e), systemic clearance (CL), volume of distribution (V_d), half-life ($T_{1/2}$), and area under the drug concentration versus time curve (AUC). Multiple blood samples are often collected to characterize the concentration–time profile, thus providing "rich" information. In this setting, NCA is often a reasonable approach for estimation of these PK parameters and includes fewer assumptions than those required by compartmental analysis. For example, evaluation of 10 subjects may suggest that a one-compartment model best predicts the PK for 3 subjects while a two-compartment model best predicts the PK for the remaining 7 subjects. In this setting, the PK modeler may force an assumption of a two-compartment model on all subjects to best explain drug disposition in the studied sample. In contrast, NCA has no explicit compartment assumptions and can be safely applied to all patients. Thus, NCA in this setting is simpler to execute. Furthermore, it will yield similar results to a properly specified compartmental analysis, especially when the PK experiment includes infusion of a drug into the bloodstream with intensive plasma or serum sampling [13]. However, a fundamental assumption of NCA is linearity, which is not true of all biological systems. For these situations, PK data are best modeled using compartmental modeling approaches with non-linear clearance terms.

Compartmental Analysis

Compartmental analysis simplifies the human biological system through its representation of the system as a series of one or more compartments with intercompartmental relationships [15]. These compartments or "tanks" are not representative of any real organs or tissues, and are often mischaracterized as such for simplicity. Fig. 9.1 illustrates one- and two-compartment models with drug input as a zero-order (fixed) input rate (R). The entry of drug into the system can be represented as a fixed rate or as a function (first, second, third … order). Communication between compartments is represented by rate constants (K) for entry or exit from these compartments. These rate constants are often assumed to be linear, permitting the system to be explained by linear differential equations. However, the rate of entry and exit can also be formulated as non-linear functions such as the Michaelis-Menten model [17]. Ultimately, the models assume homogeneous distribution within the compartment, such that the measured concentration represents an average concentration value from the sampled compartment (most often blood) [15].

Several types of compartmental models exist but are often constructed as mammillary models, composed of a common or "central" compartment that is connected to "peripheral" compartments. Compartmental modeling permits the construct of differential equations to explain the change in concentrations over time in each compartment. Although mammillary models are physiologic in their construction, it is critical to realize that concentration profiles at various sites cannot be truly actualized and only estimated through sampling of concentrations at that site [15]. While this is feasible for the central compartment, it is challenging for the peripheral compartments. Validation of "peripheral" or tissue concentrations requires

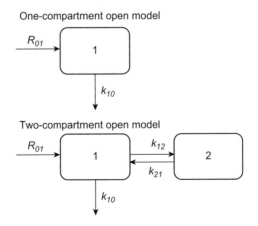

FIGURE 9.1 One and two-compartment models with drug input as a zero-order (fixed) input rate (R) with first-order elimination (k_{10}) and intercompartmental transfer rate constants (k_{12} or k_{21}).

invasive or semi-invasive measurement techniques for validation of the model [18]. However, this is often not feasible or ethical to achieve in humans. Nevertheless, compartmental analysis represents the dominant approach for PK analysis as the medium between the simplistic NCA and the more complex and multiple-assumption physiology-based pharmacokinetic (PBPK) modeling approach.

Physiology-Based Pharmacokinetic Modeling

Physiology-based pharmacokinetic modeling (PBPK) relies on blood flow rates and binding characteristics of drugs to various tissues and circulating proteins to describe the distribution of drugs between the central compartment and specific organs and tissues [14]. While intuitive, data that define the binding characteristics of drugs are often limited to plasma or serum binding data — for example, data on drug binding to endothelium compared to muscle tissue is often unknown [19]. Similarly, blood flow rates and the relationships between body size and health status on these blood flow rates must be known [20]. As expected, much of this information is very difficult to obtain empirically in humans compared to animals. As a result, PBPK approaches have been used extensively in preclinical development and are useful to explain differences in drug distribution between species [21]. The distributions of a few drugs, such as ciprofloxacin, digoxin, lidocaine and paclitaxel, have been explained in humans using PBPK models [22—24]. In this setting, PBPK models have been constructed to include key organs such as the heart, lung, liver, kidneys, muscle and adipose tissue. The remaining organs/tissues are lumped into two compartments, namely rapidly equilibrating tissue and slow equilibrating tissue. This approach leads to the construct of a six to seven "compartment"-type model with differential equations to explain the concentration—time profiles within these compartments [14]. A key criticism of this approach includes the collection of fewer data points than the number of parameters that are estimated, which reduces the reliability of the overall model. Hence, PBPK models represent an important step toward characterization of tissue-level PK, which may improve our understanding of individualized pharmacologic response [21]. However, this tool still requires refinement and is not an approach that is routinely utilized in population PK analysis for drug development [21].

Population PK Analysis

After candidate PK structural models are identified, the next step is to select a computer software program to model the data and estimate the PK parameters and their associated dispersions. The two-stage approach of PK modeling has been the traditional method for generating descriptive PK values [3]. The traditional two-stage approach first determines the PK estimates for each patient, and then uses descriptive statistics to generate the dispersion surrounding PK estimates [25]. While fitting data from an individual subject, the standard two-stage approach ignores the existence of all other individuals within the population [25]. Mean estimates of parameters are usually unbiased, but random effects (variance and covariance) are likely to be overestimated in realistic situations [26]. As a result, estimates of dispersion of model parameters and simulated drug exposures are often substantially reduced by the two-stage modeling technique.

Population pharmacokinetic (POP-PK analysis) modeling provides several distinct advantages over the standard two-stage modeling approach [25]. As stated above, its major advantage is that it deals with populations of patients rather than individual patients and aims to estimate the distribution of parameters. In other words, population pharmacokinetics explicitly estimates between-patient variability in pharmacokinetic parameters for the population pharmacokinetic model and also seeks to estimate covariance among the pharmacokinetic parameters. Another major advantage of this approach is its improved ability to estimate population pharmacokinetic parameters for subjects with limited sampling times [27−29]. In contrast to the two-stage approach, sparse concentration−time data from individuals are often sufficient to construct a useful PK model [27]. The sampling and dosing times do not have to be stringently regulated as long as the actual administration and sampling times are collected accurately. Given these strengths, use of POP-PK analysis is an especially attractive technique when employed using PK data in the less controlled clinical setting, and has become the standard pharmacokinetic methodology for estimating population pharmacokinetic parameters and associated dispersions.

Sheiner and Beal introduced the non-linear mixed effects model with first-order approximation (NONMEM) as an initial introduction into the approach of POP-PK modeling [30−32]. Since this introduction, multiple approaches and software programs have been introduced to aid POP-PK modeling, and broadly include parametric or non-parametric techniques [33−35]. Parametric POP-PK analysis assumes a specific shape to the distribution (Gaussian, log-normal, etc.) with regard to PK parameter, while non-parametric approaches do not assume a specific distribution [36]. Advocates for both models exist, and software programs that use parametric approaches presently outnumber those that utilize non-parametric approaches [37−38]. To compare the overall predictive performance of various approaches, Verme and colleagues analyzed data from a single study using seven different POP−PK modeling techniques [39]. This analysis demonstrated that no two methods yielded identical results, with an overall conclusion that favored the non-parametric approach of Schumitsky and colleagues [39]. Similarly, Bavarel *et al.* have shown non-parametric estimation methods using NONMEM VI to perform better than parametric estimation methods when using real data from 25 established models [40]. As a result, parametric POP-PK analysis is discussed, but the role of non-parametric POP-PK analysis using a non-parametric adaptive grid is described with greater emphasis.

Parametric POP-PK

With parametric population modeling, a distributional function is assigned to the parameters in the model [25]. In most cases, parameter distributions are usually assumed to be Gaussian or log-normal, and the measure of central tendency of most PK parameters is often described as an arithmetic mean. Four parametric approaches are most often utilized when conducting POP-PK analysis: (1) the standard two-stage (S2S) approach; (2) the iterative two-stage Bayesian (IT2B) approach; (3) the parametric expectation and maximization (PEM) method; and (4) the NONMEM method [37]. As described previously, the first step of the S2S approach is to define PK model parameters for each subject using a regression-based method such as non-linear least squares. Once the PK estimates for each patient are available, it uses descriptive statistics to generate the dispersion surrounding pharmacokinetic estimates; the mean and standard deviation (SD) of the estimated parameters are assumed to be normal or log-normal distributions. The IT2B approach is an extension of the two-stage approach in that it uses the mean and SD of the PK parameters from the S2S approach as an initial estimate or Bayesian priors. The individual patient data distribution is then examined using the maximum *a posteriori* probability (MAP) Bayesian procedure, which in essence draws the modal value from the posterior probability distribution for the specified parameter [41]. This iterative procedure continues until convergence is achieved. The covariance and correlation between parameters can also be included during the analysis to refine the S2S and IT2B approaches. The PEM approach is also iterative, and includes a mathematical series that computes a mathematical conditional expectation and with increasing maximization likelihood until convergence is achieved [37]. Finally, NONMEM uses a mixed effect analytical approach, which is a combination of a fixed-effects estimate and a random-effects structural model [25, 30–32, 37]. This one-stage analysis approach simultaneously estimates all parameters (e.g., mean parameters, fixed effect parameters, inter-individual variability, random residual error), including their precision. While this method is in wide use, it lacks the desirable property of mathematical consistency. Regardless, the NONMEM is currently the dominant approach in drug development due to the simplicity of the data input structure, data manipulation, and existing technical support.

Non-Parametric POP-PK

Ascribing parameters to a specific distribution is referred to as parametric analysis, while dissociation from distributional specification is referred to as non-parametric analysis [37]. This form of analysis permits the existence of multiple distributions, allowing for the identification of clustered data. In the non-parametric approach, the maximum likelihood parameter distributions obtained are discrete spikes, up to one for each subject studied in the population. The location of each spike (support point) reflects its set of estimated parameter values. The height of the spike represents the estimated probability of that individual set of estimated parameter values. The likelihood of the entire collection of support points can be computed and compared under similar conditions. No summary parameters, such as mean or standard deviation (SD), will be any more likely, given the data of dosage and serum concentrations, than the actual collection of all the estimated individual discrete points, each one having certain parameter values such as V_d and K, for example, and the estimated probability associated with each combined point of V_d and K [42].

For example, the antifungal agent voriconazole is metabolized by the cytochrome P450 2C19 (CYP2C19) isoenzyme system [43]. The CYP2C19 system is associated with genetic polymorphisms such that select proportions of a population are extensive metabolizers, heterogeneous metabolizers or poor metabolizers [43]. The proportions of these metabolizer subfamilies are known to be variable by ethnicity (whites compared to Southeast Asians) [44]. Non-parametric analysis permits the discovery of bimodal, trimodal or multimodal clearance distributions, which is very helpful when subpopulations are not suspected during the early evaluation of a NME [42]. The existence of a trimodal population clearance profile of voriconazole would be more easily detected using a non-parametric POP-PK approach compared to a parametric POP-PK approach [42].

A non-parametric expectation maximization (NPEM) method that mimics the EM approach outlined above has been developed. The NPEM method examines the patient-specific data with each iteration and creates a joint distribution that is most likely to represent the support point. In contrast, use of the EM and IT2B approaches can lead to estimation of PK parameters that are correlated when in fact no true correlation exists. However, the determination of the "true" data distribution is computationally very intensive. Leary demonstrated that a 5-parameter model in 8 subjects would require approximately 500 hours of computer time when using a 1152 processor IBM "Blue Horizon" parallel computer in order to decrease the log-likelihood from -7221.2 to -437.3. This time dependence was directly related to the grid size, which in the previous example required 40 960 000 points [42]. To overcome this problem, a new non-parametric "adaptive grid" (NPAG) was developed. The NPAG procedure begins with a smaller and coarser grid of 5000 points. Each iteration leads to the addition of grid points that improve upon the previous solution with the specific matrix of the previous grid. The consequence of this technique is a focused application of processing time on a select region with the grid that is most likely to be associated with the final solution. Finally, the Big NPAG procedure improves upon the NPAG approach by allowing for multiple inputs and outputs [45–47].

Pharmacodynamic Modeling

A key component of PK/PD systems analyses is to define a target drug exposure associated with a safety or efficacy endpoint [1]. PK/PD systems analyses have been used significantly over the past three decades to enhance antimicrobial drug development and refine the dose selection process [48]. For antimicrobials, effect is measured on both the human subject and against the microorganism [49–51]. From an antimicrobial PK/PD viewpoint, effect against the microorganism is of greatest interest and it can be measured either *in vitro* or *in vivo* [48]. The following sections outline the general approach by which *in vitro* and *in vivo* models are utilized to aid antimicrobial dose optimization in humans [49–52].

The Minimum Inhibitory Concentration

The effect of an antimicrobial against a microorganism is often measured as the inhibitory concentration associated with 50% effect (IC_{50}), the minimum inhibitory concentration (MIC), or minimum bactericidal concentration (MBC) [51, 53]. Clinically, the MIC is the PD parameter most often used to describe the relationship between antimicrobial drug and physiologic activity. The MIC is defined as the lowest or minimum antimicrobial concentration that inhibits visible microbial growth in artificial media after a fixed incubation time [54]. This is typically determined by placing a known quantity of bacteria (or other microorganism) into multiple test tubes, and then adding increasing concentrations of a particular antibiotic, typically in $\log_2$ dilution, into consecutive tubes [51, 53]. The lowest antibiotic concentration that inhibits bacterial growth is then defined as the MIC for that drug–pathogen pairing. Alternatively, agar based systems are used in conjunction with antimicrobial disks to define effect through zones of inhibition. These zones of inhibition do not readily translate to a specified concentration; however, the development of a gradient-based diffusion test, namely the Etest™, permits estimation of the MIC [55].

The Clinical Laboratory Standards Institute (CLSI) provides specific guidance on the measurement and interpretation of MIC results, including quality control approaches to ensure interlaboratory reliability [54]. The interpretive criteria are used to categorize the MIC results as susceptible, intermediate or resistant. Although these categories do not fully guarantee success or failure of an antimicrobial, they provide a qualitative estimate for these potential endpoints if the antimicrobial is used [56]. Given the widespread use of antimicrobial susceptibility testing, the MIC currently represents a reasonable metric to define antimicrobial activity [53]. However, determination of the MIC relies on two fundamental assumptions that do not mimic the clinical situation. These assumptions include a static concentration–time profile (fixed concentrations) and free drug assessment, i.e., the broth medium lacks proteins to mimic the biologic milieu [57].

In vitro PD Modeling

The limitation of MIC testing can be surmounted *in vitro* using a one-compartmental chemostat or hollow fiber model [52, 58]. This model includes a central compartment that harbors the organism in either a planktonic or a biofilm state at various starting inoculums [52, 58–61]. Drugs can be injected or pumped into the central compartment at a specified input rate. Analogously, broth is also pumped into and out of the central compartment at specified rates to generate a concentration–time profile in the central compartment that mimics human PK of the specific drug. Plasma proteins such as albumin can be added to the model to create an environment that mimics the free-drug concentration–time profile [62]. To measure changes in bacterial density over time, aliquots can then be removed from the central compartment, diluted, plated on agar and incubated [58]. The number of colony forming units (CFU)/mL can then be calculated directly and compared relative to the starting conditions by counting the number of colonies on the incubated agar plate and adjusting the count by the dilution factor. These aliquots can also be assayed for drug concentrations. Collectively, this approach affords the evaluation of an infinite number of dosing regimens that are constrained only by time and resources.

The concentration–time data collected during one-compartmental chemostat or hollow fiber model experiments can be used to quantitatively evaluate exposure–response relationships. The three most common PK/PD indices (sometimes abbreviated as PD measures) used to predict drug exposure–response relationships are (1) the ratio of the maximal free drug concentration to the MIC ($fC_{max/MIC}$), (2) the ratio of the free area under the concentration time-curve to the MIC ($fAUC_{/MIC}$), and (3) the duration of time free drug concentrations remain above the MIC ($fT_{>MIC}$) [51, 53]. Two approaches are typically used to generate a distribution of exposures. First, multiple exposures are generated against a single well-characterized organism. Second, a single exposure profile is evaluated against multiple organisms with varying MICs. Alternatively, a hybrid of the two approaches is performed. The net result of these approaches is a distribution of $fAUC_{/MIC}$, $fC_{max/MIC}$ and $fT_{>MIC}$ values than can be modeled against the change in the number of microorganisms. As shown in Fig. 9.2, the relationship between these parameters and antimicrobial effect is dependent on the drug. If the antimicrobial effect is found to be most predicted by $fT_{>MIC}$, then the antimicrobial is referred to as a time-dependent or concentration-independent drug. Alternatively, if the antimicrobial effect is found to be most predicted by $fAUC_{/MIC}$ or $fC_{max/MIC}$, then the antimicrobial is referred to as a concentration-dependent drug. The antimicrobial effect is best predicted by $fAUC_{/MIC}$ and least by $fT_{>MIC}$ based on r^2 values, suggesting that the antimicrobial in question manifests a concentration-dependent effect.

This classification is relevant to dose selection. The activity of time-dependent antibiotics is not dependent on the intensity of exposure but is a function of the duration of time concentrations above the MIC during the dosing interval. For time-dependent antibiotics like the β-lactams, concentrations do not have to remain above the MIC for the entire dosing

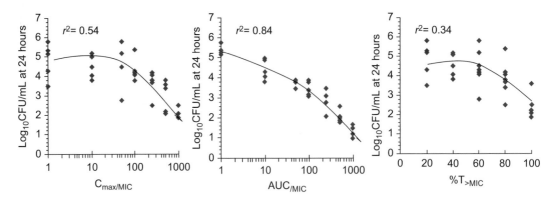

FIGURE 9.2　Colony forming units (CFU)/mL of microorganism at 24 hours (logarithmic scale) relative to three pharmacodynamic indices of the ratio of the maximum drug concentration to the minimum inhibitory concentration ($C_{max/MIC}$), ratio of the area under the concentration-time curve to the minimum inhibitory concentration ($AUC_{/MIC}$), and the percent of time during the dosing interval that the concentration exceeds the minimum inhibitory concentration (%$T_{>MIC}$).

interval, and the fraction of the dosing interval required for maximal bacterial effect varies for the different types of β-lactams [51, 63]. The use of extended infusion, continuous-infusion and oral controlled-release systems have all been used to optimize $fT_{>MIC}$ [64, 65]. In contrast, antibiotics like the aminoglycosides have concentration-dependent PK/PD [6, 66, 67]. For concentration-dependent antibiotics a dose–response relationship exists, and the therapeutic goal is to maximize exposure at the target site. Dose optimization for concentration-dependent antibiotics is achieved through use of high-dose extended interval dosing [6].

A final but critical point for evaluation of a pharmacologic response is the potential for a persistent effect despite undetectable systemic concentrations. In the case of antimicrobials, this phenomenon of persistent effect is known as the post-antibiotic effect (PAE) [68]. This phenomenon is one that is best measured *in vitro* and is highly dependent on the microorganism that is evaluated [68]. Importantly, PAE that is measured *in vitro* often underestimates the effect seen *in vivo* [68]. This underestimation is primarily a result of host immune response *in vivo*, which is ignored in most *in vitro* models.

In vivo PD Modeling

Animal infection model systems afford another opportunity to quantitatively evaluate antimicrobial exposure–response relationships. Numerous vertebrate animal models presently exist to mimic clinical infections such as skin and skin-structure infections, pneumonia, endocarditis and sepsis, to name a few [69–71]. Most infection models use rodents such as the mouse, rat, guinea pig and rabbit. As expected, "humanization" of the PK profile of drugs is not easily achieved across these species [72]. For example, the $T_{1/2}$ of an antimicrobial may be 0.5 hours in the mouse, 1 hour in the rat and 2.5 hours in the rabbit. Thus, a higher dosing frequency will be required in the mouse compared to the rabbit in order to achieve comparable PK profiles in these species. As a result, an important component for *in vivo* PD modeling is to ensure that dose regimens are designed for the specific infection model in question.

In clinical practice, a distribution of MIC values exists for a given organism and/or infection. Therefore, the final step is determining the overall PTA for the distribution of organisms encountered clinically. As previously mentioned, the PTA is determined at each MIC value within a given MIC range. Because the fraction of organisms collected at each MIC value is known, the overall or weighted PTA average can be calculated by multiplying the PTA for a specific MIC and the proportion of isolates with that MIC. This product is calculated for each MIC value within the MIC distribution. The overall PTA is then calculated by summing the products (PTA at a given MIC value × proportion of isolates with that MIC value) of the MIC values encountered within the distribution.

A key element for these simulations is the estimation of the PK parameters and their associated dispersion (variance and covariance). Pharmacokinetic data, especially for new compounds, is usually limited to data from healthy volunteer studies. Caution should be exercised when generalizing the results of volunteer studies to the population of interest. Volunteer studies are often considered as the most conservative evaluation of a new drug; volunteers are young and healthy, likely to have the highest drug clearances and shortest half-lives. However, when performing MCS, the measure of central tendency (high drug CL, short $T_{1/2}$) is only part of the story. Because MCS is explicitly creating a distribution, it is important to understand the measure of dispersion. Secondary to the limited variation surrounding PK parameters from healthy volunteer studies, it is possible that it overestimates the PTA. Ultimately, applicability to the target population must always be considered [81].

APPLIED PHARMACOKINETIC/PHARMACODYNAMIC MODELING

In recent years, the principles of PK/PD systems analyses have been used to support the approval of new antimicrobials. Telavancin and ceftaroline fosamil (a new generation of cephalosporin antibiotic) are the most recent examples of agents that have been approved by the FDA in the age of applied antimicrobial PK/PD. For each of these agents, preclinical *in vitro* and *in vivo* infection model studies were used to define the PK/PD target and population PK modeling and Monte Carlo simulations were used to select the candidate dosing regimens for Phase II and III studies. However, several antimicrobials were approved prior to the application of this science. Recent application of PK/PD principles to older but relevant antimicrobials has led to a reappraisal of their dose designs. The following section provides pharmacologic and drug-specific PK/PD information that has led to reconsideration of the dosage regimens of piperacillin/tazobactam.

Piperacillin/Tazobactam

Piperacillin/tazobactam is a β-lactam antimicrobial that is active against key nosocomial bacterial pathogens, including *Pseudomonas aeruginosa*, making it one of the most frequently used antibiotics in an empiric therapy regimen for healthcare-associated infections [87–91]. The FDA-approved dosing regimens include 30-minute infusions of 4.5 g intravenous Q6H for nosocomial pneumonia and 3.375 g IV Q6H for all other indications [50]. Unfortunately, piperacillin/tazobactam is one of the several antimicrobial agents that were developed and approved prior to our current understanding and application of PK/PD analyses. Although selection of dosing regimens for Phase III clinical trials included PK data from both healthy volunteers and infected patients [92], incorporation of the exposure–response relationship did not occur until long after FDA approval of piperacillin/tazobactam (81). Similarly, this agent's CLSI (Clinical Laboratory Standard Institute) susceptibility interpretative criteria were established prior to our current understanding of β-lactam PD properties, and susceptibility breakpoints were set much higher relative to other β-lactams [54]. For Enterobacteriaceae and *Acinetobacter baumannii* isolates, MIC values ≤ 16 mg/L are considered susceptible. The CLSI breakpoint for *P. aeruginosa* is higher, and isolates with MIC values ≤ 64 mg/L are considered susceptible [54].

Piperacillin/tazobactam, like other β-lactams, exhibits time-dependent activity, and the PD exposure that best correlates with efficacy is the $fT_{>MIC}$. *In vitro* and animal studies have demonstrated that β-lactam concentrations do not need to exceed the MIC for the entire dosing interval. Rather, free concentrations of piperacillin/tazobactam should remain above the MIC for at least 30% and 50% of the dosing interval (30% $fT_{>MIC}$ and 50% $fT_{>MIC}$) for bacteriostatic and bactericidal effects, respectively [50, 53, 93–95]. The first analysis to apply PK/PD modeling with standard doses of piperacillin/tazobactam employed a POP-PK model derived from hospitalized patients. These investigators evaluated the PTA (50% $fT_{>MIC}$) of standard FDA-approved dosing regimens against a range of MIC values commonly encountered in clinical practice (0.25–32 mg/L). The results of their PTA analysis for the MCS revealed that the FDA-approved dose of 3.375 g IV Q6H resulted in an acceptable PTA only for MIC values ≤ 8 mg/L [96]. Using the same POP-PK model, an additional analysis evaluated PTA with the nosocomial pneumonia dose of 4.5 g IV Q6H. These investigators noted a slight improvement in PD exposure against MICs = 16 mg/L (approximately 80% PTA); however, this dosage regimen remained suboptimal for MIC ≥ 32 mg/L. For MIC values = 64 mg/L, target attainment rates were < 10% [97]. The results from these evaluations are especially concerning given that the susceptibility breakpoint for *P. aeruginosa* is ≤ 64 mg/L [54].

The clinical relevance of these early PK/PD analyses showing discordance between susceptible MIC values and standard piperacillin/tazobactam doses was demonstrated in a retrospective cohort study [98]. These investigators evaluated clinical outcomes in hospitalized patients receiving appropriate empirical therapy for bacteremia due to *P. aeruginosa* between 2002 and 2006. Appropriate empirical therapy was defined as treatment (in doses appropriate for renal function as indicated by the manufacturer) initiated within 24 hours of the first positive blood culture result to which the isolate was deemed susceptible by the CLSI. Patients were stratified into two cohorts by the piperacillin/tazobactam MIC (≤ 16 mg/L versus 32–64 mg/L) and 30-day mortality rates were compared within each MIC group between those that received piperacillin/tazobactam and patients that received an alternative β-lactam susceptible to the *P. aeruginosa* isolate. The results showed significantly greater 30-day mortality when patients received piperacillin/tazobactam versus a comparator β-lactam for bacteremia due to *P. aeruginosa* with MICs of 32–64 mg/L (85.7% versus 22.2%, $P = 0.004$). In contrast, 30-day mortality rates were found to be similar between groups when the MIC was ≤ 16 mg/L (30.0% versus 20.5%, $P = 0.673$) [98].

Because of the disconnect between susceptibility breakpoints and PTA data (CLSI was unwilling to lower the breakpoint), alternative dosing schemes for optimizing $fT_{>MIC}$ for piperacillin/tazobactam were explored. For time-dependent antibiotics like piperacillin/tazobactam, a number of different dosing options are available to augment the PTA profile against a wider array of MIC values. One option is to increase the dose. However, as seen in the aforementioned MCS, increasing the dose from 3.375 g to 4.5 g had a minimal impact on the PTA profile [97]. Increasing the dosing frequency is another viable option, but is considered a second-tier option given the higher drug acquisition costs relative to the parent regimen, an increase in administration and preparation time, and a greater potential for toxicity because a higher total daily dose is given [81]. Prolonging the infusion time is another dose-optimization strategy. Intuitively, this strategy makes sense as it produces a lower C_{max} and prolongs the amount of time that drug concentrations are in excess of the MIC. Lower C_{max} values are not expected to be disadvantageous for piperacillin/tazobactam because of its time-dependent PD profile. In fact, prolonging the time that concentrations are above the MIC should yield more favorable PTA profiles [56].

The improvement in PD exposure by prolonging the infusion time was demonstrated using MCS and PK data from healthy volunteers [81]. A dosage of 3.375 g IV Q8H administered as a 4-hour infusion led to an improvement in PD target attainment as compared to the nosocomial pneumonia dose. Probability of target attainment was 92% for MICs = 16 mg/L, and 100% at lower MIC values [81]. Based on the compelling nature of this and other similar MCS studies, a number of institutions have adopted this prolonged infusion regimen into clinical practice.

Clinical application of the prolonged infusion piperacillin/tazobactam dosage regimen was first evaluated in a retrospective cohort study in patients with *P. aeruginosa* infections at Albany Medical Center Hospital, Albany, New York [79]. In February 2002, Albany Medical Center Hospital implemented an automatic substitution program to allow automatic conversion of standard intermittent infusions of piperacillin/tazobactam to the prolonged 4-hour infusion regimen of 3.375 g IV Q8H (intravenous administration every 8 h). To determine the effect of prolonged infusion, 14-day mortality rates and hospital length of stay post-culture collection were compared in patients who received the standard infusion to those who received the prolonged infusion for a *P. aeruginosa* infection, between 2000 and 2004. By limiting this analysis to *P. aeruginosa* infections, these investigators were able to evaluate outcomes in a relatively homogenous population where patients were more likely to be infected with a higher MIC pathogen and were more dependent on drug exposure for clinical success. The results showed that in critically ill patients with a high risk for mortality (Acute Physiology and Chronic Health Evaluation [APACHE] II score > 17), the prolonged infusion regimen led to significantly lower 14-day mortality rates (12.2% versus 31.6%, $P = 0.04$) and shorter lengths of stay (21 versus 38 days, $P = 0.02$) as compared to the standard infusion [82]. The results from this analysis underscore how valuable PK/PD modeling and optimizing drug exposure can be in the improvement of clinical outcomes.

It is important to note that the aforementioned MCS analyses took an expectation across all patient types and did not stratify PTA results by covariates known to modulate important PK parameters like V_d and CL. Since piperacillin/tazobactam, like other β-lactams, is primarily eliminated by the kidneys [99, 100], it is critical to understand how the PTA profile changes in patients with varying degrees of renal function. Cognizant of this clinical issue, our group first conducted a POP-PK analysis that assessed the impact of renal function on total CL. While any method to estimate a patient's renal function could have been employed as a covariate, estimates of creatinine clearance (eCL_{cr}) based on the Cockcroft-Gault equation were used since most antibiotics have renal dosage adjustments based on this formula [101]. This measure of patients' renal function was incorporated into the model by making CL from the central compartment proportional to the estimated renal function. In particular, this was accomplished by making piperacillin/tazobactam CL proportional to eCL_{cr} as follows: (CL slope $\times eCL_{cr}$) $+$ CL intercept [84]. For our model, CL slope multiplied by eCL_{cr} reflects the renal CL, and the CL intercept term reflects non-renal CL [102].

Once the model was fit to the data, our group then performed a series of Monte Carlo simulations to identify the optimal renal dose adjustment regimen for the parent piperacillin/tazobactam prolonged infusion dosing scheme (piperacillin/tazobactam 3.375 g Q8H infused over 4 hours) used at Albany Medical Center Hospital. The MCS methods used in the renal dose selection process are similar to previously described PTA analyses [81, 84]. The major distinction is in the handling of CL. In most PD profiling studies, PK parameters, including CL, are randomly selected from a multivariate distribution. These data are used to simulate the dispersion or full spread of concentration−time profiles (e.g., peak concentration, AUC) that would be seen in a large population after administration of a specific dosing regimen. From this information, the probability that the given antibiotic dosing regimen achieves the stated goal of therapy can be determined (e.g., 50% $fT_{>MIC}$, $AUC_{/MIC} > 250$). In contrast, eCL_{cr} was fixed at a predetermined level (e.g., 40 mL/min, 20 mL/min) in our MCS renal dose selection analysis [103]. By fixing eCL_{cr}, the distribution in concentration−time profiles for our candidate renal adjustment regimens was estimated at the pre-specified eCL_{cr} level, rather than across a potential continuum for the entire population. This information was then used to determine the probability that each regimen at a specified eCL_{cr} level achieved 50% $fT_{>MIC}$ for the range of MIC values deemed susceptible by the CLSI. Knowledge of both the PTA and concentration−time profiles of candidate renal dose regimens at specified CL_{cr} thresholds is critical to the renal dose selection process. In particular, it allows determination of the impact of the candidate renal dose adjustment schemes on the PTA as well as the degree of exposure just prior to the point of dose adjustment. This information can then be used to find a CL_{cr} breakpoint and dose adjustment that would leave the PTA substantially unaltered, yet not produce excessive accumulation or exposure [102].

There are two important considerations when selecting potential candidate regimens: the eCL_{cr} dose adjustment threshold and the dose alteration scheme. We limited the MCS renal dose analysis to the following two candidate regimens: (1) 3.375 g IV Q12H (4-hour infusion) at an eCL_{cr} of 40 mL/min; and (2) 3.375 g IV Q12H (4-hour infusion) at an eCL_{cr} of 20 mL/min [103]. We selected these regimens for several reasons. First, we did not want to deviate from the approved package inserts' renal dose adjustment schemes [104]. Second, a crude assessment of piperacillin CL in patients with renal impairment indicated the optimal dose adjustment was somewhere between 20 and 40 mL/min. Third, we did not have robust PK data in patients with eCL_{cr} less than 20 mL/min. Fourth, we opted to lengthen the interval rather than decrease the dose to ensure dosing consistency in clinical practice [102].

For both candidate regimens, the probability of attaining 50% $fT_{>MIC}$ was then determined for a range of MIC values encountered in clinical practice. To ensure these candidate regimens were safe and would not produce supra-therapeutic concentrations, an acceptable amount of exposure had to be established. Given that a specific exposure−toxicity relationship did not exist for piperacillin/tazobactam, we selected a target maximal exposure of $\leq$ four-fold because previous studies have not determined the safety beyond this point.

Accumulation was assessed at the eCL_{cr} level immediately prior to the dose adjustment threshold because this is the point of maximum accumulation for the parent antibiotic regimen. In particular, the degree of exposure was determined by taking the ratio of the distribution of AUC from 0 to 24 hours at steady state (AUC_{24SS}) for piperacillin/tazobactam 3.375 g IV Q8H when eCL_{cr} was fixed at 40 mL/min and 20 mL/min (eCL_{cr} dose adjustment threshold and maximum accumulation points) relative to the AUC_{24SS} distribution for the original regimen (3.375 g IV Q8H) when the eCL_{cr} was fixed at 100 mL/min [102, 103].

In the MCS analysis, both renal dose candidate regimens had a $\geq 90\%$ PTA for MIC values ≤ 4 mg/L. However, a suboptimal PTA profile was observed for MIC values > 4 mg/L for the candidate regimen adjusted at an eCL_{cr} of 40 mL/min. Similar to the aforementioned, non-renal stratified PTA analyses, the candidate regimen adjusted at an eCL_{cr} of 20 mL/min had a favorable PTA for MIC values < 16 mg/L. Not surprisingly, the improvement in PTA with the candidate regimen at an eCL_{cr} of 20 mL/min coincided with higher exposure ratios. However, the mean exposure ratio (standard deviation) was 2.0 (0.6) and nearly all of the ratios were < 3, which was acceptable per our target maximal exposure of ≤ 4. Collectively, these findings demonstrated that the candidate regimen (3.375 g IV Q12H (4-hour infusion)) at an eCL_{cr} of 20 mL/min was the optimal renal dosing adjustment scheme to incorporate into clinical practice [102, 103].

CONCLUSIONS

Selection of an optimal dose to treat an ailment is no simple task. In recent years, information regarding the covariates that influence drug exposure has been used to create mathematical models that can better predict individual-level and population level PK. Integration of PK with effect, through the science of PK/PD, has further aided our goal of discovering an optimal dose. This science has been useful for the clinical translation of preclinical and early-phase clinical trials to define doses used in Phase III clinical trials. However, in the case of antimicrobials, identification of a specific PK/PD target that is consistently predictive of an efficacious or toxic event has remained elusive. In reality, patients are a moving target with highly variable and dynamic clinical scenarios that prevent selection of a "single optimal dose" that will work for every ailment. In the case of antimicrobials, the PK/PD target is likely to be dependent on the specific bacterial pathogen. Patients' acuity of illness and immune status will also affect their ability to respond to an infection. Consequently, application of PK/PD to drive personalized medicine is a major improvement from single-sample concentration-based decisions, but still requires many years of work. Simplified mathematical algorithms that can be integrated into electronic medical systems are increasingly possible and routine on the medical ward. We expect to have electronic medical systems that can integrate microbiologic data, clinical acuity scores, and individual clinical response in the near future. This integrated system will lead to improved applicability of PK/PD principles to deliver personalized medicine.

References

[1] Gibbs JP. Prediction of exposure—response relationships to support first-in-human study design. AAPS J 2010;12:750—8.

[2] DiMasi JA, Feldman L, Seckler A, Wilson A. Trends in risks associated with new drug development: success rates for investigational drugs. Clin Pharmacol Ther 2010;87:272−7.

[3] US Department of Health and Human Services, FDA. Population Pharmacokinetics. Guidance for Industry. Whiteoak, MD: FDA; 1999.

[4] US Department of Health and Human Services, FDA. Exposure−Response Relationships − Study Design, Data Analysis, and Regulatory Applications. Guidance for Industry. Whiteoak, MD: FDA; 2003.

[5] Mager DE, Woo S, Jusko WJ. Scaling pharmacodynamics from *in vitro* and preclinical animal studies to humans. Drug Metab Pharmacokinet 2009;24:16−24.

[6] Drusano GL, Ambrose PG, Bhavnani SM, et al. Back to the future: using aminoglycosides again and how to dose them optimally. Clin Infect Dis 2007;45:753−60.

[7] US Department of Health and Human Services, FDA. Clinical Pharmacology Guidances (Drugs). Whiteoak, MD: FDA; 2011.

[8] Flegal KM, Carroll MD, Ogden CL, Curtin LR. Prevalence and trends in obesity among US adults, 1999−2008. J Am Med Assoc 2010;303:235−2341.

[9] Gilbertson DT, Liu J, Xue JL, et al. Projecting the number of patients with end-stage renal disease in the United States to the year 2015. J Am Soc Nephrol 2005;16:3736−41.

[10] WHO. United Nations Programme in HIV/AIDS: Global Facts & Figures. Geneva, Switzerland: WHO; 2009.

[11] Schwilden H, Stoeckel H, Schuttler J, Lauven PM. Pharmacological models and their use in clinical anaesthesia. Eur J Anaesthesiol 1986;3:175−208.

[12] Bradley JS, Garonzik SM, Forrest A, Bhavnani SM. Pharmacokinetics, pharmacodynamics, and Monte Carlo simulation: selecting the best antimicrobial dose to treat an infection. Pediatr Infect Dis J 2011;29:1043−6.

[13] Cobelli C, Toffolo G. Compartmental vs noncompartmental modeling for two accessible pools. Am J Physiol 1984;247:R488−96.

[14] Pang KS, Durk MR. Physiologically−based pharmacokinetic modeling for absorption, transport, metabolism and excretion. J Pharmacokinet Pharmacodyn 2011;37:591−615.

[15] Rescigno A. Compartmental analysis and its manifold applications to pharmacokinetics. AAPS J 2010;12:61−72.

[16] Boxenbaum H. Pharmacokinetics: philosophy of modeling. Drug Metab Rev 1992;24:89−120.

[17] Michaelis M, Menten ML. Die Kinetik der Invertinwirkung. Biochem 1913;49:333−69.

[18] Langer O, Muller M. Methods to assess tissue-specific distribution and metabolism of drugs. Curr Drug Metab 2004;5:463−81.

[19] Zeitlinger MA, Derendorf H, Mouton JW, et al. Protein binding: do we ever learn? Antimicrob Agents Chemother 2011;55:3067−74.

[20] Gonzalez D, Conrado DJ, Theuretzbacher U, Derendorf H. The effect of critical illness on drug distribution. Curr Pharm Biotechnol 2011 10 May [Epub ahead of print].

[21] Rowland M, Peck C, Tucker G. Physiologically-based pharmacokinetics in drug development and regulatory science. Annu Rev Pharmacol Toxicol 2011;51:45−73.

[22] Carlton LD, Pollack GM, Brouwer KL. Physiologic pharmacokinetic modeling of gastrointestinal blood flow as a rate-limiting step in the oral absorption of digoxin: implications for patients with congestive heart failure receiving epoprostenol. J Pharm Sci 1996;85:473−7.

[23] Leemann TD, Blaschke TF. Semi-quantitative simulation for reasoning about physiological models of drug kinetics and effects. Schweiz Med Wochenschr 1990;120:1849−52.

[24] Willmann S, Hohn K, Edginton A, et al. Development of a physiology-based whole-body population model for assessing the influence of individual variability on the pharmacokinetics of drugs. J Pharmacokinet Pharmacodyn 2007;34:401−31.

[25] Sheiner LB. The population approach to pharmacokinetic data analysis: rationale and standard data analysis methods. Drug Metab Rev 1984;15:153−71.

[26] Ette EI, Williams PJ. Population pharmacokinetics II: estimation methods. Ann Pharmacother 2004;38:1907−15.

[27] Drusano GL, Liu W, Perkins R, et al. Determination of robust ocular pharmacokinetic parameters in serum and vitreous humor of albino rabbits following systemic administration of ciprofloxacin from sparse data sets by using IT2S, a population pharmacokinetic modeling program. Antimicrob Agents Chemother 1995;39:1683−7.

[28] Hashimoto Y, Sheiner LB. Designs for population pharmacodynamics: value of pharmacokinetic data and population analysis. J Pharmacokinet Biopharm 1991;19:333–53.

[29] Scher HI, Jodrell DI, Iversen JM, et al. Use of adaptive control with feedback to individualize suramin dosing. Cancer Res 1992;52:64–70.

[30] Sheiner LB, Beal SL. Evaluation of methods for estimating population pharmacokinetics parameters. I. Michaelis-Menten model: routine clinical pharmacokinetic data. J Pharmacokinet Biopharm 1980; 8:553–71.

[31] Sheiner BL, Beal SL. Evaluation of methods for estimating population pharmacokinetic parameters. II. Biexponential model and experimental pharmacokinetic data. J Pharmacokinet Biopharm 1981;9:635–51.

[32] Sheiner LB, Beal SL. Evaluation of methods for estimating population pharmacokinetic parameters. III. Monoexponential model: routine clinical pharmacokinetic data. J Pharmacokinet Biopharm 1983;11:303–19.

[33] Bauer RJ, Guzy S, Ng C. A survey of population analysis methods and software for complex pharmacokinetic and pharmacodynamic models with examples. AAPS J 2007;9:E60–83.

[34] Csajka C, Verotta D. Pharmacokinetic–pharmacodynamic modelling: history and perspectives. J Pharmacokinet Pharmacodyn 2006;33:227–79.

[35] Jelliffe RW, Schumitzky A, Van Guilder M, et al. Individualizing drug dosage regimens: roles of population pharmacokinetic and dynamic models, Bayesian fitting, and adaptive control. Ther Drug Monit 1993;15:380–93.

[36] Whiting B, Kelman AW, Grevel J. Population pharmacokinetics. Theory and clinical application. Clin Pharmacokinet 1986;11:387–401.

[37] Bustad A, Terziivanov D, Leary R, et al. Parametric and nonparametric population methods: their comparative performance in analysing a clinical dataset and two Monte Carlo simulation studies. Clin Pharmacokinet 2006;45:365–83.

[38] Proost JH, Eleveld DJ. Parametric and nonparametric population methods. Clin Pharmacokinet 2006;45:851–2. author reply 852–854.

[39] Verme CN, Ludden TM, Clementi WA, Harris SC. Pharmacokinetics of quinidine in male patients. A population analysis. Clin Pharmacokinet 1992;22:468–80.

[40] Baverel PG, Savic RM, Wilkins JJ, Karlsson MO. Evaluation of the nonparametric estimation method in NONMEM VI: application to real data. J Pharmacokinet Pharmacodyn 2009;36:297–315.

[41] Jelliffe RW, Schumitzky A. Modeling, adaptive control, and optimal drug therapy. Med Prog Technol 1990;16:95–110.

[42] Jelliffe R, Schumitzky A, Bustad A, et al. Population Pharmacokinetic and Pharmacodynamic Modeling, vol. 2011. Los Angeles, CA: University of Southern California, Laboratory of Applied Pharmacokinetics; 2011.

[43] Theuretzbacher U, Ihle F, Derendorf H. Pharmacokinetic/pharmacodynamic profile of voriconazole. Clin Pharmacokinet 2006;45:649–63.

[44] Mizutani T. PM frequencies of major CYPs in Asians and Caucasians. Drug Metab Rev 2003;35:99–106.

[45] Lodise TP, Nau R, Kinzig M, et al. Pharmacodynamics of ceftazidime and meropenem in cerebrospinal fluid: results of population pharmacokinetic modelling and Monte Carlo simulation. J Antimicrob Chemother 2007;60:1038–44.

[46] Lodise Jr TP, Gotfried M, Barriere S, Drusano GL. Telavancin penetration into human epithelial lining fluid determined by population pharmacokinetic modeling and Monte Carlo simulation. Antimicrob Agents Chemother 2008;52:2300–4.

[47] Rubino CM, Ma L, Bhavnani SM, et al. Evaluation of tigecycline penetration into colon wall tissue and epithelial lining fluid using a population pharmacokinetic model and Monte Carlo simulation. Antimicrob Agents Chemother 2007;51:4085–9.

[48] Mouton JW, Ambrose PG, Canton R, et al. Conserving antibiotics for the future: new ways to use old and new drugs from a pharmacokinetic and pharmacodynamic perspective. Drug Resist Update 2011;14:107–17.

[49] Andes D, Craig WA. Animal model pharmacokinetics and pharmacodynamics: a critical review. Intl J Antimicrob Agents 2002;19:261–8.

[50] Craig WA. Pharmacokinetic/pharmacodynamic parameters: rationale for antibacterial dosing of mice and men. Clin Infect Dis 1998;26:1–10. quiz 11–12.

[51] Craig WA. Basic pharmacodynamics of antibacterials with clinical applications to the use of beta-lactams, glycopeptides, and linezolid. Infect Dis Clin North Am 2003;17:479–501.

[52] Marchbanks CR, McKiel JR, Gilbert DH, et al. Dose ranging and fractionation of intravenous ciprofloxacin against *Pseudomonas aeruginosa* and *Staphylococcus aureus* in an *in vitro* model of infection. Antimicrob Agents Chemother 1993;37:1756–63.

[53] Drusano GL. Antimicrobial pharmacodynamics: critical interactions of 'bug and drug'. Nat Rev Microbiol 2004;2:289–300.

[54] CLSI. Clinical and Laboratory Standards Institute (CLSI). Performance Standards for Antimicrobial Susceptibility Testing; Twentieth Informational Supplement CLSI Document M100-S20. 20th edn; 2010.

[55] Bolmstrom A. Susceptibility testing of anaerobes with Etest. Clin Infect Dis 1993;16(Suppl. 4):S367–70.

[56] Lodise TP, Butterfield J. Use of pharmacodynamic principles to inform beta-lactam dosing: "S" does not always mean success. J Hosp Med 2011;6(Suppl. 1):S16–23.

[57] Nightingale J. Clinical limitations of *in vitro* testing of microorganism susceptibility. Am J Hosp Pharm 1987;44:131–7.

[58] Pai MP, Samples ML, Mercier RC, Spilde MN. Activities and ultrastructural effects of antifungal combinations against simulated *Candida endocardial* vegetations. Antimicrob Agents Chemother 2008;52:2367–76.

[59] Deziel MR, Heine H, Louie A, et al. Effective antimicrobial regimens for use in humans for therapy of *Bacillus anthracis* infections and postexposure prophylaxis. Antimicrob Agents Chemother 2005;49:5099–106.

[60] Drusano GL, Okusanya OO, Okusanya A, et al. Is 60 days of ciprofloxacin administration necessary for postexposure prophylaxis for *Bacillus anthracis*? Antimicrob Agents Chemother 2008;52:3973–9.

[61] Drusano GL, Liu W, Brown DL, et al. Impact of short-course quinolone therapy on susceptible and resistant populations of *Staphylococcus aureus*. J Infect Dis 2009;199:219–26.

[62] Schmidt S, Rock K, Sahre M, et al. Effect of protein binding on the pharmacological activity of highly bound antibiotics. Antimicrob Agents Chemother 2008;52:3994–4000.

[63] Eagle H, Magnuson HJ, Fleischman R. The effect of the method of administration on the therapeutic efficacy of sodium penicillin in experimental syphilis. Bull Johns Hopkins Hosp 1946;79:168–89.

[64] Pai MP, Bruce H, Felton LA. Clinical pharmacokinetics of oral controlled-release 5-fluorocytosine. Antimicrob Agents Chemother 2010;54:1237–41.

[65] Kim A, Sutherland CA, Kuti JL, Nicolau DP. Optimal dosing of piperacillin-tazobactam for the treatment of *Pseudomonas aeruginosa* infections: prolonged or continuous infusion? Pharmacotherapy 2007;27:1490–7.

[66] Pai MP, Nafziger AN, Bertino Jr JS. Simplified estimation of aminoglycoside pharmacokinetics in underweight and obese adult patients. Antimicrob Agents Chemother 2011;55:4005–11.

[67] Kashuba AD, Bertino Jr JS, Nafziger AN. Dosing of aminoglycosides to rapidly attain pharmacodynamic goals and hasten therapeutic response by using individualized pharmacokinetic monitoring of patients with pneumonia caused by gram-negative organisms. Antimicrob Agents Chemother 1998;42:1842–4.

[68] Craig WA. Post-antibiotic effects in experimental infection models: relationship to *in-vitro* phenomena and to treatment of infections in man. J Antimicrob Chemother 1993;31(Suppl. D):149–58.

[69] Craig WA, Andes DR. *In vivo* pharmacodynamics of ceftobiprole against multiple bacterial pathogens in murine thigh and lung infection models. Antimicrob Agents Chemother 2008;52:3492–6.

[70] Meers P, Neville M, Malinin V, et al. Biofilm penetration, triggered release and *in vivo* activity of inhaled liposomal amikacin in chronic *Pseudomonas aeruginosa* lung infections. J Antimicrob Chemother 2008;61:859–68.

[71] Hershberger E, Coyle EA, Kaatz GW, et al. Comparison of a rabbit model of bacterial endocarditis and an *in vitro* infection model with simulated endocardial vegetations. Antimicrob Agents Chemother 2000;44:1921–4.

[72] Ring BJ, Chien JY, Adkison KK, et al. PhRMA CPCDC initiative on predictive models of human pharmacokinetics, part 3: comparative assessment of prediction methods of human clearance. J Pharm Sci 2011;100:4090–110.

[73] Haller I. Evaluation of ciprofloxacin alone and in combination with other antibiotics in a murine model of thigh muscle infection. Am J Med 1987;82:76–9.

[74] Pearsall NN, Lagunoff D. Immunological responses to *Candida albicans*. I. Mouse-thigh lesion as a model for experimental candidiasis. Infect Immun 1974;9:999–1002.

[75] van der Voet GB, Mattie H, van Furth R. The antibacterial activity of combinations of mecillinam and ampicillin *in vitro* and in normal and granulopenic mice. Scand J Infect Dis 1983;15:91–6.

[76] Burkhardt O, Kumar V, Katterwe D, et al. Ertapenem in critically ill patients with early-onset ventilator-associated pneumonia: pharmacokinetics with special consideration of free-drug concentration. J Antimicrob Chemother 2007;59:277–84.

[77] Preston SL, Drusano GL, Berman AL, et al. Pharmacodynamics of levofloxacin: a new paradigm for early clinical trials. J Am Med Assoc 1998;279:125—9.
[78] Roberts JA, Kirkpatrick CM, Lipman J. Monte Carlo simulations: maximizing antibiotic pharmacokinetic data to optimize clinical practice for critically ill patients. J Antimicrob Chemother 2011;66:227—31.
[79] McGregor JC, Rich SE, Harris AD, et al. A systematic review of the methods used to assess the association between appropriate antibiotic therapy and mortality in bacteremic patients. Clin Infect Dis 2007;45:329—37.
[80] Cardone KE, Lodise TP, Patel N, et al. Pharmacokinetics and pharmacodynamics of intravenous daptomycin during continuous ambulatory peritoneal dialysis. Clin J Am Soc Nephrol 2011;6:1081—8.
[81] Lodise TP, Lomaestro BM, Drusano GL. Application of antimicrobial pharmacodynamic concepts into clinical practice: focus on beta-lactam antibiotics: insights from the Society of Infectious Diseases Pharmacists. Pharmacotherapy 2006;26:1320—32.
[82] Lodise Jr TP, Lomaestro B, Drusano GL. Piperacillin-tazobactam for *Pseudomonas aeruginosa* infection: clinical implications of an extended-infusion dosing strategy. Clin Infect Dis 2007;44:357—63.
[83] Lodise TP, Patel N, Renaud-Mutart A, et al. Pharmacokinetic and pharmacodynamic profile of ceftobiprole. Diagn Microbiol Infect Dis 2008;61:96—102.
[84] Lodise Jr TP, Pypstra R, Kahn JB, et al. Probability of target attainment for ceftobiprole as derived from a population pharmacokinetic analysis of 150 subjects. Antimicrob Agents Chemother 2007;51:2378—87.
[85] Lodise Jr TP, Rhoney DH, Tam VH, et al. Pharmacodynamic profiling of cefepime in plasma and cerebrospinal fluid of hospitalized patients with external ventriculostomies. Diagn Microbiol Infect Dis 2006;54:223—30.
[86] Lodise TP, Sorgel F, Melnick D, et al. Penetration of meropenem into epithelial lining fluid of patients with ventilator-associated pneumonia. Antimicrob Agents Chemother 2011;55:1606—10.
[87] Solomkin JS, Mazuski JE, Bradley JS, et al. Diagnosis and management of complicated intra-abdominal infection in adults and children: guidelines by the Surgical Infection Society and the Infectious Diseases Society of America. Clin Infect Dis 2010;50:133—64.
[88] Niederman MS, Craven DE, Bonten MJ, et al. Guidelines for the management of adults with hospital-acquired, ventilator-associated, and healthcare-associated pneumonia. Am J Respir Crit Care Med 2005;171:388—416.
[89] Lipsky BA, Berendt AR, Deery HG, et al. Diagnosis and treatment of diabetic foot infections. Clin Infect Dis 2004;39:885—910.
[90] Mermel LA, Allon M, Bouza E, et al. Clinical practice guidelines for the diagnosis and management of intravascular catheter-related infection: 2009 Update by the Infectious Diseases Society of America. Clin Infect Dis 2009;49:1—45.
[91] Freifeld AG, Bow EJ, Sepkowitz KA, et al. Clinical practice guideline for the use of antimicrobial agents in neutropenic patients with cancer: 2010 update by the infectious diseases society of america. Clin Infect Dis 2011;52:e56—93.
[92] Perry CM, Markham A. Piperacillin/tazobactam: an updated review of its use in the treatment of bacterial infections. Drugs 1999;57:805—43.
[93] Craig WA, Andes D. Pharmacokinetics and pharmacodynamics of antibiotics in otitis media. Pediatr Infect Dis J 1996;15:255—9.
[94] Leggett JE, Ebert S, Fantin B, Craig WA. Comparative dose—effect relations at several dosing intervals for beta-lactam, aminoglycoside and quinolone antibiotics against gram-negative bacilli in murine thigh-infection and pneumonitis models. Scand J Infect Dis Suppl 1990;74:179—84.
[95] Leggett JE, Fantin B, Ebert S, et al. Comparative antibiotic dose—effect relations at several dosing intervals in murine pneumonitis and thigh-infection models. J Infect Dis 1989;159:281—92.
[96] Lodise Jr TP, Lomaestro B, Rodvold KA, et al. Pharmacodynamic profiling of piperacillin in the presence of tazobactam in patients through the use of population pharmacokinetic models and Monte Carlo simulation. Antimicrob Agents Chemother 2004;48:4718—24.
[97] DeRyke CA, Kuti JL, Nicolau DP. Reevaluation of current susceptibility breakpoints for Gram-negative rods based on pharmacodynamic assessment. Diagn Microbiol Infect Dis 2007;58:337—44.
[98] Tam VH, Gamez EA, Weston JS, et al. Outcomes of bacteremia due to *Pseudomonas aeruginosa* with reduced susceptibility to piperacillin-tazobactam: implications on the appropriateness of the resistance breakpoint. Clin Infect Dis 2008;46:862—7.

[99] Auclair B, Ducharme MP. Piperacillin and tazobactam exhibit linear pharmacokinetics after multiple standard clinical doses. Antimicrob Agents Chemother 1999;43:1465–8.

[100] Batra VK, Morrison JA, Lasseter KC, Joy VA. Piperacillin kinetics. Clin Pharmacol Ther 1979;26:41–53.

[101] Cockcroft DW, Gault MH. Prediction of creatinine clearance from serum creatinine. Nephron 1976;16:31–41.

[102] Patel N, Scheetz MH, Drusano GL, Lodise TP. Determination of antibiotic dosage adjustments in patients with renal impairment: elements for success. J Antimicrob Chemother 2010;65:2285–90.

[103] Patel N, Scheetz MH, Drusano GL, Lodise TP. Identification of optimal renal dosage adjustments for traditional and extended-infusion piperacillin-tazobactam dosing regimens in hospitalized patients. Antimicrob Agents Chemother 2010;54:460–5.

[104] Leary R, Jelliffe R, Schumitzky A, van Guilder M. An adaptive grid non-parametric approach to pharmacokinetic and dynamic (pk/pd) population models. In: 14th IEEE Symposium on Computer-Based Medical Systems. Bethesda; MD: 2001. pp. 389–394.

Guidelines for the Monitoring of Vancomycin, Aminoglycosides and Certain Antibiotics

Ronald W. McLawhon

Department of Pathology, University of California, San Diego School of Medicine,
La Jolla, CA

Therapeutic Drug Monitoring: Newer Drugs and Biomarkers
DOI: 10.1016/B978-0-12-385467-4.00010-5

INTRODUCTION

Antibiotics represent a diverse group of chemotherapeutic agents with activity against microorganisms such as bacteria, fungi or protozoa. The first effective antibiotic discovered was penicillin. Since the discovery of penicillin more than 100 antibiotics have been developed and are currently used in medicine. Antibiotics can be classified based on their chemical structures. Alternatively, antibiotics can be categorized on the basis of their target specificity: narrow-spectrum antibiotics target particular types of bacteria, such as gram-negative or gram-positive bacteria, while broad-spectrum antibiotics can be effective against a wide range of bacteria [1–3]. In addition, antibiotics can be broadly classified as either bactericidal or bacteriostatic, based on their mechanism of action [1, 4]. Bactericidal agents typically kill bacteria directly, whereas bacteriostatic agents prevent cell growth and division, although there can be considerable overlap of these classifications depending on the drug and organism. Antibiotics can also be classified on the basis of their mechanism of action. There are five major mechanisms by which an antibiotic exerts its pharmacological action: inhibition of cell wall synthesis, inhibition of bacterial protein synthesis, alteration of bacterial cell wall, inhibition of bacterial nucleic acid synthesis, and antimetabolite activities.

Inhibition of bacterial cell wall formation is probably the most common mechanism by which an antibiotic kills bacteria or inhibits bacterial growth. Antibiotics which interfere with cell-wall synthesis are beta-lactam antibiotics, including penicillins, cephalosporins, vancomycin, etc., while antibiotics such as clindamycin, chloramphenicol, lincomycin and macrolide antibiotics interfere with protein synthesis of bacteria by binding to the 50S ribosomal unit. Antibiotics that interfere with bacterial protein synthesis by binding to the 30S ribosomal unit are tetracycline and aminoglycosides. Sulfonamides and trimethoprim kills bacteria by inhibiting folate synthesis. Antibacterial effects of metronidazole, quinolones and novobiocin are due to their capability of interfering with bacterial DNA synthesis, while rifampin interferes with bacterial RNA synthesis. Both polymyxin B and gramicidin kill bacterial by interfering with cell membrane function [1]. In Table 10.1, antibiotics are classified based on their mechanism of action.

Typically, minimum inhibitory concentration (MIC) and minimum bactericidal concentration are used to measure *in vitro* activity of an antimicrobial, and provide excellent indicators of antimicrobial potency [2]. As such, antibiotics can be further characterized as either concentration-dependent (for which achieving a large post-dose concentration to MIC ratio appears important) or concentration-independent/time-dependent (where efficacy is related to maintaining the overall concentration above the MIC). Antibiotics such as beta-lactams (penicillins, cephalosporins, carbapenems and monobactams), clindamycin, macrolides (erythromycin and clarithromycin), etc., can be effective in eradicating bacteria because these antibiotics can bind to microorganisms for a long time; these antibiotics are referred to as time-dependent antibiotics. The inhibitory effects are observed for these antibiotics if drug concentration exceeds MIC. For antibiotics which are involved in concentration-dependent killing (aminoglycosides and quinolones), the peak/MIC ratio is crucial for eradication of the bacteria [2].

Therapeutic ranges and dosage regimen can be based theoretically on a drug's known pharmacokinetics and pharmacodynamics [2–6]; thus in some clinical situations direct monitoring of drug concentrations within serum, plasma or other body fluids may be warranted. The side

TABLE 10.1 Classification of Antibiotics Based on Chemical Structure

Chemical structure	Example of drugs
Aminoglycoside	Amikacin*, gentamicin*, kanamycin*, neomycin, netilmicin*, streptomycin, tobramycin*
Glycopeptides	Vancomycin*
Beta-lactam	Penicillin G, penicillin V, ampicillin, carbenicillin, dicloxacillin, nafcillin, oxacillin, piperacillin, temocillin, ticarcillin
Cephalosporins	Cefadroxil, cefazolin, ceflatonin, cephalexin, cefixime, cefdinir, cefditoren, cefoperazone, cefotaxime, cefepime
Carbapenem	Ertapenem, doripenem, meropenem
Macrolide	Azithromycin, clarithromycin, dirithromycin, erythromycin, roxithromycin, troleandomycin
Monobactam	Aztreonam
Polypeptides	Bacitracin, colistin, polymyxin B
Oxazolidinones	Linezolid, quinupristin/dalfopristin
Quinolones	Ciprofloxacin, enoxacin, gatifloxacin, lomefloxacin. moxifloxacin, ofloxacin, norfloxacin, levofloxacin
Sulfonamides	Mafenide, sulfacetamide, sulfadiazine, sulfamethoxazole, sulfanilamide, sulfisoxazole, trimethoprim
Tetracycline	Doxycycline, minocycline, oxytetracycline, tetracycline

*Therapeutic drug monitoring is essential to avoid drug toxicity.

effects and toxicity of antibiotic therapy [1, 6, 7] range from fever, nausea, vomiting and diarrhea to severe allergic reactions. Additional serious and irreversible complications, such as nephrotoxicity and ototoxicity, can be observed with drugs like vancomycin and aminoglycosides. When these agents are used, peak and trough concentrations should be closely monitored due to their narrow therapeutic index and serious risks of toxicity to the host [5, 7]. Other antibiotics are rarely measured in routine clinical practice, due to wider therapeutic indices and lower toxicity risks and complications. However, these risks can increase considerably in certain clinical situations (e.g., decreased renal clearance with kidney failure) and therapeutic monitoring may be beneficial.

Aminoglycosides and vancomycin are the most frequently assessed antibiotics in today's clinical laboratories, due to the need for close monitoring and the widespread availability and application of commercially available immunoassays. Most other antibiotics require more complex and specialized chromatographic methods — including gas liquid chromatography (GC) with or without mass spectrometry, high performance liquid chromatography

(HPLC) or liquid chromatography/mass spectrometry (LC/MS) — for quantitation of drug concentrations; as such, therapeutic monitoring of these antibiotics is rarely performed except when there are exceptional clinical indications. This chapter reviews the monitoring of vancomycin and aminoglycosides [5, 7, 8], as well as the potential need for and various methods for evaluating several other classes of common antibiotics that are less frequently monitored today.

VANCOMYCIN: OVERVIEW

Vancomycin is a tricyclic glycopeptide isolated from *Streptomyces orientalis*, which has time-dependent bacteriocidal activity against susceptible gram-positive organisms. The structure of vancomycin is given in Fig. 10.1. Vancomycin is a relatively large molecule with a molecular weight of 1456 Da; its primary mode of action interferes with cell-well biosynthesis and it is widely used to treat infections caused by *Streptococcus viridans*, coagulase negative *staphylococci, Enterococcus* species and *Staphylococcus aureus* [1, 5–8].

More recently, vancomycin has received considerable attention and has become the primary drug of choice against the growing problem of community- and hospital-acquired methicillin-resistant *Staphylococcus aureus* (MRSA) as well as US 300, a community-associated

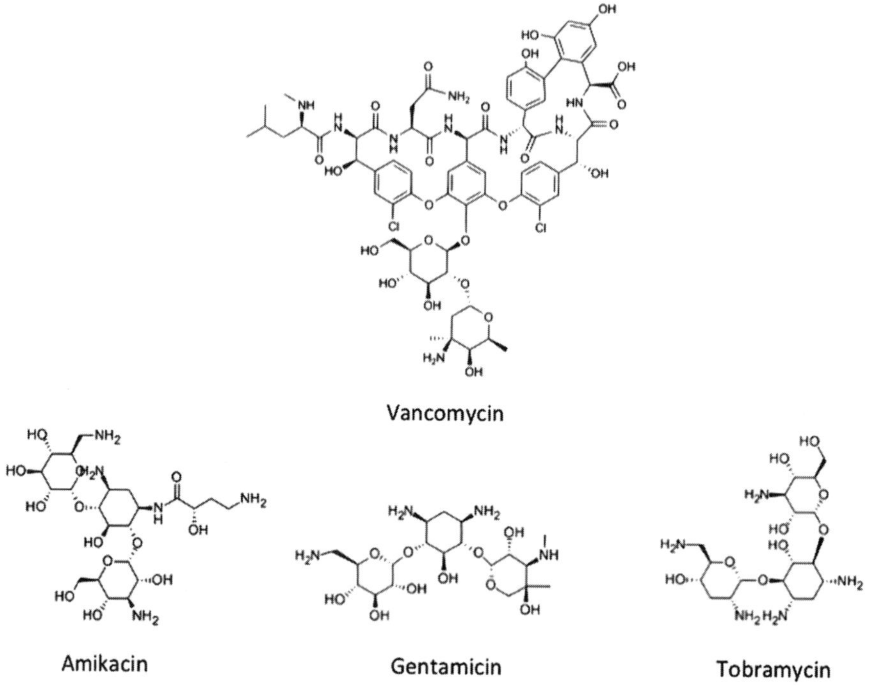

Vancomycin

Amikacin   Gentamicin   Tobramycin

FIGURE 10.1   Chemical structures of vancomycin and the major aminoglycide antibiotics (amikaci, tobramycin and gentimicin).

strain of MRSA. Hota *et al.* reported that in the year 2000 there were 75 cases of MRSA per 100 000 people, rising to a rate of 396 cases per 100 000 people. In addition, the number of serious MRSA infections increased from 5 cases per 100 000 people to 17 cases per 100 000 people. However, infection due to the US 300 strain was negatively associated with severity of the disease indicating that this strain is less virulent than other MRSA strains [9]. With greater and more widespread clinical use of vancomycin, vancomycin-resistant enterococcal infections emerged and have risen dramatically, and are increasingly recognized to be a major infection control problem amongst both hospitalized and institutionalized (long-term care) patient populations. Gould commented that the clinical utility of vancomycin is under serious threat due to the increased number of strains with reduced or intermediate suscep-tibility to vancomycin [10].

Vancomycin Pharmacokinetics and Pharmacodynamics

Oral vancomycin is poorly absorbed, and a major clinical indication for oral vancomy-cin therapy is treating *Clostridium difficile* infection. However, for treating life-threatening bacterial infections vancomycin is administered intravenously. Due to its poor absorption, variable distribution and narrow therapeutic index, quantitative measurement of both trough and peak concentrations of this bacteriocidal agent has been recommended and routinely performed [5–7] for decades, primarily to assess both therapeutic benefit and toxicity — most notably, ototoxicity (long-term vestibular and sensory damage) and nephrotoxicity. Vancomycin is protein bound in serum or plasma primarily to albumin, in a variable amount. The protein-bound fraction is estimated to be approximately 55%, although reports have ranged from 10–82% in some studies. As free vancomycin is considered to be active, interpretation of serum or plasma drug levels may be dependent on protein binding and correlates with albumin concentrations [11, 12]. Vancomycin distri-bution is complex [12], but for the purpose of monitoring serum concentrations and adjusting dosage a one-compartment model has been typically used clinically. Two- and three-compartment models may be better predictors of the concentration–time profile. Distribution half-life is 0.5–1 hour in most patients, with a volume of distribution of 0.39–0.9 L/kg; this, however, may be prolonged in renal failure patients. Additional factors that can affect vancomycin distribution and penetration into tissues and fluids include protein binding, tissue type, tissue perfusion, degree of tissue inflammation, and diabetes, among others.

Vancomycin is eliminated principally by glomerular filtration and drug clearance, and also closely correlates with creatinine clearance. Small amounts are also eliminated by renal tubular secretion and through the biliary tract. Drug half-life increases as glomerular filtra-tion declines [13]. Certain age-groups (neonates, children) and patient populations (burn victims, obese adults) have been observed to exhibit differences in the elimination and distri-bution of vancomycin when compared to normal adults [14, 15].

Vancomycin demonstrates time-dependent killing of bacteria. By keeping vancomycin concentrations above the minimum inhibitory concentration (MIC), optimization of bacterial killing at the site of the infection is achieved. Maximal bacterial killing is obtained by keeping the free vancomycin concentration at four times the vancomycin MIC [11]. Vancomycin MIC for various organisms has been reported in detail elsewhere [11, 16]. Vancomycin typically displays concentration-independent activity (as best documented against *Staphylococcus aureus*), with the area under the concentration curve (AUC) divided by the MIC as the primary predictive pharmacodynamic parameter for efficacy. Some pharmacodynamics studies have shown that maintaining area under the concentration curve above the MIC (AUC_{24}/MIC) of 400 or 125 is associated with a greater chance of treating *Staphylococcus aureus* pneumonia or *Enterococcus faecium* infections, respectively [17, 18]. As such, when the AUC_{24}/MIC increases, the patient may need to be exposed to higher concentrations of vancomycin.

To achieve this pharmacokinetic/pharmacodynamic target, it is now widely felt by consensus expert committees [19] that larger vancomycin doses and high trough serum concentrations may be required. Although vancomycin administration is associated with some adverse effects, the potential benefit of increased drug dosage is worth the risk of mostly reversible adverse events.

Therapeutic Drug Monitoring of Vancomycin and Recommended Guidelines

The primary premise for monitoring and adjustment of serum vancomycin concentrations is based on the perceived need to achieve serum concentrations at some multiple above the minimum inhibitory concentration (MIC) for the offending organisms while avoiding potential adverse effects. For almost four decades of clinical practice, monitoring vancomycin concentrations in serum or plasma consisted of measuring peak and trough levels during intermittent dosing. The desired range has been traditionally specified at 20–40 μg/mL for peak concentrations and 10–15 μg/mL for trough concentrations, but these values were based less on clinical efficacy and more on achievable serum concentrations with standard dosing protocols [11, 20]. Although increasing trough vancomycin concentration to 15–20 μg/mL has been proposed, this proposal has not currently been supported by clinical trials. Therefore, alternative therapy should be considered in patients with methicillin-resistant *Staphylococcus aureus* infection if the MIC of vancomycin is 2 mg/L or higher, because increasing the dosage to achieve a higher trough vancomycin concentration may also increase the potential of vancomycin toxicity. Currently, the risk of vancomycin therapy is considered as minimal if the dosage is 1 g (15 μmg/kg) every 12 h, but a higher rate of nephrotoxicity is encountered at a dosage of 4 g/day or higher [21]. The relationship between serum concentrations and treatment success or failure in serious *Staphylococcus aureus* infections has been clearly established (failure rates exceeding 60% for *S. aureus* displaying a vancomycin MIC value of 4 mg/L), prompting recommendations to lower the breakpoint for susceptibility from 4 to 2 mg/L by the Clinical and Laboratory Standards Institute and the Food and Drug Administration in 2006 and 2008, respectively. Recently, a number of studies have established a relationship between vancomycin treatment failures and infections in patients with methicillin-resistant *S. aureus* displaying a MIC at 2 mg/L (2 μg/mL) or more. Taking into account other variables, for most gram-positive organisms that have MIC values of 1 μg/mL the desired trough concentration should be at least 8–10 μg/mL. For treatment of *S. aureus* pneumonia, additional recommendations have been made for trough concentrations of 10–15 μg/mL, with endocarditis, osteomyelitis and meningitis requiring higher trough concentrations [11, 19]. Patel *et al.* studied the pharmacodynamic profile of the more intensive dosing of vancomycin, ranging from 0.5 mg intravenously every 12 h to 2 g every 12 h, to treat methicillin-resistant *Staphylococcus aureus* infection using Monte

Carlo simulation. At a MIC of 2 mg/L, even the most aggressive vancomycin dosing regimen considered (2 g every 12 h) only yielded a probability of target attainment (PTA) of 57% while generating a nephrotoxicity probability above 35%. However, at MICs less than 1 mg/L, all subjects with trough vancomycin concentrations between 15 and 20 μg/mL showed a PTA of 100%. The authors concluded that vancomycin may not be useful for treating serious methicillin-resistant *Staphylococcus aureus* infection with MIC values exceeding 1 mg/L. Because an AUC/MIC ratio of 400 or higher is the target associated with efficacy, incorporating AUC (area under the serum drug concentration curve) in routine therapeutic drug monitoring of vancomycin could be useful [22]. For all practical purposes, trough serum vancomycin concentrations are now viewed as the most accurate and practical method of monitoring the effectiveness of vancomycin. Trough serum concentrations should be obtained just before the fourth dose, at steady-state conditions.

Available evidence does not support monitoring of peak serum vancomycin concentrations to decrease the frequency of toxicity [19]. Depending on the variable definitions of nephrotoxicity with vancomycin, the incidence is still relatively low, estimated at about 5% [23]. There are limited data suggesting a direct causal relationship between toxicity and specific serum vancomycin concentrations. There are also conflicting data characterized by confounding nephrotoxic agents and the inability to examine the time sequence of events surrounding changes in renal function secondary to vancomycin exposure. A patient should be considered to have vancomycin-induced nephrotoxicity only if multiple (at least two or three consecutive) high serum creatinine concentrations are observed during vancomycin therapy.

Monitoring of trough serum vancomycin concentrations is also useful in those individuals receiving aggressive therapy to achieve sustained trough serum concentrations of 15–20 μg/mL, (which is higher than the recommended level) or who are at high risk of toxicity, as in patients receiving concurrent treatment with other nephrotoxins such as aminoglycosides, amphotericin B and vasopressors. However, monitoring of serum vancomycin concentrations to prevent ototoxicity is discouraged, because this toxicity is rarely associated with monotherapy and does not correlate with serum vancomycin concentrations. Monitoring may be more important when other ototoxic agents, such as aminoglycosides, are co-administered. Therapeutic monitoring of vancomycin is also recommended (Table 10.2) for patients with unstable renal function (either deteriorating or significantly improving function) and for patients receiving prolonged courses of therapy (greater than 5 days or more). Currently, frequent monitoring for short-course therapy (< 5 days) is not recommended [11, 19–21].

Reliable, inexpensive and easy to perform homogeneous and heterogeneous immunoassays [5, 7, 8] for vancomycin (as well as aminoglycosides) are commercially available in a variety of different formats and are frequently offered in many clinical laboratories today, as they are readily adapted to existing instrumentation (including high-throughput, random access, automated chemistry and immunoassay analyzers). While high-performance liquid chromatography (HPLC) methods for separation and quantitation of aminoglycosides and vancomycin have been developed [24, 25], the availability of sensitive and precise immunoassays has led to them largely supplanting chromatographic methods as the latter rarely offer any additional analytical and clinical advantages for serum and plasma measurements in most patients. HPLC and, more recently, liquid chromatography combined with mass

TABLE 10.2   Current Guidelines for Monitoring of Vancomycin

TIME OF SAMPLING RELATIVE TO DOSE

- Peak concentration obtained 30–60 min after a 30-min infusion (NB: peak concentrations have not been shown to correlate well with efficacy or toxicity and are not recommended according to American Society of Health-System Pharmacists, and the Society of Infectious Diseases Pharmacists consensus document)
- Trough concentration obtained within 30 min before the next dose
- Trough levels should be at steady state (24–30 hours after initiation of therapy in patients with normal renal function; approximately fourth or fifth dose in adults)

RECOMMENDED FREQUENCY OF SAMPLING

- Patients for whom vancomycin is not currently recommended include:
  - Adults < 60 years with normal body weight and stable renal function
  - Short course of therapy (< 5 days)
- Patients for whom trough vancomycin concentrations should be obtained at steady state:
  - Patients receiving vancomycin therapy for longer than 5 days
  - All patients with renal impairment (creatinine clearance < 40 mL/min)
  - Patients with changing renal function > 0.5 mg/mL or > 50% over baseline
  - Special patient populations who have altered renal clearance and/or altered volume distribution
    - Elderly ≥ 60 years
    - Burn
    - Obesity
    - Cancer
    - Pediatric and neonates
  - Concomitant therapy with nephrotoxic drugs
    - Aminoglycosides
    - Amphotericin B
    - Loop diuretics
    - Vasopressors
    - Other (ACE inhibitors, IV contrast)
- Patients who require more frequent monitoring to achieve goal concentrations and prevent toxicity
  - Higher dose of vancomycin to penetrate site of infection, treatment of more serious life-threatening infections, or extended duration therapy
    - Endocarditis
    - Meningitis
    - Osteomyelitis
    - Pneumonia
    - Sepsis

spectrometry or tandem mass spectrometry (LC/MS or LC/MS/MS) applications are most widely used when analysis is required on a particular biological matrix of the specimen for which immunoassay is inappropriate or unsuitable, including human body fluid and tissue extracts as well as biological and pharmaceutical preparations. In addition, certain analytical biases and potential inaccuracies have been reported with some immunoassay methods in specific clinical situations, and chromatographic separation may be preferred as the method of choice to resolve such diagnostic dilemmas. Although LC/MS methods [26, 27] offer enhanced sensitivity, linearity, precision, and accuracy compared to either immunoassay or conventional HPLC, they have been slow to be adopted due to the investment costs associated with the acquisition of instrumentation and operation compared to other available methods.

AMINOGLYCOSIDES: OVERVIEW

Aminoglycosides are small, hydrophilic, and constitute one of the oldest classes of antibiotics. Streptomycin was the first aminoglycoside discovered, in 1914, and represents just one of a large class of antibiotics that share in common the general structure of two or more amino-sugars joined by a glycosidic linkage to either hexose or aminoglycitol [1, 28]. Aminoglycosides are polycationic inhibitors of the 30S ribosomal subunit that interferes with protein synthesis and disrupts cell membrane transport and cell permeability. These drugs are most commonly used for the treatment of life-threatening systemic infections with gram-negative bacilli such as *Escherichia coli*, *Klebsiella pneumoniae*, *Proteus mirabilis* and *Pseudomonas aeruginosa* [1]. The drugs are among the most effective front-line chemotherapeutic agents used in the management of aerobic gram-negative bacteremia, causing concentration-dependent bacterial cell death (strongly associated with peak serum or plasma levels) regardless of the size of the bacterial load [11, 29].

While many aminoglycoside antibiotics have been developed and marketed worldwide over the years, the ones most commonly used in the US today are amikacin, gentamicin and tobramycin. Due to their known toxicity, which is similar to that of vancomycin (i.e., nephrotoxicity and ototoxicity), the use of this class of antibiotics has been largely reserved for treating the most serious infections, which may explain the low incidence of drug resistance seen thus far in comparison to many other more commonly used antibiotics. Other aminoglycosides, such as streptomycin and kanamycin, have been shown to be effective in the treatment of mycobacterial infections, and will be discussed later in this chapter.

Aminoglycosides: Pharmacokinetics and Pharmacodynamics

Aminoglycosides are poorly absorbed via the oral route, and are usually administered parenterally for treatment of systemic infections. All drugs in this class of antibiotics demonstrate similar volumes of distribution and overall kinetics, with elimination half-lives of 2—3 hours [11, 28, 29]. The volume of distribution of aminoglycosides is similar to extracellular fluid volume. These drugs exhibit little protein binding ($< 10\%$), and distribution can be increased, with corresponding decrease in peak levels measured in serum or plasma, in patients with fever and sepsis.

The major route of elimination for aminoglycosides is through the kidney, and these drugs remain essentially (85—95%) unchanged. Patients with impaired renal function and elderly patients eliminate aminoglycosides more slowly, and have longer drug half-lives, when compared to the normal adult population [30—32]. In contrast, children and patients with fever have shorter drug half-lives and lower concentrations of some aminoglycosides, particularly gentamicin. Patients with other conditions, such as cystic fibrosis, may also have lower serum or plasma concentrations due to increased renal clearance combined with larger volumes of distribution.

Aminoglycosides exhibit concentration-dependent bacteriocidal activity. Two predictors [11, 33] seem to be most closely correlated with efficacy: the AUC at 24 hours to MIC ratio (AUC_{24}/MIC) and the ratio of peak aminoglycoside concentration (C_{max}) to MIC. The C_{max}/MIC ratio of 8–10 should be targeted for successful therapy with aminoglycosides, and the C_{max} can be established from known MIC data. Because clearance of aminoglycosides is proportional to glomerular filtration rate, patients with renal impairment may be more susceptible to aminoglycoside toxicity due to reduced clearance of aminoglycosides. For these patients, expansion of dosing frequency has been recommended. On the other hand, shorter dosing frequency may be needed for patients with higher clearance of aminoglycosides — for example, burn patients. The goal of dosing is to achieve maximum antimicrobial effect from these drugs. Rea *et al.*, based on their study of 102 critically ill patients receiving aminoglycosides (211 aminoglycoside serum levels studied), commented that the majority of critically ill patients did not reach the pharmacodynamic target of C_{max} to MIC of 10 or above from initial standard dosage aminoglycosides because the probability of reaching the pharmacodynamic target was only 20% with a standard 7-mg/kg dosage of gentamicin and 40% with a 7-mg/kg dosage of tobramycin. This may be due to a larger volume of distribution in these critically ill patients than reported in the literature. The authors recommended that after the first standard 7-mg/kg dosage of gentamicin or tobramycin the C_{max} should be measured and the MIC of the pathogen determined, with adjustment of subsequent dosage to achieve the pharmacodynamic target in critically ill patients [34].

As mentioned previously, the two major toxicities of aminoglycosides are similar to vancomycin; namely, nephrotoxicity and ototoxicity. Nephrotoxicity is seen in 15–17% of patients, and ototoxicity in 20–25% of patients. The risks increase considerably with prolonged therapy over 7 days in duration, or in combination with other agents such as vancomycin, cyclosporine, tacrolimus, cisplatin, furosemide or cephalosporin antibiotics. Sustained peak concentrations of 15–20 µg/mL are associated with nephrotoxicity, while levels > 16 µg/mL are associated with ototoxicity [30, 35]. Nephrotoxicity risks have been reported to increase in some patients with chronic liver disease and hypoalbuminemia. A less commonly encountered toxicity is neuromuscular blockade, and aminoglycoside levels should be closely monitored when being co-administered with neuromuscular blocking agents [11].

Monitoring of Aminoglycosides and Recommended Guidelines

Aminoglycosides are characterized by high clinical effectiveness in the treatment of infection with gram-negative bacilli, but the main drawback is occurrence of toxicity in a number of patients, which can be minimized by routine therapeutic drug monitoring. Therapeutic monitoring of aminoglycosides is dependent on the type of dosing scenario that is used: traditional dosing, once daily (extended) dosing or synergy dosing [36–38]. The primary purpose of monitoring in each case is to attain the desired therapeutic concentrations and avoid toxic serum concentrations. Studies have clearly demonstrated that therapeutic drug monitoring of aminoglycosides, if administered in multiple doses, is cost-effective and useful in maximizing the efficacy of aminoglycosides and at the same time reducing incidences of drug toxicity. However, the requirement for therapeutic drug monitoring of aminoglycosides if administered as a once-daily dosage has not been clearly demonstrated [39]. Like vancomycin, monitoring is probably unnecessary for the majority of patients, if aminoglycoside therapy is of only short duration (3 days or less).

Traditional dosing is intermittent dosing, occurring two to three times per day, until serum concentration targets are attained. Peak concentrations are measured in serum or plasma specimens collected approximately 30–60 minutes after a 30-min infusion of drug, whereas trough concentrations are collected approximately 30 minutes prior to the next dose. Steady-state levels are reached after four or five half-lives. Once steady-state and desired concentrations are attained, monitoring of trough levels should be performed at least weekly unless renal function is unstable or other nephrotoxic drugs are included. Typically, peak and trough concentrations of 5–10 μg/mL and < 2 μg/mL, respectively, for both gentamicin and tobramycin are desired in order to treat life-threatening infections, whereas peak levels of 20–35 μg/mL and trough levels of 4–8 μg/mL are desired for amikacin [11, 33, 36]. These targets can vary (increase or decrease) depending on the type of infection being treated. Lower peak (15–25 μg/mL) and trough (1–4 μg/mL) concentrations may be desirable in treating less severe infections.

Once-daily (or extended) dosing requires the administration of a large dose of aminoglycoside, once each day. It has advantages and disadvantages, and may be contraindicated in patients with endocarditis, burns, cystic fibrosis or enterococcal infections, and in children less than 12 years of age. For patients with significant renal dysfunction, dosage may be administered every 36–48 hours. For once-daily dosage of aminoglycosides, monitoring peak concentration is generally redundant because the desired peak concentration can be easily achieved. However, for a patient where the volume of distribution could be significantly different than normally expected − for example, critically ill patients, burn patients, etc. − measuring peak concentration may have some merit even with a once-daily dosing protocol. Moreover, when following a single-dose protocol of aminoglycosides the trough concentration could be below the detection limit of the assay and trough concentration determination may not be useful. Therefore, for once-daily dosage of aminoglycosides there is no universally accepted guideline for monitoring. For the 36- to 48-hour dosing interval in renally compromised patients, trough concentration monitoring has been suggested to ensure administration of another dosage does not cause aminoglycoside toxicity. Several nomograms have been published to aid dosing of aminoglycosides. These nomograms include MacGowan and Reeves, Begg and Nicolau nomograms. Another approach is to use Bayesian adaptive feedback software by a skilled pharmacologist to facilitate achievement of a C_{max}/MIC ratio of 8–10 and AUC targets of 70–120 mg·h/L over 24 hours [40]. In general, the once-daily dosage of aminoglycosides provides a longer time of administration until the threshold of nephrotoxicity is reached compared to multiple daily dosing. However, regarding ototoxicity, no dosing protocol appears to be less toxic [41].

The use of aminoglycosides synergistically with other antibiotics is a common practice in treating gram-negative and gram-positive bacterial infections. For gram-negative infections, monitoring should occur as described for the traditional dosing approach. With aminoglycoside dosing for gram-positive infections, lower doses will be required and minimal monitoring is recommended. In these instances only trough levels should be monitored, as peak concentrations should not be excessive − typically, for a drug like gentamicin, trough concentration should be maintained at 0.5–1 μg/mL. With aminoglycoside therapy, other tests should be monitored; serum creatinine should be measured at least twice weekly, with vestibular function/hearing tests also being indicated during prolonged courses of therapy (7—14 days). Suggested therapeutic ranges of vancomycin, aminoglycosides and selected antibiotics are given in Table 10.3.

Commonly used aminoglycosides can be readily monitored in serum or plasma using commercially available homogeneous or heterogeneous automated immunoassays [5—8], with turnaround times of less than an hour. Rarely would HPLC [42, 43] or LC/MS [44, 45] methods be routinely employed; these are usually reserved for cases where drug levels are measured in atypical specimen matrices or if any concern is raised about drug impurities,

TABLE 10.3   Therapeutic Range of Various Commonly Monitored Aminoglycosides
and Vancomycin

Antibiotic	Therapeutic range, µg/mL
AMINOGLYCOSIDES	
Amikacin	20—35 µg/mL (peak)
	< 4—8 µg/mL (trough)
Gentamicin	5—10 µg/mL (peak)
	< 2 µg/mL (trough)
Tobramycin	5—10 µg/mL (peak)
	< 2 µg/mL (trough)
GLYCOPEPTIDES	
Vancomycin	20—40 µg/mL (peak)
	5—15 µg/mL (trough)
OTHER ANTIBIOTICS	
Chloramphenicol	5—20 µg/mL (trough)
(Neonates)	3.5—13.9 µg/mL (trough)
Ciprofloxacin	3—5 µg/mL (peak)
	0.5—3 µg/mL (trough)
Cefazolin	60—120 µg/mL (peak)
ANTITUBERCULOSIS	
Isoniazid	3—6 µg/mL (2-h peak), daily dosage
	9—18 µg/mL (2-h peak), bi-weekly dosage
Rifampin	8—24 µg/mL (2-h peak), daily or bi-weekly
Ethambutol	2—6 µg/mL (2-h peak)
Pyrazinamide	20—50 µg/mL (2-h peak)
Rifabutin	0.3—0.9 µg/mL (2-h peak)

complex parent compounds, metabolites, or biases/interferences with the more commonly used immunoassay techniques.

THERAPEUTIC DRUG MONITORING OF BETA-LACTAM ANTIBIOTICS

The beta-lactam antibiotics penicillins and cephalosporins are still the most widely-used group of antibiotics available, with penicillin being one of the oldest commercially available antibiotics. These drugs are part of a broad class of antimicrobial agents know as beta-lactam antibiotics [1], as they share a beta-lactam ring nucleus as part of their core molecular structure. The drugs [1, 4] are bactericidal, and act to disrupt the synthesis of the peptidoglycan layer of bacterial cell walls and cell-wall structural integrity. Beta-lactam antibiotics interfere with the final transpeptidation step and competitively inhibit crosslinking of peptidoglycan.

Penicillins, such as Penicillin G, Penicillin V, amoxicillin, nafcillin and ampicillin, are used for the treatment of gram-positive infections [1, 5, 7] such as *Staphylococcus* species, *Streptococcus pneumoniae*, beta-hemolytic strains of *Streptococcus*, and *Enterococcus faecalis.* These drugs may be used alone or in preparations that include beta-lactamase inhibitors, such as clavulanic acid, tazobactam and sulbactam, for the treatment of penicillin-resistant organisms.

Several generations (first through fifth) of cephalosporin antibiotics have now been developed and are widely prescribed, with an increasingly broader spectrum of action against both gram-negative and gram-positive organisms [1]. First-generation cephalosporins (e.g., cephazolin) are predominantly active against gram-positive bacteria, and successive generations have increased activity against gram-negative bacteria (albeit often with reduced activity against gram-positive organisms). Later generations of cephalosporins, such as cefaclor, ceftazidime, ceftriaxone and cefazolin, are effective against organisms including *Proteus mirabilis*, *Klebsiella* species, *Enterobacter aerogenes*, *Haemophilus influenzae* and *Pseudomonas aeruginosa*.

Beta-lactam antibiotics (both penicillins and cephalosporins) have wide therapeutic indices and dose-dependent toxicity. As such, routine therapeutic drug monitoring is not indicated in most patients [5—7]. Adverse drug reactions [1] with beta-lactam antibiotics include diarrhea, nausea, rash, urticaria, fever, vomiting, erythema and dermatitis. Allergic hypersensitivity occurs in up to 10% patients, with anaphylaxis as a rare complication (most frequently with penicillins). Monitoring adequacy of blood concentration may be beneficial, especially in patients with kidney failure, where renal clearance of the drug is compromised, or to assess overall patient compliance. In general, antibiotic levels for these will need to be above a certain minimum concentration (e.g., 3 µg/mL), but no additional benefit will be derived with concentrations even slightly above that range (e.g., 6—9 µg/mL), depending on the drug used.

Currently, there is no commercially available immunoassay for monitoring any drug of this class and all currently available methods are based on chromatography, mostly HPLC combined with ultraviolet detection (UV). Samanidou *et al.* reviewed over 80 reports of analysis of beta-lactam antibiotics using HPLC, and 76% of all reports used UV detection [46]. Mascher and Kikuta described a method for determination of amoxicillin in human serum and plasma by HPLC and on-line post-column derivatization [47]. Newer LC/MS methods with electrospray ionization have been developed to quantitate various penicillins and cephalosporins in serum or plasma, and are extremely powerful – resolving multiple drugs in a single analytical run, with limits of quantitation reported down to 0.1 ng/mL and improved precision with CVs of 3% [48–51].

THERAPEUTIC DRUG MONITORING OF SULFONAMIDES AND TRIMETHOPRIM

Sulfonamides (sometimes called simply sulfa drugs), along with penicillin, are among the oldest and, historically, most widely prescribed chemotherapeutic agents for the treatment of infectious diseases. This large and diverse group of antimicrobial agents (which include sulfamethoxazole, sulfisoxazole, sulfadiazine and many others) act as competitive inhibitors of dihydropteroate synthetase, a key enzymatic step in folate synthesis [1, 7], to exhibit a bacteriostatic rather than bactericidal effect [1, 4] by interfering with normal cell division.

Organisms susceptible to sulfonamides include group A *Streptococcus, Streptococcus pneumoniae, Haemophilus influenzae, Haemophilus ducreyi, Vibrio cholerae, Chlamydia trachomatis,* some strains of *Bacillus anthracis* and *Corynebacterium diphtheriae,* and *Brucella, Yersinia, Nocardia,* and *Actinomyces* species. These broad-spectrum agents are most frequently used in the prophylaxis and treatment of urinary tract infections, and in some cases (sulfapyridine), have been found effective in the treatment of dermatitis herpetiformis and inflammatory bowel disease [1, 7].

Trimethoprim is another bacteriostatic antibiotic, mainly used in the prophylaxis and treatment of urinary tract infections, that acts by interfering with the action of bacterial dihydrofolate reductase [1]. While used as a monotherapy, trimethoprim has been commonly used in prescription combination (Bactrim, Septra) with the sulfonamide antibiotic sulfamethoxazole. This co-trimoxazole therapy results in an in a synergistic antibacterial effect by inhibiting successive steps in the pathway of folate synthesis. Sulfamethoxazole-trimethoprim preparations are effective for treatment of infections due to chlamydia, susceptible strains of *Enterobacteriaceae* species such as *Escherichia coli, Klebsiella* species, *Morganella morganii, Proteus mirabilis* and *Proteus vulgaris,* in addition to gram-positive cocci such as *Staphylococcus pyogenes, Streptococcus pyogenes, Streptococcus pneumoniae* and *Streptococcus viridans.*

The primary indication for therapeutic monitoring is to assess therapeutic dosing, particularly in patients with renal disease. The toxicity in renal disease is often characterized by formation of sulfonamide crystals [1, 7] in the kidney resulting in calculi development, and is concentration-dependent (usually with prolonged serum concentrations in excess of 125 μg/mL). Because trimethoprim (used in either monotherapy or co-trimoxazole therapy) similarly has a wide therapeutic index and dose-dependent toxicity [1, 5], routine drug monitoring is not warranted, except again in patients with evidence of renal failure. For other drugs in this class, like sulfapyridine, high levels can also, rarely, cause agranulocytosis and leukopenia in some patients, and may be another indication for therapeutic monitoring.

The most commonly used method for assaying sulfonamides, either alone or in combination with trimethoprim, is HPLC [52]. More recently, a solid phase extraction LC/MS method has been developed for simultaneous quantitation of sulfonamides and trimethoprim that is six-times more sensitive than conventional HPLC-UV and has broader applications for use in a wide range of biological fluids [53].

THERAPEUTIC DRUG MONITORING OF CHLORAMPHENICOL AND TETRACYCLINE

Chloramphenicol and tetracycline are bactericidal agents that inhibit protein synthesis [1, 7]; their effects are dependent on the relative toxicity against the microorganism versus that on the host [1, 5–7]. Chloramphenicol acts by binding to the 50S ribosomal subunit of bacteria mRNA and inhibits protein synthesis in prokaryotic organisms, whereas tetracycline (and related drugs such as doxycycline) inhibits the action of the prokaryotic 30S ribosome by binding the 16S rRNA and thereby blocking the aminoacyl-tRNA. In eukaryotic cells, toxicity of tetracycline and its analogs may be related to inactivation of mitochondrial 30S ribosomes.

Chloramphenicol is typically used [1, 7] against gram-negative bacteria such as *Haemophilus influenzae*, *Neisseria meningitidis*, *Neisseria gonorrhoeae*, *Salmonella typhi*, *Brucella* species, *Bordetella pertussis*, *Vibrio cholerae* and *Shigella* species. Due to its side effects, tetracycline's primary use is now limited to the treatment of acne vulgaris and rosacea. Another analog, doxycycline, is most frequently used to treat chronic prostatitis, sinusitis, syphilis, chlamydia, pelvic inflammatory disease, acne and rosacea, as well as *Yersinia pestis* (the infectious agent of bubonic plague), Lyme disease, ehrlichiosis and Rocky Mountain spotted fever.

Host toxicity with chloramphenicol therapy [1, 7] may be manifested as blood dyscrasias or, less commonly, cardiovascular collapse; both show a modest relationship to blood concentration [2, 6]. The therapeutic range of chloramphenicol is usually considered as 5–20 μg/mL in adults, but in neonates the suggested therapeutic range is 3.5 –13.9 μg/mL due to significantly reduced protein binding of chloramphenicol in neonates compared to adults (average 32.4% protein binding in neonates compared to average 53.1% protein binding in adults). Patients with liver cirrhosis also show a lower protein binding (average of 42.2%) than normal adults [54]. Usually, anemia, characterized by maturation arrest in the marrow, is seen with serum concentrations in excess of 25 μg/mL. Cardiovascular collapse, which occurs primarily in newborns, has been observed with serum chloramphenicol concentrations >50 μg/mL.

Tetracycline and related drugs are also used widely in clinical practice, but therapeutic drug monitoring of these antibiotics is not needed. These drugs are currently only rarely monitored, using reversed phase HPLC techniques and simple organic extraction in the presence of an internal standard and ultraviolet detection. However, chloramphenicol monitoring may have some clinical utility due to its toxic nature [55]. A solid phase extraction of the sample followed by LC/MS separation and quantitation of various tetracycline analogs has been described, but the method was applied to environmental monitoring [56] and its clinical utility has not been established.

THERAPEUTIC DRUG MONITORING OF QUINOLONES

Quinolones, also known as fluoroquinolones, are a group of bactericidal antibiotics that are increasingly prescribed among inpatient and outpatient populations, largely due to their broad-spectrum actions against both gram-positive and gram-negative bacteria [1]. These agents function by inhibiting DNA gyrase, a type II topoisomerase, and topoisomerase, which is an enzyme necessary to separate replicated DNA and that thereby interferes with cell division. Drugs in this class include levofloxacin and ciprofloxacin, and may be administered via intravenous and oral routes.

Levofloxacin and ciprofloxacin are effective [1] in treating infections (particularly tenacious and recurring respiratory tract infections) caused by gram-positive pathogens (*Streptococcus pneumoniae* and *Streptococcus pyogeneses*, with some activity against *Staphylococcus aureus* and *Enterococcus faecalis*), gram-negative pathogens (*Escherichia coli*, *Haemophilus influenzae*, *Moraxella catarrhalis*, *Klebsiella pneumoniae* and *Pseudomonas aeruginosa*) and atypical pathogens (*Chlamydia pneumoniae*, *Mycoplasma pneumoniae* and *Legionella pneumophila*). Ciprofloxacin has also been increasingly used for treatment of both complicated and uncomplicated urinary tract infections, as resistance has emerged to many primary therapeutic agents such as sulfonamides and penicillins.

Toxicities [1] may include diarrhea, gastrointestinal upset, allergic reactions and phototoxicity. Central nervous system (CNS) effects such as agitation, restlessness, anxiety and nightmares can also occur. QT prolongation has also been observed, and rare cases of *torsades de pointes*, an uncommon type of ventricular tachycardia, have been reported. Achilles tendon rupture due to fluoroquinolone use is typically associated with renal failure. Therapeutic monitoring of these drugs is not usually required. The tentative therapeutic range of ciprofloxacin is considered to be 3–5 µg/mL (peak concentration). The pharmacodynamic target for ciprofloxacin has been defined as a 24-hour area under the plasma concentration time curve (AUC) to MIC ratio of over 125 for bacterial eradication, and the peak concentration should be 10 times the MIC. Van Zanten *et al.* reported that if the MIC is 0.125 µg/mL, then with a ciprofloxacin dosage of 400 mg twice a day 100% of patients can reach a AUC/MIC ratio over 125 and C_{max}/MIC ratio over 10; however, if MIC is 2 µg/mL, then 0% of patients achieve the target AUC/MIC or C_{max}/MIC. Therefore, higher dosage of ciprofloxacin, such as 1200 g daily, may be needed for intensive care unit patients where MIC exceeds 0.25 C_{max}/MIC [57].

Current methods for quantitation of quinolones in serum or plasma are based on simple liquid–liquid extraction techniques followed by analysis using HPLC-UV. These methods [58, 59] typically span the clinically relevant range, although imprecision tolerances have been found to be somewhat higher than with other HPLC methods for antibiotics.

THERAPEUTIC DRUG MONITORING OF MACROLIDES

The macrolides are a unique class of antibiotics whose activity stems from the presence of a macrolide ring, a large macrocyclic lactone ring to which one or more deoxy-sugars, usually cladinose and desosamine, may be attached. Erythromycin was one of the first drugs of this type used in clinical practice, but subsequent broader-spectrum drugs, such as clarithromycin and azithromycin, have been developed more recently and are widely utilized. Like chloramphenicol, the action of these antimicrobial agents is inhibiting bacterial protein biosynthesis by binding reversibly to the subunit 50S of the bacterial ribosome and preventing translocation of peptidyl tRNA [1]. Consequently, drugs in this class are primarily bacteriostatic, but can also be bacteriocidal when used in high concentrations.

The antimicrobial spectrum of macrolides is broader than that of penicillins (and comparable to many late-generation cephalosporins); therefore, macrolide antibiotics have been successfully used as a substitute in treating patients with a known penicillin allergy. Macrolide antibiotics are most frequently used to treat infections of the upper and lower respiratory tract, and skin and soft tissue infections [1]. They have been found to be particularly effective against beta-hemolytic streptococci, pneumococci, staphylococci and enterococci, in addition to many atypical respiratory pathogens such as *Mycoplasma pneumoniae* and *Legionella pneumophila*. Nonetheless, they have also been used to treat chlamydia, syphilis, acne, gonorrhea and non-gonococcal cystitis, as well as certain mycobacterial and rickettsial infections.

Most common side effects are minimal and non-life-threatening, including gastrointestinal symptoms (diarrhea, nausea, abdominal pain and vomiting), headaches, dizziness, nervousness, rashes and occasional facial swelling. Adverse reactions with macrolide antibiotics are relatively rare, and most do not require discontinuance of drug or routine therapeutic monitoring of drug concentrations in serum or plasma [1, 5]. However, serious allergic and dermatologic reactions have been reported with some drugs in this class, with the most serious and potentially life-threatening cases being toxic epidermal necrolysis and Stevens-Johnson syndrome (clarithromycin).

Macrolide antibiotics, such as erythromycin, azithromycin, and clarithromycin, can be quantitated in serum or plasma, after solid phase or organic extraction, using HPLC techniques with ultraviolet, electrochemical or fluorescence detection methods [60−63]. Sensitive methods using LC/MS have also been introduced in recent years, which eliminate time-consuming pretreatment and derivatization steps and show greater reproducibility and less interference than the more conventional HPLC methods [62, 63].

THERAPEUTIC DRUG MONITORING OF ANTIMYCOBACTERIAL AGENTS

Antimycobacterial, or antituberculosis, agents represent a diverse group of structurally-unrelated compounds that includes rifampin, isoniazid, ethambutol, streptomycin, amikacin and kanamycin. Other antibiotics may be added to the drug therapy if needed; for example, a fluoroquinolone. Each of these agents has very different and unique biological mechanisms of biological action [1], yet, when used alone or in combination, these drugs have historically proven to be clinically effective in the acute treatment and long-term public health management of *Mycobacterium* infections, such as tuberculosis and leprosy [1, 5]. Antimycobacterial agents are most commonly prescribed today in multidrug combinations [1] due to the frequent emergence of resistance, which is often seen as a consequence of poor patient compliance and incomplete treatment of active infections during the long course of treatment required with most therapeutic regimens.

Rifampin inhibits DNA-dependent RNA polymerase in bacterial cells by binding its beta-subunit, and thus prevents RNA transcription and subsequent translation to proteins. In contrast, isoniazid and ethambutol separately exert their bacteriostatic effects through different molecular mechanisms by interfering with the synthesis of the mycolic acid−peptidoglycan complex in the cell wall to increase overall cell permeability. Streptomycin, amikacin and kanamycin are aminoglycoside antibiotics that interfere with protein synthesis and alter cell membrane transport, with a similar net effect of increasing overall cell permeability as well.

The most serious adverse and toxic side effects have been observed with rifampin and isoniazid − most notably, hepatitis and jaundice (with liver failure in severe cases) and sideroblastic anemia [1, 5]. Other milder side effects include flushing, pruritus, rash, redness and watering of eyes, as well as gastrointestinal and central nervous system disturbances and general flu-like symptoms. As observed with most other bacteriostatic agents, toxicity with these drugs is independent of drug concentration. Serious drug toxicity was reported in one 37-year-old woman who received ethambutol 825 mg, isoniazid 225 mg, rifampicin 450 mg and pyrazinamide 1200 mg and had serious impairment in her vision. The authors commented that ethambutol and isoniazid are notorious for causing visual impairment [64].

Although antimycobacterial agents are generally not subject to therapeutic drug monitoring, treatment failure may result from subtherapeutic drug concentrations. Peloquin commented that therapeutic drug monitoring may not be needed for otherwise healthy individuals who are responding to standard four-drug treatment regimens for tuberculosis, but therapeutic drug monitoring is useful in patients who are slow to respond to therapy or are at a higher risk of drug–drug interactions. Early intervention based on therapeutic drug monitoring is useful for these patients to avoid development of drug resistance. When only one specimen is obtained for therapeutic drug monitoring, a 2-h post-dosage specimen is appropriate for isoniazid, rifampin, ethambutol and pyrazinamide. Unfortunately, 2-hour post-dosage concentration may not differentiate between delayed absorption and malabsorption, and for that purpose a 6-h post-dose specimen can be collected and analyzed. Prompt analysis of the specimen is necessary as these drugs are not stable in serum at room temperature, although rifampin is stable at room temperature for more than 6 hours [65]. Babalik *et al.* reported that 60% of 20 patients receiving antituberculosis drugs in their study showed a below therapeutic drug concentration. The authors commented that drug levels were below therapeutic ranges in patients with active tuberculosis, particularly in patients with HIV infection or other comorbidities [66]. Fahimi *et al.* reported that 37.8% of the patients they studied had subtherapeutic levels of plasma isoniazid. The authors recommended therapeutic drug monitoring of isoniazid especially in patients with inadequate clinical response or experiencing toxicity to isoniazid [67].

Currently, there are no commercially available immunoassays for therapeutic drug monitoring of antituberculosis drugs. Therefore, chromatographic methods are only available for the determination of serum or plasma concentrations of these drugs using reversed phased HPLC, with no pretreatment following deproteinization of serum or plasma, or by gas chromatography/mass spectometry (GC/MS) techniques [68–71]. Both methods appear to provide acceptable reproducibility, accuracy and limits of quantitation, with little or no upfront intervention. Recently, Fox *et al.* described a simple HPLC method combined with UV detection for determination of rifampicin and its metabolite desacetyl rifampicin in human plasma [72].

CONCLUSIONS

Today, therapeutic monitoring of antibiotic concentrations in blood and other body fluids remains largely reserved for vancomycin and the aminoglycosides, which are often used to treat the most serious and life-threatening infections. Drugs in these classes typically have narrow therapeutic indices, and drug levels have to be closely followed to optimize therapy and prevent the serious and irreversible complications of nephrotoxicity and ototoxicity. Even with short duration therapy (typically 3 days or less), recent guidelines now suggest routine therapeutic monitoring may not be warranted for these antibiotics, except in exceptional clinical circumstances or with prior history of adverse reactions. In contrast, the majority of other antibiotics have wider therapeutic margins and lower toxicity risks at the dosages prescribed, and typically do not require routine monitoring of drug concentrations in serum or plasma for appropriate patient management. When clinical practice guidelines or other preexisting conditions warrant (e.g., kidney failure, crystalluria, etc.), a wide range of antibiotics can be monitored using established immunoassay and/or chromatographic (HPLC, GC, GC/MS or LC/MS) techniques available in most tertiary care hospital and clinical reference laboratories.

References

[1] Section VIII. Chemotherapy of microbial diseases. In: L. Brunton, J. Lazo, K. Parker, editors. Goodman & Gilman's The Pharmacological Basis of Therapeutics, 11th ed. New York, NY: Graw-Hill Professional, p. 1141–294.

[2] Dawson SJ, Reeves DS. Therapeutic monitoring, the concentration–effect relationship and impact on the clinical efficacy of antibiotic agents. J Chemother 1997;9(Suppl.1):84–92.

[3] Spanu T, Santangelo R, Andreotti F, et al. Antibiotic therapy for severe bacterial infections: correlation between the inhibitory quotient and outcome. Intl J Antimicrob Agents 2004;23:120–8.

[4] Rhee KY, Gardiner DF. Clinical relevance of bacteriostatic versus bactericidal activity in the treatment of gram-positive bacterial infections. Clin Infect Dis 2004;39:755–6.

[5] Klein RD, Edberg SC. Applications, significance of, and methods for the measurement of antimicrobial concentrations in human body fluids. In: Lorian V, editor. Antibiotics in Laboratory Medicine. 5th edn. Philadelphia, PA: Lippincott Williams & Wilkins; 2005. p. 290–364.

[6] Schentag JJ, Meager AK, Jelliffe RW. Aminogly cosideo. In: Burton ME, Shaw LM, Schentag JJ, Evans WE, editors. Applied Pharmacokinetics & Pharmacodynamics, Principles of Therapeutic Drug Monitoring. Baltimore, MD: Lippincott Williams & Wilkins; 2006. p. 285–353.

[7] Moyer TP. Therapeutic drug monitoring. In: Burtis CA, Ashwood ER, editors. Tietz Textbook of Clinical Chemistry and Molecular Diagnostics. 4th edn. Philadelphia, PA: WB Saunders Company; 2005. p. 1237–85.

[8] Dasgupta A, Datta P. Analytical techniques for measuring concentrations of therapeutic drugs in biological fluids. In: Dasgupta A, editor. Handbook of Drug Monitoring Methods. Totowa, NJ: Humana Press Inc.; 2007. p. 67–86.

[9] Hota B, Lyles R, Rim J, et al. Predictors of clinical virulence in community-onset methicillin resistant *Staphylococcus aureus* infections: the importance of US300 and pneumonia. Clin Infect Dis 2011;53:757–65.

[10] Gould IM. Is vancomycin redundant for serious staphylococcal infection? Intl J Antimicrob Agents 2010;36(Suppl. 2):S55–57.

[11] Dean R, Dasgupta A. Therapeutic drug monitoring of vancomycin and aminoglycoside antibiotics with guidelines. In: Dasgupta A, editor. Chromatographic Techniques for Therapeutic Drug Monitoring. Boca Raton, FL: CRC Press Inc.; 2010. p. 323–40.

[12] Rybak MJ. The pharmacokinetic and pharmacodynamic properties of vancomycin. Clin Infect Dis 2006;42:S35–39.

[13] Rodvold KA, Blum RA, Fischer JH, et al. Vancomycin pharmacokinetics in patients with various states of renal dysfunction. Antimicrob Agents Chemother 1988;32:848–52.

[14] De Hoog M, Mouton JW, van der Anker JN. Vancomycin pharmacokinetics and administration regimens in neonates. Clin Pharmacokinet 2004;43:417–40.

[15] Garrelts JC, Peterie JD. Altered vancomycin dose vs. serum concentration relationship in burn patients. Clin Pharmacol Ther 1988;44:9–13.

[16] Draghi DC, Benton BM, Krause KM, et al. Comparative surveillance study of telavancin activity against recently collected gram-positive clinical isolates from across the United States. Antimicrob Agents Chemother 2008;52:2382–8.

[17] Moise-Broder PA, Forrest A, Birmingham MC, Schentag JJ. Pharmacodynamics of vancomycin and other antimicrobials in patients with *Staphylococcus aureus* lower respiratory tract infections. Clin Pharmacokinet 2004;43:925–42.

[18] Lodise TP, Graves J, Evans A, et al. Relationship between vancomycin MIC and failure among patients with methicillin resistant *Staphylococcus aureus* bacteremia treated with vancomycin. Antimicrob Agents Chemother 2008;52:3315–20.

[19] Rybak MJ, Lomaestro BM, Rotscahfer JC, et al. Vancomycin therapeutic guidelines: A summary of consensus recommendations from the Infectious Diseases Society of America, the American Society of Health-System Pharmacists, and the Society of Infectious Diseases Pharmacists. Clin Infect Dis 2009;49:325–7.

[20] Kritzis MD, Goldstein FW. Monitoring of vancomycin serum levels for treatment of staphylococcal infections. Clin Microbiol Infect 2006;42:92–5.

[21] Rybak MJ, Lomaestro BM, Rotschafer JC, et al. Therapeutic monitoring of vancomycin in adults summary of consensus recommendations from the American Society of Health-System Pharmacists, the Infectious Disease Society of America, and the Society of Infectious Diseases Pharmacists. Pharmacotherapy 2009;29:1275–9.

[22] Patel N, Pai MP, Rodvold KA, et al. Vancomycin: we can't get there from here. Clin Infect Dis 2011; 52:969–74.

[23] Rybak MJ, Albrecht LM, Boike, Chandrasekar PH. Nephrotoxicity for vancomycin, alone and with an aminoglycoside. J Antimicrobiol Chemother 1990;25:679–87.

[24] Jehl F, Corinne Gallion C, Robert C, et al. Determination of vancomycin in human serum by high-pressure liquid chromatography. Antimicrob Agents Chemother 1985;27:503–7.

[25] Furuta I, Kitahashi T, Kuroda T, et al. Rapid serum vancomycin assay by high-performance liquid chromatography using a semipermeable surface packing material column. Clin Chim Acta 2000;301:31–9.

[26] Zhang T, Watson DG, Azike C, et al. Determination of vancomycin in serum by liquid chromatography-high resolution full scan mass spectrometry. J Chromatogr B Analyt Technol Biomed Life Sci 2007;857:352–6.

[27] Cass RT, Villa JS, Karr DE, Schmidt Jr DE. Rapid bioanalysis of vancomycin in serum and urine by high-performance liquid chromatography tandem mass spectrometry using on-line sample extraction and parallel analytical columns. Rapid Commun Mass Spectrom 2001;15:406–12.

[28] Lortholary O, Tod M, CohenY, Petijean O. Aminoglycosides. Med Clin North Am 1995;79:761–87.

[29] Turnidge J. Pharmacodynamics and dosing of aminoglycosides. Infect Dis Clin North Am 2003;17:503–28.

[30] Bujik SE, Mouton JW, Gyssens IC, et al. Experience with a once daily dosing program in critically ill patients. Intensive Care Med 2002;28:936–42.

[31] Nagai T, Takano M. Molecular aspect of renal handling of aminoglycosides and strategies for preventing nephrotoxicity. Drug Metab Pharmacokinetic 2004;19:159–70.

[32] Matzke GR, Jameson JJ, Halstenson CE. Gentamicin disposition in young and elderly patients with various degrees of renal function. J Clin Pharmacol 1987;27:216–20.

[33] Moore RD, Lietman PS, Smith CR. Clinical response to aminoglycoside therapy: importance of the ratio of pick concentration to minimum inhibitory concentration. J Infect Dis 1987;155:93–9.

[34] Rea RS, Capitano B, Bies R, et al. Suboptimal aminoglycoside dosing in clytically ill patients. Ther Drug Monit 2008;30:674–8.

[35] Black RE, Lau WK, Weinsten RJ, et al. Ototoxicity of amikacin. Antimicrob Agents Chemother 1976;9:956–61.

[36] McCormack JP, Jewsson PJ. A critical reevaluation of the "therapeutic range" of aminoglycosides of aminoglycosides. Clin Infect Dis 1992;14:230–9.

[37] Drusano GL, Ambrose PG, Bhavani SM, et al. Back to the future: using aminoglycosides again and how to dose them optimally. J Infect Dis 2007;155:93–9.

[38] Freeman CD, Nicholau DP, Belliveau PP, Nightingale CH. One daily dosing of aminoglycosides review and recommendations for clinical practice. J Antimicrob Chemother 1997;39:677–86.

[39] Venisse N, Boulamery A. Level of evidence for therapeutic drug monitoring of aminoglycosides. Therapie 2011;66:39–44.

[40] Roberts JA, Norris R, Paterson DL, Martin JH. Therapeutic drug monitoring of aminoglycosides. Br J Clin Pharmcol 2011. August 10 [e-pub ahead of print].

[41] Pagkalis S, Mantadakis E, Mavrons MN, et al. Pharmacological considerations for the proper clinical use of aminoglycosides. Drugs 2011;71:2277—94.

[42] Soltes L. Aminoglycoside antibiotics — two decades of their HPLC bioanalysis. Biomed Chromatogr 1999;13:3—10.

[43] Isoherrane N, Soback S. Determination of gentamicin C1, C1a, and C2 in plasma and urine by HPLC. Clin Chem 2000;46:837—42.

[44] Kim BH, Lee SC, Lee HJ, Ok JH. Reversed-phase liquid chromatographic method for the analysis of aminoglycoside antibiotics using pre-column derivatization with phenylisocyanate. Biomed Chromatogr 2003;17:396—403.

[45] Concepcion Lecaroz C, Miguel A, Campanero MA, et al. Determination of gentamicin in different matrices by a new sensitive high-performance liquid chromatography-mass spectrometric method. J Antimicrob Chemother 2006;58:557—63.

[46] Samanidou VF, Evaggelopoulou EN, Papadoyannis IN. Development of a validated HPLC method for determination of four penicillin antibiotics in pharmaceuticals and human biological fluids. J Sep Sci 2006;29:1550—60.

[47] Mascher HJ, Kikuta C. Determination of amoxicillin in human serum and plasma by high-performance liquid chromatography and on-line postcolumn derivatization. J Chromatogr A 1998;812:221—6.

[48] Viberg A, Sandström M, Britt S, Jansson B. Determination of cefuroxime in human serum or plasma by liquid chromatography with electrospray tandem mass spectrometry. Rapid Commun Mass Spectrom 2008;18:707—10.

[49] Heller DN, Smith ML, Chiesa OA. LC/MS/MS measurement of penicillin G in bovine plasma, urine, and biopsy samples taken from kidneys of standing animals. J Chromatogr B Analyt Technol Biomed Life Sci. 2005;830:91—9.

[50] Becker M, Erhard Z, Petz M. Residue analysis of 15 penicillins and cephalosporins in bovine muscle, kidney and milk by liquid chromatography-tandem mass spectrometry. Analyt Chimica Acta 2004;520:19—32.

[51] Heller DN, Smith ML, Albert CO. Confirmatory assay for the simultaneous detection of penicillins and cephalosporins in milk using liquid chromatography/tandem mass spectrometry. Rapid Commun Mass Spectrom 2000;15:1404—9.

[52] DeAngelis DV, Wooley JL, Sigel CW. High performance liquid chromatographic assay for the simultaneous measurement of trimethoprim and sulfamethoxazole in plasma or urine. Ther Drug Monit 1990; 12:382—92.

[53] Bedora DCG, Gonçalvesa TM, Ferreiraa ML, et al. Simultaneous determination of sulfamethoxazole and trimethoprim in biological fluids for high-throughput analysis: Comparison of HPLC with ultraviolet and tandem mass spectrometric detection. J Chromatogr B 2008;863:46—54.

[54] Koup JR, Lau AH, Brodsky B, Slaughter RL. Chloramphenicol pharmacokinetics in hospitalized patients. Antimicrob Agents Chemother 1979;15:651—7.

[55] Koup R, Brodsky B, Alan Lau A, Beam Jr TR. High-performance liquid chromatographic assay of chloramphenicol in serum. Antimicrob Agents Chemother 1978;14:439—43.

[56] Zhu J, Snow DD, Cassada DA, et al. Analysis of oxytetracycline, tetracycline, and chlortetracycline in water using solid phase extraction and liquid chromatography—tandem mass spectrometry. J Chromatogr A 2001;928:177—86.

[57] Van Zanten AR, Polderman KH, van Geijlswijk IM, et al. Ciprofloxacin pharmacokinetics in critically ill patients: a prospective cohort study. J Crit Care 2008;23:422—30.

[58] Srinivas N, Narasu L, Shankar BP, Mullangi R. Development and validation of a HPLC method for simultaneous quantitation of gatifloxacin, sparfloxacin and moxifloxacin using levofloxacin as internal standard in human plasma: application to a clinical pharmacokinetic study. Biomed Chromatogr 2008;22:1288—95.

[59] Chamseddin C, Jira TH. Comparison of the chromatographic behavior of levofloxacin, ciprofloxacin, and moxifloxacin on various HPLC phases. Pharamazie 2011;66:244—8.

[60] Stubbs C, Haigh JM, Kanfer I. Determination of erythromycin in serum and urine by high-performance liquid chromatography with ultraviolet detection. J Pharmaceut Sci 2006;74:1126—8.

[61] Bahramia G, Mirzaeeib S, Kiania A. High performance liquid chromatographic determination of azithromycin in serum using fluorescence detection and its application in human pharmacokinetic studies. J Chromatogr B 2005;820:277—81.

[62] Fouda HG, Schneider RP. Quantitative determination of the antibiotic azithromycin in human serum by high performance liquid chromatography (HPLC)-atmospheric pressure chemical ionization mass spectrometry: correlation with a standard HPLC electrochemical method. Ther Drug Monit 1995;17:179—83.

[63] Barrett B, Bořek-Dohalský V, Fejt P, et al. Validated HPLC-MS-MS method for determination of azithromycin in human plasma. Anal Bioanal Chem 2005;383:210—7.

[64] Ayanniyi AA, Ayanniyi RO. A 37-year-old woman presenting with impaired visual function during antituberculosis drug therapy: a case report. J Med Case Reports 2011;15:317.

[65] Peloquin CA. Therapeutic drug monitoring in the treatment of tuberculosis. Drugs 2002;62:2169—83.

[66] Babalik A, Babalik A, Mannix S, et al. Therapeutic drug monitoring in the treatment of active tuberculosis. Can Respir J 2011;18:225—9.

[67] Fahimi F, Kobarfard F, Tabarsu P, et al. Isoniazid blood levels in patients with pulmonary tuberculosis at a tuberculosis referral center. Chemotherapy 2011;57:7—11.

[68] Holdiness MR. Chromatographic analysis of antituberculosis drugs in biological samples. J Chromatogr 1985;340:321—59.

[69] Malone RS, Fish DN, Spiegel DM, et al. The effect of hemodialysis on isoniazid, rifampin, pyrazinamide, and ethambutol. Am J Respir Crit Care Med 1999;159:1580—4.

[70] Unsalan S, Sancar M, Bekce B, et al. Therapeutic monitoring of isoniazid, pyrazinamide and rifampicin in tuberculosis patients using LC. Chromatographia 2005;61:595—8.

[71] Calleri E, De Lorenzi E, Furlanetto S, et al. Validation of a RP-LC method for the simultaneous determination of isoniazid, pyrazinamide and rifampicin in a pharmaceutical formulation. J Pharm Biomed Anal. 2002;29:1089—96.

[72] Fox D, O'Connor R, Mallon P, McMohon G. Simultaneous determination of efavirenz, rifampicin, and its metabolites desacetyl rifampicin levels in human plasma. J Pharm Biomed Anal 2011;56:785—91.

Challenges in Therapeutic Drug Monitoring of Digoxin and Other Anti-Arrhythmic Drugs

Amitava Dasgupta

Department of Pathology and Laboratory Medicine, University of Texas-Houston, Houston, TX

OUTLINE

Therapeutic Drug Monitoring: Newer Drugs and Biomarkers
DOI: 10.1016/B978-0-12-385467-4.00011-7

INTRODUCTION

Despite the introduction of many new anti-arrhythmic drugs in the last century, cardiac glycosides such as digoxin and digitoxin are still used in clinical practice. Digitalis glycosides derived from foxglove plants were used for medicinal purposes as early as the 16th century, and this plant was listed in the *London Pharmacopeia* in 1661. However, due to lack of knowledge of its proper use, reports of treatment failures and toxicities resulted in removal of digitalis from the Pharmacopeia in 1745. William Withering's classical description of the effects of digitalis was then published in 1785. He treated many patients with congestive heart failure successfully with digitalis, and also recorded digitalis toxicity systematically. Today, digoxin isolated from a species of foxglove plant *Digitalis lantana* is a widely prescribed drug in the United States, while digitoxin prepared from the foxglove plant *Digitalis purpurea* is used less frequently in the United States [1].

Digoxin can be administered acutely or long term, orally or intravenously, and is safe and beneficial in treating both acute and chronic heart failure [2]. Digoxin, digitoxin, ouabain and related compounds act by inhibiting the Na, K-ATPase pump that generates a sodium and potassium gradient across the plasma membrane and drives many important physiological activities. The amino acids that constitute the ouabain binding site are highly conserved across the evolutionary spectrum, probably because of its role in maintaining essential physiological functions of the body [3]. The major pharmacological action of digitalis, including its positive inotropic effect, is due to its inhibition of Na, K-ATPase, which eventually increases cellular calcium, and also the release of calcium during depolarization, thus increasing myocardial contractility. Digitalis also increases the refractory period and decreases impulse velocity in certain myocardial tissues (such as the AV node). The electrophysiological properties of digitalis are reflected in ECGs by shortening of the QT interval. A wide variety of placebo-controlled trials have unequivocally confirmed that therapy with digoxin can improve symptoms, exercise tolerance and quality of life in patients suffering from mild to severe heart failure. Unlike some other newer cardioactive agents with positive inotropic properties, digoxin does not increase all-cause mortality from heart failure. In addition, digoxin therapy is also associated with reduction in the rate of hospitalization due to heart failure. American College of Cardiology/American Heart Association consensus guidelines recommend that digoxin should be considered for the outpatient treatment of all patients with persistent symptoms of heart failure; digoxin may be used after emergent treatment of heart failure; and the dosage of digoxin should be 0.125—0.25 mg in the majority of patients, with the lowest dosage being used in patients over 70 years of age. In addition, the guidelines also state that although digoxin toxicity is encountered at a serum digoxin level > 2 ng/mL, it may occur at lower digoxin levels if hypokalemia, hypomagnesemia or hypothyroidism coexists. In addition, drugs such as quinidine, verapamil, spironolactone, flecainide and amiodarone may increase serum digoxin levels, causing toxicity. In addition, the guidelines also specify where digoxin use is inappropriate [4].

Due to its narrow therapeutic range, monitoring of serum or plasma digoxin levels is essential for patient management. Although digoxin is more widely used than digitoxin in clinical practice, Bussey *et al.* reported that a therapeutic concentration of digoxin was only reached in 5 out of 15 patients, while therapeutic digitoxin levels were achieved in 14 out of 15 patients. The authors concluded that therapeutic serum concentrations can be achieved more easily and frequently with digitoxin than digoxin without compromising the patient's congestive heart failure status [5].

Although therapeutic drug monitoring of digoxin is probably one of the most commonly ordered tests in many clinical laboratories, therapeutic drug monitoring of several anti-arrhythmic drugs is also required. In general, anti-arrhythmic drugs can be classified under four broad categories, and monitoring of some members of individual groups is clinically useful [6]. Various classes of anti-arrhythmic drugs including drugs that require therapeutic drug monitoring are listed in Table 11.1.

TABLE 11.1 Common Anti-Arrhythmic Drugs Indicating Which Agents Require Therapeutic Drug Monitoring

Drug class	Mechanism of action	Drug	TDM needed?	Therapeutic range
IA	Moderate sodium channel blocker	Procainamide	Yes	4.0–10.0 µg/mL
		Quinidine	Yes	2.0–5.0 µg/mL
		Disopyramide	Yes	1.5–5.0 µg/mL
				2.0–5.0 µg/mL[a,b]
IB	Weak sodium channel blocker	Lidocaine	Yes	1.5–5.0 µg/mL
		Mexiletine	Yes	0.5–2.0 µg/mL
				1.0–2.0 µg/mL[a]
				0.8–2.0 µg/mL[b]
IC	Strong sodium channel blocker	Flecainide	Yes	0.2–1.0 µg/mL
		Tocainide	Yes	5.0–12.0 µg/mL
		Propafenone	Yes	0.4–3.0 µg/mL
				0.5–2.0 µg/mL[a,b]
II	β-adrenoceptor blockers (β-blockers)	Atenolol	No	
		Propranolol	Yes	50.0–100.0 ng/mL
		Esmolol	No	
		Timolol	No	
		Metoprolol	No	
		Bisoprolol	No	
		Labetalol	No	
		Pindolol	No	
		Nadolol	No	

(Continued)

TABLE 11.1 Common Anti-Arrhythmic Drugs Indicating Which Agents Require Therapeutic Drug Monitoring—cont'd

Drug class	Mechanism of action	Drug	TDM needed?	Therapeutic range
III	Potassium channel blocker	Amiodarone	Probably	1.0–2.5 µg/mL
		Sotalol	Probably	0.5–2.0 µg/mL
				1.0–4.0 µg/mL[a]
		Ibutilide	No	
		Dofetilide	No	
IV	Calcium channel blockers	Diltiazem	No	
		Verapamil	Probably	50–200 ng/mL
Other	Na, K-ATPase	Digoxin	Yes	0.8–1.8 ng/mL

Therapeutic range (no mark) suggested by various published papers as well as by the [a]ARUP Reference Laboratory, Salt Lake City, UT and [b]Mayo Medical Laboratory Rochester, MN, two national reference laboratories affiliated with medical centers.

CHALLENGES IN THERAPEUTIC DRUG MONITORING OF DIGOXIN

Compared to other anti-arrhythmic drugs, digoxin serum drug concentrations are 100- to 1000-fold lower in the therapeutic range because digoxin's therapeutic range is 0.6–1.5 ng/mL while most other anti-arrhythmic drugs are present in microgram per milliliter concentrations during therapy. Immunoassays are commonly used in clinical laboratories for therapeutic drug monitoring of digoxin, and such assays are subject to interferences from both endogenous and exogenous substances; in general, digoxin immunoassays suffer from more interferences than immunoassays for any other therapeutic drug. For example, let's assume that 100 ng/mL of a cross-reactive substance with only 2% cross-reactivity with digoxin immunoassay is present in a patient's specimen submitted for therapeutic drug monitoring of digoxin. Further, we assume that this cross-reactant falsely increases the serum digoxin level and such interference has an additive effect on serum digoxin measurement. Therefore, if the true digoxin concentration in a patient is 1 ng/mL which is therapeutic, the observed digoxin value in the presence of this cross-reactant would be 3 ng/mL, because 100 ng/mL of this cross-reactant with 2% cross-reactivity would contribute a 2-ng/mL false digoxin reading. This is a very serious interference issue, because if the dosage of digoxin is reduced based on this falsely elevated digoxin value then the patient may receive only a subtherapeutic level of digoxin, causing treatment failure. On the other hand, if this cross-reactive substance has even 10% cross-reactivity with the procainamide assay and assuming again 100 ng/mL of this substance is present in a specimen submitted to the laboratory for therapeutic drug monitoring of procainamide, then this cross-reactant would falsely increase procainamide concentration by 10 ng/mL. If the true procainamide concentration is 5 µg/mL, then this value would be falsely increased to only 5. 010 µg/mL — a non-significant increase.

Digoxin immunoassays may be affected by digoxin metabolites, endogenous digoxin-like immunoreactive substances, or a variety of drugs and metabolites, including spironolactone, potassium canrenoate and their common metabolite canrenone. In addition, certain Chinese medicines such as Chan Su, Lu-Shen-Wan and oleander containing herbal supplements may interfere with serum digoxin measurements using various immunoassays. Various factors that affect digoxin immunoassays are listed in Table 11.2.

Effect of Digoxin Metabolites on Digoxin Immunoassays

The major metabolites of digoxin are digoxigenin, digoxigenin monodigitoxoside, digoxigenin bisdigitoxoside and dihydrodigoxin. There is a wide variation in cross-reactivity of digoxin metabolites with digoxin immunoassays because various assays differ in antibody specificity. In general, digoxin concentrations in serum obtained by more specific analytical techniques such as high-performance liquid chromatography (HPLC) tend to be lower than the corresponding digoxin concentrations obtained by immunoassay, due to metabolite cross-reactivity. Miller *et al.* reported that digoxigenin has 0.7% cross-reactivity with the ACS assay (Ciba-Corning Diagnostics, now SIEMENS Medical Diagnostic Solution), 103%

TABLE 11.2   Various Factors that Affect Digoxin Immunoassays

Factors	Comments
Digoxin metabolites	Digoxigenin bisdigitoxoside and Digoxigenin monodigitoxoside metabolites usually show more cross-reactivity than digitoxigenin and other metabolites. Metabolite cross-reactivities vary widely with antibody specificity.
DLIS	Endogenous digoxin-like immunoreactive substances (DLIS) affect polyclonal-based assays but have minimal interference with more specific monoclonal antibody-based digoxin assays. The MEIA (microparticle enzyme immunoassay, Abbott Laboratories) showed negative interference. Monitoring free digoxin eliminates this interference.
Spironolactone	Negative interference with MEIA assay and positive bias with certain digoxin assays, but low-dose therapy with spironolactone does not affect any digoxin assay. The spironolactone metabolite canrenone demonstrates more interference than spironolactone. Monitoring free digoxin also may eliminate this interference.
Potassium canrenoate	Not used in the United States, but this drug and its metabolite significantly affect various digoxin assays. Negative interference of potassium canrenoate and its metabolite canrenone with MEIA digoxin assay is particularly problematic because clinicians may increase the digoxin dose without recognizing this negative interference and such an increase in digoxin dosage may cause a serious adverse reaction.
Digibind	Fab fragment of antidigoxin antibody used in treating life-threatening digoxin overdose. Digibind interferes with various digoxin immunoassays. Therefore, during therapy with Digibind or (more recently introduced) DigiFab, free digoxin should be monitored.
Chan Su, Lu-Shen-Wan	Chan Su and Lu-Shen-Wan contain bufalin as an active component which interferes with both polyclonal and monoclonal antibody-based digoxin immunoassays due to structural similarity with digoxin.
Oleander	Oleander contains oleandrin which, due to structural similarity with digoxin, interferes with both polyclonal and monoclonal antibody-based digoxin assays.

cross-reactivity with the Stratus™ assay (Baxter Corporation, now Dade-Behring, Deerfield, IL) and 153% cross-reactivity with the Magic™ digoxin assay (Ciba-Corning) [7]. Solnica compared the performance of the FPIA digoxin assay (Abbott Laboratories) and dry chemistry enzyme assay (EIA) on the Vitros 950 analyzer (Johnson and Johnson, Rochester, NY), and observed that the EIA demonstrated significantly higher analytical digoxin concentrations bias than the FPIA assay. The mean value of digoxin in sera of 88 patients as measured by the EIA was 1.3 ng/mL compared to the mean value of 1.1 ng/mL as obtained by the FPIA. The author speculated that the mouse antibody of the EIA assay may be affected by the presence of HAMA (human antimouse antibody) in some serum specimens causing falsely elevated results. The author also commented that HPLC combined with mass spectrometry is the reference method [8]. Tzou et al. compared a chromatographic method for measuring serum digoxin concentration with a commercially available immunoassay (the ACA® digoxin assay, DuPont) and concluded that digoxin values obtained by the immunoassay compared well with values obtained by the chromatographic method in patients with cardiovascular disease but without renal disease, liver disease or diabetes. However, for patients with renal disease, liver disease or diabetes, the immunoassay significantly overestimated digoxin values (in the range of 0.3–1.1 ng/ml) compared to the chromatographic method [9].

Effect of DLIS on Digoxin Immunoassays

The presence of digoxin-like immunoreactive substances (DLIS), the endogenous equivalent of digitalis, was first described in a volume-expanded dog in 1980 [10]. Later, many investigators confirmed the presence of endogenous DLIS in serum and other biological fluids in volume-expanded patients, including patients with uremia, liver disease or essential hypertension, transplant recipients, and women with eclampsia as well as pregnant women [11, 12]. The exact biological role of DLIS has not been fully understood, but in general these endogenous factors can inhibit Na, K-ATPase and be considered as a type of natriuretic hormone [13]. These compounds have a steroid-like structure [14].

The highest magnitudes of interferences with serum digoxin measurement in the presence of elevated concentrations of DLIS were reported in digoxin radioimmunoassays (RIA) and fluorescence polarization immunoassays (FPIA, Abbott Laboratories, Abbot Park, IL) [15]. Saccois et al., in 1996, reported that the EMIT® 2000 immunoassay (enzyme multiplied immunoassay technique, Syva Corporation) had minimal interference with DLIS compared to a RIA digoxin assay (Amerlex™ 125I assay) and the FPIA digoxin assay as assessed by analyzing cord blood samples of neonates, which contain high amounts of DLIS [16]. Fortunately, RIA digoxin assays were discontinued in the 1990s, while, more recently, Abbott Laboratories has also discontinued manufacturing the FPIA digoxin assay for application on the TDX analyzer. Although DLIS causes positive interference with some digoxin immunoassays, the MEIA (Microparticle Enzyme Immunoassay) digoxin assay marketed by Abbott Laboratories for application on the AxSYM analyzer showed negative interference. However, taking advantage of strong protein binding of DLIS and only 25% protein binding of digoxin, interference of DLIS in the MEIA assay can be eliminated by monitoring the free digoxin concentration in protein-free ultrafiltrate. Due to the high concentration of digoxin in protein-free ultrafiltrate (approximately 75% of total digoxin concentration), immunoassays designed for total digoxin can also be used for measuring free drug digoxin. Lack of protein in the ultrafiltrate does not affect free digoxin measurement. In a clinical laboratory, protein-free ultrafiltrate is usually prepared by centrifuging serum for approximately 20–25 minutes in a Centrifree Micropartition filter with a molecular cut-off of 30 000 Da [17]. Valdes and his colleagues first reported strong protein binding of DLIS [18]. Taking advantage of the strong protein binding of DLIS, other investigators also reported that interference of DLIS in serum digoxin measurement can be eliminated by monitoring the free digoxin concentration [19]. Newer, more specific monoclonal antibody-based digoxin assays are virtually free from DLIS interferences. Nevertheless, due to its narrow therapeutic range, discordance in digoxin values measured using two different assays may occur. Jones and Morris analyzed digoxin values in 36 plasma samples by sending aliquots to two different laboratories using different digoxin immunoassays (CEDIA DRI digoxin assay, Microgenics Corporation, Fremont, CA, and DGNA® digoxin assay, Dade Behring, now Siemens Diagnostics, Deerfield, CA). The authors observed clinically significant discordance in 39% of these samples, and commented that DLIS interference may explain only some of the discordance [20].

Heterophilic Antibody and Digoxin Measurement

The presence of human anti-animal antibodies, especially those directed against the mouse, in serum may cause interference with certain immunoassays. The clinical use of mouse monoclonal antibodies for radioimaging and treatment for certain cancers may cause the accumulation of human antimouse antibodies (HAMA). Anti-animal antibodies are also found in veterinarians, farm workers or people with pets due to their exposure to animals, and these antibodies are broadly classified as heterophilic antibodies. The presence of heterophilic antibodies in serum may interfere with sandwich assays designed for measuring relatively large molecules such as hCG (human chorionic gonadotropin). Bonetti *et al.* described a case where serum myoglobin concentration was falsely increased after using an immunoassay (Beckman Access® assay), due to the presence of heterophilic antibodies [21]. Usually, heterophilic antibodies do not affect competitive assays used for determining concentrations of small molecules, such as in many therapeutic drugs. Nevertheless, Liendo *et al.* described a case of a patient with cirrhotic liver disease and atrial fibrillation who was treated with spironolactone and digoxin and showed an elevated digoxin concentration of 4.2 ng/mL. He was asymptomatic, and despite discontinuation of both drugs showed persistent digoxin values of over 3.0 ng/mL for approximately 5 weeks. The authors ruled out DLIS, digoxin antibodies and spironolactone as potential sources of the observed interference. Because both ultrafiltration and treating with protein A markedly lowered digoxin values, the authors concluded that the interference was due to heterophilic antibodies in the serum. Protein A can selectively remove heterophilic antibodies (IgG class) by forming a complex. In addition, due to their high molecular weight (approximately 150 000 Da), heterophilic antibodies are absent in the protein-free ultrafiltrate which usually utilizes a filter with a molecular weight cut-off of 30 000 Da [22].

Effect of Digibind™ and DigiFab™ on Serum Digoxin Measurement

Digibind and DigiFab are Fab fragments of antidigoxin antibody used in treating a life-threatening acute digoxin overdose. Digibind, the first antidote available for treating digoxin overdose, has been available in the United States since 1986 (Glaxo Wellcome Inc.), and more recently, in 2001, the Food and Drug Administration of the United States (FDA) approved DigiFab for treating digoxin overdoses. Digibind is produced by immunizing sheep with digoxin–human albumin conjugate followed by isolation of digoxin-specific antibody from the blood and papain digestion to generate the Fab fragment of the antibody. The Fab fragment of the antidigoxin antibody is then further purified. DigiFab is prepared by injecting sheep with digoxin-dicarboxymethylamine, a digoxin analog, followed by isolation of antidigoxin antibody from the blood, papain digestion, and then purification of the Fab fragment using affinity chromatography. The molecular weight of DigiFab (46 000 Da) is similar to the molecular weight of Digibind (46 200 Da). Usually the Digibind dosage is 80 times the digoxin body burden; if neither the dose ingested nor the plasma digoxin concentration is known, then 380 mg of Digibind is usually injected into the patient. The half-life of the Fab fragment in humans is 12–20 hours, but this may be prolonged in patients with renal failure [23]. Digibind and DigiFab are equivalent in their digoxin-binding capacity. Moreover, both compounds are capable of binding endogenous DLIS [24].

In addition to digoxin, Digibind demonstrates the ability to neutralize cardenolide that is glycosylated in position 3 (digitoxin and ouabain) with a similar potency, regardless of substitutions in the steroid part of the molecule. Therefore, Digibind is effective in treating plant poisoning with foxglove, which contains various cardiac glycosides. Rich *et al.* demonstrated successful treatment of a 22-year-old man with Digibind who was overdosed intentionally with a homemade foxglove extract [25]. In addition, Digibind is capable of neutralizing both cardiac glycosides and respective aglycons – for example oleandrin, the active component of oleander extract – and is effective in treating life-threatening oleander toxicity [26]. Moreover, Digibind may be effective in treating Chan Su overdose – Chan Su being a Chinese medicine containing bufalin and other cardioactive steroids from the bufadienolide class – but the efficacy of Digibind in treating Chan Su poisoning is poor compared to its efficacy in treating digoxin overdose. This is due to the poor specificity of Digibind to neutralize cinobufagin and cinobufatolin, which are also constituents of Chan Su, as is toad venom [27].

Both Digibind and DigiFab interfere with serum digoxin measurement using immunoassays. The magnitude of interference depends on the assay design and the specificity of the antidigoxin antibody. The microparticle enzyme immunoassay of digoxin (MEIA on the AxSYM analyzer, Abbott Laboratories, Abbott Park, IL) as well as the Stratus digoxin assay demonstrated digoxin values which were higher than measured free digoxin concentration in the presence of Digibind [28]. McMillin *et al.* studied the effect of Digibind and DigiFab on 13 different digoxin immunoassays. Positive interference in the presence and absence of digoxin was observed with Digibind and DigiFab, although the magnitude of interference was somewhat less with DigiFab. The magnitude of interference varied significantly with each method, while the IMMULITE®, Vitros®, Dimension® and Access® digoxin methods showed the highest interference. Minimal interferences were observed with FPIA, MEIA, SYNCHRON and CEDIA methods. The authors also commented that monitoring free digoxin (in the protein-free ultrafiltrate) eliminates this interference because both Digibind and DigiFab, due to their approximate molecular weight of 46 000 Da, are absent in protein-free ultrafiltrate [29]. Digibind and DigiFab do not interfere with serum digoxin measurement using a chromatographic method, such as liquid chromatography combined with mass spectrometry. Kanno *et al.* described a method for simultaneous analysis of digoxin, digitoxin and related compounds using liquid chromatography combined with tandem mass spectrometry [30]. Oiestad *et al.* also described a liquid chromatography-tandem mass spectrometry (LC-MS/MS) method for digoxin and digitoxin in whole blood for autopsy cases. Samples were prepared by liquid–liquid extraction using ethyl acetate/heptane/dichloromethane (3 : 1 : 1 by volume), and chromatographic separations were achieved by using a C-18 reverse-phase column. Mass detection was performed by positive ion mode electrospray on ammonium adducts, and deuterated digoxin (digoxin-d3) was used as the internal standard [31]. However, chromatographic methods are rarely used in clinical laboratories, although forensic toxicology laboratories and crime laboratories involved in death investigations are equipped with such analyzers.

Effect of Spironolactone and Related Drugs in Therapeutic Drug Monitoring of Digoxin

Spironolactone is a competitive aldosterone antagonist which blocks the binding of aldosterone to the renal receptor, causing sodium loss and potassium retention, and acts as a diuretic. This drug is used clinically in treating primary aldosteronism, essential hypertension, congestive heart failure and edema. After oral administration, spironolactone is rapidly and extensively metabolized to several metabolites, including canrenone, which is an active metabolite. Potassium canrenoate is also metabolized to canrenone, but this drug is not approved for clinical use in the United Sates. Because of the structural similarity between spironolactone and related compounds with digoxin, these substances interfere with serum digoxin assays, especially assays utilizing polyclonal antibodies against digoxin. This may be troublesome because spironolactone is often used with digoxin, especially in treating patients with congestive heart failure. Although positive interference of spironolactone and canrenone in the radio-immunoassay for digoxin was reported as early as 1974 [32], currently radioimmunoassays are not used in clinical laboratories. Morris *et al.* reported positive interference of spironolactone in digoxin measurement using the fluorescence polarization immunoassay (FPIA, Abbott Laboratories) [33], but this assay is no longer commercially available. Another report discussed two cases where cross-reactivity of potassium canrenoate with digoxin assay caused clinical problems and recommended use of the OPUS digoxin assay, which showed minimum cross-reactivity with potassium canrenoate [34]. Steimer *et al.* reported, for the first time, the negative interference of canrenone in serum digoxin measurement using microparticle enzyme immunoassay (MEIA, Abbott laboratories). Misleading subtherapeutic concentrations of digoxin as measured on several occasions led to falsely guided digoxin dosing, resulting in serious digoxin toxicity in the patients [35]. Later, Steimer *et al.* published a follow-up study, reporting that spironolactone, potassium canrenoate and their common metabolite canrenone can cause both positive interference and negative interference in serum digoxin measurements using immunoassays. Positive interference was observed using FPIA, aca® (Dade Behring, Deerfield, IL) or Elecsys® (Roche Diagnostics, Indianapolis, IN). Digoxin values are falsely lower (negative interference) if measured by MEIA, IMx® (both from Abbott Laboratories) and Dimension digoxin assays (Dade Behring, Deerfield, IL). The magnitude of interference was more significant with potassium canrenoate, where concentration of its metabolite canrenone could be significantly higher compared to spironolactone therapy. The authors observed a 42% decline in the expected value of serum digoxin in the presence of 3125 ng/ml of canrenoate using MEIA, 78% decline using Dimension, and 51% decrease using IMx. A positive bias was observed with aca (0.7 ng/ml), TDx (0.62 ng/ml) and Elessys (0.58 ng/ml). EMIT 2000, Tina-Quant (Roche Diagnostics, Indianapolis, IN) and the Vitros digoxin assay did not demonstrate any such interference [36]. Howard *et al.* showed that low-dose spironolactone (up to 25 mg per day) as used for oral therapy did not cause clinically significant negative interference in the MEIA digoxin assay on the AxSYM analyzer by comparing results with the EMIT assay, which is free from spironolactone interference [37]. However, with a higher spironolactone dose, such as 200 mg per day, significant interference may be observed with the MEIA assay [38]. The relatively new digoxin assays manufactured by the Abbott Laboratories for application on ARCHITECT clinical chemistry platforms (*c*Dig, particle enhanced turbidimetric inhibition immunoassay, PETINIA) and ARCHITECT immunoassay platforms (*i*Dig, chemiluminescent microparticle immunoassay, CMIA) are completely free from such interferences [39]. Chemical structures of spironolactone and digoxin are given in Fig. 11.1.

Effect of Herbal Supplements on Digoxin Immunoassays

In the United States, complementary and alternative medicines are classified as dietary supplements and marketed pursuant to the Dietary Supplement Health and Education Act of 1994. Complementary and alternative medicines, including Ayurvedic medicines, are becoming increasingly popular in the United States, Europe and other parts of the world. Interestingly, herbal supplements only interfere with digoxin immunoassays, and the magnitude of interference depends on the antibody-specificity of the assay. In general, polyclonal antibody-based digoxin immunoassays are more affected by these supplements than are specific monoclonal antibody-based digoxin immunoassays. Significant interferences of the Chinese medicines Chan Su, Lu-Shen-Wan and oleander-containing herbal products with various digoxin assays have been reported.

Chan Su is prepared from the dried white secretion of the auricular glands and the skin glands of Chinese toads (*Bufo melanostictus* Schneider or *Bufo bufo gargarzinas* Gantor) and

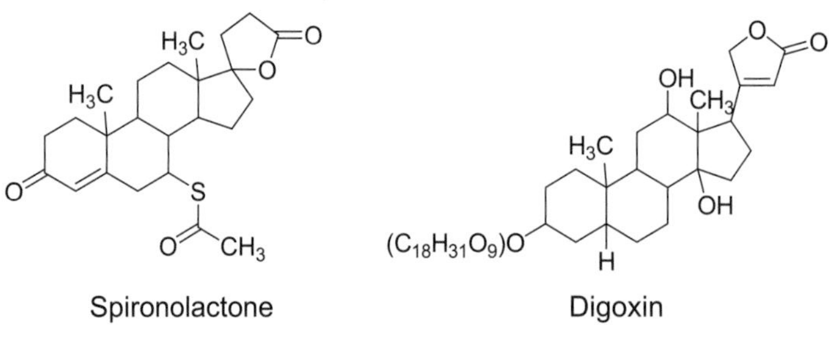

Spironolactone   Digoxin

FIGURE 11.1 Chemical structures of digoxin and spironolactone.

used for treating various heart diseases in traditional Chinese medicine. Bufalin, the active component of Chan Su, is responsible for interference with various digoxin assays due to structural similarity with digoxin. The interference of Chan Su and Lu-Shen-Wan in serum digoxin measurement can be positive (falsely elevated digoxin concentrations) or negative (falsely lowered digoxin concentrations) depending on the assay design. Although the Beckman assay (Synchron LX system, Beckman Coulter) and Roche assay (Tina-Quant) showed positive interference in the presence of Chan Su, the MEIA (microparticle enzyme immunoassays) digoxin assay on the AxSYM platform (Abbott Laboratories) showed negative interference of Chan Su in serum digoxin measurement. However, the components of Chan Su responsible for digoxin-like immunoreactivity are significantly bound to serum proteins ($>90\%$) and are virtually absent in the protein-free ultrafiltrate. Therefore, measuring free digoxin concentration in the protein-free ultrafiltrate could be used in order to mostly eliminate the interference of Chan Su in serum digoxin measurements [40].

Oleanders are evergreen ornamental shrubs that grow in the Southern parts of the United States, from Florida to California, and in Australia, India, Sri Lanka, China and other parts of the world. There are two major varieties of oleander tree. The pink oleander plant (*Nerium oleander*) grows widely in the Southern parts of the United States and has beautiful pink flowers; the yellow oleander tree (*Thevetia peruviana*) is common throughout much of the tropics and subtropics. All parts of both types of oleander plants are toxic, and the toxic effect may occur after exposure to a small amount of the plant; ingestion of even a single leaf may be fatal, especially in children. Boiling or drying the plant does not inactivate the toxins. Many cardenolides have been isolated from yellow oleander, including thevetin A, thevetin B (major components), peruvoside, neriifolin, thevetoxin, ruvoside and theveridoside. These cardenolides have structural similarity with digoxin, and cross-react with antidigoxin antibodies utilized in digoxin immunoassays. Oleandrin, the active component of pink oleander, also has structural similarity with digoxin and interferes with digoxin immunoassays. Eddleston *et al.* reported a mean apparent serum digoxin concentration of 1.49 nmol/L (1.16 ng/mL) in patients who were poisoned with yellow oleander but were eventually discharged from hospital. Severe toxicity from oleander resulted in a mean apparent serum digoxin concentration of 2.83 nmol/L (2.21 ng/mL) as measured by the FPIA digoxin assay [41]. Although the FPIA digoxin assay demonstrated the highest cross-reactivity with pink oleander extract as well as oleandrin, this assay is no longer commercially available. The Beckman digoxin assay on SYNCHRON LX as well as the turbidimetric assay on the ADVIA 1650 analyzer (Bayer Diagnostics) also showed significant interference with oleander, although the magnitude of interference was approximately 65% less with both the Beckman assay and the turbidimetric assay compared with the FPIA assay. The chemiluminescent assay (Bayer Diagnostics, now Siemens), is virtually free from interference of oleander. Although oleander causes positive interference with most digoxin assays, the MEIA digoxin assays (Abbott Laboratories) demonstrated negative interference [42]. The chemical structures of bufalin and oleandrin are given in Fig. 11.2.

There is one case report in the literature of interference of Siberian ginseng in serum digoxin measurement. A 74-year-old man had a steady serum digoxin level of 0.9–2.2 ng/ml for 10 years. His serum digoxin increased to 5.2 ng/ml on one occasion after taking Siberian ginseng. Although the level was toxic, the patient did not experience any signs or symptoms of digoxin toxicity. After the patient stopped taking Siberian ginseng, his digoxin level

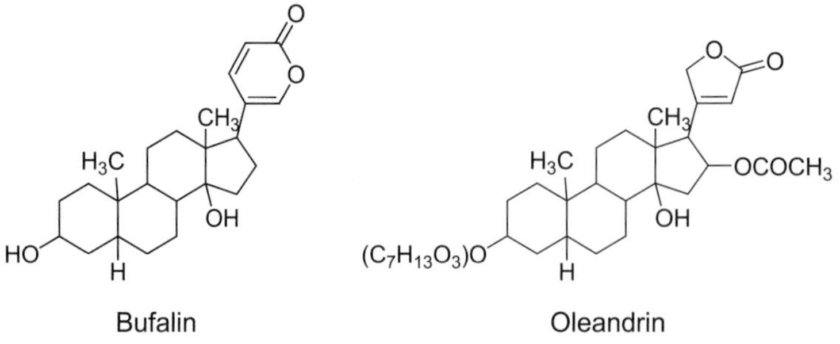

FIGURE 11.2 Chemical structures of bufalin and oleandrin.

Bufalin

Oleandrin

returned to normal [43]. However, in our experience Siberian ginseng only has very modest interference with the fluorescence polarization immunoassay (FPIA) and has no effect on other digoxin assays investigated. Therefore, it is possible that the Siberian ginseng ingested by this patient was mislabeled and the plant was probably from a digitalis group of plants.

THERAPEUTIC DRUG MONITORING OF OTHER ANTI-ARRHYTHMIC DRUGS

Other than digoxin, several other anti-arrhythmic drugs also require therapeutic drug monitoring. Immunoassays are commercially available for therapeutic drug monitoring of lidocaine, procainamide (along with its active metabolite N-acetylprocainamide), quinidine and disopyramide. These immunoassay methods include enzyme multiplied immunoassays (EMIT), cloned donor enzyme immunoassays (CEDIA), chemiluminescence and electro-chemiluminescence immunoassays as well as immunoturbidimetry assays. In most cases, these immunoassays are easy to perform and are capable of producing rapid results. In addition these assays are reliable and, unlike digoxin immunoassays, are rarely affected by interferences. In the past 30 years several next-generation cardioactive drugs have been developed and introduced into the market, which are now widely prescribed. Many of these drugs are preferred because of their broad and diverse therapeutic benefits, but therapeutic drug monitoring may be required for some of them. The drugs where therapeutic drug monitoring may be of value include amiodarone, flecainide, tocainide, mexiletine and verapamil. The chemical structures of these drugs are given in Fig. 11.3. The major challenge in monitoring these drugs is unavailability of any FDA-approved immunoassays. At present, the only methods that are available for therapeutic drug monitoring of these drugs are chromatographic techniques — gas-liquid chromatography (GC) with various types of detectors as well as mass spectrometry (MS), high-performance liquid chromatography (HPLC), or liquid chromatography/mass spectrometry (LC/MS) as well as liquid chromatography combined with tandem mass spectrometry (LC/MS/MS). Unfortunately, chromatographic methods for therapeutic drug monitoring are available only in large medical centers, academic medical centers and reference laboratories due to the complexity of these methods. Therefore, small and medium medical centers are unable to offer therapeutic drug monitoring of these drugs

FIGURE 11.3 Chemical structures of amiodarone, flecainide, tocainide, mexiletine and verapamil.

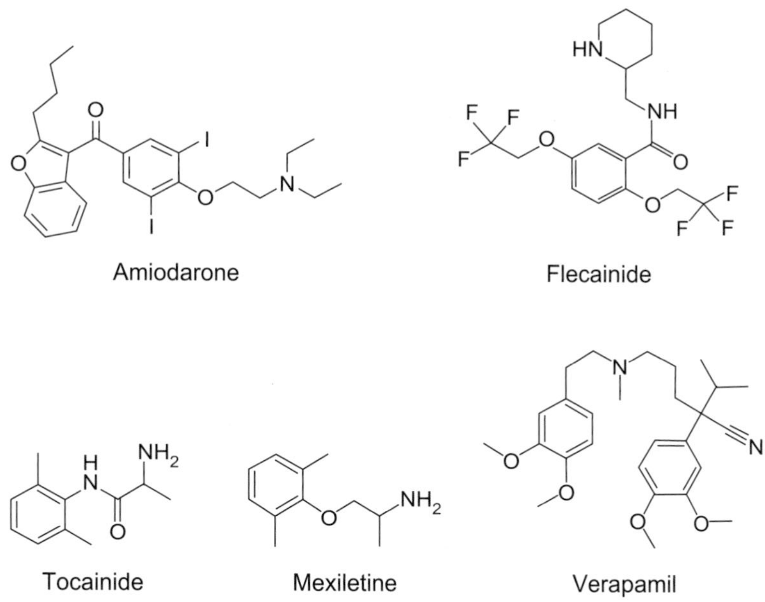

Amiodarone

Flecainide

Tocainide

Mexiletine

Verapamil

on a routine basis, which could be problematic if a patient is showing an adverse drug reaction to any of these cardioactive drugs. Lee *et al.* described a case of a severe mexiletine-induced hypersensitivity reaction in an 82-year-old man which was accompanied by fever, cough, generalized erythematous rash and eosinophilic pneumonia [44]. Supratherapeutic flecainide plasma concentration due to interaction with paroxetine was associated with delirium in a 69-year-old female. The cause of the elevated flecainide concentration was impaired metabolism due to inhibition of CYP2D6 activity by paroxetine. The authors commented that therapeutic drug monitoring of flecainide is essential to avoid such adverse drug reactions due to drug–drug interaction [45].

Other challenges involved in therapy with cardioactive drugs include administration of certain drugs as a racemic mixture. In addition, for certain drugs the concentrations of both the parent drug and the active metabolite must be considered. Moreover, for drugs such as disopyramide, lidocaine and quinidine, which are strongly bound to serum protein, free drug monitoring could be more useful than traditionally monitored total drug concentration (free drug + protein-bound drug). These factors are summarized in Table 11.3.

Challenges in Monitoring Class IA Anti-Arrhythmic Drugs

Therapeutic drug monitoring of the Class IA anti-arrhythmic drugs quinidine, procainamide and disopyramide is essential because these drugs have a low toxic to therapeutic ratio and their use is associated with several serious adverse drug reactions. In addition, drug overdose may be potentially lethal. Quinidine syncope (a transient loss of consciousness due to paroxysmal ventricular tachycardia, sometimes the torsade de pointe type) may

TABLE 11.3 Cardioactive Drugs which are either Administered as Racemic Mixture and/or are Strongly Protein Bound and also Require Therapeutic Drug Monitoring

Drug	Administered as racemic?	Active metabolite	Protein binding	Free drug monitoring?
CLASS IA				
Disopyramide	Yes	Yes	65%	No
Procainamide	No	Yes	10–20%	No
Quinidine	No	Yes	80–90%	Yes
CLASS IB				
Lidocaine	No	Yes	70–80%	Yes
Mexiletine	Yes	No	50–70%	No
CLASS IC				
Flecainide	Yes	No	40%	No
Tocainide	Yes		10–20%	No
Propafenone	No	Yes	85–95%	Not established
CLASS II				
Propranolol	Yes	Yes	90%	Not established
CLASS III				
Amiodarone	No	Yes	95%	Not established
Sotalol	Yes	No	< 10%	No
CLASS IV				
Verapamil	Yes	No	90%	Not established

even occur with a therapeutic dose, often with the initiation of therapy and within the first few days. Procainamide can cause a hypersensitivity reaction as well as electrophysiological changes including QRS prolongation. Disopyramide has a negative inotropic effect, which may cause a serious adverse drug reaction in a patient with pre-existing left ventricular dysfunction. Renal dysfunction may cause accumulation of procainamide and its active metabolite N-acetylprocainamide, causing severe toxicity [46].

Procainamide is 50% cleared by the kidney and the other 50% is metabolized to N-acetylprocainamide, an active metabolite. Martin *et al.* reported that ofloxacin, a fluoroquinolone antibiotic, inhibits renal clearance of procainamide and increases area under the curve of procainamide by 27% and peak plasma concentration by 21%. Interestingly, ofloxacin did not interfere with renal clearance of N-acetylprocainamide. The authors recommended close monitoring of procainamide plasma concentrations during therapy with ofloxacin [47]. Immunoassays are available for accurate determination of both procainamide and N-acetylprocainamide concentrations in serum or plasma, and such immunoassays correlate well with liquid chromatographic methods [48].

Quinidine is an optical isomer of the antimalarial drug quinine. Quinidine immunoassays are robust and stereospecific because quinine does not interfere with immunoassays for quinidine [49]. Although the therapeutic range of quinidine is considered to be 2–5 µg/mL, an altered therapeutic range of quinidine after myocardial infarction and cardiac surgery has been reported. Quinidine is strongly bound to serum alpha-1-acid glycoprotein, an acute phase reactant, and its concentration is elevated after myocardial infarction. Garfinkel *et al.* reported a case of a woman who suffered from myocardial infarction after cardiac surgery and showed a high fraction of alpha-1-acid glycoprotein (228 mg/dL); she experienced no toxicity from quinidine despite a high quinidine level of 11 µg/mL. This was due to a very small amount of free fraction of quinidine (0.032), and her free quinidine concentration was not elevated [50]. McCollam *et al.* reported that the concentration of alpha-1-acid glycoprotein may remain elevated in serum for at least 28 days after atrial fibrillation and flutter, resulting in a relative reduction of free quinidine fraction by up to 32%. Therefore, the therapeutic range of total quinidine may be misleading in these patients [51]. Digoxin– quinidine interaction is also an important consideration for therapeutic drug monitoring of both quinidine and digoxin. An increase in serum digoxin concentration occurs in 90% of patients given quinidine. On average, the serum digoxin concentration doubles during treatment with therapeutic doses of quinidine because quinidine impairs renal clearance of digoxin and may also decrease its volume of distribution. Therefore, dosage adjustments based on therapeutic drug monitoring of both digoxin and quinidine are needed to avoid adverse drug reactions [52].

Disopyramide is administered as a racemic mixture. Although both optical isomers (*R* and *S*) act similarly in the prolongation of the effective refractory period, the anticholinergic activity of the *S*-isomer is three to four times more than that of the *R*-isomer. In addition, most of the negative inotropic effect associated with administration of the racemic mixture can be avoided by using the *S*-isomer alone [53]. Disopyramide is also strongly bound to serum proteins, including alpha-1-acid glycoprotein, and significant changes in protein binding after myocardial infarction, acute renal failure, cancer and inflammatory disease may complicate the interpretation of serum or plasma disopyramide concentrations based on the therapeutic range of 1.5–5.0 µg/mL for the total drug. Caplin *et al.* reported that the binding of disopyramide increased from 80% to 87% from day 1 to day 5 after myocardial infarction due to an increase in the alpha-1-acid glycoprotein concentration from 1.04 gm/L on day 1 to 1.80 gm/L on day 5. Because only free disopyramide is pharmacologically active, monitoring of free levels is useful in such patients [54]. Echizen *et al.* reported that free disopyramide concentrations were significantly less in patients with cancer or inflammatory disease compared to healthy subjects. This was related to an increase in the concentration of alpha-1-acid glycoprotein, which also binds disopyramide. The authors concluded that therapeutic range of disopyramide in patients with cancer or inflammatory disease should be higher than the generally recognized therapeutic range of 1.5–5.0 µg/mL [55].

Disopyramide is metabolized to mono-*N*-dealkyldisopyramide, an active metabolite. In patients with chronic renal failure, plasma concentrations of both disopyramide and its active metabolite rise after oral administration of the drug every 8–12 hours and it is important to monitor concentration of the active metabolite due to its accumulation in these patients [56]. There is no immunoassay for measuring concentration of the active metabolite in serum or plasma. Wang *et al.* described a chromatographic method for simultaneous measurement of both disopyramide and its active metabolite in human serum using chlorodisopyramide as the internal standard [57].

Challenges in Monitoring Class IB Anti-Arrhythmic Drugs

Therapeutic drug monitoring of the Class IB anti-arrhythmic drugs lidocaine and mexiletine is recommended. Lidocaine cannot be given orally due to first-pass metabolism, and must be given by the intravenous route. If lidocaine therapy is continued for a short time, therapeutic drug monitoring may not be needed; however, if treatment is continued beyond 24 hours then therapeutic drug monitoring is recommended in order to avoid adverse drug effects. Immunoassays are available for therapeutic drug monitoring of lidocaine, which are robust and mostly free from interferences.

Lidocaine is metabolized to monoethylglycinexylidide and glycinexylidide, both pharmacologically active but less active than the parent drug. The major initial metabolite of lidocaine, monoethylglycinexylidide, can be used for assessment of hepatic function in transplantation, and in critical care medicine. Because of the relatively high excretion ratio, this liver function test depends not only on hepatic metabolic capacity but also on hepatic blood flow. For determination of the monoethylglycinexylidide concentration in serum, both chromatographic methods (gas chromatography and high-performance liquid chromatography) and the fluorescence polarization immunoassay are available. Although chromatographic methods are free from interference, immunoassay showed cross-reactivity with 3-hydroxy monoethylglycinexylidide [58].

Lidocaine is strongly bound to serum alpha-1-acid glycoprotein, and concentration of this acute-phase reactant increases in renal disease, hepatic dysfunction and myocardial infarction, and in patients taking classical anticonvulsants. Therefore, the pharmacologically free fraction of lidocaine may be reduced in these patients, requiring higher total lidocaine serum levels than the recommended lidocaine therapeutic range of 1.5–5.0 µg/mL. Because the usual therapeutic range of lidocaine does not apply in these patients, especially patients after myocardial infarction, free lidocaine monitoring is recommended [59].

Mexiletine has similar electrophysiological properties to lidocaine, but can be administered orally because it does not undergo significant first-pass metabolism like lidocaine. The bioavailability of mexiletine is over 90% and plasma protein binding is approximately 70%. The elimination half-life is 10 hours, but this drug is extensively metabolized by the liver, with more than 11 metabolites identified. Various pathophysiological parameters affect the disposition of mexiletine, and, due to overlapping concentrations between the therapeutic and toxic ranges, therapeutic drug monitoring is recommended. Myocardial infarction, therapy with opioid analgesics, and antacids all reduce the rate of absorption of mexiletine after oral administration, while metoclopramide enhances its absorption. Rifampin, phenytoin and cigarette-smoking enhance the elimination of mexiletine, whereas ciprofloxacin, propafenone and liver cirrhosis decrease its elimination. Factors affecting the elimination of mexiletine may be clinically important, and dosage adjustments are often necessary [60]. Again therapeutic drug monitoring can be useful for dosage adjustment. Mexiletine is administered as a racemic mixture, but the R-isomer demonstrates higher anti-arrhythmic potency than the S-isomer. The S-isomer concentration in the serum, based on area under the curve, is greater than that of the R-isomer due to enhanced clearance of the

R-isomer in the urine [61]. Usually, chromatographic methods are employed for monitoring mexiletine without resolving optical isomers. However, a chiral column can be used for determination of mexiletine enantiomers in plasma [62].

Challenges in Monitoring Class IC Anti-Arrhythmic Drugs

Flecainide, tocainide and propafenone are Class IC anti-arrhythmic drugs which are good candidates for therapeutic drug monitoring. Flecainide has electrophysiologic properties similar to lidocaine, procainamide and quinidine, and produces a dose-dependent decrease in intracardiac conduction as well as being capable of suppressing recurrence of ventricular tachycardia. However, due to its toxicity and overlapping therapeutic and toxic concentrations, flecainide is mostly reserved for use in patients who failed to respond to other sodium channel blockers. This drug is also contraindicated for use in patients with sick sinus syndrome and myocardial infarction. Death can occur from acute hypotension, respiratory failure and asystole [63]. Flecainide is administered as a racemic mixture, and has a bioavailability of approximately 70%. Flecainide undergoes stereoselective hepatic metabolism, with the R-isomer being metabolized by CYP2D6. Therefore, poor metabolizers due to genetic polymorphism of CYP2D6 may be more susceptible to flecainide toxicity, and careful monitoring of flecainide is important to avoid such adverse effects. Flecainide also demonstrates large variability between a given dosage and serum drug level, and a toxic level can be observed even after a therapeutic dosage. Therefore, therapeutic drug monitoring is essential [64]. Currently there is no commercially available immunoassay for therapeutic drug monitoring of flecainide, and the most widely accepted and reliable method for analysis of flecainide in serum and plasma is high-performance liquid chromatography with ultraviolet or fluorescence detection. Flecainide and its metabolites, m-O-dealkylated flecainide and the m-O-dealkylated lactam of flecainide, can be reliably separated and measured with these techniques. For example, Doki et al. reported simultaneous determination of serum flecainide and its metabolites using C-18 reverse phase column and fluorescence detection after extracting flecainide and its metabolites from serum using ethyl acetate [65].

Tocainide, which is also administered as a racemic mixture, shares electrophysiological properties with lidocaine, but has the advantage of being administered orally and has a relatively long half-life in the circulation (13—16 hours). This drug acts to reduce the amplitude and rate of depolarization of the cardiac action potential by decreasing the refractory period, and has proven most useful in the treatment of life-threatening ventricular arrhythmias associated with prolonged QT intervals. Tocainide is minimally protein bound, and undergoes renal clearance without significant first-pass metabolism. Therapeutic monitoring of serum and plasma levels of tocainide is performed to determine the optimal dose and dose interval, and, more importantly, is used in patients who have congestive heart failure and severe renal dysfunction where the clearance half-life of this drug is increased significantly. Toxicity occurs at concentrations greater than 15 μg/mL, and ranges from gastrointestinal and central nervous disturbances to cardiopulmonary depression (including arrest) and the rare complications of leukopenia, agranulocytosis and pulmonary fibrosis [66]. Currently there is no immunoassay available for therapeutic drug monitoring of tocainide, and chromatographic techniques are used for determining serum or plasma levels of the drug. Although enantiomeric separation of tocainide is not necessary for therapeutic drug monitoring, Carr et al.

described a stereospecific high-performance liquid chromatographic determination of tocainide in human plasma after extraction and derivatization with S-(+)-1-(1-naphthyl) ethylisocynate and fluorescence detection [67].

Propafenone is another Class IC anti-arrhythmic drug that is structurally similar to flecainide and has beta-adrenergic receptor-blocking and minor calcium channel antagonist activities. Propafenone is currently used for the treatment of supraventricular tachyarrhythmias, premature ventricular contractions and ventricular tachycardia. Propafenone undergoes significant first-pass metabolism, with a half-life of approximately 6 hours. Its clinical efficacy appears to be related to formation of 5-hydroxypropanfenone, an active metabolite with a half-life that is two to four times longer than that of the parent compound. Therapeutic monitoring of propafenone is useful to determine patient's compliance, as well as for assessing adverse and toxic effects, such as hypersensitivity reactions, lupus-like syndrome, agranulocytosis, central nervous system (CNS) disturbances such as dizziness amd lightheadedness, gastrointestinal upset, a metallic taste and bronchospasm [66]. Therapeutic concentrations tend to be in the range of 0.5–2.0 μg/mL, with toxicity observed at levels greater than 2.0 μg/mL. Quantitation of both propafenone and the 5-hydroxypropanfenone can be simply and reliably performed by using a HPLC-UV method following a liquid–liquid extraction with n-butyl chloride or methylene chloride [68].

Challenges in Monitoring Class II and Class III Anti-Arrhythmic Drugs

Class II anti-arrhythmic agents are beta-blockers which show wide therapeutic range, and therapeutic drug monitoring is usually not recommended except in the case of propranolol. However, therapeutic drug monitoring is indicated for the Class III anti-arrhythmic drugs amiodarone and sotalol. Nevertheless, therapeutic drug monitoring of the beta-blocker propranolol may be useful under certain circumstances — for example, patients with liver cirrhosis or portal hypertension. The starting dose should also be low [69]. Although therapeutic drug monitoring is rarely conducted for other beta-blockers, Umezawa *et al.* described a liquid chromatography combined with tandem mass spectrometric assay for simultaneous determination of four beta-blockers (acebutolol, labetalol, metoprolol and propranolol) using direct injection of a crude plasma sample [70].

Amiodarone is most commonly used to treat supraventricular and life-threatening ventricular arrhythmias. This drug is 95% protein bound, undergoes renal clearance and has a long, multiphasic elimination of up to 53 days. When long-term therapy with amiodarone is initiated, the dosage should be kept at the minimum effective level, especially in patients also taking digoxin and warfarin. Sometimes the interaction of amiodarone with other drugs may not be obvious clinically until several weeks after initiation of therapy [71]. Amiodarone is also associated with thyroid dysfunction, due to its high iodine content. Although most patients remain euthyroid, amiodarone-induced thyrotoxicosis and amiodarone-induced hypothyroidism may occur depending on the iodine status of the patient and history of prior thyroid disease. Screening for thyroid disease prior to initiation of amiodarone therapy and periodic monitoring of thyroid function during therapy is recommended [72]. Despite severe adverse effects, routine monitoring of serum or plasma concentrations of amiodarone and its potentially active metabolite N-desethyl-amiodarone is not commonly performed. Typical clinical indications for laboratory analysis are to monitor patient compliance and adequacy of blood concentrations (usually above 1.0 μg/mL), or when signs and symptoms of toxicity are manifested. The current methodology that is most widely employed is high-performance liquid chromatography with ultraviolet (UV), fluorescence, or chemiluminescence detection, and using rapid and simple liquid extraction techniques. Ou *et al.* described a liquid chromatographic technique for determination of amiodarone and its metabolite in human serum using HPLC and UV detection [73].

Sotalol is a beta-adrenoreceptor blocker drug that also has Class III anti-arrhythmic properties and has been prescribed to patients with ventricular, atrial and supraventricular arrhythmias. During the first week of treatment, adverse effects arise more frequently as a consequence of the prolongation of QT interval. Much like amiodarone, the current methodology that is most widely employed is HPLC with ultraviolet or fluorescence detection following liquid—liquid or solid phase extraction. Although sotalol is administered as a racemic mixture, for therapeutic drug monitoring separation of enantiomers is not usually performed. However, de Cunha *et al.* described determination of both *R* and *S* isomers in human plasma after extraction and derivatization with (−) menthylcloformate and analysis by a reverse phase C-18 column and fluorescence detection [74]. Therapeutic range of sotalol is considered to be 0.5—2.0 μg/mL and toxicity may be encountered in some patients especially QRS prolongation over a serum level of 2.55 μg/mL [64].

CHALLENGES IN MONITORING CLASS IV ANTI-ARRHYTHMIC DRUGS

Verapamil, a Class IV anti-arrhythmic drug, is a voltage-dependent calcium channel blocker that is used extensively in the treatment of a wide range of cardiovascular disorders. Verapamil decreases impulse conduction through the AV node, and has proven particularly effective in protecting the ventricles from supraventricular tachyarrhythmias (atrial arrhythmia, atrial flutter, and paroxysmal supraventricular tachycardia). Due to its additional vasodilatory actions on vascular smooth muscle, the drug is also used for treatment of stable and unstable angina pectoris, preservation of ischemic myocardium, hypertension, congestive heart failure, migraine headaches and Raynaud's phenomenon. Verapamil is metabolized by *N*-demethylation to its active metabolite, norverapamil, which is usually found in similar concentrations to the parent drug after the steady state is reached. This drug undergoes first-pass metabolism in the liver and is cleared from the circulation by the kidneys. Therefore, decreased clearance, and increased bioavailability, volume of distribution and half-life may be observed in patients with severe hepatic dysfunction. Serum concentrations of verapamil (ranging from 50 to 250 ng/mL) appear to correlate well with cardiac response, and are most frequently monitored to ensure optimal dosing and levels are achieved to assess the potential toxic side effects. There is no immunoassay for therapeutic drug monitoring of verapamil, but both verapamil and its active metabolite norverapamil can be measured in serum or plasma using either gas chromatography or high-performance liquid chromatography. Chytil *et al.* described a liquid chromatography combined with tandem mass spectrometric method for determination of both verapamil and doxazosin in human serum using trimipramine-d3 as the internal standard [75].

CHROMATOGRAPHIC METHODS FOR DETERMINING MULTIPLE ANTI-ARRHYTHMIC DRUGS SIMULTANEOUSLY

There are published methods for the simultaneous determination of multiple anti-arrhythmic drugs in a single run, and such techniques are valuable for reference laboratories as well as academic medical center-based hospital laboratories. In one report the authors measured 12 anti-arrhythmic drugs (amiodarone, aprindine, disopyramide, flecainide, lidocaine, lorcainide, mexiletine, procainamide, propafenone, sotalol, tocainide and verapamil) using HPLC after solid phase extraction of these drugs from human plasma. Because most anti-arrhythmic drugs are basic in nature, good absorption on the extraction columns was obtained by alkalinization except in the cases of aprindine (extracted at neutral pH) and amiodarone (extracted at pH 3.5) [76]. Li *et al.* described a liquid chromatography combined with a tandem mass spectrometric method for simultaneous determination of 10 anti-arrhythmic drugs (diltiazem, amiodarone, mexiletine, propranolol, sotalol, verapamil, bisoprolol, metoprolol, atenolol and carvedilol) in human plasma using a reverse phase C-18 column [77]. However, liquid chromatography combined with mass spectrometric methods may show inaccuracy for determination of various drugs and metabolites which are small molecules. The inaccuracy may be related to the ionization process in the mass spectrometer, or the matrix effect during ionization affecting the analyte and the internal standard differently, or can be associated with the process of ion selection. However, most inaccuracies can be controlled by sufficient liquid chromatographic separation-based sample workup prior to mass spectrometric analysis. Therefore, liquid chromatography combined with tandem mass spectrometric methods should undergo rigorous and systematic validation before application for analysis of specimens collected from patients [78].

CONCLUSIONS

Digoxin is one of the most commonly monitored anti-arrhythmic drugs in clinical laboratories and immunoassays are commonly used for its monitoring. Digoxin immunoassays are affected by a variety of endogenous and exogenous factors. Immunoassays for other anti-arrhythmic drugs are less affected. For newer anti-arrhythmic drugs immunoassays are not available, and only chromatographic techniques can be applied for therapeutic monitoring of these drugs. Therefore, small and medium clinical laboratories are unable to offer these tests in-house, and specimens must be referred to a reference laboratory for analysis.

References

[1] Bessen HA. Therapeutic and toxic effects of digitalis: William Withering 1785. J Emerg Med 1986;4:243–8.
[2] Gheorghiade M, Harinstein ME, Filippatos GS. Digoxin for the treatment of chronic and acute heart failure. Acute Cardiac Care 2009;11:83–7.
[3] Lingrel JB. The physiological significance of the cardiotonic steroid/ouabain binding site of the Na, K-ATPase. Annu Rev Physiol 2010;72:395–412.
[4] Dec GW. Digoxin remains useful in the management of chronic heart failure. Med Clin North Am 2003;87:317–37.

[5] Bussey HI, Hawkins DW, Gaspard JJ, Walsh RA. A comparative trail of digoxin and digitoxin in the treatment of congestive heart failure. Pharmacotherapy 1988;8:235—40.

[6] Campbell TJ, Williams KM. Therapeutic drug monitoring of antiarrhythmic drugs. Br J Clin Pharmacol 1998;46:307—19.

[7] Miller JJ, Straub RW, Valdes R. Digoxin immunoassays with cross-reactivity of digoxin metabolites proportional to their biological activities. Clin Chem 1994;40:1898—903.

[8] Solnica B. Comparison of serum digoxin concentration monitored by fluorescence polarization immunoassay on the TDxFLx and dry chemistry enzyme immunoassay on the Vitros 950. Clin Chem Lab Med 2004;42:958—64.

[9] Tzou MC, Reuning RH, Sams RA. Quantitation of interference in digoxin immunoassay in renal, hepatic and diabetic disease. Clin Pharm Ther 1997;61:429—41.

[10] Gruber KA, Whitaker JM, Buckalew VM. Endogenous digitalis-like substances in plasma of volume expanded dogs. Nature 1980;287:743—5.

[11] Craver JL, Valdes R. Anomalous serum digoxin concentration in uremia. Ann Intern Med 1983;98:483—4.

[12] Jortani SA, Valdes Jr R. Digoxin and its related endogenous factors. Crit Rev Clin Lab Sci 1997;34:225—74.

[13] Dasgupta A, Yeo K, Malik S, et al. Two novel endogenous digoxin-like immunoreactive substances isolated from human plasma ultrafiltrate. Biochem Biophys Res Comm 1987;148:623—8.

[14] Qazzaz HM, Valdes R. Simultaneous isolation of endogenous digoxin-like immunoreactive factor, ouabain-like factor, and deglycosylated congeners from mammalian tissue. Arch Biochem Biophys 1996;328:193—200.

[15] Dasgupta A. Therapeutic drug monitoring of digoxin: impact of endogenous and exogenous digoxin-like immunoreactive factors. Toxicol Rev 2006;25:273—81.

[16] Saccoia NC, Hackett LP, Morris RG, Ilett KF. Enzyme-multiplied immunoassay (EMIT 2000) digoxin assay compared with fluorescence polarization immunoassays and amerlex 125I radioimmunoassay at two Australian centers. Ther Drug Monit 1996;18:672—7.

[17] Dasgupta A, Trejo O. Suppression of total digoxin concentration by digoxin-like immunoreactive substances in the MEIA digoxin assay: elimination of interference by monitoring free digoxin concentrations. Am J Clin Pathol 1999;111:406—10.

[18] Valdes R, Graves SW. Protein binding of endogenous digoxin-like immunoreactive factors in human serum and its variation with clinical condition. J Clin Endocrinol Metab 1985;60:1135—43.

[19] Christenson RH, Studenberg SD, Beck-Davis SS, Sedor FA. Digoxin-like immunoreactivity eliminated from serum by centrifugal ultrafiltration before fluorescence polarization immunoassay of digoxin. Clin Chem 1987;33:606—8.

[20] Jones TE, Morris RG. Discordant results from real-world patient samples assayed for digoxin. Ann Pharmacother 2008;42:1797—803.

[21] Bonetti A, Monica C, Bonaguri C, et al. Interference by heterophilic antibodies in immunoassays: wrong increase of myoglobin values. Acta Biomed 2008;79:140—3.

[22] Liendo C, Ghali JK, Graves SW. A new interference in some digoxin assays: anti-murine heterophilic antibodies. Clin Pharmacol Ther 1996;60:593—8.

[23] Flanagan RJ, Jones AL. Fab antibody fragments: some applications in clinical toxicology. Drug Saf 2004;27:1115—33.

[24] Pullen MA, Harpel MR, Danoff TM, Brooks DR. Comparison of non-digitalis binding properties of digoxin specific Fab using direct binding methods. J Immunol Methods 2008;336:235—41.

[25] Rich SA, Libera JM, Locke RJ. Treatment of foxglove extracts poisoning with digoxin specific Fab treatments. Ann Emerg Med 1993;22:1904—7.

[26] Camphausen C, Hass NA, Mattke AC. Successful treatment of oleander intoxication (cardiac glycoside) with digoxin specific Fab antibody fragment in a 7-year-old child: case report and review of literature. Z Kardiol 2005;94:817—23.

[27] Brubacher JR, Lachmanen D, Ravikumar PR, Hoffman RS. Efficacy of digoxin specific Fab fragments (Digibind) in the treatment of toad venom poisoning. Toxicon 1999;37:931—42.

[28] Rainey P. Digibind and free digoxin [Letter]. Clin Chem 1999;45:719—20.

[29] McMillin GA, Qwen W, Lambert TL, et al. Comparable effects of DIGIBIND and DigiFab in thirteen digoxin immunoassays. Clin Chem 2002;48:1580—4.

[30] Kanno S, Watanabe K, Yamagishi I, et al. Simultaneous analysis of cardiac glycoside in blood and urine by thermo responsive LC-MS-MS. Anal Bioanal Chem 2011;339:1141—9.

[31] Oiestad EL, Johansen U, Stokke Opdal M, et al. Determination of digoxin and digitoxin in whole blood. J Anal Toxicol 2009;33:372—8.

[32] Huffman DH. The effects of spironolactone and canrenone in digoxin radioimmunoassay. Res Comm Chem Pathol Pharmacol 1974;9:787—90.

[33] Morris RG, Frewin DB, Taylor WB, et al. The effect of renal and hepatic impairment and of spironolactone on serum digoxin assay. Eur J Clin Pharmacol 1988;34:233—9.

[34] Okazaki M, Tanigawara Y, Kita T, et al. Cross-reactivity of TDX and OPUS immunoassay system for serum digoxin determination. Ther Drug Monit 1997;19:657—62.

[35] Steimer W, Muller C, Eber B, Emmanuilidis K. Intoxication due to negative canrenone interference in digoxin drug monitoring [Letter]. Lancet 1999;354:1176—7.

[36] Steimer W, Muller C, Eber B. Digoxin assays: frequent, substantial and potentially dangerous interference by spironolactone, canrenone and other steroids. Clin Chem 2002;48:507—16.

[37] Howard G, Barclay M, Florkowski C, et al. Lack of clinically significant interference by spironolactone with the AxSYM digoxin II assay. Ther Drug Monit 2003;25:112—3.

[38] Steimer W. Lack of critically significant interference by spironolactone with the AxSYM digoxin II assay only applies to low dose therapy with spironolactone [Letter]. Ther Drug Monit 2003;25:484—5.

[39] DeFrance A, Armbruster D, Petty D, et al. Abbott ARCHITECT clinical chemistry and immunoassay systems — digoxin assays are free of interferences from spironolactone, potassium canrenoate and their common metabolite canrenone. Ther Drug Monit 2011;33:128—31.

[40] Chow L, Johnson M, Wells A, Dasgupta A. Effect of the traditional Chinese medicine Chan Su, Lu-Shen-Wan, DanShen and Asian ginseng on serum digoxin measurement by Tina-Quant (Roche) and Synchron LX system (Beckman) digoxin immunoassays. J Clin lab Anal 2003;17:22—7.

[41] Eddleston M, Ariaratnam CA, Sjostrom L, et al. Acute yellow oleander (*Thevetia peruvica*) poisoning: cardiac arrhythmias, electrolyte disturbances, and serum cardiac glycoside concentrations on presentation to hospital. Heart 2000;83:310—306.

[42] Dasgupta A, Datta P. Rapid detection of oleander poisoning by using digoxin immunoassays: comparison of five assays. Ther Drug Monit 2004;26:658—63.

[43] McRae S. Elevated serum digoxin levels in a patient taking digoxin and Siberian ginseng. Can Med Assoc J 1996;155:293—5.

[44] Lee SP, Kim SH, Kim TH, et al. A case of mexiletine induced hypersensitivity syndrome presenting an eosinophilic pneumonia. J Korean Med Sci 2010;25:148—51.

[45] Tsao YY, Gugger JJ. Delirium in a patient with toxic flecainide plasma concentrations: the role of a pharmacokinetic drug interaction with paroxetine. Ann Pharamcother 2009;43:1366—9.

[46] Kim SY, Benowitz NL. Poisoning due to class 1A antiarrhythmic drugs. Quinidine, procainamide and disopyramide. Drug Saf 1990;5:393—420.

[47] Martin DE, Shen J, Griener J, et al. Effects of ofloxacin on the pharmacokinetics and pharmacodynamics of procainamide. J Clin Pharamcol 1996;36:85—91.

[48] Pape BE. Enzyme immunoassay, liquid chromatography and spectrofluorometry compared for the determination of procainamide and N-acetylprocainamide. J Anal Toxicol 1982;6:44—8.

[49] Paul A, Wells A, Dasgupta A. Stereospecificity of antibody: quinine, the optical isomer of quinidine and anti-malarial drug chloroquine do not cross-react with quinidine immunoassay. Ther Drug Monit 2000;22: 174—6.

[50] Garfinkel D, Mamelok RD, Blaschke TF. Altered therapeutic range for quinidine after myocardial infarction and cardiac surgery. Ann Intern Med 1987;107:48—50.

[51] McCollam PL, Crouch MA, Watson JE. Altered protein binding of quinidine in patients with atrial fibrillation and flutter. Pharamcother 1997;17:753—9.

[52] Bigger Jr JT, Leahey Jr EB. Quinidine and digoxin: an important interaction. Drugs 1982;24:229—39.

[53] Lima JJ, Boudoulas H. Stereoselective effects of disopyramide enantiomers in humans. J Cardiovas Pharamcol 1987;9:594—600.

[54] Caplin JL, Johnston A, Hamer J, Camm AJ. The acute changes in serum binding of disopyramide and flecainide after myocardial infarction. Eur J Clin Pharmacol 1985;28:253—5.

[55] Echizen H, Saima S, Umeda N, Ishizaki T. Altered protein binding of disopyramide in plasma from patients with cancer and inflammatory disease. Ther Drug Monit 1987;9:272—8.

[56] Nagura Y, Kuno T, Yanai M, et al. Pharmacokinetics and optimum dose of disopyramide in patients with chronic renal failure. Nippon Jinzo Gakkai Shi 1991;33:539−43.

[57] Wang LH, Kushida K, Ishizaki T. Use of silica gel with aqueous elute for simultaneous high-performance liquid chromatographic assay of disopyramide and mono-N-dealkyldisopyramide. Ther Drug Monit 1986;8:85−9.

[58] Oellerich M, Armstrong V. The MEGX test: a tool for the real time assessment of hepatic function. Ther Drug Monit 2001;23:81−92.

[59] Shand DG. Alpha-1-acid glycoprotein and plasma lidocaine binding. Clin Pharamcokinetic 1984;9(Suppl. 1): 27−31.

[60] Labbe L, Turgeon J. Clinical pharmacokinetics of mexiletine. Clin Phramacokinetic 1999;37:361−84.

[61] Grech-Belanger O, Turgeon J, Gilbert M. Stereoselective disposition of mexiletine in man. Br J Clin Pharamcol 1986;21:481−7.

[62] Lanchote VL, Bonato PS, Dreossi SA, et al. High-performance liquid chromatographic determination of mexiletine enantiomers in plasma and indirect enantioselective separation. J Chromatogr B Biomed Appl 1996;685:281−9.

[63] Winkelmann B, Leinberger H. Life-threatening flecainide toxicity. A pharmacodynamic approach. Ann Intern Med 1987;106:807−14.

[64] Jurgens G, Graudal NA, Kampman JP. Therapeutic drug monitoring of antiarrhythmic drugs. Clin Pharamcokinetic 2003;42:647−63.

[65] Doki K, Homma M, Kuga K, et al. Simultaneous determination of serum flecainide and its metabolites by using high-performance liquid chromatography. J Pharmaceutic Biomed Anal 2004;35:1307−12.

[66] Darbar R, Roden DM. The future of antiarrhythmic drugs. Curr Opin Cardiol 2006;21:361−7.

[67] Carr RA, Foster RT, Freitag D, Pasutto FM. Stereoselective high-performance liquid chromatographic determination of tocainide. J Chromatogr 1991;566:155−62.

[68] Hoyer GL. A HPLC method for the quantitation of propafenone and 5-hydroxy propafenone. Chromatographia 1988;25:1034−8.

[69] Arthur MJ, Tanner AR, Patel C, et al. Pharmacology of propranolol in patients with cirrhosis and portal hypertension. Gut 1985;26:14−9.

[70] Umezawa H, Lee XP, Arima Y, et al. Simultaneous determination of beta blockers in human plasma using liquid chromatography-tandem mass spectrometry. Biomed Chromatogr 2008;22:702−11.

[71] Siddoway LA. Amiodarone: guidelines for use and monitoring. Am Fam Physician 2003;68:2189−96.

[72] Padmanabjan H. Amiodarone and thyroid dysfunction. South Med J 2010;103:922−30.

[73] Ou CN, Rogneurud CL, Doung LT, Frawley VL. Liquid chromatographic determination of amiodarone and N-desmethylamiodarone in serum. Clin Chem 1990;36:532−4.

[74] Da Cunha LC, Gondim FA, de Paola AA, et al. An improved HPLC fluorescence stereoselective method for analysis of (+) S and (−)R sotalol enantiomers in plasma samples. Boll Chim Farm 2001;140:448−54.

[75] Chytil L, Strauch B, Cvacka J, et al. Determination of doxazosin and verapamil in human serum by fast LC-MS/MS: application to document non compliance in patients. J Chromatogr B Analyt Technolol Biomed Life Sci 2010;878:3167−73.

[76] Verbesselt R, Tjandramaga TB, De Schepper PJ. High-performance liquid chromatographic determination of 12 antiarrhythmic drugs in plasma using solid phase column extraction. Ther Drug Monit 1991;13:157−65.

[77] Li S, Liu G, Jia J, et al. Simultaneous determination of ten antiarrhythmic drugs and a metabolite in human plasma by liquid chromatography-tandem mass spectrometry. J Chromatogr B Analyt Tecnhol Biomed Life Sci 2007;847:174−81.

[78] Vogeser M, Seger C. Pitfalls associated with the use of liquid chromatography-tandem mass spectrometry in clinical laboratory. Clin Chem 2010;56:1234−44.

Therapeutic Drug Monitoring of Classical and Newer Anticonvulsants

Matthew Luke

University of New Mexico, Alberquerque, NM

OUTLINE

Therapeutic Drug Monitoring: Newer Drugs and Biomarkers
DOI: 10.1016/B978-0-12-385467-4.00012-9

INTRODUCTION

Epilepsy, or recurrent abnormal discharges of the central nervous system, has a wide spectrum from severe debilitating convulsions to only slight neuronal disturbances that are sometimes not even noticed by the affected individual themselves. Individual medications used for this purpose are generally known as anti-epileptic drugs (AEDs). The goal of AED therapy is to eliminate or reduce these unwanted neuronal discharges. Fourteen new AEDs have been introduced since 1975, when the Anticonvulsant Drug Development Program began screening for compounds that would improve upon the existing drugs. These new drugs, which are often referred to as second-generation AEDs, include eslicarbazepine acetate, felbamate, gabapentin, lacosamide, lamotrigine, levetiracetam, oxcarbazepine, pregabalin, rufinamide, stiripentol, tiagabine, topiramate, vigabatrin and zonisamide.

PATHOPHYSIOLOGY OF EPILEPSY

Individual abnormal neuronal discharges are termed seizures. Epilepsy is a central nervous system disorder that is characterized by a recurrent abnormal discharge of neurons. Epilepsy is reported to occur in 0.5% of the population during their lifetime [1]. Epilepsy can be further classified by clinical features as well as findings on electroencephalographs. A simple classification scheme divides seizures into three main categories. These categories include partial seizures, generalized seizures and unclassified seizures, with the unclassified seizures including neonatal seizures and infantile spasms. Partial seizures are localized to specific discrete areas of the central nervous system, and can be simple or complex. A seizure episode is termed as simple seizure if consciousness is not affected, and complex if consciousness is affected. Partial seizures can evolve into generalized seizures but are classified as a partial seizure as this was the initial evolution of the seizure. Generalized seizures can also be further classified as absence, tonic—clonic, tonic, atonic and myoclonic. Distinction of the seizure types is important as it can have implications in the treatment, prognosis and identification of the potential causative insult within the central nervous system.

Treatment includes identification of the possible underlying cause of the seizures, and, if correctable, steps are undertaken to eliminate such cause. If a reversible cause for the seizures is not identified and the seizures continue then treatment is usually required, and consists of one or multiple of the many AEDs. Ideally, monotherapy would be the best choice; however, nearly all of the newer AEDs have been approved for use in the United States as an adjunct or add-on therapy. Monotherapy has the benefit of avoiding potential AED drug interactions, especially enzyme-inducing drugs which can alter levels of other drugs when their dosing is either increased or decreased [2]. Many additional factors need to be taken into account when choosing an initial AED on which to start the patient. These include the patient's type of seizure or syndrome, risk of seizure recurrence, additional patient conditions, the side-effect profile of the AED, and the patient's view of the situation [3, 4].

Sufficient concentrations of these drugs need to reach their site of action at the central nervous system neurons where the abnormal discharges originate. The level of the AED needs to be kept at a low enough level so as to avoid cellular disturbances due to drug toxicity, or other undesirable side effects from the drug. Complaints of side effects can be quite common. One community-based study showed 60% of patients on AEDs had side effects that they personally rated at a level of at least moderate/serious in nature, in at least three of the following areas: general CNS issues (fatigue, headache and dizziness), motor problems, gastrointestinal complaints, cognition, visual, mood, cosmetic and insomnia [5].

Finding an appropriate dose of the specific AED that stops or decreases the unwanted neuronal discharges, but without reaching drug levels that cause toxicity, is the goal of treatment. Following clinical practices of increasing the dosage of the AED until the seizures stop, up to the maximum recommended dosage, or until toxicity is identified, can be problematic. Specifically, three concerns are identified by a subcommission paper from the International League Against Epilepsy (ILAE) [6]. First, seizures rarely occur on a frequent specific interval. Thus the absence of seizures maybe part of the normal course of the disease, and not due to the AED. Only long-term seizure control can signify appropriate treatment. If the dosage is subtherapeutic and seizures are infrequent, the patient could be on this subtherapeutic dosage of medication for extended periods of time. Secondly, side effects of the therapy may be difficult to differentiate from the seizure disorder itself, especially if it is part of a syndrome. This difficulty is exemplified in the instance where a patient is placed on an AED to stop the seizures but there is a paradoxical increase in seizure activity. This event can occur while at potentially therapeutic levels of an AED, although it is more likely with supratherapeutic doses [7, 8]. Thirdly, the level of an AED, while useful, is only a guideline, and cannot give precise information as to the course of the seizure disorder. No commonly available laboratory tests are available to ensure clinical efficacy or to warn of impending side effects.

ANTI-EPILEPTIC DRUG MONITORING

Levels of the AED in the blood, serum or plasma, and in certain cases the saliva, can be used to ensure appropriate dosing of medication for the individual patient in treating epilepsy. This type of information initially became available in the 1960s, when methods were first developed to measure serum concentrations of classical AEDs [9]. These drug levels are then compared to reference levels that have been derived from collective data from multiple studies. Some problems, especially with the newer AEDS, are that studies have few patients, or patients come from subgroups that include those who have more resistant epilepsy, in that they have failed previous therapy with other AEDs.

Laboratory testing for AED levels needs to be done on a regular interval. However, it is important for the clinician to treat the patient rather than a laboratory result. One can misconstrue that to be effective in treating patients one must maintain the level of the drug within a suggested reference range. It is important to remember that this is only a suggested range, and the individual patient may become seizure-free at a serum level of medication that is below the lower end of the generally accepted reference range. In the initial work in determining a target range for phenytoin, 25% of patients improved at a level below 10 mg/L (10 μg/mL) but the currently generally accepted range today for this AED is between 10 and 20 mg/L (10–20 μg/mL) [9]. At the opposite end of the spectrum, some patients may continue to have seizures when the level of drug is near or even above the upper limit of a reference range. Although seizures in some patients may be controlled with AED concentrations below the reference range, side effects, which become more common above the therapeutic range, may occur in other patients despite an AED concentration within the therapeutic range.

It may be best to consider these AED reference ranges in terms of probabilities and as such to use them only as a guideline. Reference ranges should never be considered as an absolute, as it signifies a combination of probability charts. Below the lower limit of the reference range there is a low probability that the AED will be clinically effective. As the level increases from the low end of the reference range to the high end, the probability of clinical efficacy continually increases. Even beyond the upper limit of the reference range there continues to be a slow increase of probable clinical efficacy. However, the probability of AED toxicity often rapidly increases at the upper limit of the reference range and beyond the range. Some investigators have suggested that there should be no lower limit on the therapeutic range of an AED, with the thought that if the seizures can be controlled then any level of the AED is acceptable. As up to 30% of seizures are mild and self-limiting, with an additional 30% essentially controlled with AED therapy that will remit over time [10], some of the patients controlled on low levels of an AED may represent those that could come off of their AED medication completely and continue to do fine.

The concept of probabilities has given rise to the idea of an "individual therapeutic concentration" for AEDs [11]. This allows for the identification of an ideal level of an AED that effectively treats the patient without any toxicity. Once this clinical goal has been obtained, the corresponding AED level can be identified. Should the clinical picture change, current AED levels could be compared to the previously determined "individual therapeutic concentration" and appropriate corrections should be made. Important issues that could negate such a program would include potential alteration of the active or free concentration of the drug due to alteration in protein levels or protein binding, worsening of the disease, and new drug–drug interactions [6].

INDICATIONS FOR MEASURING A DRUG LEVEL

Measuring of AED therapy is often done without clear-cut indications, which adds to the medical costs as well as patient inconvenience. In studies with rigid indications for when testing for AED levels is appropriate, up to two-thirds of requests have been deemed to be inappropriate [12]. In a prospective 2-year study of 116 patients with partial or idiopathic generalized non-absence epilepsy, no significant clinical differences were found when monitoring these patients using clinical grounds alone versus using therapeutic drug monitoring to keep the serum level of the AED within a reference range [13]. The authors did acknowledge that therapeutic drug monitoring would have a place in specific patients and situations. Several prominent organizations have stated that no monitoring for a stable patient is indicated except if there are clinical indications for measurement of individual therapeutic concentration.

Situations that may be appropriate for therapeutic drug monitoring include identification of non-adherence or non-compliance, suspected toxicity or overdose, phenytoin dose adjustment, management of pharmacokinetics interactions, and specific clinical conditions [14]. Several issues present themselves under the pharmacokinetics interactions. Protein binding of the AED is an issue; as only the free or unbound drug is metabolically active, variation of this protein binding and variation in the amount of protein can significantly alter the amount of free drug. AEDs with high levels of protein binding, such as phenytoin, may benefit from free drug monitoring. Variation of protein binding can also be altered by uremia as well as other drugs and substances that would compete for protein binding sites.

Other pharmacokinetic issues that must be accounted for include the fact that the AED may have multiple metabolites each with varying degrees of effect both within the realm of treating the neuronal discharges and also within the spectrum of toxicity. The route in which the drug is metabolized or excreted could affect its levels, especially if the patient has concomitant disease of the organ mainly responsible for such clearance, such as hepatic or renal dysfunction. Hepatic isoenzyme involvement in metabolism must also be accounted for especially if there is induction or inhibition of the isoenzymes.

Monitoring of AEDs During Pregnancy

Adequately controlling seizures during pregnancy while using the lowest possible dosage of an AED is a prevailing concept [15–17].This allows for a reduction of the potential unwanted outcomes associated with exposure of the fetus to AEDs that may include birth defects, intrauterine growth retardation and developmental delays after birth [18]. On the other hand, the pregnant woman must not be undertreated, as seizures during pregnancy increase the risk for maternal death and may result in spontaneous abortion or still birth [19]. Obtaining a pre-pregnancy baseline to be used as an individual reference level as previously described may be helpful in guiding treatment during pregnancy when the AED pharmacokinetics of protein binding, absorption, drug metabolizing capacity and glomerular filtration rate are altered along with changes in plasma volumes [20, 21].

Changes in the plasma levels of lamotrigine during gestation have been well documented and show a significant decrease in concentration [22]. Several studies have shown significant alterations of lamotrigine clearance that begin within the first trimester and continue to increase until the thirty-second gestational week [23, 24]. These changes were more marked on those women on lamotrigine monotherapy as opposed to those treated with concomitant AED enzyme-inducing therapy. Other second-generation AEDs with likely gestational changes in drug levels include oxcarbazepine and levetiracetam [25]. Monitoring post-delivery drug levels for a period of 2 weeks is also suggested for those who had gestational dosage adjustment.

THERAPEUTIC DRUG MONITORING OF CLASSICAL AEDS

Some of the anti-epileptic drug treatments include drugs such as carbamazepine, phenobarbital, phenytoin and valproic acid. An additional AED is primidone, which is a pro-drug that is metabolized into phenobarbital but also has AED activity itself. These drugs have been classified as classical or first-generation AEDs, and some have been used for over 100 years — such as bromide, which was first used in the 1850s, and phenobarbital, which was introduced in 1912 and is still extensively used today. These classical AED have various properties that are more likely to require therapeutic drug monitoring (TDM) during their use than the more newly developed second-generation AEDs. Table 12.1 includes parameters of the more commonly used classic anti-epileptic drugs

Some of the properties of the classic AEDs include their metabolism by the cytochrome P450 enzymes and uridine diphosphate glucuronyl enzymes. These enzymes transform classical AEDs into inactive metabolites, with specific isoenzymes being important for specific drugs [26]. The cytochrome P450 enzymes can be induced or upregulated by carbamazepine, phenobarbital, phenytoin and primidone, or can be inhibited as with valproic acid. These variations can significantly add to changes in the individual drug levels in patients. The isoenzymes have individual polymorphisms which can further alter levels of the drug, and with phenytoin could alter the needed dosage of medication by at least a factor of two [27]. Autoinduction, where the drug itself induces its own metabolism, as found with carbamazepine, can delay the time for a drug to reach steady-state levels.

The free or unbound drug is the portion of the drug that is freely able to move to its site of action in the central nervous system. That portion of the drug bound to protein has little clinical effect, and is less important when measuring amounts of drug in the blood. As the amount of protein binding decreases the pharmacologically active free percentage increases, and small changes in protein binding can have significant effects on the free concentration of the drug. This is particularly apparent with phenytoin, which is 90% bound to protein, and monitoring of free drug is especially useful. Valproic acid is also highly bound, 90—95% to protein; however, due to a lack of correlation of blood levels to the clinical effect and to concentrations of the drug in the brain, the monitoring of free levels, which can be difficult, is not always helpful [28]. Partitioning of the drug between free and bound states can be altered by pregnancy, aging, liver disease, uremia, burns, changes in pH of the blood, and other drugs that competitively bind at the same site. These issues, as well as hypoalbuminemia, need to be taken into consideration when comparing free and total drug concentration and assessing adequacy of treatment.

The presence of drug metabolites can interfere with the measurement of drug levels. Ideally, if a drug was excreted in an unchanged form in the urine all activity of the drug could be ascribed to the parent compound. In the case of metabolites, they may be

TABLE 12.1 Properties of Classic Anti-Epileptic Drugs

Drug	Oral bioavailability (%)	Time to peak concentration (hour)	Serum protein binding (%)	Adult half-life (hours)	Reference range in serum
Carbamazepine	75—85	4—8	76	12—17 on stable dosing	4—12 μg/mL
Clonazepam	> 95	1—4	85	18—50	10—75 ng/mL
Ethosuximide	> 90	1—4	0	40—60	40—100 μg/mL
Phenobarbital	> 95	0.5—4	55	53—140	15—40 μg/mL
Phenytoin	> 80	1—12	90	Drug-level dependent	10—20 μg/mL
Valproic acid	> 90	3—6	90	13—19	50—100 μg/mL

inactive or have varying degrees of activity, and may cause interference with accurately measuring drug levels. Several of the newer AED drugs are excreted in urine as unchanged drugs.

NEWER ANTICONVULSANTS

At the beginning of 1975 a systematic program was instituted by the National Institute of Neurological Disorders and Stroke to discover new AEDs. This program, identified as the Anticonvulsant Screening Program, screens chemical compounds through a blinded competitively evaluated process using consistent methodologies. The success of this program can be attested through the development of 14 second-generation AEDs that as a group have advantages over the first generation. These second-generation AEDs have various mechanisms of neuronal action that include alteration in specific subtypes of GABA (gamma-aminobutyric acid) or glutamate receptor responses, modulation of ion-specific channels, and alteration of neurotransmitter release and uptake [29]. Some of the AEDs have multiple modes of action, with the end goal of all being to inhibit the abnormal discharge of neurons.

The following sections highlight the properties of the drugs that are important when therapeutically monitoring drugs, and include such items as protein binding, percentage of bioavailability, metabolism and excretion, method of action, more frequently encountered side effects, and suggested reference ranges. Additional detailed information can be found in several review articles that include those about the newer anti-epileptic medications from 2010 [30], a combination of new and old anti-epileptic medications from 2004 [31], and a review of new anti-epileptic drugs from the (2007) 8th Eilat Conference [32]. Chemical structures of the drug are shown in Fig. 12.1 and pharmacokinetic parameters of these drugs are shown in Table 12.2.

THERAPEUTIC DRUG MONITORING OF ESLICARBAZEPINE ACETATE

One of the newer AEDs to be approved in 2009 for use in Europe is eslicarbazepine acetate, and it is still in Phase III clinical trials in the United States. It is a pro-drug used for the treatment of refractory partial-onset seizures in adults [33]. Eslicarbazepine acetate is thought to work through preferential binding to the inactivated state of the sodium channels as opposed to the resting state of the sodium channels [34]. Eslicarbazepine acetate is rapidly converted by a liver esterase into licarbazepine in unequal amounts of R and S enantiomers. The $S(+)$ enantiomer (licarbazepine but also referred to as eslicarbazepine) predominates that of the $R(-)$ enantiomer, with 96%–97% being the former [35]. Another minor metabolite from eslicarbazepine acetate is the AED drug in its own right, oxcarbazepine [32]. The chemical structure of eslicarbazepine acetate is similar to carbamazepine but different at the 10,11-position so that the toxic epoxide of carbamazepine-10,11 does not form [36]. Neither food nor hepatic failure causes significant alterations in the previously mentioned pharmacokinetics [37, 38].

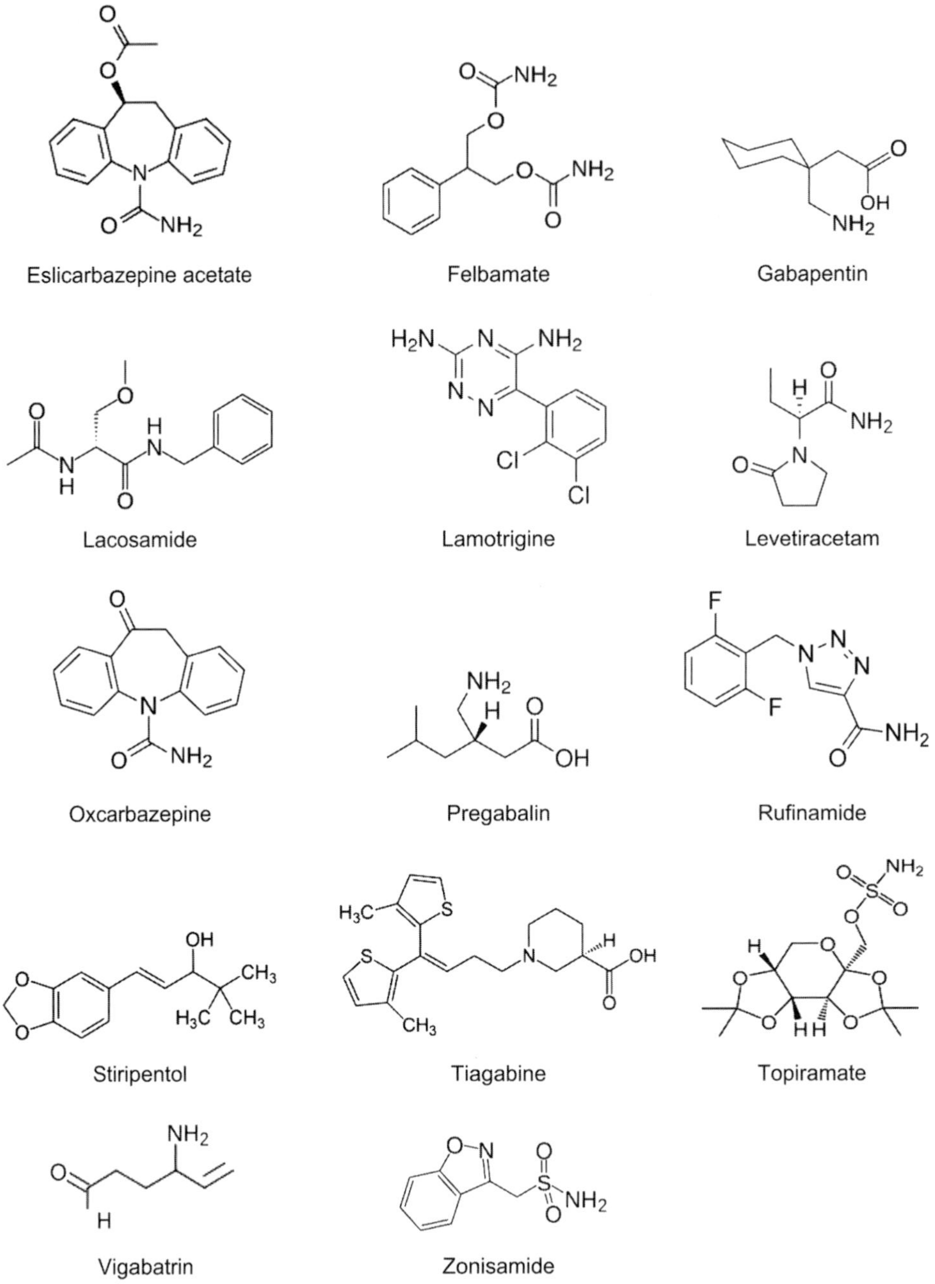

FIGURE 12.1 Chemical structure of the second-generation anti-epileptic drugs.

TABLE 12.2 Properties of Second-Generation Anti-Epileptic Drugs

Drug	Approval year in US	Time to peak concentration after oral dosing (hours)	Serum protein binding (%)	Half-life (hours)	Serum reference range
Eslicarbazepine acetate	Approved in Europe 2008	<3	30	17–18	Not established
Felbamate	1993	2–6	20–25	15–23	30–60 µg/mL[a]
Gabapentin	1993	2–3	5–9	6	12–20 µg/mL[a] 2–10 µg/mL[b] 2–20 µg/mL[b]
Lacosamide	2008	1–4	15	13	5–10 µg/mL[a]
Lamotrigine	1994	1–3	55	25	3–14 µg/mL[a,c] 2.5–15 µg/mL
Levetiracetam	1999	1	<1	6–8	10–37 µg/mL[a] 12–46 µg/mL[b]
MHD active drug of Oxcarbazepine	2000	4–6	30–40	8–10	15–35 µg/mL[a,c]
Pregabalin	2004	1–2	0	6–7	2.8–8.3 µg/mL[a]
Rufinamide	2008	5–6	34	6–10	4.7–28.2 µg/mL[a]
Stiripentol	Not FDA approved yet	1–2	99	NA	4–22 µg/mL[a]
Tiagabine	1997	1–2	96	5–9	20–200 ng/mL[a]
Topiramate	1996	2–4	19–23	13–17	5–20 µg/mL 2–20 µg/mL[b]
Vigabatrin	2009	1–2	0	5–6	1–36 µg/mL
Zonisamide	2000	2–5	40–60	50–70	10–38 µg/mL 10–40 µg/mL[b]

[a]Reference range cited in the text with appropriate literature reference.
[b]Reference range suggested by Mayo Medical Reference Laboratory at Rochester, MN.
[c]Reference range suggested by the ARUP National Reference Laboratory at Salt Lake City, UT.

Eslicarbazepine acetate has no significant protein binding [32] and an effective half-life of 17–18 hours [35]. The maximum concentrations of eslicarbazepine acetate are reached with 3 hours of oral dosing [39]. Eslicarbazepine acetate may be more favorable than the use of oxcarbazepine when comparing the side-effect profile, as the active metabolites of these two pro-drugs are the same [33]. Because of the favorable pharmacokinetics of this drug, therapeutic drug monitoring is not required unless under special circumstances such as questionable compliance or unexpected toxicity. Different assay methods have the ability to identify both enantiomers, while other methods will only identify the eslicarbazepine.

THERAPEUTIC DRUG MONITORING OF FELBAMATE

Felbamate is one of the second-generation AEDs that was approved in 1993 for the treatment of partial seizures and as an adjunctive therapy in seizures associated with Lennox-Gastaut syndrome in children. It is thought to exert its effects through both a sodium channel antagonist as well as inhibiting calcium channels and N-methyl-D-aspartate receptors. It also affects the GABA receptors through a weak barbiturate-like action [40]. After a year of widespread use of the drug a small number of cases of liver failure and aplastic anemia were associated with it. The deaths of 23 persons led to a significant limitation of the use of felbamate, although the drug continues to be on the market today [41–43]. A reactive atropaldehyde has been postulated as a metabolite that is responsible for both of the severe side effects, but has yet to be directly related [44].

Felbamate is absorbed in 2–6 hours and has about 90% bioavailability. The drug is approximately 20–25% bound to albumin [6]. Paths of elimination of the drug include both hepatic and renal, with 50–60% being hepatic and 40–60% renal [45]. There is also a clearance difference with regards to age, with the older age population having reduced clearance. The half-life of the drug varies between 15 and 23 hours [46]. For those on monotherapy, serum values of between 30 and 60 mg/L (30 and 60 µg/mL) are associated with a reduction of seizures [47]. The drug has hepatic cytochrome metabolism by CYP3A4 and CYP2E1, and its clearance is increased up to 40% when given with inducers of these isoenzymes such as carbamazepine, phenytoin and phenobarbital [45, 48]. The variable effect with adjunctive therapy, variation in clearance based upon age and the fact that most of the deadly side effects occur within 3 months of beginning drug therapy may give utility to monitoring felbamate, especially early on in treatment.

MONITORING OF GABAPENTIN

Gabapentin was approved for use in 1994 as an adjunctive drug for the treatment of partial seizures. Although its chemical structure is related to GABA, it is neither a GABA agonist nor a precursor to GABA. It was designed to be a GABA mimetic with lipophilic properties to help it cross the blood–brain barrier [49]. The exact mechanism of action is not clearly understood but may be related to its association with an alpha-2-delta subunit of L-type voltage-regulated calcium channels [50]. It is also used for multiple additional conditions many of which are related to various types of pain. Gabapentin is absorbed through the L-amino acid transport system, reaching maximum levels 2–3 hours after dosing [51]. Information on bioavailability is conflicting, with variations attributed to higher dosing levels and increased dosing frequency [52]. Significant intra-individual bioavailability has also been reported, with some of this being attributable to sex differences with females having higher variability than males [53]. However, other studies have not shown these differences in bioavailability related to sex [54] and higher levels of dosing, although many of the subjects in the latter study never reached high levels of dosing as the symptoms were controlled at lower doses of gabapentin [55].

Many of the other parameters of gabapentin are favorable; these include no protein binding, no metabolism with the drug being cleared through renal excretion in an unchanged state, and it not being known to interact with other AEDs [56]. The half-life in healthy subjects is 6 hours [54], and would be longer in those with renal impairment. There is a wide variance in the range of suggested therapeutic levels of the drug, with some proposing up to 61 mg/L (61 µg/mL), however a more modest range of 12−20 mg/L (12−20 µg/ml) is suggested [57]. The favorable pharmacokinetics of this drug make therapeutic monitoring for other than general accepted principles unnecessary; however, the variability of bioavailability and its use in renal impaired patients may be an additional reason for monitoring this drug.

THERAPEUTIC DRUG MONITORING OF LACOSAMIDE

Lacosamide is one of the newest approved AEDs, having been approved in late 2008 for the adjunctive treatment of partial onset seizures in patients over the age of 16. Research suggests that lacosamide, a functionalized amino acid analog, has several modes of action. The first is the selective modulation of the slow inactivation sodium channel as opposed to the more commonly modulated fast inactivation sodium channel. A second proposed method of action is its binding and modulation of the collapsin response mediator protein-2 [58−60]. In one of the larger studies of the drug, involving over 400 participants taking it, lacosamide showed highly favorable pharmacokinetics to include an oral bioavailability approaching 100% with little alteration when taken with food, and protein binding of less than 15% which decreases the risk of displacement drug interactions [61]. The half-life of lacosamide is 13 hours [62]. Variation in the pharmacokinetics has shown low intra- and inter-patient variability [58]. Common side effects associated with lacosamide therapy were mostly CNS (central nervous system) and GI (gastrointestinal) related, and more common as the medication dose increased [63].

The elimination pharmacokinetics include minimal first-pass metabolism with 40% being eliminated by renal excretion. The predominate metabolite produced by CYP2C19 demethylation has no activity and is also cleared through renal excretion [64].

The predictable pharmacokinetics of this drug with little variability makes therapeutic monitoring for other than general accepted principles unnecessary. No commonly agreed upon reference levels for the drug are described, but a suggested range is 5−10 mg/L (5−10 µg/mL) [30].

THERAPEUTIC DRUG MONITORING OF LAMOTRIGINE

Lamotrigine is an anti-epileptic drug that was approved in 1994 for the adjuvant treatment of partial seizures. It has multiple mechanisms of action, to include inhibition of voltage-sensitive sodium channels, modulation of neurotransmitter release, and stabilization of neuronal membranes [32]. It may also have an effect on the calcium channels, which may enhance its anti-epileptic properties [65]. Lamotrigine also has indications for use in bipolar I disorder, and is used to delay the time to occurrence of mood episodes [66].

Lamotrigine is quickly absorbed after oral dosing, with high bioavailability and peak concentration of the drug being reached in 1−3 hours [67]. The drug is 55% bound to plasma proteins and when used as monotherapy has a half-life of around 25 hours [68].

The half-life is greatly influenced by co-administration of other drugs. When given with a cytochrome P450 enzyme-inducing drug, such as carbamazepine, phenobarbital or phenytoin, the half-life is reduced to about 15 hours; when given with valproate (an enzyme inhibitor) the half-life is increased to approximately 50 hours [69]. Lamotrigine is metabolized mostly through glucuronidation to an inactive metabolite and then excreted in the urine, with approximately 90% of the drug being excreted through this mechanism [70]. Drug levels do not consistently predict clinical response [71]. A proposed reference range of 3−14 mg/L (3−14 µg/mL) has gained acceptance, but this range has significant overlap with drug levels associated with toxicity [72].

One serious side effect of lamotrigine therapy is a rash, which occurs in about 10% of patients [73]. This rash varies in severity, but can necessitate discontinuation of the drug. Rapid induction of therapy and concomitant use of valproate are likely associations [74], and may be related to valproate lengthening the half-life of lamotrigine. The use of oral contraceptives can cause a 50% decrease in the plasma level of lamotrigine, and levels can rise significantly again when oral contraceptives are withdrawn [75]. Other factors that can add to individual variability of lamotrigine levels include pregnancy, age, race, and other medications [18, 69, 76, 77].

Many of the features of lamotrigine lend themselves to making therapeutic drug monitoring beneficial. These include the significant individual variability of the levels of drug for a given dosage of the medication, with much of this variability being attributed to induction or inhibition of lamotrigine metabolism with wide alterations in its half-life [78]. The previously mentioned factors also cause wide fluctuations of drug levels. Additionally, side effects of the drug occur with increased frequency at the upper end of the therapeutic range.

THERAPEUTIC DRUG MONITORING OF LEVETIRACETAM

Levetiracetam is an anti-epileptic drug that was approved in 1999 for the adjuvant treatment of partial seizures in adults [79]. It has a unique mechanism of action in that it binds to the synaptic vesicle glycoprotein 2A (SV2A) which is involved in vesicle exocytosis [80]. This SV2A protein has several polymorphisms as well as two other isoforms, SV2B and SV2C, but the anti-epileptic effect appears to be related only to the SV2A isoform without regard to any polymorphism [81]. Levetiracetam has a favorable safety profile that has led at least one researcher to proclaim this AED to be the closest thing to the ideal AED [82]. Levetiracetam is rapidly and almost completely absorbed over a wide range of oral doses [83]. The co-consumption of food with levetiracetam does not significantly alter the rate or extent of the absorption of the drug. The mixing of the drug in an enteral nutrition formula did cause a slight but insignificant increase in time to peak serum concentration [84].

Levetiracetam is not metabolized by the hepatic P450 cytochrome system. About two-thirds of the drug is excreted unchanged in the urine, with most of the remainder being excreted in the urine as an inactive metabolite L057 which is formed by enzymatic hydrolysis of the acetamide group. There are a few other minor inactive metabolites which are also excreted in the urine, and less than 1% of the drug is excreted in the feces [85]. Levetiracetam is not protein bound and has linear pharmacokinetics, and in the adult population has a half-life of 6−8 hours with a slightly longer half-life in the elderly [86].

Levetiracetam has been successfully used in combination with other anti-epileptic drugs, and potentiates the protective effects of these drugs without additional toxicity [87]. This benefit has been attributed to the novel mechanism of action, lack of protein binding, and lack of hepatic metabolism which decreases the chance for pharmacokinetic interactions. At drug levels 5 times greater than the therapeutic level, levetiracetam was found to have no inhibitory effect on 11 different drug metabolizing enzymes [83].

Measuring of levetiracetam serum levels is performed mainly for standard indications and for monitoring of levels in the elderly or those adults with impaired renal function of this nearly exclusive renal excreted drug. Potential monitoring of this drug during the third trimester of pregnancy may be beneficial [88]. Clearance of levetiracetam is increased in children, with one study showing an approximate 30–40% increase in clearance of the drug in 6- to 12-year-olds [89]. Whole blood samples have B esterase activity that will slowly metabolize the levetiracetam, causing artifactually low levels, and therefore prompt separation of whole blood into serum or plasma is needed [90]. A tentative target range for levetiracetam is 10–37 mg/L (10–37 µg/mL) [31].

THERAPEUTIC DRUG MONITORING OF OXCARBAZEPINE

Oxcarbazepine has been approved for use in the United States since 2000. It is an analog of carbamazepine. Oxcarbazepine is quickly reduced to an active compound, 10-hydroxy-10, 11-dihydrocarbazepine, also known as monohydroxy derivative (MHD). The parent compound is also active, but is found in the blood at concentrations low enough that it is excluded when therapeutically monitoring oxcarbazepine use. There are other metabolites as well, which include a glucuronide, but they are without anti-epileptic activity. MHD is chimeric and forms enantiomers which are the same as those formed by the activation of the pro-drug eslicarbazepine acetate, a previously discussed AED [29]. As opposed to the eslicarbazepine acetate ratio of the S to R enantiomers of 20 : 1, the ratio of enantiomers of oxcarbazepine is not as disparate. Oxcarbazepine has a worse side-effect profile than that of eslicarbazepine acetate, and this has been attributed by some to the increased levels of the R enantiomer [33].

The active component of the drug, MHD, reaches peak serum concentration in 4–6 hours, has a half life of 8–10 hours and is excreted in the urine along with its inactivate glucuronide conjugate at rates corresponding to creatinine clearance [91]. There are pharmacokinetic differences in people with mild to moderate hepatic impairment and pregnancy that increase the clearance of the drug [92]. Dosing may need to be adjusted in pregnancy and those with hepatic and renal impairment. An accepted range for the level of drug is 15–35 mg/L (15–35 µg/mL) [93].

THERAPEUTIC DRUG MONITORING OF PREGABALIN

Pregabalin is a drug that is structurally similar to gabapentin, which itself was designed to be a GABA mimetic drug that would more easily disseminate into the central nervous system. Pregabalin is an additional alkylated analog of GABA that hoped to further improve on the properties of gabapentin [49]. It was approved for use by the FDA in 2004 for adjunctive treatment of partial seizures in epilepsy. It is thought to work through its binding to the alpha-2-delta subunits of voltage-gated calcium channels, with decreased neurotransmitter release and thus a reduction of nerve activity [94]. It also has other indications for use, including diabetes-associated neuropathic pain [95], post-herpetic neuralgia [96] and fibromyalgia [97].

The pharmacokinetics of pregabalin are very favorable, and include negligible metabolism with more than 98% of the drug being excreted unchanged in the urine, no binding to plasma proteins, no hepatic metabolism or induction or inhibition of liver enzymes, rapid and near complete absorption when taken orally in a fasting state, and a half-life of 6.3 hours [98]. The oral clearance of pregabalin is proportional to creatinine clearance and is not altered by variables including sex, race, age, co-administration of other AEDs, or dosing schemes [99]. Drug interaction studies showed no significant changes in pharmacokinetics in those with partial epilepsy in combination therapy with carbamazepine, phenytoin, lamotrigine or valproate [100].

The lack of interaction with other drugs and the uniform renal clearance give little use for the application of TDM other than standard indications. Given the half-life of 6.3 hours and the dosing frequency of up to three times a day, missed doses within the past 2 days could alter the interpretation of blood levels of pregabalin. Timing of the blood draw relative to the last dose of medication would also be important. Pregabalin could be a good choice of drug for those with hepatic failure and for patients with renal impairment. Algorithms for altering of daily dosage and dosing frequency are available [101]. A suggested drug range for trough pregabalin levels is recommended to be between 2.8 and 8.3 mg/L (2.8−8.3 µg/mL) [102], and has generally been accepted by others [6].

THERAPEUTIC DRUG MONITORING OF RUFINAMIDE

Rufinamide is a newer drug approved in 2008 for the adjunctive treatment of seizures associated with Lennox-Gastaut syndrome in those aged 4 years and older. Its exact mechanism of action is unknown, but it is thought to work through the inhibition of voltage-gated sodium channels [103]. The drug is well absorbed after oral ingestion with a bioavailability of between 70−85%, with increased absorbance when taken with food and decreased absorption at increasing dosages of medication [104]. Rufinamide is predominately metabolized through carboxylesterase enzymatic hydrolysis to an inactive metabolite that is excreted mainly in urine and a smaller fraction in the feces; < 4% of the drug remains unchanged and this is excreted roughly half through urine and half through feces [105]. Cytochrome P450 inducers such as phenobarbital, primidone, phenytoin and carbamazepine increase the clearance of rufinamide; this is actually due to secondary induction of carboxylesterase activity by these drugs (106).

The half-life of rufinamide is approximately 6−10 hours and there is protein binding of 34% [107]. The low renal involvement in clearing the unchanged drug means fewer changes in dosing levels for the patient with renal impairment. The level of rufinamide is higher in children than in an adult at comparable body-weight doses, and is increased with valproic acid co-administration [108]. The need for therapeutic drug monitoring comes mainly from variability of bioavailability, especially at higher dosing levels, and the variation caused by induction of the carboxylesterase activity and concomitant AED therapy. Although not approved by the FDA for use in partial seizures, the estimated concentration of this drug in those receiving benefit from the drug for partial seizures and on recommended therapeutic dosages ranged from 4.7–28.2 mg/L (4.7–28.2 µg/mL) [109].

THERAPEUTIC DRUG MONITORING OF STIRIPENTOL

Stiripentol has been approved for use as an orphan drug in the adjunctive treatment of the childhood epilepsy syndrome known as severe myoclonic epilepsy in infancy, or Dravet syndrome [110]. Stiripentol is thought to work by several mechanisms, to include acting directly on GABA (A) receptors through positive allosteric modulation, which gives it its independent activity [111]. Stiripentol also alters the metabolism of other drugs through its effect on cytochrome P450 modulation, which enhances its antiseizure properties when combined with other AED drugs. Both *in vitro* and *in vivo* studies showed that stiripentol reduced the CYP3A4 biotransformation of carbamazepine and could shorten the time to reach the optimum dose or prolong the dosing interval of carbamazepine [112]. In a study of 97 children with epilepsy the more common side effects included anorexia, weight loss, drowsiness and ataxia, some of which were improved by lowering the dose of co-medication. Other side effects included hyper- and hypotonia, nausea and vomiting, oculomotor disorders and neutropenia, which were more likely when two or more AEDs were used in conjunction with stiripentol [113].

The kinetics of orally dosed stiripentol includes rapid absorption with plasma levels peaking approximately 1.5–2.0 hours after dosing. There is non-linear clearance of the drug with decreasing clearance while increasing the dosage, consistent with Michaelis-Menten kinetics [114]. Urinary clearance of the unchanged drug is less than 4%, and 16–22% is excreted in the urine as conjugates [115]. Stiripentol is highly protein bound at 99%, leaving only the unbound 1% of the drug able to act on the GABA receptors [115]. Because of the non-linear kinetics, high protein binding and alteration of other AEDs, monitoring this drug is important and monitoring the free drug should also be considered, although no mechanism for such monitoring has been published. In one study in children aged 6–16 years, serum levels of stiripentol in the order of 4–22 mg/L were achieved to decrease the frequency of their seizures, although all of the subjects were on concomitant AED drugs. Two of the three subjects with concentrations of stiripentol above 22 mg/L (22 µg/mL) had side effects [116]. This suggestion of a low therapeutic to toxic range would be another reason to monitor this specific drug.

THERAPEUTIC DRUG MONITORING OF TIAGABINE

Tiagabine has enhanced lipophilic properties that allow it to cross the blood–brain barrier [31]. It was approved in 1997 for the treatment of partial seizures in patients 12 years and older. It is thought to work by inhibiting the uptake of gamma-aminobutyric acid (GABA), an inhibitory neurotransmitter [117]. Three multicenter studies showed a clinically significant response rate in patients, but in no study was this rate greater than one-third of the patients [118–120]. Also limiting the use of this drug is its association with non-convulsive status epilepticus [121–124].

The pharmacokinetics of tiagabine include linear kinetic characteristics and near complete absorption from oral dosing, and it undergoes extensive oxidative metabolism with less than 1% of the drug excreted unchanged in the urine [125]. Tiagabine is highly protein bound, at 96% [126], and concomitant administration with valproic acid, another highly protein-bound drug, can lead to increased free concentration of tiagabine *in vitro*. The half-life of tiagabine is variable, depending on the co-administration of enzyme-inducing drugs and hepatic status. In those patients not on enzyme inducers the half-life is 5–9 hours; in those on enzyme inducers the half-life is 2–4 hours [127], and in those patients with hepatic dysfunction the half-life is 12–16 hours [128].

The high protein binding and high variability of hepatic metabolism of tiagabine make therapeutic monitoring of this drug highly useful. The proposed therapeutic range varies, with 20–200 ng/mL being more common [6, 30], and comes from a study [120] where the average 1-hour post-dosing measurements of tiagabine in patients at the high and low therapeutic doses were 38 and 140 ng/mL, respectively. In this same study, trough levels were significantly lower; thus, most values would be expected to be at the lower end of the range. Although tiagabine is highly protein bound, no mechanism for measuring free tiagabine levels was identified.

THERAPEUTIC DRUG MONITORING OF TOPIRAMATE

Topiramate is a novel sulfamate-substituted monosaccharide AED that has multiple mechanisms of action, to include blockade of voltage-sensitive sodium channels, enhancement of GABA activity at some of the GABA-A receptors, modulation of AMPA receptor subtypes, and inhibiting carbonic anhydrase isoenzymes [129]. This AED was first approved in 1996 for the adjuvant treatment of partial and general seizures in those aged 2 years and older [130]. It is also indicated for the prophylaxis of migraine headaches in adults, and has gained approval for monotherapy in patients 2 years and older with partial onset or primary generalized tonic–clonic seizures [131]. Topiramate is rapidly absorbed within 2–4 hours after oral dosing with a bioavailability of greater than 80% [6]. Consumption of food can delay the absorption of the drug by about 2 hours, but has little effect on its bioavailability [132]. Protein binding of the drug is not significant, and the drug is 13–17% bound to plasma proteins [133]. There is additional binding of the drug to erythrocytes, most likely due to the carbonic anhydrase present in the cells; this binding is high affinity but low capacity [6]. Due to this erythrocyte binding of the drug, whole blood is not recommended for monitoring levels and serum or plasma should be used.

The half-life of topiramate is 19–23 hours, and most of the drug is excreted unchanged in the urine. Approximately 20% is metabolized by the liver when induction of hepatic enzymes is not an issue, but the percentage of hepatic metabolism is significantly altered by other drugs, including AEDs [134]. When topiramate is co-administered with enzyme-inducing AEDs to include phenytoin and carbamazepine, its clearance rate doubles, the serum concentration is reduced by a factor of two, and the half-life is reduced by a factor of two to 10–12 hours [135]. Co-administration with valproate also decreased the serum concentration of topiramate by about 10–15% [6, 136].

Children metabolize topiramate faster than adults, and this increased clearance is additive to the effect of AED enzyme inducers. As the drug is significantly cleared by renal excretion, dosing modification in renal impairment would be warranted [134]. A generally accepted reference range for topiramate is 5–20 mg/L (5–20 μg/mL). Besides standard indications therapeutic drug monitoring may be considered for drug–drug interactions, especially when used in conjunction with first-generation AEDs.

THERAPEUTIC DRUG MONITORING OF VIGABATRIN

Vigabatrin is a drug approved in the United States in 2009 for adjunctive therapy for refractory complex partial seizures. The drug exerts its effect through irreversible binding to GABA transaminase, which is an enzyme that breaks down the GABA neurotransmitter [137]. During the drug's development it was found to cause a progressive and permanent bilateral concentric visual field constriction such that its use was restricted in a special distribution program. This visual field loss was found in 44% of people exposed to vigabatrin, and is related to cumulate dosing as well as age [138]. Its pharmacokinetic profile is favorable as it has high bioavailability, negligible protein binding, primary renal elimination, minimal drug interaction and a half life of 5–6 hours [139].

The drug is supplied as a racemic mixture of both the $S(+)$ and $R(-)$ enantiomers, with only the $S(+)$ moiety having clinical activity [140]. The pharmacokinetics of the two enantiomers in single-dose studies are mostly similar, with differences mainly being in time to peak concentration and renal clearance [141]. One study of chronic over-dosage with renal failure showed a preponderance of the inactive enantiomer in the serum. Therapeutic monitoring is limited due to the irreversible binding of the drug, which causes lack of correlation of current drug level with drug effect, and suggested target range levels are wide at 1–36 mg/L (1–36 μg/mL) [31]. Drug levels may be helpful when monitoring for compliance and over-dosage, but otherwise have little utility [142].

THERAPEUTIC DRUG MONITORING OF ZONISAMIDE

Zonisamide is approved for use as an adjunctive therapy for partial seizures in epilepsy. It is also in trial for other indications to include migraine headaches and Parkinson's disease. It is a sulfonamide derivative that has been approved for use in the United States since 2000. Zonisamide acts through multiple different mechanisms, including alteration of sodium and calcium channels and altering levels of neurotransmitters (GABA). In addition, zonisamide has neuroprotective attributes [143]. The drug has mostly favorable pharmacokinetics, to include no active metabolites, protein binding of 40–60%, bioavailability of 100% and a half-life of 50–70 hours [31].

After its rapid absorption the drug undergoes a variety of metabolic alterations. About 20% of the drug undergoes acetylation, and 50% is reduced through a hepatic CYP3A4 process which is then further modified by glucuronidation before renal excretion.

The 30% remainder of the drug is excreted in the urine in an unchanged state [144]. Because half of the inactivation of this drug occurs through a CYP3A4 process, any inducer or inhibitor of this enzyme could cause alteration of the half-life. This half-life alteration occurs when it is co-administered with phenytoin and carbamazepine, with a reduction of half-life to 27 hours and 36 hours, respectively [145]. Suggested therapeutic drug levels were initially placed in a range of 20–30 mg/L (20–30 µg/mL) as levels above the upper end of 30 mg/L had an increased risk of toxicity [146]; however, newer ranges now extend from 10–38 mg/L (10–38 µg/mL) [31].

One zonisamide monotherapy study with dosing based on weight in children aged 3 months to 15 years showed an increasing plasma level of the drug with age, and suggests dose adjustments in children based on their age [147]. Zonisamide is taken up by red blood cells, but this uptake is saturated at therapeutic concentration of the drug [145]. Due to this higher accumulation of zonisamide in red blood cells, whole blood is not recommended for monitoring levels and serum or plasma should be used. Therapeutic monitoring could be considered while on drugs altering CYP3A4, and in children, in addition to the standard reasons for monitoring drugs.

ANALYTICAL METHODS FOR MONITORING OF AEDS

Radioimmunoassay was one of the earliest commercially assays available for therapeutic drug monitoring of classical anticonvulsants. These methods required radioactive isotopes, and the regulatory and safety precautions needed did not lead to widespread acceptance of this technique. Today, immunoassay testing such as enzyme multiplied immunoassay technique and fluorescence polarization immunoassay, cloned enzyme donor immunoassay (CEDIA), chemiluminescent assay, etc., are widely used for the classical AEDs. These tests can be scaled to small hospital laboratories and they can also be automated. However, only a few of the second-generation AEDs have immunoassay testing available; these include lamotrigine [148], topiramate [149], and zonisamide [150].

The second-generation AEDs are analyzed in serum or plasma using chromatographic techniques; gas chromatography (GC) and high-performance liquid chromatography (HPLC). The detection system for HPLC could be ultraviolet detection (UV) or mass spectrometry (including tandem mass spectrometry). These relatively more expensive and more complex testing mechanisms relegate testing to large hospital laboratories or a reference laboratory for analysis, and smaller local laboratories are unable to offer these tests. High-performance liquid chromatography with tandem mass spectrometry gives very high sensitivity and selectivity in quantifying gabapentin, lacosamide, lamotrigine, levetiracetam, oxcarbazepine, pregabalin and topiramate [30]. These chromatographic methods have the additional advantage of being able to measure multiple AEDs concurrently. Kim reported a liquid chromatography combined with tandem mass spectrometric protocol for simultaneous analysis of nine anti-epileptic drugs and active metabolites of carbamazepine (carbamazepine 10, 11-epoxide) in human plasma. These drugs included gabapentin, levetiracetam, valproic acid, lamotrigine, carbamazepine, zonisamide, oxcarbazepine, topiramate and phenytoin. Protein precipitation in plasma specimens was achieved by using acetonitrile, and supernatant was subjected to chromatographic analysis using a reverse phase C-18 column. The authors claimed that the method is useful in identification and quantitation of AEDs in patients undergoing mono- or polytherapy for epilepsy [151]. Capillary electrophoresis methods are also being developed with the potential to perform testing in smaller local laboratories as costs are decreased and automation is possible.

Saliva could be used as a specimen for testing. This non-invasive mechanism of collection could facilitate collections, especially in the pediatric population. It could also facilitate specimen collection shortly after a seizure event to be able to relate the AED level to the time when seizure activity occurred. These specimens could be collected by the patient and sent for testing through the United States Postal Service, as there is sufficient stability of the AEDs [152]. For salivary levels of drug to give meaningful information they must have some consistent relationship to the serum level. This appears to be the case for levetiracetam [153] and topiramate [154], but there is conflicting information for lamotrigine [155, 156].

CONCLUSION

The routine monitoring of classical or first-generation AEDs is a widely accepted practice. Fourteen new AED drug have been approved since 1993, including eslicarbazepine acetate, felbamate, gabapentin, lacosamide, lamotrigine, levetiracetam, oxcarbazepine, pregabalin, rufinamide, stiripentol, tiagabine, topiramate, vigabatrin and zonisamide. The utility of therapeutic drug monitoring in this group of drugs has not been clearly established or defined. Monitoring of drug levels clearly has purpose in establishing patient compliance with taking medication, suspected drug overdose, measuring of free drug when the drug is highly bound and the amount of protein binding is altered, and in establishing an individual therapeutic concentration. There are additional individual clinical situations that benefit from monitoring of drug levels. These situations can be identified by knowledge of the pharmacokinetics and pharmacodynamics of the AEDs as well as the clinical aspects of the patient.

References

[1] Shorvon SD. Epidemiology, classification, natural history, and genetics of epilepsy. Lancet 1990;336:93–6.
[2] Faught E. Monotherapy in adults and elderly persons. Neurology 2007;69:S3–9.
[3] Stephen LJ, Brodie MJ. Selection of antiepileptic drugs in adults. Neurol Clin 2009;27:967–92.
[4] Holland KD. Efficacy, pharmacology, and adverse effects of antiepileptic drugs. Neurol Clin 2001;19:313–45.
[5] Carpay JA, Aldenkamp AP, van Donselaar CA. Complaints associated with the use of antiepileptic drugs: results from a community-based study. Seizure 2005;14:198–206.
[6] Patsalos PN, Berry DJ, Bourgeois BF, et al. Antiepileptic drugs — best practice guidelines for therapeutic drug monitoring: a position paper by the subcommission on therapeutic drug monitoring, ILAE Commission on Therapeutic Strategies. Epilepsia 2008;49:1239–76.
[7] Schachter SC. Iatrogenic seizures. Neurol Clin 1998;16:157–70.
[8] Perucca E, Gram L, Avanzini G, Dulac O. Anti-epileptic drugs as a cause of worsening seizures. Epilepsia 1998;39:5–17.
[9] Buchthal F, Svensmark O. Aspects of the pharmacology of phenytoin (dilantin) and phenobarbital relevant to their dosage in the treatment of epilepsy. Epilepsia 1960;1:373–84.
[10] Shorvon SD. The epidemiology and treatment of chronic and refractory epilepsy. Epilepsia 1996; 37(Suppl. 2):S1–3.

[11] Perucca E. Is there a role for therapeutic drug monitoring of new anticonvulsants? Clin Pharmacokinet 2000;38:191−204.

[12] Walters RJ, Hutchings AD, Smith DF, Smith PE. Inappropriate requests for serum anti-epileptic drug levels in hospital practice. QJM 2004;97:337−41.

[13] Jannuzzi G, Cian P, Fattore C, et al. A multicenter randomized controlled trial on the clinical impact of therapeutic drug monitoring in patients with newly diagnosed epilepsy. The Italian TDM Study Group in Epilepsy. Epilepsia 2000;41:222−30.

[14] Smellie WS, McNulty CA, Collinson PO, et al. Best practice in primary care pathology: review 12. J Clin Pathol 2010;63:330−6.

[15] Yerby MS, Friel PN, McCormick K. Anti-epileptic drug disposition during pregnancy. Neurology 1992;42:12−6.

[16] Commission on Genetics, Pregnancy and the Child, International League against Epilepsy. Guidelines for the care of women of childbearing age with epilepsy. Epilepsia 1993;34:588−9.

[17] Committee on Educational Bulletins of the American College of Obstetricians and Gynecologists. Seizure disorders in pregnancy: ACOG Educational Bulletin No. 231, December 1996. Intl J Gynaecol Obstet 1997;56:279−86.

[18] Tomson T, Perucca E, Battino D. Navigating toward fetal and maternal health: the challenge of treating epilepsy in pregnancy. Epilepsia 2004;45:1171−5.

[19] EURAP Study Group. Seizure control and treatment in pregnancy: observations from the EURAP Epilepsy Pregnancy Registry. Neurology 2006;66:354−60.

[20] Perucca E, Crema A. Plasma protein binding of drugs in pregnancy. Clin Pharmacokinet 1982;7:336−52.

[21] Yerby MS, Friel PN, McCormick K, et al. Pharmacokinetics of anticonvulsants in pregnancy: alterations in plasma protein binding. Epilepsy Res 1990;5:223−8.

[22] Ohman I, Vitols S, Tomson T. Lamotrigine in pregnancy: pharmacokinetics during delivery, in the neonate, and during lactation. Epilepsia 2000;41:709−13.

[23] Tran TA, Leppik IE, Blesi K, et al. Lamotrigine clearance during pregnancy. Neurology 2002;59:251−5.

[24] Pennell PB, Newport DJ, Stowe ZN, et al. The impact of pregnancy and childbirth on the metabolism of lamotrigine. Neurology 2004;62:292−5.

[25] Tomson T, Dahl ML, Kimland E. Therapeutic monitoring of antiepileptic drugs for epilepsy. Cochrane Database Syst Rev 2007:CD002216.

[26] Johannessen SI, Landmark CJ. Antiepileptic drug interactions − principles and clinical implications. Curr Neuropharmacol 2010;8:254−67.

[27] Hung CC, Lin CJ, Chen CC, et al. Dosage recommendation of phenytoin for patients with epilepsy with different CYP2C9/CYP2C19 polymorphisms. Ther Drug Monit 2004;26:534−40.

[28] Anderson GD. Pharmacokinetic, pharmacodynamic, and pharmacogenetic targeted therapy of antiepileptic drugs. Ther Drug Monit 2008;30:173−80.

[29] Rogawski MA. Diverse mechanisms of anti-epileptic drugs in the development pipeline. Epilepsy Res 2006;69:273−94.

[30] Krasowski MD. Therapeutic drug monitoring of the newer anti-epilepsy medications. Pharmaceuticals (Basel) 2010;3:1909−35.

[31] Neels HM, Sierens AC, Naelaerts K, et al. Therapeutic drug monitoring of old and newer anti-epileptic drugs. Clin Chem Lab Med 2004;42:1228−55.

[32] Bialer M, Johannessen SI, Kupferberg HJ, et al. Progress report on new antiepileptic drugs: a summary of the Eighth Eilat Conference (EILAT VIII). Epilepsy Res 2007;73:1−52.

[33] Prunetti P, Perucca E. New and forthcoming anti-epileptic drugs. Curr Opin Neurol 2011;24:159−64.

[34] Bonifacio MJ, Sheridan RD, Parada A, et al. Interaction of the novel anticonvulsant, BIA 2-093, with voltage-gated sodium channels: comparison with carbamazepine. Epilepsia 2001;42:600−8.

[35] Almeida L, Falcao A, Maia J, et al. Single-dose and steady-state pharmacokinetics of eslicarbazepine acetate (BIA 2-093) in healthy elderly and young subjects. J Clin Pharmacol 2005;45:1062−6.

[36] Almeida L, Soares-da-Silva P. Eslicarbazepine acetate (BIA 2-093). Neurotherapeutics 2007;4:88−96.

[37] Almeida L, Potgieter JH, Maia J, et al. Pharmacokinetics of eslicarbazepine acetate in patients with moderate hepatic impairment. Eur J Clin Pharmacol 2008;64:267−73.

[38] Maia J, Vaz-da-Silva M, Almeida L, et al. Effect of food on the pharmacokinetic profile of eslicarbazepine acetate (BIA 2-093). Drugs R&D 2005;6:201−6.

[39] Almeida L, Minciu I, Nunes T, et al. Pharmacokinetics, efficacy, and tolerability of eslicarbazepine acetate in children and adolescents with epilepsy. J Clin Pharmacol 2008;48:966–77.

[40] Chang HR, Kuo CC. Molecular determinants of the anticonvulsant felbamate binding site in the N-methyl-D-aspartate receptor. J Med Chem 2008;51:1534–45.

[41] Kaufman DW, Kelly JP, Anderson T, et al. Evaluation of case reports of aplastic anemia among patients treated with felbamate. Epilepsia 1997;38:1265–9.

[42] Pellock JM. Felbamate. Epilepsia 1999;40(Suppl. 5):S57–62.

[43] Pellock JM, Faught E, Leppik IE, et al. Felbamate: consensus of current clinical experience. Epilepsy Res 2006;71:89–101.

[44] Kapetanovic IM, Torchin CD, Thompson CD, et al. Potentially reactive cyclic carbamate metabolite of the antiepileptic drug felbamate produced by human liver tissue in vitro. Drug Metab Dispos 1998;26:1089–95.

[45] White JR, Leppik IE, Beattie JL, et al. Long-term use of felbamate: clinical outcomes and effect of age and concomitant antiepileptic drug use on its clearance. Epilepsia 2009;50:2390–6.

[46] Palmer KJ, McTavish D. Felbamate. A review of its pharmacodynamic and pharmacokinetic properties, and therapeutic efficacy in epilepsy. Drugs 1993;45:1041–65.

[47] Sachdeo R, Kramer LD, Rosenberg A, Sachdeo S. Felbamate monotherapy: controlled trial in patients with partial onset seizures. Ann Neurol 1992;32:386–92.

[48] Glue P, Banfield CR, Perhach JL, et al. Pharmacokinetic interactions with felbamate. In vitro–in vivo correlation. Clin Pharmacokinet 1997;33:214–24.

[49] Dworkin RH, Kirkpatrick P. Pregabalin. Nat Rev Drug Discov 2005;4:455–6.

[50] Striano P, Striano S. Gabapentin: a Ca2+ channel alpha 2-delta ligand far beyond epilepsy therapy. Drugs Today (Barc) 2008;44:353–68.

[51] Johannessen SI, Battino D, Berry DJ, et al. Therapeutic drug monitoring of the newer antiepileptic drugs. Ther Drug Monit 2003;25:347–63.

[52] Gidal BE, DeCerce J, Bockbrader HN, et al. Gabapentin bioavailability: effect of dose and frequency of administration in adult patients with epilepsy. Epilepsy Res 1998;31:91–9.

[53] Gidal BE, Radulovic LL, Kruger S, et al. Inter- and intra-subject variability in gabapentin absorption and absolute bioavailability. Epilepsy Res 2000;40:123–7.

[54] Boyd RA, Turck D, Abel RB, et al. Effects of age and gender on single-dose pharmacokinetics of gabapentin. Epilepsia 1999;40:474–9.

[55] Berry DJ, Beran RG, Plunkeft MJ, et al. The absorption of gabapentin following high dose escalation. Seizure 2003;12:28–36.

[56] McLean MJ. Clinical pharmacokinetics of gabapentin. Neurology 1994;44:S17–22. discussion S31–12.

[57] Lindberger M, Luhr O, Johannessen SI, et al. Serum concentrations and effects of gabapentin and vigabatrin: observations from a dose titration study. Ther Drug Monit 2003;25:457–62.

[58] Doty P, Rudd GD, Stoehr T, Thomas D. Lacosamide. Neurotherapeutics 2007;4:145–8.

[59] Beyreuther BK, Freitag J, Heers C, et al. Lacosamide: a review of preclinical properties. CNS Drug Rev 2007;13:21–42.

[60] Beydoun A, D'Souza J, Hebert D, Doty P. Lacosamide: pharmacology, mechanisms of action and pooled efficacy and safety data in partial-onset seizures. Expert Rev Neurother 2009;9:33–42.

[61] Ben-Menachem E, Biton V, Jatuzis D, et al. Efficacy and safety of oral lacosamide as adjunctive therapy in adults with partial-onset seizures. Epilepsia 2007;48:1308–17.

[62] Hovinga CA. SPM-927 (Schwarz Pharma). IDrugs 2003;6:479–85.

[63] Halasz P, Kalviainen R, Mazurkiewicz-Beldzinska M, et al. Adjunctive lacosamide for partial-onset seizures: Efficacy and safety results from a randomized controlled trial. Epilepsia 2009;50:443–53.

[64] Halford JJ, Lapointe M. Clinical perspectives on lacosamide. Epilepsy Curr 2009;9:1–9.

[65] Stefani A, Spadoni F, Siniscalchi A, Bernardi G. Lamotrigine inhibits Ca2+ currents in cortical neurons: functional implications. Eur J Pharmacol 1996;307:113–6.

[66] Calabrese JR, Bowden CL, Sachs G, et al. A placebo-controlled 18-month trial of lamotrigine and lithium maintenance treatment in recently depressed patients with bipolar I disorder. J Clin Psychiatry 2003;64:1013–24.

[67] Johannessen SI, Tomson T. Pharmacokinetic variability of newer antiepileptic drugs: when is monitoring needed? Clin Pharmacokinet 2006;45:1061–75.

[68] Rambeck B, Wolf P. Lamotrigine clinical pharmacokinetics. Clin Pharmacokinet 1993;25:433–43.

[69] Hussein Z, Posner J. Population pharmacokinetics of lamotrigine monotherapy in patients with epilepsy: retrospective analysis of routine monitoring data. Br J Clin Pharmacol 1997;43:457–65.

[70] Cohen AF, Land GS, Breimer DD, et al. Lamotrigine, a new anticonvulsant: pharmacokinetics in normal humans. Clin Pharmacol Ther 1987;42:535–41.

[71] Bartoli A, Guerrini R, Belmonte A, et al. The influence of dosage, age, and comedication on steady state plasma lamotrigine concentrations in epileptic children: a prospective study with preliminary assessment of correlations with clinical response. Ther Drug Monit 1997;19:252–60.

[72] Morris RG, Black AB, Harris AL, et al. Lamotrigine and therapeutic drug monitoring: retrospective survey following the introduction of a routine service. Br J Clin Pharmacol 1998;46:547–51.

[73] Calabrese JR, Sullivan JR, Bowden CL, et al. Rash in multicenter trials of lamotrigine in mood disorders: clinical relevance and management. J Clin Psychiatry 2002;63:1012–9.

[74] Guberman AH, Besag FM, Brodie MJ, et al. Lamotrigine-associated rash: risk/benefit considerations in adults and children. Epilepsia 1999;40:985–91.

[75] Sabers A, Buchholt JM, Uldall P, Hansen EL. Lamotrigine plasma levels reduced by oral contraceptives. Epilepsy Res 2001;47:151–4.

[76] Battino D, Croci D, Granata T, et al. Single-dose pharmacokinetics of lamotrigine in children: influence of age and antiepileptic comedication. Ther Drug Monit 2001;23:217–22.

[77] Kaufman KR, Gerner R. Lamotrigine toxicity secondary to sertraline. Seizure 1998;7:163–5.

[78] May TW, Rambeck B, Jurgens U. Serum concentrations of lamotrigine in epileptic patients: the influence of dose and comedication. Ther Drug Monit 1996;18:523–31.

[79] Klitgaard H. Levetiracetam: the preclinical profile of a new class of antiepileptic drugs? Epilepsia 2001;42(Suppl. 4):13–8.

[80] Lynch BA, Lambeng N, Nocka K, et al. The synaptic vesicle protein SV2A is the binding site for the anti-epileptic drug levetiracetam. Proc Natl Acad Sci USA 2004;101:9861–6.

[81] Lynch JM, Tate SK, Kinirons P, et al. No major role of common SV2A variation for predisposition or levetiracetam response in epilepsy. Epilepsy Res 2009;83:44–51.

[82] Akiyama T, Otsubo H. Antiepileptic drugs in North America. Brain Nerve 2010;62:519–26.

[83] Patsalos PN. Pharmacokinetic profile of levetiracetam: toward ideal characteristics. Pharmacol Ther 2000;85:77–85.

[84] Fay MA, Sheth RD, Gidal BE. Oral absorption kinetics of levetiracetam: the effect of mixing with food or enteral nutrition formulas. Clin Ther 2005;27:594–8.

[85] Radtke RA. Pharmacokinetics of levetiracetam. Epilepsia 2001;42(Suppl. 4):24–7.

[86] Patsalos PN. Clinical pharmacokinetics of levetiracetam. Clin Pharmacokinet 2004;43:707–24.

[87] Kaminski RM, Matagne A, Patsalos PN, Klitgaard H. Benefit of combination therapy in epilepsy: a review of the preclinical evidence with levetiracetam. Epilepsia 2009;50:387–97.

[88] Abou-Khalil B. Levetiracetam in the treatment of epilepsy. Neuropsychiatr Dis Treat 2008;4:507–23.

[89] Pellock JM, Glauser TA, Bebin EM, et al. Pharmacokinetic study of levetiracetam in children. Epilepsia 2001;42:1574–9.

[90] Patsalos PN, Ghattaura S, Ratnaraj N, Sander JW. In situ metabolism of levetiracetam in blood of patients with epilepsy. Epilepsia 2006;47:1818–21.

[91] Tecoma ES. Oxcarbazepine. Epilepsia 1999;40(Suppl. 5):S37–46.

[92] Mazzucchelli I, Onat FY, Ozkara C, et al. Changes in the disposition of oxcarbazepine and its metabolites during pregnancy and the puerperium. Epilepsia 2006;47:504–9.

[93] May TW, Korn-Merker E, Rambeck B. Clinical pharmacokinetics of oxcarbazepine. Clin Pharmacokinet 2003;42:1023–42.

[94] Fink K, Dooley DJ, Meder WP, et al. Inhibition of neuronal Ca(2+) influx by gabapentin and pregabalin in the human neocortex. Neuropharmacology 2002;42:229–36.

[95] Bril V, England J, Franklin GM, et al. Evidence-based guideline: Treatment of painful diabetic neuropathy: report of the American Academy of Neurology, the American Association of Neuromuscular and Electro-diagnostic Medicine, and the American Academy of Physical Medicine and Rehabilitation. Neurology 2011;76:1758–65.

[96] Dworkin RH, Corbin AE, Young Jr JP, et al. Pregabalin for the treatment of postherpetic neuralgia: a randomized, placebo-controlled trial. Neurology 2003;60:1274–83.

[97] Pauer L, Winkelmann A, Arsenault P, et al. An international, randomized, double-blind, placebo-controlled, phase III Trial of pregabalin monotherapy in treatment of patients with fibromyalgia. J Rheumatol 2011;8:2643–52.

[98] Ben-Menachem E. Pregabalin pharmacology and its relevance to clinical practice. Epilepsia 2004; 45(Suppl. 6):13–8.

[99] Bockbrader HN, Burger P, Knapp L, Corrigan BW. Population pharmacokinetics of pregabalin in healthy subjects and patients with chronic pain or partial seizures. Epilepsia 2011;52:248–57.

[100] Brodie MJ, Wilson EA, Wesche DL, et al. Pregabalin drug interaction studies: lack of effect on the pharmacokinetics of carbamazepine, phenytoin, lamotrigine, and valproate in patients with partial epilepsy. Epilepsia 2005;46:1407–13.

[101] Randinitis EJ, Posvar EL, Alvey CW, et al. Pharmacokinetics of pregabalin in subjects with various degrees of renal function. J Clin Pharmacol 2003;43:277–83.

[102] Berry D, Millington C. Analysis of pregabalin at therapeutic concentrations in human plasma/serum by reversed-phase HPLC. Ther Drug Monit 2005;27:451–6.

[103] White HS, Franklin MR, Kupferberg HJ, et al. The anticonvulsant profile of rufinamide (CGP 33101) in rodent seizure models. Epilepsia 2008;49:1213–20.

[104] Wier HA, Cerna A, So TY. Rufinamide for pediatric patients with Lennox-Gastaut syndrome: a comprehensive overview. Paediatr Drugs 2011;13:97–106.

[105] Perucca E, Cloyd J, Critchley D, Fuseau E. Rufinamide: clinical pharmacokinetics and concentration–response relationships in patients with epilepsy. Epilepsia 2008;49:1123–41.

[106] Wheless JW, Vazquez B. Rufinamide: a novel broad-spectrum antiepileptic drug. Epilepsy Curr 2010; 10:1–6.

[107] Arroyo S. Rufinamide. Neurotherapeutics 2007;4:155–62.

[108] May TW, Boor R, Rambeck B, et al. Serum concentrations of rufinamide in children and adults with epilepsy: the influence of dose, age, and comedication. Ther Drug Monit 2011;33:214–21.

[109] Brodie MJ, Rosenfeld WE, Vazquez B, et al. Rufinamide for the adjunctive treatment of partial seizures in adults and adolescents: a randomized placebo-controlled trial. Epilepsia 2009;50:1899–909.

[110] Chiron C. Current therapeutic procedures in Dravet syndrome. Dev Med Child Neurol 2011;53(Suppl. 2): 16–8.

[111] Fisher JL. The anti-convulsant stiripentol acts directly on the GABA(A) receptor as a positive allosteric modulator. Neuropharmacology 2009;56:190–7.

[112] Cazali N, Tran A, Treluyer JM, et al. Inhibitory effect of stiripentol on carbamazepine and saquinavir metabolism in human. Br J Clin Pharmacol 2003;56:526–36.

[113] Perez J, Chiron C, Musial C, et al. Stiripentol: efficacy and tolerability in children with epilepsy. Epilepsia 1999;40:1618–26.

[114] Levy RH, Loiseau P, Guyot M, et al. Stiripentol kinetics in epilepsy: nonlinearity and interactions. Clin Pharmacol Ther 1984;36:661–9.

[115] Levy RH, Lin HS, Blehaut HM, Tor JA. Pharmacokinetics of stiripentol in normal man: evidence of nonlinearity. J Clin Pharmacol 1983;23:523–33.

[116] Farwell JR, Anderson GD, Kerr BM, et al. Stiripentol in atypical absence seizures in children: an open trial. Epilepsia 1993;34:305–11.

[117] Adkins JC, Noble S. Tiagabine. A review of its pharmacodynamic and pharmacokinetic properties and therapeutic potential in the management of epilepsy. Drugs 1998;55:437–60.

[118] Kalviainen R, Brodie MJ, Duncan J, et al. A double-blind, placebo-controlled trial of tiagabine given three-times daily as add-on therapy for refractory partial seizures. Northern European Tiagabine Study Group. Epilepsy Res 1998;30:31–40.

[119] Sachdeo RC, Leroy RF, Krauss GL, et al. Tiagabine therapy for complex partial seizures. A dose-frequency study. The Tiagabine Study Group. Arch Neurol 1997;54:595–601.

[120] Uthman BM, Rowan AJ, Ahmann PA, et al. Tiagabine for complex partial seizures: a randomized, add-on, dose–response trial. Arch Neurol 1998;55:56–62.

[121] Jette N, Cappell J, VanPassel L, Akman CI. Tiagabine-induced nonconvulsive status epilepticus in an adolescent without epilepsy. Neurology 2006;67:1514–5.

[122] Balslev T, Uldall P, Buchholt J. Provocation of non-convulsive status epilepticus by tiagabine in three adolescent patients. Eur J Paediatr Neurol 2000;4:169–70.

[123] Kellinghaus C, Dziewas R, Ludemann P. Tiagabine-related non-convulsive status epilepticus in partial epilepsy: three case reports and a review of the literature. Seizure 2002;11:243–9.

[124] Koepp MJ, Edwards M, Collins J, et al. Status epilepticus and tiagabine therapy revisited. Epilepsia 2005;46:1625–32.

[125] Gustavson LE, Mengel HB. Pharmacokinetics of tiagabine, a gamma-aminobutyric acid-uptake inhibitor, in healthy subjects after single and multiple doses. Epilepsia 1995;36:605–11.

[126] Perucca E, Bialer M. The clinical pharmacokinetics of the newer antiepileptic drugs. Focus on topiramate, zonisamide and tiagabine. Clin Pharmacokinet 1996;31:29–46.

[127] So EL, Wolff D, Graves NM, et al. Pharmacokinetics of tiagabine as add-on therapy in patients taking enzyme-inducing antiepilepsy drugs. Epilepsy Res 1995;22:221–6.

[128] Lau AH, Gustavson LE, Sperelakis R, et al. Pharmacokinetics and safety of tiagabine in subjects with various degrees of hepatic function. Epilepsia 1997;38:445–51.

[129] Latini G, Verrotti A, Manco R, et al. Topiramate: its pharmacological properties and therapeutic efficacy in epilepsy. Mini Rev Med Chem 2008;8:10–23.

[130] LaRoche SM, Helmers SL. The new antiepileptic drugs: scientific review. J Am Med Assoc 2004;291:605–14.

[131] Glauser TA, Dlugos DJ, Dodson WE, et al. Topiramate monotherapy in newly diagnosed epilepsy in children and adolescents. J Child Neurol 2007;22:693–9.

[132] Doose DR, Walker SA, Gisclon LG, Nayak RK. Single-dose pharmacokinetics and effect of food on the bioavailability of topiramate, a novel antiepileptic drug. J Clin Pharmacol 1996;36:884–91.

[133] Langtry HD, Gillis JC, Davis R. Topiramate. A review of its pharmacodynamic and pharmacokinetic properties and clinical efficacy in the management of epilepsy. Drugs 1997;54:752–73.

[134] Garnett WR. Clinical pharmacology of topiramate: a review. Epilepsia 2000;41(Suppl. 1):S61–5.

[135] Britzi M, Perucca E, Soback S, et al. Pharmacokinetic and metabolic investigation of topiramate disposition in healthy subjects in the absence and in the presence of enzyme induction by carbamazepine. Epilepsia 2005;46:378–84.

[136] Rosenfeld WE, Liao S, Kramer LD, et al. Comparison of the steady-state pharmacokinetics of topiramate and valproate in patients with epilepsy during monotherapy and concomitant therapy. Epilepsia 1997;38:324–33.

[137] Rimmer E, Kongola G, Richens A. Inhibition of the enzyme, GABA-aminotransferase in human platelets by vigabatrin, a potential antiepileptic drug. Br J Clin Pharmacol 1988;25:251–9.

[138] Maguire MJ, Hemming K, Wild JM, et al. Prevalence of visual field loss following exposure to vigabatrin therapy: a systematic review. Epilepsia 2010;51:2423–31.

[139] Gidal BE, Privitera MD, Sheth RD, Gilman JT. Vigabatrin: a novel therapy for seizure disorders. Ann Pharmacother 1999;33:1277–86.

[140] Rey E, Pons G, Richard MO, et al. Pharmacokinetics of the individual enantiomers of vigabatrin (gamma-vinyl GABA) in epileptic children. Br J Clin Pharmacol 1990;30:253–7.

[141] Haegele KD, Schechter PJ. Kinetics of the enantiomers of vigabatrin after an oral dose of the racemate or the active S-enantiomer. Clin Pharmacol Ther 1986;40:581–6.

[142] Patsalos PN. New antiepileptic drugs. Ann Clin Biochem 1999;36(Pt. 1):10–9.

[143] Biton V. Clinical pharmacology and mechanism of action of zonisamide. Clin Neuropharmacol 2007;30:230–40.

[144] Sills G, Brodie M. Pharmacokinetics and drug interactions with zonisamide. Epilepsia 2007;48:435–41.

[145] Baulac M. Introduction to zonisamide. Epilepsy Res 2006;68(Suppl. 2):S3–9.

[146] Wilensky AJ, Friel PN, Ojemann LM, et al. Zonisamide in epilepsy: a pilot study. Epilepsia 1985;26:212–20.

[147] Miura H. Zonisamide monotherapy with once-daily dosing in children with cryptogenic localization-related epilepsies: clinical effects and pharmacokinetic studies. Seizure 2004;13(Suppl. 1):S17–23. discussion S24–15.

[148] Westley IS, Morris RG. Seradyn quantitative microsphere system lamotrigine immunoassay on a Hitachi 911 analyzer compared with HPLC-UV. Ther Drug Monit 2008;30:634–7.

[149] Snozek CLH, Rollins LA, Peterson PW, Langman LJ. Comparison of a new serum topiramate immunoassay to fluorescence polarization immunoassay. Ther Drug Monit 2010;32:107–11.

[150] Kalbe K, Nishimura S, Ishii H, et al. Competitive binding enzyme immunoassay for zonisamide, a new antiepileptic drug, with selected paired-enzyme labeled antigen and antibody. Clin Chem 1990;36:24–7.

[151] Kim KB, Seo KA, Kim SE, et al. Simple and accurate quantitative analysis of ten antiepileptic drugs in human plasma by liquid chromatography/tandem mass spectrometry. J Pharm Biomed Anal 2011;56:771–7.

[152] Jones MD, Ryan M, Miles MV, et al. Stability of salivary concentrations of the newer antiepileptic drugs in the postal system. Ther Drug Monit 2005;27:576—9.

[153] Mecarelli O, Li Voti P, Pro S, et al. Saliva and serum levetiracetam concentrations in patients with epilepsy. Ther Drug Monit 2007;29:313—8.

[154] Miles MV, Tang PH, Glauser TA, et al. Topiramate concentration in saliva: an alternative to serum monitoring. Pediatr Neurol 2003;29:143—7.

[155] Malone SA, Eadie MJ, Addison RS, et al. Monitoring salivary lamotrigine concentrations. J Clin Neurosci 2006;13:902—7.

[156] Ryan M, Grim SA, Miles MV, et al. Correlation of lamotrigine concentrations between serum and saliva. Pharmacotherapy 2003;23:1550—7.

Challenges in Therapeutic Drug Monitoring of Classical Tricyclic and Newer Antidepressants

Analytical and Pharmacogenetics Considerations

Uttam Garg, Angela Ferguson

Children's Mercy Hospitals and Clinics, University of Missouri, Kansas City, MO

OUTLINE

Therapeutic Drug Monitoring: Newer Drugs and Biomarkers
DOI: 10.1016/B978-0-12-385467-4.00013-0

INTRODUCTION

Depression is one of the most common and widespread psychiatric disorders. It is estimated that 10−20% of adults in the United States experience depression in their lifetime, and 3% of the population is depressed at any given time. The patients with depression are at a greater risk of suicide and development of many other serious illnesses, such as cardiovascular disease and myocardial infarction. Antidepressants are frequently prescribed for the treatment of depression.

Over the decades a number of antidepressants have been developed for the treatment of depression. Monoamine oxidase inhibitors (MAOIs) were the first group of antidepressants that were discovered in the early 1950s. Tricyclic antidepressants (TCAs) were discovered in the late 1950s and 1960s. MAOIs and TCAs are generally referred to as first-generation antidepressants or classical antidepressants. Due to the many side effects of MAOIs and TCAs, the search for safer antidepressants continued. Since the 1980s, many other antidepressants that are safer than MAOIs and TCAs have been discovered and received FDA (Federal Drug Administration of the United States Government) approval. These newer antidepressants include selective serotonin reuptake inhibitors (SSRIs), serotonin−norepinephrine reuptake inhibitors (SNRIs), tetracyclic antidepressants and other atypical non-cyclic compounds. Although newer antidepressants have higher margins of safety, some of these drugs still need monitoring for many reasons, including narrow therapeutic range and side effects, compliance issues, drug−drug interactions and pharmacogenetics variations.

Therapeutic drug monitoring (TDM) of antidepressants is performed by immunoassays and chromatographic methods. Immunoassays are rapid and easy to perform and are available for the measurement of TCAs. However, immunoassays are non-specific, and many drugs cause false-positive TCA results. Chromatographic methods, though cumbersome and not routinely available in many clinical laboratories, are preferred due to their higher specificity and versatility. Chromatographic methods are the only methods for the measurement of most new antidepressants.

TRICYCLIC ANTIDEPRESSANTS

Tricyclic antidepressants were discovered in the 1950s and 1960s. Still widely used, until the 1980s TCAs were the major pharmacological agents for the treatment of endogenous depression. In addition to their use as antidepressants, TCAs are used in the treatment of many other disorders, including enuresis, chronic pain, fibromyalgia, obsessive-compulsive disorder, attention-deficit hyperactivity disorder, migraine prophylaxis and school phobia [1, 2]. Commonly used TCAs are amitriptyline, clomipramine, desipramine, doxepin, imipramine, nortriptyline, protriptyline and trimipramine. When administered orally, TCAs are almost completely absorbed through the intestinal tract and reach peak concentrations within 2−12 hours. TCAs undergo significant first-pass metabolism with a bioavailability of approximately 40−80%. They are highly lipophilic and have a very high volume of distribution (~15−30 L/kg) and protein binding of > 90%. Demethylation and hydroxylation are two major pathways for the metabolism of TCAs. Monodemethylation of tertiary amine TCAs leads to formation of secondary amines which are also pharmacologically active.

Hydroxy-metabolites are less active than parent drugs, are inactivated by glucuronidation and excreted in urine, and are generally not monitored. However, their monitoring may be warranted in specific situations such as renal impairment, where these metabolites may accumulate to significant concentrations. Some pharmacokinetic properties of commonly used TCAs are shown in Table 13.1. The values provided are approximate, and may vary due to many factors, such as genetic variations, drug–drug interactions, and renal and hepatic function.

The exact mechanism of action of TCAs is not well understood. At least in part, they act by inhibiting the presynaptic norepinephrine and serotonin uptake. Since many other drugs that inhibit norepinephrine and serotonin uptake are not antidepressants, such as amphetamines and cocaine, it is postulated that the mechanism of TCAs is more complicated. Common side effects of TCAs include dry mouth, constipation and urinary retention. Some patients may develop serious side effects such as blurred vision, respiratory depression, hypotension, cardiac arrhythmias and seizures.

Analytical Considerations in the Assay of TCAs

Like most drugs, therapeutic ranges for TCAs are based on the trough drug levels. Therefore, samples should be drawn before the next dose. Since TCAs are very lipophilic, the samples should not be drawn in serum or plasma gel separator tubes [3]. It has been shown that if the samples are collected in gel separator tubes, more than 40% of the drug can be lost. Once the proper sample has been drawn, and serum or plasma separated, TCAs are stable for 1 week at room temperature, for up to 4 weeks at 4 °C and for > 1 year at -20 °C [4].

Commonly used techniques for the assays of TCAs are immunoassays and chromatographic techniques. Both techniques have advantages and disadvantages. Assays are available in qualitative, semiquantitative and quantitative formats. It is important to look at patient care needs before selecting a specific method.

TABLE 13.1 Pharmacokinetic Properties of Tricyclic Antidepressants (TCAs)

Parent drug	Active metabolite	Major metabolizing enzyme (s)	Oral bioavailability	Average half-life (hours)	V_d (L/kg)	Therapeutic range (ng/mL)	Toxic level (ng/mL)
Amitriptyline	Nortriptyline	2D6	50	21	15	120–250[a]	> 500[a]
Desipramine	NA	2D6	40	20	42	75–300	> 500
Doxepin	Nordoxepin	2D6,1A2,3A4	27	17	20	150–250[a]	> 500[a]
Imipramine	Desipramine	2D6, 2C19	40	12	18	150–250[a]	> 500[a]
Nortriptyline	NA	2D6	50	30	18	50–150	> 500
Protriptyline	NA	2D6	75	80	13	70–250	> 500
Trimipramine	NA	2D6,2C19,3A4	50	27	32	100–250	> 500

V_d, Volume of distribution; NA, No significant active metabolite.
[a]Total concentration of parent and active metabolite.

Immunoassays for the Measurement of TCAs

Immunoassays are available in different formats for the measurement of individual drugs or TCAs as a group. Depending on the assay, they provide qualitative, semiquantitative or quantitative results. The advantages of immunoassays include smaller sample volume, easy assay performance and rapid turnaround time. These advantages are particularly useful in overdose situations when rapid turnaround time is desired and quantitative results are not that important.

The major disadvantage of TCAs immunoassays is lack of specificity due to interference from many therapeutic drugs. False-positive results can lead to misdiagnosis and mistreatment of a patient. The situation of a false positive can be more serious in a child where child abuse or neglect can be suspected. Therefore, the results of immunoassays should be interpreted with caution, and alongside the patient's clinical and medication history. Many drugs, including carbamazepine, quetiapine, phenothiazines, diphenhydramine, cyproheptadine and cyclobenzaprine, are shown to cause false-positive results with various TCAs immunoassays. Structures of a few TCAs and drugs which interfere in their immunoassays are shown in Fig. 13.1.

Carbamazepine, which is structurally close to TCAs, has been reported to cause false-positive results in TCA immunoassays [5–8]. Two patients with a history of carbamazepine ingestion tested positive for TCAs by FPIA immunoassay with apparent concentrations of 80 and 130 ng/mL. The samples tested negative by HPLC [5]. A 16-year-old girl with a history of seizures and being treated with carbamazepine tested positive for TCAs by immunoassay. ECG showed no evidence of TCA toxicity, and the investigation showed that the positive TCA result was due to carbamazepine [6]. The carbamazepine metabolite iminostilbene has been shown to cause false-positive TCA results on a Triage Panel Immunoassay System [8]. Carbamazepine interferes at a statistically significant level with serum fluorescence-polarized immunoassay assays, and in a dose-dependent fashion [7].

Quetiapine, an antipsychotic drug that is structurally related to TCAs, has been found to interfere in TCA immunoassays [9–13]. A 34-year-old patient who was prescribed quetiapine tested positive for TCAs by immunoassay [13]. Since the patient was not on TCAs, interference by quetiapine was suspected. Various concentrations ranging from 1–10 µg/mL were tested. Cross-reactivity of quetiapine was 4.3%, whereas olanzapine, another antipsychotic, did not cross-react. In another study, three TCA immunoassays, Microgenics®, Syva® Rapid Test and Biosite Triage®, were tested for quetiapine interference [11]. Quetiapine solution and blood and urine samples from patients were tested. Syva and Microgenics immunoassays, but not the Triage immunoassay, tested positive with patient samples. Also, Syva and Microgenics immunoassays were positive at quetiapine levels of 100 µg/mL and 10 µg/mL, respectively, whereas the Triage immunoassay was negative up to 1000 µg/mL. False-positive results by quetiapine in Abbott Laboratories fluorescence polarization TCAs immunoassay have also been shown [10, 12]. Other drugs such as phenothiazines, cyclobenzaprine and cyproheptadine that have a tricyclic ring have been shown to cause false-positive results on TCA immunoassays. False-positive TCA results due to thioridazine [14], chlorpromazine and trimeprazine [15] have been reported. Although most of the interferences are in immunoassays, false elevations of imipramine and desipramine by HPLC (cyanopropyl column) have

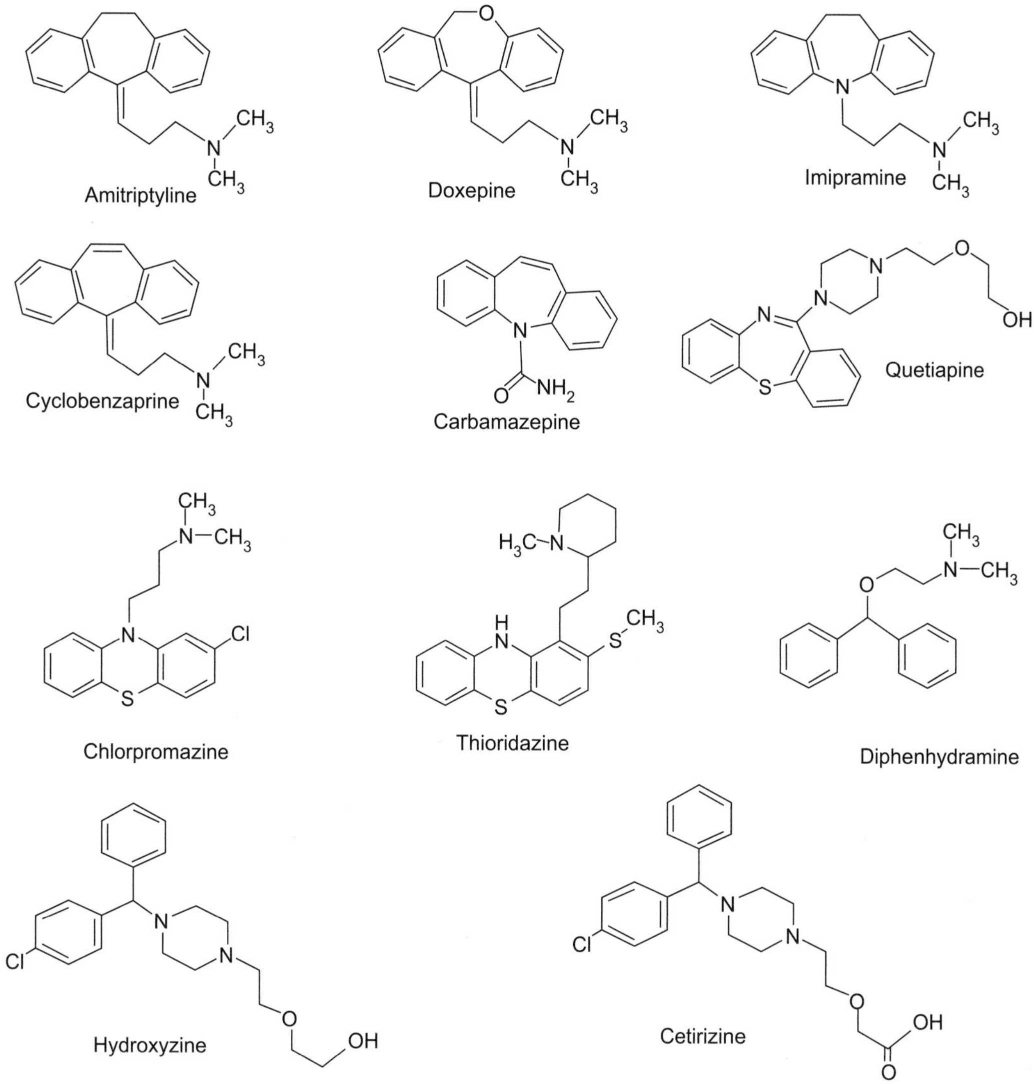

FIGURE 13.1 Chemical structures of some TCAs and drugs interfering in their immunoassays.

been reported [16]. Cyclobenzaprine and its major metabolite norcyclobenzaprine, which differ from amitriptyline and nortriptyline only by the presence of a double bond in the cycloheptane ring, are known to interfere with TCA immunoassays [17] and HPLC. A review on cyclobenzaprine interference in TCA assay has been published [18]. Case reports and *in vitro* studies have shown that cyproheptadine and its metabolite cause false-positive TCA immunoassays [19,20]. Interestingly, many other drugs which are structurally quite different from TCAs have been shown to interfere with TCA immunoassays. A 21-year-old female who ingested 2 g of diphenhydramine tested positive on an EMIT TCA assay [21]. Interferences in fluorescence polarization immunoassays by hydroxyzine and cetirizine have also been reported [22].

There have been several publications on estimating or eliminating interferences. In a fluorescence polarization immunoassay (FPIA), Dasgupta *et al.* [23] proposed a mathematical model for the estimation of TCA concentration in the presence of carbamazepine. A method has been described for removing phenothiazine interference in TCA immunoassays [24]. With Abbott FPIA, this method allowed an accurate quantification of the TCAs in the presence of 1000 ng/mL chlorpromazine or desmethylchlorpromazine.

Chromatographic Methods for the Measurement of TCAs

As discussed above, immunoassays for TCAs are non-specific and many drugs interfere in these assays. Furthermore, tertiary amine TCAs are metabolized to secondary amines that are also active. Therefore, measurement of both parent drug and metabolites is desirable. Chromatographic methods are preferred since they are more specific and can measure parent drug and metabolites simultaneously. However, chromatographic methods are technically demanding and frequently not available on an urgent basis.

Gas chromatography (GC) and high-performance liquid chromatography (HPLC) are the commonly used techniques for the measurement of TCAs. Thin-layer chromatography, which is used in broad-spectrum drug screening, can reliably identify TCAs. Before analysis by chromatographic methods, TCAs are extracted from a sample using liquid—liquid or solid phase extraction. Liquid—liquid extraction generally involves alkalization of sample and extraction of drugs in organic solvents. The extract is concentrated and injected into the GC. Sometimes additional steps are used to reduce interferences and increase sensitivity. One common step used to clean the extract is back extraction. In back extraction, TCAs from the organic solvents are back-extracted in acidic aqueous medium such as dilute hydrochloric acid. The acidic extract is then alkalinized and re-extracted in an organic solvent. Sometimes samples are derivatized to increase the sensitivity and specificity. This may be particularly important in the analysis of secondary amine and hydroxy metabolites that are more polar and are difficult to subject to chromatographic analysis without derivatization. Commonly used derivatives include trifluoroacetyl, heptafluorobutyryl, 4-carbethoxyhexafluorobutyryl chloride, fluoracyl and silane. Since liquid—liquid extraction is non-specific, it generates a lot of organic solvent waste and is less clean. Solid phase extraction is sometimes used to overcome these problems [25—28].

Gas chromatography equipped with a capillary column and coupled with flame ionization, nitrogen phosphorus or mass spectrometer detectors is commonly used for the screening and quantification of TCAs [29—34]. The capillary columns are typically 10- to 30-m fused silica columns with non-polar to intermediate polarity. Due to its increased specificity, the mass spectrometer detector is preferred over flame ionization or nitrogen phosphorus detectors. GC-MS analysis is performed using either the electron impact mode or the chemical ionization mode. Although electron impact ionization is more commonly used, the chemical ionization mode is gaining popularity due to its higher sensitivity and selectivity. When a mass spectrometer is used, it is operated in full-spectrum acquisition mode or selected-ion monitoring mode. The full-spectrum acquisition mode is preferred

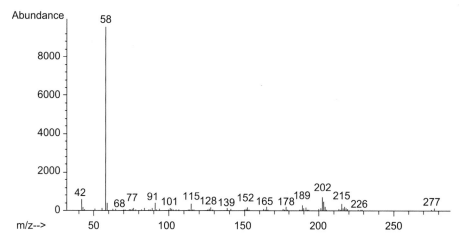

FIGURE 13.2   GC-MS electron impact mass spectrum of amitriptyline.

for identification and the selected-ion monitoring mode is preferred for quantification due to increased sensitivity. The full ion spectrum of amitriptyline is shown as an example (Fig. 13.2). In recent years, gas chromatography-tandem mass spectrometry (GC-MS-MS) methods that provide better sensitivity and selectivity than GC-MS instruments have become available.

Gas chromatography (GC) provides fairly good separation of primary amine TCAs. However, polar secondary amines and hydroxy metabolites generally require derivatization before analysis by GC. Since these issues can be resolved by HPLC, it has become a method of choice for the assay of TCAs. Based on current College of American Pathologist (CAP) proficiency surveys, HPLC with UV detector is the most commonly used method for the quantification of TCAs. A number of HPLC methods with UV detection for the assay of TCAs have been published [35–39]. A typical HPLC method for TCAs involves a stationary phase such as C18, C8, phenyl and CN; a mobile phase such as phosphate or acetate buffers in organic solvents such as acetonitrile and methanol; and a UV or mass spectrometer detector. UV is perhaps the most commonly used detector, but the mass spectrometer is gaining popularity. Like GC, HPLC may not separate all the TCAs of interest and can pose problems in HPLC methods with the UV detector. Also, certain drugs may co-elute in HPLC — for example, cyclobenzaprine and amitriptyline are structurally closely related and may co-elute. However, a diode array detector can be used to distinguish these drugs. These issues can also be overcome by the use of HPLC-MS or HPLC-MS-MS [34, 40–42]. For example, an atmospheric pressure chemical ionization tandem mass-spectrometry method for the simultaneous assay of amitriptyline, nortriptyline, doxepin, dosulepin, dibenzepin, opipramol and melitracen has been published [43]. Another HPLC-MS-MS method for the simultaneous determination of TCAs, non-TCAs and monoamine oxidase inhibitors — amitriptyline, clomipramine, trimipramine, and imipramine, doxepin, mianserin, maprotiline, dosulepin, amoxapine and their active metabolites desipramine, nortriptyline, dimethyl-clomipramine, and nordoxepin, toloxatone and moclobemide — has been published [44]. A recent method describes the simultaneous assay of many antipsychotics and antidepressants [40].

Challenges in Therapeutic Drug Monitoring of TCAs

TCAs exhibit a number of side effects through inhibition of cholinergic, histaminic and α_1-adrenergic receptors. Anticholinergic effects of TCAs include dry mouth, urinary retention, constipation, dry eyes, dry nose, decreased sweating and hyperthermia. Cardiac effects include inhibition of the fast sodium channels in the His-Purkinje system, and the atrial and ventricular myocardium. These effects are similar to Class 1A anti-arrhythmic drugs such as quinidine. The conduction abnormalities are seen in ECG as widening of the QRS, PR and QT intervals. These conduction abnormalities, along with TCAs' inhibitory effect on peripheral α_1-adrenergic receptors, may lead to severe hypotension. TCAs should be avoided in patients with pre-existing cardiac conduction problems due to risk of development of atrioventricular heart block. CNS effects due to inhibition of antihistaminic, anticholinergic and GABA-A receptors include mental status changes such as obtundation, delirium and seizures.

Many factors, including a narrow therapeutic window, high cardiac and CNS (central nervous system) toxicity, high intra- and inter-individual variability and non-compliance, justify therapeutic drug monitoring of TCAs. However, due to poor correlation between the drug levels and clinical response, the value of TDM has been questioned. This is particularly true in overdose situations. Some argue that ECG changes, particularly in overdose situations, correlate better with TCA toxicity than blood concentrations. Nevertheless, despite these arguments, the measurement of TCA levels is unequivocally useful in specific situations such as to monitor patient compliance, achieve target concentrations based on the patient's clinical response, and assess metabolic differences due to age, gender and genetic variations. The other factors that justify TDM for TCAs include significant variation in bioavailability among different brands and change in patient's other characteristics, such as weight loss/gain, smoking and exercise [4, 45–50].

A number of studies in the literature justify TDM of TCAs based on the reasons listed above. For example, Preskorn *et al.* showed that metabolism of TCAs varies significantly with age. The authors found significant inter-individual variations in concentrations of imipramine and its metabolite desipramine in hospitalized children; the steady-state concentrations varied 12- and 72-fold, respectively [45]. Also, there are significant differences in TCAs metabolism among different races and ethnic groups. African-Americans and Japanese metabolize TCAs significantly more slowly than Caucasians; Asians and Hispanics respond to lower doses of TCAs due to hypersensitivity receptors [46]. Drug–drug interactions and genetic variations are other major causes that justify TDM of TCAs. For example, CYP2D6, a major isoenzyme of the cytochrome P450 family of drug-metabolizing enzymes, is involved in the metabolism of TCAs. Co-administration of drugs that inhibit or induce CYP2D6 activity could affect the levels of TCAs. CYP2D6 inhibitors include amiodarone, bupropion, celecoxib, chlorpromazine, cimetidine, citalopram, doxorubicin, haloperidol, methylphenidate, quinidine, ranitidine, ritonavir, terbinafine, ticlopidine and histamine H1 receptor antagonists [4, 49]. Drugs that induce CYP2D6 include carbamazepine, phenobarbital, phenytoin and rifampin, and decrease TCA blood concentrations.

Furthermore, comparison of TCA doses based on clinical judgment and blood levels found that treating depression based on therapeutic drug monitoring of TCAs was superior to clinical judgment [48, 51, 52].

NEWER ANTIDEPRESSANTS

Although even in the 1980s TCAs remained the major pharmacological agents for the treatment of depression, due to their antihistaminic, anticholinergic and other toxic effects newer non-tricyclic antidepressants have been developed. Sometimes these newer antidepressants are referred to as second- and third-generation antidepressants. These drugs include the monoamine reuptake inhibitors amoxapine and maprotiline; the serotonin reuptake inhibitor trazodone; bupropion, which inhibits reuptake of norepinephrine and dopamine; and duloxetine, venlafaxine and mirtazapine, which inhibit reuptake of both serotonin and norepinephrine (SNRIs). Another category of newer antidepressants is selective serotonin uptake inhibitors (SSRIs). Due to their higher efficacy, tolerability and safety and low toxicity, SSRIs have become the first-line and most commonly used antidepressants in the United States [53, 54]. However, the efficacy of SSRIs has been disputed. A recent meta-analysis concluded that the magnitude of benefit of antidepressant medication compared with placebo increases with the severity of depression symptoms and may be minimal or non-existent, on average, in patients with mild or moderate symptoms. However, for patients with very severe depression, the benefit of medications over placebo is substantial [55].

The FDA-approved SSRIs include citalopram, escitalopram, fluoxetine, fluvoxamine, paroxetine and sertraline. Fluoxetine was the first SSRI approved by the FDA for the treatment of depression. In addition to its use as an antidepressant, fluoxetine is used for the treatment of bulimia and obsessive-compulsive disorder (OCD). Similarly, other SSRIs are used for disorders other than depression. Citalopram is used in the treatment of dementia, smoking cessation, ethanol abuse and OCD; fluvoxamine is used for the treatment of OCD in children ≥ 8 years of age and adults [53], and panic disorder and anxiety disorders in children [56]; sertraline is used for the treatment of OCD, panic disorder, post-traumatic stress disorder, premenstrual dysphoric disorder and social anxiety disorder. Paroxetine, which was first approved by the FDA for the treatment of social phobia and generalized anxiety disorder, is now approved for the treatment of post-traumatic stress disorder, panic disorder with or without agoraphobia, and OCD in adults [53]. It is also used in the treatment of eating disorders, impulse control disorders, self-injurious behavior and premenstrual disorders [56].

The major mechanism of action of SSRIs is through inhibition of serotonin uptake by the presynaptic serotonin reuptake pump and interaction with serotonin receptors (5-HT$_{1A}$, 5-HT$_2$, and 5-HT$_3$) to cause a pharmacological response. However, it appears that additional mechanisms are involved in the actions of SSRIs. The inhibition of serotonin reuptake happens soon after SSRI treatment, whereas the therapeutic effects take 3—8 weeks [57]. Pharmacokinetic properties, including absorption, distribution, metabolism and elimination of SSRIs, are fairly well understood [58, 59]. After oral intake, SSRIs are well absorbed in the gastrointestinal tract and reach the peak plasma levels within 1—8 hours. Their absorption is not affected by food. SSRIs are metabolized in the liver and may inhibit hepatic cytochrome P450 enzymes that metabolize other medications, thereby causing drug—drug interactions.

SSRIs are much safer than TCAs and MAOIs, and rarely cause fatality or serious sequelae. As an example, 31–32% of patients with TCA overdoses require intubation, compared to 4–6% of SSRI overdoses [57]. Also, SSRIs are safer than SNRIs. Furthermore, SSRIs have wider toxic indexes: ingestion of up to 30 times the daily dose typically produces minor or no symptoms, while ingestion of 50–75 times the daily dose can cause vomiting, mild CNS depression, or tremor. Most fatalities occur with extremely high doses or in the presence of other drugs such as ethanol or benzodiazepines [57].

The most common side effect of SSRIs is serotonin syndrome, characterized by agitation, hyperthermia, tachycardia, and neuromuscular disturbance including rigidity [60]. SSRIs rarely cause serotonin syndrome by themselves. However, co-administration of SSRIs with other drugs can cause severe serotonin syndrome. Most severe cases of serotonin syndrome are caused by co-administration of monoamine oxidase inhibitors (MAOIs). Therefore, co-administration of SSRIs and MAOIs is highly contradicted. Co-administration of SSRIs and many drugs, including tramadol, sibutramine, meperidine, sumatriptan, lithium, St John's wort, gingko biloba and atypical antipsychotic agents, can also lead to serotonin syndrome [61]. The other major concern of SSRIs is increased suicidal thinking in children. The FDA black-box warning for SSRIs includes the risk of suicidal thinking and behavior in children and adolescents with major and other depressive disorders. Some pharmacokinetic properties of SSRIs and other non-TCAs are given in Table 13.2.

Analytical and Therapeutic Drug Monitoring Considerations for Non-TCAs

For the most part, immunoassays are not available for the assay of non-TCAs. Chromatographic methods such as gas or liquid chromatography are frequently used for the measurement of non-TCAs [62–65]. The GC-MS methods for the analysis of non-TCAs are very similar to those for TCAs, and involve similar capillary columns and liquid–liquid or solid phase extraction. Methods are available for the assay of individual drugs or the simultaneous determination of many drugs. For example, Wille *et al.* [63] reported a GC-MS method for the simultaneous analysis of 13 new-generation antidepressants (venlafaxine, fluoxetine, viloxazine, fluvoxamine, mianserin, mirtazapine, melitracen, reboxetine, citalopram, maprotiline, sertraline, paroxetine and trazodone) along with their eight metabolites (O-desmethylvenlafaxine, norfluoxetine, desmethylmianserin, desmethylmirtazapine, desmethylcitalopram, didesmethylcitalopram, desmethylsertraline and m-chlorophenylpiperazine). The extract was suitable for both GC and HPLC. Recently, a GC-MS method for simultaneous assay of TCAs and non-TCAs has been published [33]. As described in analysis of TCAs, mass spectrometers can be operated in selected-ion monitoring mode, or full spectra can be obtained. As an example, the full ion spectrum of fluoxetine is shown in Fig. 13.3.

Since many non-TCAs, such as trazodone and nefazodone, are heat labile and many need derivatization before analysis, HPLC is preferred over GC for the analysis of many non-TCAs. Commonly used HPLC methods involve a non-polar stationary phase (C18 or C8) and a moderately polar mobile phase. However, since some metabolites are polar, the use of a weakly hydrophobic stationary phase such as CN or short alkyl chain may provide better chromatographic separation. A number of HPLC methods for the determination of SSRIs and other non-TCAs have been described [66]. HPLC coupled with a UV detector had been the most common method for the determination of non-TCAs. An example HPLC

TABLE 13.2 Pharmacokinetic Properties of Non-Tricyclic Antidepressants

Parent drug	Active metabolite	Major metabolizing enzyme(s)	Oral bioavailability	Average half-life (hours)	V_d (L/kg)	Average protein binding	Therapeutic range (ng/mL)	Toxic level (ng/mL)
Amoxapine	8-Hydroxyamoxapine	2D6	90	10	1	90	200–400[b]	>600[b]
Bupropion	Hydroxybupropion[a]	2B6	90	15	45	85	25–100	>400
Citalopram	Norcitalopram[a]	2C19	80	30	14	50	40–100	>250
Duloxetine	NA	2D6, 1A2	90	12	23	90	20–80	Not known
Escitalopram	Desmethylcitalopram[a]	2C19, 3A4	90	30	15	55	50–100	Not known
Fluoxetine	Norfluoxetine	2C9,2D6	100	60	50	94	300–1000[b]	>2000[b]
Fluvoxamine	NA	1A2, 2D6	95	23	25	77	20–400	Not known
Maprotiline	NA	2D6	100	33	24	88	150–300	>1000
Mirtazapine	Normirtazapine	1A2, 2D6	90	30	12	85	4–40	Not known
Paroxetine	NA	2D6	90	22	15	95	20–200	>800
Sertraline	Norsertraline[a]	2D6, 2C19	90	28	20	98	30–200	>500
Trazodone	NA	3A4	80	9	1	90	800–1600	>5000
Venlafaxine	O-desmethylvenlafaxine	2D6, 3A4	90	5	7	27	250–500[b]	>1000[b]

[a]Significantly less active metabolite than the parent drug.
[b]Total concentration of parent and active metabolite.
V_d, Volume of distribution.

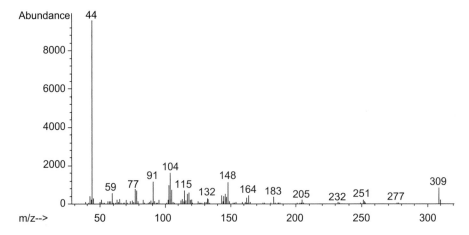

FIGURE 13.3   GC-MS electron impact mass spectrum of fluoxetine.

chromatogram of fluoxetine and non-fluoxetine is shown in Fig. 13.4. However, for many non-TCAs HPLC with UV may not be sensitive enough. Other detection methods involving fluorescence, electrochemical and mass detectors have been developed over the years. Due to their increased sensitivity and selectivity, LC-MS or LC-MS-MS have gained popularity for the assays of antidepressants [40, 66–68].

As described above, SSRIs are very safe and, unlike TCAs, do not require therapeutic drug monitoring on a regular basis. However, therapeutic drug monitoring is useful in achieving target concentrations based on the patient's clinical response, and to account for metabolic differences due to age, gender and genetic variations. Since SSRIs rarely cause serious toxicity, laboratory monitoring for other drugs and organ function markers may be helpful.

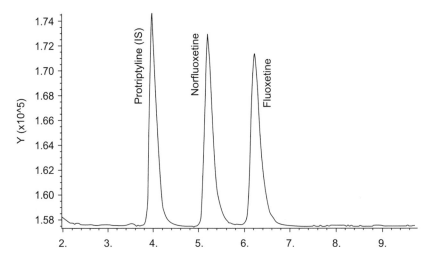

FIGURE 13.4   HPLC chromatogram of fluoxetine and norfluoxetine involving solid phase extraction, C8 column and UV detection at 230 nm.

PHARMACOGENETICS CONSIDERATIONS IN TDM OF ANTIDEPRESSANTS

In recent years it has become clear that pharmacogenetics plays an important role in drug metabolism and therapeutic drug monitoring. It is estimated that 30–60% of patients do not respond to standard drug therapy [69], and pharmacogenetic variability might be partially responsible for the lack of response in these patients. For antidepressants, 30–50% of patients do not respond to an initial treatment regime, and since efficacy can only be determined after several weeks of drug therapy, this can increase the time the patient experiences depressive symptoms [70, 71]. Since optimizing the dose of antidepressants is difficult due to several factors, such as slow onset of action of the drugs, unpredictable clinical effects with plasma concentration correlating poorly with clinical efficacy, side effects that mimic the symptoms of the disease that is being treated and variability in drug metabolism [72, 73], it has been proposed that having the patient's genetic information could help guide in the selection of an antidepressant that would be optimally metabolized by that patient, leading to fewer side effects and possibly a better therapeutic response.

Role of CYP2D6 Polymorphism

The CYP2D6 isoenzyme is almost entirely responsible for the metabolism of tricyclic antidepressants [74], and the CYP2D6 genotype has been shown to predict clearance of antidepressants such as desipramine, fluvoxamine, mexiletine and nortriptyline [75, 76]. In a large meta-analysis looking at the effects of genotype on dosing of antidepressants, it was estimated that for many drugs the dose required for extensive metabolizers (EMs) would need to be double the dose given to poor metabolizers (PMs) [77]. A patient genotyped as a CYP2D6 ultra-metabolizer (UM) can require a 10-fold larger dose of nortriptyline than a PM to achieve similar plasma drug levels [78]. In a separate study, a UM phenotype was shown to be 10 times more likely in patients who are non-responders to antidepressant therapy than in those who do respond [79]. A pilot study done in a group of patients that were classified as treatment-refractory showed that patients with a CYP2D6 duplication and a UM genotype had significantly higher worse week scores when assessed by the Hamilton Depression Rating Scale [79]. This was hypothesized to be a result of the patients metabolizing the drug at a higher rate and not maintaining appropriate drug levels.

While many studies report that knowledge of CYP2D6 genotype can predict plasma levels of antidepressants, other studies have not successfully been able to predict treatment response. A study of 136 depressed inpatients on a variety of antidepressants underwent weekly plasma concentration measurements and assessments of their illness severity and treatment response [80]. Those patients who were PMs and those taking drugs that inhibited CYP2D6 activity had plasma concentrations of drug significantly higher than the drug-specific median. Five of the six patients who genotyped as PMs also experienced side effects, but no relationship between genotype and treatment response was found in this study. Another study of 100 depressed patients being treated with venlafaxine examined the ratios of the major metabolite to parent drug, and those patients with decreased ratios had at least one deficient CYP2D6 allele, while patients with a gene duplication had increased ratios [81]. Patients classified as PMs had significantly more side effects when compared to EMs and

UMs; however, no significant difference in therapeutic efficiency was reported between the groups.

CYP2D6 has not been shown to be involved in the metabolism of SSRIs [74]. A study done in 246 elderly patients with major depression taking the SSRI paroxetine found no difference in severity of adverse events, daily dose achieved, dosing compliance or frequency of discontinuation between patients classified as CYP2D6 EMs or UMs and those classified as intermediate or PMs [82]. Patients in the same study taking mirtazapine, a drug that is not an SSRI and is partially metabolized by CYP2D6, also did not show any differences between genotypes, implying that other enzymes are able to compensate for reduced CYP2D6 activity.

In 2005, the FDA approved the first pharmacogenetic test, the AmpliChip™ CYP450, which tests for the presence of CYP2D6 and CYP2C19 alleles [83]. Other companies have developed CYP genotyping tests, and single gene sequencing is available at many clinical laboratories as well [83]. The combination of CYP2D6 genotyping and traditional TDM could be useful for determining adverse drug reactions due to poor metabolism of antidepressants, as well as treatment failure due to ultra rapid metabolism [73]. However, only 10–15% of cases show a direct link between the effect of a specific drug treatment and genotype [74].

Is knowledge of a patient's CYP2D6 genotype useful in clinical practice? A retrospective study looked at all requisitions for CYP2D6 genotyping over an 11-year period to see if the genotype of individual patients could explain their abnormal drug metabolism [84]. Patients were sorted into groups based on whether or not the drug they were taking was metabolized by CYP2D6, and compared to a control group. A majority of the patients in the study group (72%) were taking psychopharmacological drugs, including TCAs or SSRIs. The results indicate that the majority of patients who underwent testing had a normal CYP2D6 genotype (EM), in spite of the clinical suspicion of altered CYP2D6 metabolism. In patients found to have a PM phenotype, the genotyping result was consistent with the clinical suspicion 63% of the time. In 25% of cases, the patient was suspected to have an UM phenotype but genotyped as a PM. A possible explanation for this seemingly paradoxical finding could be that patients who are PM fail to take the medication due to experiencing side effects, resulting in low serum drug levels. The study concludes that there is poor correlation between CYP2D6 genotype and clinical suspicion of a patient's phenotype. To date, no large, randomized prospective study examining genotype-specific dosing of antidepressants has been published, due to a lack of understanding of the relationship between drug response and dose given and the requirement for a large population of patients in monotherapy that would be necessary for such a clinical study [72]. Currently, pharmacogenetic testing for CYP2D6 is the only test that is widely used in clinical practice, but only to optimize dose to prevent drug toxicity. Using genotype information to predict treatment response has not proven successful, despite extensive study.

Role of Polymorphism of 2C9

The metabolism of antidepressants by CYP2C9 has not been as extensively studied as the other CYP alleles. Most of the studies that have been done compare CYP2C9 genotype to plasma drug levels, but do not have data with regard to clinical outcome [80, 85, 86]. One small study looked at the effect of CYP2C9 genotype in a group of patients on maintenance treatment with fluoxetine for major depression [86]. Patients who were genotyped as homozygous CYP2D6 EMs with the CYP2C9*1 allele had a lower concentration of one fluoxetine enantiomer (R-fluoxetine) when compared to other CYP2C9 genotypes. This was in agreement with a separate study examining the role of CYP2C9 in patients at steady-state treatment with fluoxetine [85]. The study also showed a significant relationship between higher plasma concentrations of fluoxetine and patients with the CYP2C9*3 allele, which is known to have lower activity [86]. However, in a separate study of 136 depressed inpatients on a variety of second-generation antidepressants, CYP2C9 genotype had no influence on the plasma concentration of drug [80].

Role of Polymorphism of 2C19

Similar to the other CYP alleles, most of the studies attempting to correlate CYP2C19 genotype with phenotype have found that while the genotype can give an indication of plasma drug concentration, it does not predict treatment response. CYP2C19 PMs are hypothesized to have poor tolerance for drugs that are demethylated by CYP2C19 such as TCAs citalopram, escitalopram and sertraline [83]. A study involving 136 depressed inpatients showed a low mean plasma concentration of drug in patients who were genotyped as EMs, but this had no relevance to the patient's response to treatment [80]. A similar study examining homozygous carriers of a non-functional allele of CYP2C19 showed a 42% decrease in the clearance of the citalopram when compared to carriers of the wild-type allele [87]. In spite of this relationship between genotype and drug metabolism, a large prospective trial showed no significant correlation between genotype and tolerance of citalopram [88]. The Sequenced Treatment Alternatives to Relieve Depression (STAR*D) trial involved 4041 subjects who were taking citalopram, and was designed to assess effectiveness of antidepressant treatments and determine outcomes over 12 weeks. At the end of the trial, neither dose of medication nor ability to remain on the medication and participate in the trial correlated with CYP2C19 genotype. Plasma citalopram levels were not obtained from any of the patients, so the study was not able to correlate patient drug metabolism to genotype, and medication compliance also could not be assessed.

SSRI Receptor

Selective serotonin reuptake inhibitors (SSRIs) are the most commonly prescribed antidepressants, as described earlier [53, 54]. Several studies have examined polymorphisms in the serotonin receptor locus, HTR2A, to investigate if there is a correlation between treatment response or side effects and patient genotype. In a study of elderly patients with major depression taking paroxetine, medication intolerance was strongly associated with HTR2A genotype [82]. Patients with the HTR2A 102 C/C SNP had significantly more discontinuations due to adverse reactions when compared to patients with T/C and T/T genotypes, and the severity of side effects in the C/C patients was greater as well. These differences in tolerance were not seen when genotypes were compared in the group taking mirtazapine, which is partially metabolized by CYP2D6. In a separate study of the STAR*D trial participants, a significant association was found between a variation of HTR2A and treatment outcome, which was the first time an association with response to an antidepressant had been reported [89]. Carriers of the A allele of the rs7997012 intronic SNP (single nucleotide polymorphism) had a 16–18% reduction in absolute risk of being a non-responder to citalopram. Treatment effectiveness was scored by response, remission and a change in the final symptom score. Additionally, the allele that was associated with better treatment outcome was six times more frequent in white patients than in black patients, who had less favorable treatment outcomes overall in this study. Of interest, this study did not identify the functional variants of HTR2A that had previously been published, but an intronic variant of unknown functional significance.

A recent meta-analysis that analyzed pharmacogenetic studies on both antidepressant response and side effects included several serotonin-related genes [90]. A better treatment response was seen in those patients with the serotonin transporter gene promoter allele 5-HTTLPR-1. The serotonin-1A receptor HTR1A-1019G/G and the serotonin-2A receptor HRT2A -1438G/G (102C/C) alleles also contributed to a better treatment response, but this effect was only seen in Asian populations. Fewer side effects were seen with the 5-HTTLPR-1 and HTRA2-1438A (102T) alleles as well. While the significant affects seen in this analysis are modest, this result is not unexpected when analyzing a complicated phenotype such as depression.

Genome-Wide Association Studies

While quite a bit has been learned about the pharmacogenetics of depression through the studies of the different CYP alleles and other genes, much about the mechanism of action of antidepressants is still not understood. There are several possible reasons for lack of progress in this area. The heritability of depression is less than 40%, which implies that it is a very complex disorder [91], and it can be difficult to properly assess the pharmacological phenotype to ensure that genotypic differences will be revealed [92]. The presence of a strong placebo effect in clinical trials for antidepressants may also confound categorization of the drug's effect.

Several groups have undertaken genome-wide association studies (GWAS) to find other genetic variants to gain a better understanding of antidepressant action and better predict patient responses. The Genome-Based Therapeutic Drugs for Depression (GENDEP) project was a 12-week partially randomized pharmacogenetic study with 811 moderately to severely depressed patients who received either escitalopram (SSRI) or nortriptyline (TCA) [93]. This study was specifically designed as a pharmacogenetic study, so the subjects were all of European Caucasian descent to minimize ethnic heterogeneity. Treatment outcome was assessed as a change in depression severity over a 12-week period, and associations were examined between 72 candidate genes as well as 500 000 common genetic variants. None of the 72 candidate genes, which were selected due to published associations with antidepressant action, showed a significant pharmacogenetic association. The results from the GWAS portion of the study were slightly more encouraging, showing a significant association of a marker in the uranyl 2-sulphotransferase gene and response to nortriptyline, and an association with a marker in the interleukin-11 gene and a response to escitalopram.

Two separate GWAS studies were conducted by Ising and colleagues [94] in patients from the Munich Antidepressant Response Signature (MARS) project and separate pooled samples from a German replication study, but no SNPs were identified that met the criteria for genome-wide significance. The results from these studies demonstrate the multifactorial nature of the antidepressant response, and emphasize that many genes play a role in determining if a specific treatment is effective for a specific patient.

CONCLUSIONS

In conclusion, depression remains a major health problem. A number of therapeutic drugs are available for the treatment of depression. TCAs were the main therapeutic drugs until the 1980s. Although still widely used for depression and many other indications, TCAs have been replaced by SSRIs as the first-line antidepressive drugs. Immunoassays and chromatographic methods are widely used for the measurement of these antidepressants. Analytical considerations for the assay of antidepressants are important, since these methods pose a number of challenges. Therapeutic drug monitoring of antidepressants is important due to many factors, including drug toxicity, patient compliance, age, race, drug–drug interactions and pharmacogenetics variability. Using pharmacogenetics to personalize antidepressant therapy is still in the early phase of implementation, and its current clinical usefulness appears to be in optimizing dosing to avoid side effects and prevent toxicity rather than to predict a therapeutic response.

References

[1] Sindrup SH, Otto M, Finnerup NB, Jensen TS. Antidepressants in the treatment of neuropathic pain. Basic Clin Pharmacol Toxicol 2005;96:399–409.

[2] Hauser W, Bernardy K, Uceyler N, Sommer C. Treatment of fibromyalgia syndrome with antidepressants: a meta-analysis. J Am Med Assoc 2009;301:198–209.

[3] Dasgupta A, Yared MA, Wells A. Time-dependent absorption of therapeutic drugs by the gel of the Greiner Vacuette blood collection tube. Ther Drug Monit 2000;22:427–331.

[4] Linder MW, Keck Jr PE. Standards of laboratory practice: antidepressant drug monitoring. National Academy of Clinical Biochemistry. Clin Chem 1998;44:1073–84.

[5] Chattergoon DS, Verjee Z, Anderson M, et al. Carbamazepine interference with an immune assay for tricyclic antidepressants in plasma. J Toxicol Clin Toxicol 1998;36:109–13.

[6] Fleischman A, Chiang VW. Carbamazepine overdose recognized by a tricyclic antidepressant assay. Pediatrics 2001;107:176–7.

[7] Saidinejad M, Law T, Ewald MB. Interference by carbamazepine and oxcarbazepine with serum- and urine-screening assays for tricyclic antidepressants. Pediatrics 2007;120:e504–509.

[8] Tomaszewski C, Runge J, Gibbs M, et al. Evaluation of a rapid bedside toxicology screen in patients suspected of drug toxicity. J Emerg Med. 2005;28:389–94.

[9] Chathanchirayil SJ. False positive urine drug screening for tricyclic antidepressants in patients taking quetiapine. Aust N Z J Psychiatry 2011;45:792.

[10] Caravati EM, Juenke JM, Crouch BI, Anderson KT. Quetiapine cross-reactivity with plasma tricyclic antidepressant immunoassays. Ann Pharmacother 2005;39:1446–9.

[11] Hendrickson RG, Morocco AP. Quetiapine cross-reactivity among three tricyclic antidepressant immunoassays. J Toxicol Clin Toxicol 2003;41:105–8.

[12] Schussler JM, Juenke JM, Schussler I. Quetiapine and falsely elevated nortriptyline level. Am J Psychiatry 2003;160:589.

[13] Sloan KL, Haver VM, Saxon AJ. Quetiapine and false-positive urine drug testing for tricyclic antidepressants. Am J Psychiatry 2000;157:148–9.

[14] Ryder KW, Glick MR. The effect of thioridazine on the Automatic Clinical Analyzer serum tricyclic antidepressant screen. Am J Clin Pathol 1986;86:248–9.

[15] Benitez J, Dahlqvist R, Gustafsson LL, et al. Clinical pharmacological evaluation of an assay kit for intoxications with tricyclic antidepressants. Ther Drug Monit 1986;8:102—5.

[16] Maynard GL, Soni P. Thioridazine interferences with imipramine metabolism and measurement. Ther Drug Monit 1996;18:729—31.

[17] Wong EC, Koenig J, Turk J. Potential interference of cyclobenzaprine and norcyclobenzaprine with HPLC measurement of amitriptyline and nortriptyline: resolution by GC-MS analysis. J Anal Toxicol 1995;19:218—24.

[18] Van Hoey NM. Effect of cyclobenzaprine on tricyclic antidepressant assays. Ann Pharmacother 2005;39:1314—7.

[19] Wians Jr FH, Norton JT, Wirebaugh SR. False-positive serum tricyclic antidepressant screen with cyproheptadine. Clin Chem 1993;39:1355—6.

[20] Yuan CM, Spandorfer PR, Miller SL, et al. Evaluation of tricyclic antidepressant false positivity in a pediatric case of cyproheptadine (periactin) overdose. Ther Drug Monit 2003;25:299—304.

[21] Sorisky A, Watson DC. Positive diphenhydramine interference in the EMIT-st assay for tricyclic antidepressants in serum. Clin Chem 1986;32:715.

[22] Dasgupta A, Wells A, Datta P. False-positive serum tricyclic antidepressant concentrations using fluorescence polarization immunoassay due to the presence of hydroxyzine and cetirizine. Ther Drug Monit 2007;29:134—9.

[23] Dasgupta A, McNeese C, Wells A. Interference of carbamazepine and carbamazepine 10,11-epoxide in the fluorescence polarization immunoassay for tricyclic antidepressants: estimation of the true tricyclic antidepressant concentration in the presence of carbamazepine using a mathematical model. Am J Clin Pathol 2004;121:418—25.

[24] Adamczyk M, Fishpaugh JR, Harrington CA, et al. Immunoassay reagents for psychoactive drugs. Part 3. Removal of phenothiazine interferences in the quantification of tricyclic antidepressants. Ther Drug Monit 1993;15:436—9.

[25] Lee XP, Hasegawa C, Kumazawa T, et al. Determination of tricyclic antidepressants in human plasma using pipette tip solid phase extraction and gas chromatography-mass spectrometry. J Sep Sci 2008;31:2265—71.

[26] de la Torre R, Ortuno J, Pascual JA, et al. Quantitative determination of tricyclic antidepressants and their metabolites in plasma by solid phase extraction (Bond-Elut TCA) and separation by capillary gas chromatography with nitrogen-phosphorous detection. Ther Drug Monit 1998;20:340—6.

[27] Lee XP, Kumazawa T, Sato K, Suzuki O. Detection of tricyclic antidepressants in whole blood by headspace solid phase microextraction and capillary gas chromatography. J Chromatogr Sci 1997;35:302—8.

[28] Uddin MN, Samanidou VF, Papadoyannis IN. Bio-sample preparation and analytical methods for the determination of tricyclic antidepressants. Bioanalysis 2011;3:97—118.

[29] Van Brunt N. Application of new technology for the measurement of tricyclic antidepressants using capillary gas chromatography with a fused silica DB5 column and nitrogen phosphorus detection. Ther Drug Monit 1983;5:11—37.

[30] Bredesen JE, Ellingsen OF, Karlsen J. Rapid isothermal gas—liquid chromatographic determination of tricyclic antidepressants in serum with use of a nitrogen-selective detector. J Chromatogr 1981;204:361—7.

[31] Dorrity Jr F, Linnoila M, Habig RL. Therapeutic monitoring of tricyclic antidepressants in plasma by gas chromatography. Clin Chem 1977;23:1326—8.

[32] Martinez MA, Sanchez de la Torre C, Almarza E. A comparative solid phase extraction study for the simultaneous determination of fluvoxamine, mianserin, doxepin, citalopram, paroxetine, and etoperidone in whole blood by capillary gas-liquid chromatography with nitrogen-phosphorus detection. J Anal Toxicol 2004;28:174—80.

[33] Winecker RE. Quantification of antidepressants using gas chromatography-mass spectrometry. Methods Mol Biol 2010;603:45—56.

[34] Breaud AR, Harlan R, Di Bussolo JM, et al. A rapid and fully-automated method for the quantitation of tricyclic antidepressants in serum using turbulent-flow liquid chromatography-tandem mass spectrometry. Clin Chim Acta 2010;411:825—32.

[35] Theurillat R, Thormann W. Monitoring of tricyclic antidepressants in human serum and plasma by HPLC: characterization of a simple, laboratory developed method via external quality assessment. J Pharm Biomed Anal 1998;18:751—60.

[36] Queiroz RH, Lanchote VL, Bonato PS, et al. de Carvalho D. Simultaneous HPLC analysis of tricyclic antidepressants and metabolites in plasma samples. Pharm Acta Helv 1995;70:181—6.

[37] Dorey RC, Preskorn SH, Widener PK. Results compared for tricyclic antidepressants as assayed by liquid chromatography and enzyme immunoassay. Clin Chem 1988;34:2348−51.

[38] Mercolini L, Mandrioli R, Finizio G, et al. Simultaneous HPLC determination of 14 tricyclic antidepressants and metabolites in human plasma. J Sep Sci 2010;33:23−30.

[39] Malfara WR, Bertucci C, Costa Queiroz ME, et al. Reliable HPLC method for therapeutic drug monitoring of frequently prescribed tricyclic and nontricyclic antidepressants. J Pharm Biomed Anal 2007;44:955−62.

[40] Hasselstrom J. Quantification of antidepressants and antipsychotics in human serum by precipitation and ultra high pressure liquid chromatography-tandem mass spectrometry. J Chromatogr B Analyt Technol Biomed Life Sci 2011;879:123−8.

[41] Breaud AR, Harlan R, Kozak M, Clarke W. A rapid and reliable method for the quantitation of tricyclic antidepressants in serum using HPLC-MS/MS. Clin Biochem 2009;42:1300−7.

[42] de Castro A, Concheiro M, Quintela O, et al. LC-MS/MS method for the determination of nine antidepressants and some of their main metabolites in oral fluid and plasma. Study of correlation between venlafaxine concentrations in both matrices. J Pharm Biomed Anal 2008;48:183−93.

[43] Kollroser M, Schober C. Simultaneous determination of seven tricyclic antidepressant drugs in human plasma by direct-injection HPLC-APCI-MS-MS with an ion trap detector. Ther Drug Monit 2002;24:537−44.

[44] Titier K, Castaing N, Le-Deodic M, et al. Quantification of tricyclic antidepressants and monoamine oxidase inhibitors by high-performance liquid chromatography-tandem mass spectrometry in whole blood. J Anal Toxicol 2007;31:200−7.

[45] Preskorn SH, Bupp SJ, Weller EB, Weller RA. Plasma levels of imipramine and metabolites in 68 hospitalized children. J Am Acad Child Adolesc Psychiatry 1989;28:373−5.

[46] Ziegler VE, Biggs JT. Tricyclic plasma levels. Effect of age, race, sex, and smoking. J Am Med Assoc 1977;238:2167−9.

[47] Ciraulo DA, Barnhill JG, Jaffe JH. Clinical pharmacokinetics of imipramine and desipramine in alcoholics and normal volunteers. Clin Pharmacol Ther 1988;43:509−18.

[48] Muller MJ, Dragicevic A, Fric M, et al. Therapeutic drug monitoring of tricyclic antidepressants: how does it work under clinical conditions? Pharmacopsychiatry 2003;36:98−104.

[49] Wilkinson GR. Drug metabolism and variability among patients in drug response. N Engl J Med 2005;352:2211−21.

[50] Garg U. Pitfalls in measuring antidepressant drugs. In: Dasgupta A, editor. Handbook of Drug Monitoring Methods: Therapeutics and Drugs of Abuse. Totowa, NJ: Humana Press; 2008. p. 133−63.

[51] Pfuhlmann B, Gerlach M, Burger R, et al. Therapeutic drug monitoring of tricyclic antidepressants in everyday clinical practice. J Neural Transm Suppl 2007:287−96.

[52] Wille SM, Cooreman SG, Neels HM, Lambert WE. Relevant issues in the monitoring and the toxicology of antidepressants. Crit Rev Clin Lab Sci 2008;45:25−89.

[53] Ables AZ, Baughman III OL. Antidepressants: update on new agents and indications. Am Fam Physician 2003;67:547−54.

[54] Pacher P, Kecskemeti V. Trends in the development of new antidepressants. Is there a light at the end of the tunnel? Curr Med Chem 2004;11:925−43.

[55] Fournier JC, DeRubeis RJ, Hollon SD, et al. Antidepressant drug effects and depression severity: a patient-level meta-analysis. J Am Med Assoc 2010;303:47−53.

[56] Lacy CF, Armstrong LL, Goldman MP, Lance LL. Lexi-Comp's Drug Information Handbook. Hudson, OH: Lexi-Comp; 2006.

[57] Ganetsky M. Selective Serotonin Reuptake Inhibitor Poisoning. Waltham, MA: UpToDate; 2011.

[58] Caccia S. Metabolism of the newer antidepressants. An overview of the pharmacological and pharmacokinetic implications. Clin Pharmacokinet 1998;34:281−302.

[59] Preskorn SH. Clinically relevant pharmacology of selective serotonin reuptake inhibitors. An overview with emphasis on pharmacokinetics and effects on oxidative drug metabolism. Clin Pharmacokinet 1997; 32(Suppl. 1):1−21.

[60] Evans RW. The FDA alert on serotonin syndrome with combined use of SSRIs or SNRIs and Triptans: an analysis of the 29 case reports. MedGenMed 2007;9:48.

[61] Garg U. Therapeutic drug monitoring of antidepressants. In: Hammett-Stabler CA, Dasgupta A, editors. Therapeutic Drug Monitoring Data. Washington, DC: AACC Press; 2007. p. 107−28.

[62] Wille SM, Van Hee P, Neels HM, et al. Comparison of electron and chemical ionization modes by validation of a quantitative gas chromatographic-mass spectrometric assay of new generation antidepressants and their active metabolites in plasma. J Chromatogr A 2007;1176:236—45.

[63] Wille SM, Maudens KE, Van Peteghem CH, Lambert WE. Development of a solid phase extraction for 13 "new" generation antidepressants and their active metabolites for gas chromatographic-mass spectrometric analysis. J Chromatogr A 2005;1098:19—29.

[64] Bickeboeller-Friedrich J, Maurer HH. Screening for detection of new antidepressants, neuroleptics, hypnotics, and their metabolites in urine by GC—MS developed using rat liver microsomes. Ther Drug Monit 2001;23:61—70.

[65] Namera A, Watanabe T, Yashiki M, et al. Simple analysis of tetracyclic antidepressants in blood using headspace-solid phase microextraction and GC-MS. J Anal Toxicol 1998;22:396—400.

[66] Plenis A, Baczek T. Modern chromatographic and electrophoretic measurements of antidepressants and their metabolites in biofluids. Biomed Chromatogr 2011;25:164—98.

[67] Sauvage FL, Gaulier JM, Lachatre G, Marquet P. A fully automated turbulent-flow liquid chromatography-tandem mass spectrometry technique for monitoring antidepressants in human serum. Ther Drug Monit 2006;28:123—30.

[68] Castaing N, Titier K, Receveur-Daurel M, et al. Quantification of eight new antidepressants and five of their active metabolites in whole blood by high-performance liquid chromatography-tandem mass spectrometry. J Anal Toxicol 2007;31:334—41.

[69] Spear BB, Heath-Chiozzi M, Huff J. Clinical application of pharmacogenetics. Trends Mol Med 2001;7:201—4.

[70] de Leon J, Susce MT, Johnson M, et al. DNA microarray technology in the clinical environment: the AmpliChip CYP450 test for CYP2D6 and CYP2C19 genotyping. CNS Spectr 2009;14:19—34.

[71] Doris A, Ebmeier K, Shajahan P. Depressive illness. Lancet 1999;354:1369—75.

[72] Kirchheiner J, Seeringer A, Viviani R. Pharmacogenetics in psychiatry — a useful clinical tool or wishful thinking for the future? Curr Pharm Des 2010;16:136—44.

[73] Gervasini G, Benitez J, Carrillo JA. Pharmacogenetic testing and therapeutic drug monitoring are complementary tools for optimal individualization of drug therapy. Eur J Clin Pharmacol 2010;66:755—74.

[74] Ingelman-Sundberg M. Pharmacogenetics of cytochrome P450 and its applications in drug therapy: the past, present and future. Trends Pharmacol Sci 2004;25:193—200.

[75] Ingelman-Sundberg M. Human drug metabolising cytochrome P450 enzymes: properties and polymorphisms. Naunyn Schmiedebergs Arch Pharmacol 2004;369:89—104.

[76] Ingelman-Sundberg M, Oscarson M, McLellan RA. Polymorphic human cytochrome P450 enzymes: an opportunity for individualized drug treatment. Trends Pharmacol Sci 1999;20:342—9.

[77] Kirchheiner J, Nickchen K, Bauer M, et al. Pharmacogenetics of antidepressants and antipsychotics: the contribution of allelic variations to the phenotype of drug response. Mol Psychiatry 2004;9:442—73.

[78] Dalen P, Dahl ML, Bernal Ruiz ML, et al. 10-Hydroxylation of nortriptyline in white persons with 0, 1, 2, 3, and 13 functional CYP2D6 genes. Clin Pharmacol Ther 1998;63:444—52.

[79] Kawanishi C, Lundgren S, Agren H, Bertilsson L. Increased incidence of CYP2D6 gene duplication in patients with persistent mood disorders: ultrarapid metabolism of antidepressants as a cause of nonresponse. A pilot study. Eur J Clin Pharmacol 2004;59:803—7.

[80] Grasmader K, Verwohlt PL, Rietschel M, et al. Impact of polymorphisms of cytochrome-P450 isoenzymes 2C9, 2C19 and 2D6 on plasma concentrations and clinical effects of antidepressants in a naturalistic clinical setting. Eur J Clin Pharmacol 2004;60:329—36.

[81] Shams ME, Arneth B, Hiemke C, et al. CYP2D6 polymorphism and clinical effect of the antidepressant venlafaxine. J Clin Pharm Ther 2006;31:493—502.

[82] Murphy Jr GM, Kremer C, Rodrigues HE, Schatzberg AF. Pharmacogenetics of antidepressant medication intolerance. Am J Psychiatry 2003;160:1830—5183.

[83] de Leon J, Armstrong SC, Cozza KL. Clinical guidelines for psychiatrists for the use of pharmacogenetic testing for CYP450 2D6 and CYP450 2C19. Psychosomatics 2006;47:75—85.

[84] Vetti HH, Molven A, Eliassen AK, Steen VM. Is pharmacogenetic CYP2D6 testing useful? Tidsskr Nor Laegeforen 2010;130:2224—8.

[85] LLerena A, Dorado P, Berecz R, et al. Effect of CYP2D6 and CYP2C9 genotypes on fluoxetine and norfluoxetine plasma concentrations during steady-state conditions. Eur J Clin Pharmacol 2004;59:869—73.

[86] Scordo MG, Spina E, Dahl ML, et al. Influence of CYP2C9, 2C19 and 2D6 genetic polymorphisms on the steady-state plasma concentrations of the enantiomers of fluoxetine and norfluoxetine. Basic Clin Pharmacol Toxicol 2005;97:296—301.

[87] Yin OQ, Wing YK, Cheung Y, et al. Phenotype—genotype relationship and clinical effects of citalopram in Chinese patients. J Clin Psychopharmacol 2006;26:367—72.

[88] Peters EJ, Slager SL, Kraft JB, et al. Pharmacokinetic genes do not influence response or tolerance to citalopram in the STAR*D sample. PLoS One 2008;3:e1872.

[89] McMahon FJ, Buervenich S, Charney D, et al. Variation in the gene encoding the serotonin 2A receptor is associated with outcome of antidepressant treatment. Am J Hum Genet 2006;78:804—14.

[90] Kato M, Serretti A. Review and meta-analysis of antidepressant pharmacogenetic findings in major depressive disorder. Mol Psychiatry 2010;15:473—500.

[91] Sullivan PF, Neale MC, Kendler KS. Genetic epidemiology of major depression: review and meta-analysis. Am J Psychiatry 2000;157:1552—62.

[92] Malhotra AK. The pharmacogenetics of depression: enter the GWAS. Am J Psychiatry 2010;167:493—5.

[93] Uher R, Perroud N, Ng MY, et al. Genome-wide pharmacogenetics of antidepressant response in the GENDEP project. Am J Psychiatry 2010;167:555—864.

[94] Ising M, Lucae S, Binder EB, et al. A genomewide association study points to multiple loci that predict antidepressant drug treatment outcome in depression. Arch Gen Psychiatry 2009;66:966—75.

Therapeutic Drug Monitoring of Selected Anticancer Drugs
Pharmacogenomics Issues

Michael C. Milone

Department of Pathology and Laboratory Medicine,
University of Pennsylvania School of Medicine, Philadelphia, PA

Therapeutic Drug Monitoring: Newer Drugs and Biomarkers
DOI: 10.1016/B978-0-12-385467-4.00014-2

291

INTRODUCTION

Drug therapy has long been practiced in a personalized fashion, where physicians tailor therapies to meet the special needs and values of their patients. In cancer therapy, where the risks of therapy are often high with efficacy that may be quite low, individualization of therapy is tantamount. The first decision often centers on whether to use a particular anti-cancer drug. Should erlotinib be first-line therapy in a 60-year-old male with a 20 pack-year smoking history and a less curable (T2N1) non-small cell lung cancer? Should the 40-year-old female patient with a 0.5-cm adenocarcinoma of the breast and negative lymph nodes receive adjuvant therapy with tamoxifen following resection? After the oncologist and patient have weighed all available evidence regarding treatment risks and benefits and made the decision to use a drug, the oncologist must then further adjust the dose and schedule of drug therapy according to a number of factors, such as age, weight and renal function, that affect the efficacy and toxicity of therapy. Despite this personalized tailoring, most anticancer agents still have a relatively low success rate. The poor success is likely multifaceted; however, variation in human physiology and tumor biology unquestionably makes large contributions to treatment failure.

Genetic factors are increasingly being recognized as important variables affecting the pharmacokinetic and pharmacodynamic variation of many drugs. Techniques for DNA genotyping, gene expression profiling and deep genome sequencing have exploded over the past decade, as discussed in Chapter 7. These technologies are leading us into a new era of personalized medicine, where there is great hope for highly specific, genetically tailored therapy. Cancer chemotherapy is leading the way. Several genetic and other biomarker tests have been introduced over the past decade for anticancer agents, with some becoming part of the standard of care for these drugs. This chapter will focus upon the most promising tests for "personalization" of anticancer drugs, and discuss some of the challenges to implementing these tests in a routine clinical setting.

TRADITIONAL THERAPEUTIC DRUG MONITORING FOR ANTICANCER DRUGS

Unlike other areas of pharmacology, traditional therapeutic drug monitoring (TDM) has been applied in a very limited fashion to anticancer drugs. In the US, only busulfan and methotrexate are routinely monitored in the clinical setting.

Monitoring of Methotrexate

Methotrexate (4-amino-10-methylpteroylglutamic acid) is an antimetabolite used for treating a wide range of neoplastic and non-neoplastic disorders. In some cases, such as rheumatologic disease, methotrexate is administered chronically at a low dose. It has been well established that life-threatening toxicity from methotrexate correlates with the dose and serum concentration reached with a particular dose; however, the duration of exposure to high concentrations is more important than the concentration. It is therefore possible to capitalize upon this pharmacodynamics behavior by subjecting patients to a short exposure of very high concentrations of methotrexate. This promotes the beneficial uptake of the drug into cells and compartments unaffected by lower doses of methotrexate, provided the unwanted toxic effects of methotrexate are countered sufficiently with the reduced folate, leucovorin (folinic acid, citrovorum factor) [1]. This "rescue" therapy with leucovorin permits methotrexate doses that would otherwise be lethal, and renders the therapy relatively free of toxicity; however, use of high-dose therapy with leucovorin rescue is not without its challenges. Insufficient leucovorin therapy following high-dose methotrexate can lead to significant, irreversible toxicity and a fatal outcome [2].

Most individuals eliminate methotrexate predictably, but methotrexate elimination can be prolonged in some individuals, placing them at high risk for severe toxicity and/or death if leucovorin rescue therapy is prematurely discontinued. Methotrexate concentration monitoring is a standard component of high-dose methotrexate treatment. High-dose methotrexate treatment regimens vary in the dose and duration of methotrexate infusions; however, the approach to using methotrexate serum concentration monitoring is generally the same with leucovorin therapy typically initiated 24–48 hours after the start of methotrexate. Methotrexate levels, most commonly determined using simple, rapid immunoassay techniques, are measured starting 24 hours after the initiation of methotrexate. Measurements are continued daily, with the leucovorin dose adjusted according to measured drug concentrations and established nomograms. Methotrexate monitoring is generally continued until the concentration falls below a 50-nmol/L threshold concentration, at which point leucovorin is discontinued. Use of this simple concentration-monitoring scheme reduces the incidence of severe, life-threatening toxicity from high-dose methotrexate therapy [3–10], and demonstrates the tremendous impact that a TDM program can have on drug therapy.

Monitoring of Busulfan

In contrast to methotrexate, in which TDM is used to control rescue therapy rather than adjust drug dosage, high-dose busulfan therapy represents a more traditional use of TDM in applied pharmacokinetics. Busulfan is primarily used as part of the myeloablation regimen in combination with cyclophosphamide, fludarabine or total body irradiation for hematopoietic stem cell transplantation. Busulfan therapy is complicated by significant inter-patient variability in pharmacokinetic behavior. The coefficient of variation (%CV) for busulfan area under the concentration–time curve (AUC) has been reported to be 23% [11] and 25% [12] for the oral and IV formulations, respectively. Age, obesity, underlying disease and organ dysfunction also exert a significant influence on observed clearance for busulfan. Children under the age of 6 typically display more than twice the average clearance of 2.5 ml/min·kg reported for adults [13, 14]. While the AUC variability for busulfan is not as high as that observed with other drugs, the observed variability is nevertheless clinically relevant. Several studies have identified a pharmacodynamic relationship between exposure to busulfan and both its toxicity and efficacy. The risk of toxicity due to busulfan (veno-occlusive disease or pulmonary toxicity) rises significantly with a steady-state concentration (C_{ss}) that exceeds 900–1025 ng/ml [15–18]. In contrast, the risk of relapse in patients undergoing hematopoietic stem cell transplant for chronic myelogenous leukemia rises substantially with a C_{ss} of < 917 ng/ml, indicating that a very narrow therapeutic range of exposure exists for this drug [19].

Control of busulfan exposure within this tight range requires an accurate and precise estimate of exposure. In order to achieve this level of accuracy and precision, a pharmacokinetic (PK) study using extensive sampling is often necessary. Early approaches used non-compartmental analysis with estimation of AUC using the trapezoidal rule. Although this approach was effective, fitting the concentration data to a one-compartment, first-order PK model by non-linear regression has become the preferred method for estimating the C_{ss} or AUC for a dose interval. Dosing of busulfan is usually performed every 6 hours over 4 days for a total of 16 doses. As a result, a study is typically performed following the first dose, and the results are promptly reported in order to effect a dose adjustment as early as possible in the course of the treatment regimen. However, the completion and reporting of a busulfan pharmacokinetic study is not a simple task. A variety of chromatographic methods are used for measurement of busulfan in plasma, with GC-MS (gas chromatography combined with mass spectrometry) generally the preferred method. Given the complexity of this analytical method, onsite testing is not always available. Sample extraction and analysis also usually require several hours to complete for a single patient. Nevertheless, using the above labor-intensive TDM approach with dose adjustment, exposures that are within < 10% of the target exposure are possible, and toxicity can be avoided without a compromise in efficacy [15, 16, 18–20].

NEWER APPROACHES TO PERSONALIZED DOSING AND TREATMENT WITH ANTICANCER AGENTS: PHARMACOGENETICS

With the advent of the Human Genome Project and the increasingly robust technology for DNA sequencing and genotyping, personalized genomics and biomarkers have become the "holy grail" of modern anticancer therapy. While there still may be a role for traditional PK monitoring of many anticancer agents, genetics and other biomarkers offer a number of real advantages. Most notably, genomics, especially constitutional genomics, permits the ability to test patients prior to administration of a drug, with the potential to avoid early adverse events. It also offers the possibility to assess factors influencing the pharmacodynamic behavior of a drug, such as a drug's receptor or transporters that control access of the drug to its site of action. Neither of these factors can be assessed by traditional TDM using drug concentrations in blood. In the oncology realm, it is also well established that cancer is a genetic disease. A number of genetic events underlie the transformation of normal cells to cancer, and these events affect the responsiveness of an individual tumor to chemotherapy. Genetic and molecular analysis of tumors provides at least one approach to providing more individualized chemotherapy to patients; however, there are novel issues surrounding tumor genetics when compared to evaluating the constitutional (or germline) genetics of the tumor's "host".

Constitutional Genetics versus Tumor Genetics

While common technologies may be used to evaluate genetic variability, the analysis of constitutional and tumor genetics each offers unique challenges that must be well understood in order to practically and safely apply this information to the care of patients.

Constitutional genetic factors contribute to the pharmacokinetic (PK) and pharmacodynamic (PD) variability of most drugs. Inherited polymorphisms have been described in the drug transporters and enzymes mediating Phase I biotransformation reactions and Phase II conjugation reactions [21–24]. Some of these polymorphisms affect the expression and/or function of these transporters and enzymes, leading to differences in drug absorption, distribution, metabolism and elimination. Unfortunately, while a plethora of studies demonstrate associations between individual polymorphisms and the PK/PD variability of many drugs, few studies have successfully demonstrated a clinically meaningful benefit to prospective use of genetic information to enhance drug efficacy or reduce drug toxicity. There are many reasons for the failure of a pharmacogenetic test. The complex, multigenic nature of drug metabolism is part of the problem. The cytochrome P450 enzyme system illustrates some of the challenges to using constitutional genetic information in pharmacogenetically-guided drug therapy. Multiple genes encode the cytochrome P450 mixed function oxidase family of enzymes (CYP enzymes). Numerous polymorphisms in CYP enzymes exist. Some of these polymorphisms are relatively frequent in some ethnic populations, and some are completely absent in others. Thus, a genetic test developed and proven useful in one patient population may be useless in another. The genetics of drug-metabolizing enzymes is also complex. Consider the CYP3A enzymes, which metabolize more than 50% of clinically useful drugs. CYP3A activity has been reported to vary from 30-fold to more than 100-fold between individuals [25]. The CYP enzymes show constitutive and inducible expression in diverse tissues, especially the liver and intestines. The expression level and pattern varies with age, gender, diet and concomitant drug therapy, and epistatic factors such as genetic variability in steroid receptors interact with environmental factors to produce an individual CYP3A metabolism phenotype. Some drugs also inhibit the enzymatic activity of CYP isoenzymes. Due to the similarity between CYP enzymes, a drug may also undergo CYP-mediated oxidative metabolism by more than one CYP family member, such as the overlapping substrate specificities of CYP3A4 and CYP3A5. The overlapping metabolism of CYP3A4 and CYP3A5 along with the inducible and variable nature of expression for both enzymes produces very complex genetic interactions for this important enzyme system [26]. Despite these challenges, genetic polymorphisms that influence the toxicity and efficacy of clinically important drugs have been described, and information regarding CYP2D6, uridine diphosphate glucuronosyltransferase 1 family polypeptide 1 (UGT1A1), vitamin K epoxide reductase complex subunit 1 (VKORC1), CYP2C19 and thiopurine methyl transferase (TPMT) genetics is currently included in the labeling for some drugs [27].

Unlike constitutional genetics, analyzing the genetics of a cancer is a far more complicated matter. The cells within a cancer may harbor genetic variation that is distinct from the normal cells of the individual. These genetic alterations may not only contribute to the development and progression of cancer, but also affect the response of a cancer to drug therapy. Tumors are also complex tissues. In addition to the cancer cells that harbor oncogenic, genetic changes, normal fibroblasts, macrophages, vascular endothelial cells and other cell types are often present within a tumor. These stromal elements are essential to formation and survival of the tumor, and their abundance relative to the transformed cells of the cancer varies widely between different cancers as well as within an individual tumor. Even the cancer cells, despite a clonal origin, may vary genetically within a given tumor, and between a primary tumor and a metastatic tumor [28, 148].

The significant heterogeneity within a tumor therefore challenges genetic analysis. This is especially true when the analysis must be performed on small samples such as a needle core biopsy, where sampling errors may be severe. Performing the analysis therefore requires the expertise of a pathologist to ensure selection of appropriate material for analysis. The processing of tissues in standard formalin fixative also poses problems for some analyses in comparison to the specimens typically employed for constitutional genetic testing. An in-depth analysis of epidermal growth factor receptor (EGFR) mutations in BR21 trial (BR21 is the trial code), which demonstrated a much higher rate of rare mutations compared with similar trials, revealed that fixation led to deamination of cytosine and mutation artifacts in low-concentration DNA specimens [29].

PHARMACOGENETIC CONSIDERATIONS FOR SPECIFIC ANTICANCER AGENTS

Chemotherapy with several anticancer drugs may benefit from pharmacogenomics testing. In this section of the chapter the current knowledge of such testing is discussed.

Mercaptopurine Class of Drugs

Originally developed in the 1950s for their potent cytotoxic activity, the thiopurine drugs 6-mercaptopurine, azathioprine (azo precursor to 6-mercaptopurine) and 6-thioguanine represent a class of drugs that are used today to treat cancer (such as pediatric acute lymphoblastic leukemia) along with rheumatologic disease, inflammatory bowel disease and solid organ transplant rejection. These agents derive their potent pharmacologic activity from the dependence of normal and malignant lymphocytes on purine metabolism for robust proliferation and function. Following the bio-activation of 6-mercaptopurine and 6-thioguanine through phospho-ribosylation via hypoxanthine-guanine phosphoribosyl-transferase (HGPRT) and conversion to 6-thioguanine nucleotides, these thiol-containing nucleotides are readily incorporated into DNA (Fig. 14.1). Cell death by apoptosis ensues due to failure of base mismatch repair induced by the "false" nature of these thioguanine nucleotides. Incorporation into RNA and inhibition of purine biosynthesis are likely to further contribute to the cytotoxic effect of these compounds. In addition to the cytotoxic activity of these drugs, guanine nucleotides also play important roles in T-lymphocyte development, activation and function through their role in the regulation of small GTPase proteins (a large family of hydrolase enzymes that can bind and hydrolyze guanosine triphosphate) like Ras and Rap1. Interruption of these latter signal transduction pathways may contribute to the immunosuppressive effects of 6-mercaptopurine and azathioprine.

Myelosuppression represents the most pronounced toxicity associated with the thiopurine drugs. The dose-dependence of myelosuppression is well recognized; however, some individuals are much more sensitive to the myelosuppressive effects of 6-mercaptopurine and azathioprine than others. The pharmacokinetic behavior of 6-mercaptopurine and azathioprine are characterized by poor oral bioavailability ($< 25\%$) with a relatively short half-life ($t_{1/2}$) of approximately 50 minutes. The clearance of 6-mercaptopurine is variable, and is mediated primarily via two enzymatic pathways: (1) oxidation to thiouric acid by xanthine

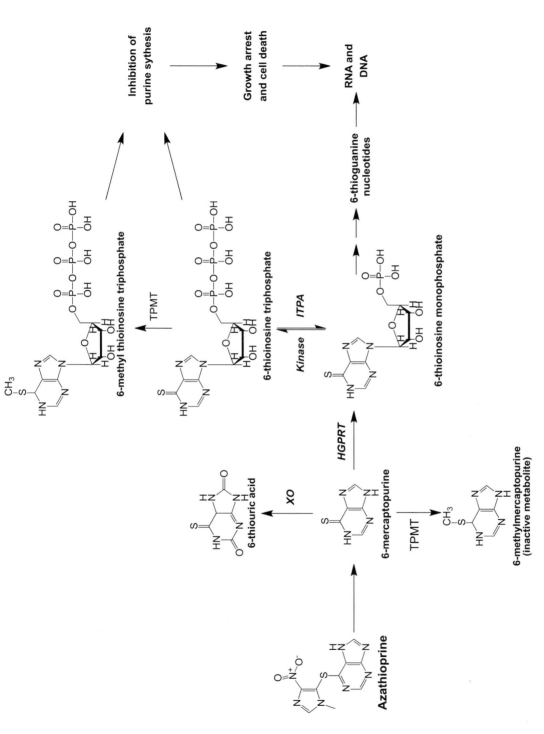

FIGURE 14.1 Thiopurine metabolism. The thiopurine drugs azathioprine, mercaptopurine and 6-thioguanine undergo metabolism within the normal salvage and catabolism pathways for purine nucleotides. TPMT, thiopurine methyltransferase; XO, xanthine oxidase; HGPRT, hypoxanthine-guanine phosphoribosyltransferase; ITPA, inosine triphosphate pyrophosphatase.

oxidase, and (2) *S*-methylation via thiopurine *S*-methyltransferase (TPMT). Xanthine oxidase contributes significantly to the poor bioavailability of 6-mercaptopurine and azathioprine through first-pass metabolism within the intestines and liver. Inhibition of xanthine oxidase via allopurinol leads to a five-fold increase in 6-mercaptopurine bioavailability. In contrast, allopurinol exhibits little effect on 6-mercaptopurine pharmacokinetics in plasma, suggesting that the contribution of xanthine oxidase to metabolism once the drug is absorbed is negligible [30].

The large inter-individual variability in sensitivity to toxicity noted with these drugs has led to the search for genetic factors that might contribute to the pharmacokinetic and pharmacodynamics variation of these drugs. TPMT-mediated metabolism appears to be the principle mechanism for plasma clearance of 6-mercaptopurine. Studies in the 1980s demonstrated that Caucasian individuals could be classified into three categories of TPMT activity based upon enzymatic assays of TPMT in red blood cell lysates, with frequencies suggestive of a monogenic inherited trait in Hardy-Weinberg equilibrium [31]. Individuals with the lowest TPMT activity, approximately 0.3% of Caucasians, exhibit approximately 10-fold higher erythrocyte 6-thioguanine nucleotide concentrations compared with the majority of individuals with "wild-type" enzymatic activity following 6-mercaptopurine therapy [32]. All individuals with the lowest TPMT phenotype suffer severe toxicity associated with doses of 6-mercaptopurine derived from population-based PK/PD studies. Individuals with intermediate activity (~11% in Caucasian populations) also demonstrate higher levels of erythrocyte 6-thioguanine nucleotide concentrations that are intermediate between individuals with wild-type and low activity. The pharmacodynamics effects of this intermediate phenotype are still relevant, with 30−60% of heterozygous individuals experiencing significant 6-mercaptopurine-associated toxicity requiring dose reductions [32, 33]. These findings support the importance of TPMT as the principle mechanism for 6-mercaptopurine and azathioprine clearance, and they further suggest that pre-treatment recognition of individuals in the reduced metabolism category will benefit from a dose-reduction in 6-mercaptopurine or azathioprine. Although TMPT activity is associated with the toxicity of these drugs, TPMT may only explain approximately a third of the toxicity [34]. Additional polymorphisms in genes such as inosine triphosphate phosphorylase (*ITPA*) also appear to contribute to the toxicity of these drugs [35]. Much less is known about the relationship between TPMT activity and 6-thioguanine pharmacokinetics or pharmacodynamics; however, the dependence of 6-thioguanine nucleotide on TPMT for methylation leading to inactivation (Fig. 14.1) suggests that 6-thioguanine PK should be well correlated with TPMT phenotype [36].

Identification of individuals with reduced TPMT activity can be accomplished via measurement of TPMT enzymatic activity in red blood cell lysates as used in the early original studies described above; however, a number of potential confounding variables limit the sensitivity and specificity of this testing. Erythrocyte TPMT enzymatic activity varies with the age of the red blood cells (RBC) [37]. Processes that alter normal RBC turnover and the average age of RBCs may therefore contribute significant, non-genetic variability to TPMT activity analysis. Activity measurements are further complicated by transfusion, which will most likely provide RBCs with normal TPMT activity.

Due the limitations of erythrocyte (red blood cells) TPMT activity testing, genetic testing has been advocated as an alternative to phenotypic testing. Currently, over 21 different genetic changes that can contribute to reduced or absent TPMT activity have been identified. Studies in Caucasian populations have revealed that more than 90% of low activity alleles are due to three relatively common variants, designated *TPMT *2*, *TPMT *3A* and *TPMT *3B*. Many commercial laboratories currently offering *TPMT* genotype testing limit their testing to only these common alleles. Due to genetic differences among ethnic populations, these commercial *TPMT* genotype tests may therefore miss a considerable proportion of deficient alleles in individuals, particularly individuals of non-Caucasian ancestry [38–41]. Testing platforms that permit detection of all identified alleles have been described [42], but these methods have not been widely deployed to date.

Given the limitation of both methods of testing, the method of choice for detection of TPMT deficiency still remains somewhat unclear. The method chosen will likely depend upon a number of factors, such as access to testing, prior transfusion of the patient and, of course, cost. A systematic review of the literature by Donnan *et al.* evaluated 26 separate English-language articles reporting on the performance characteristics (sensitivity and specificity) of genotypic or phenotypic testing for detection of TPMT deficiency [43]. A range of different genotypic and phenotypic methods has been employed, and most genotyping studies included the common TPMT alleles in testing; however, the variant alleles observed more frequently in non-Caucasian populations were not consistently included. Studies were also small and generally underpowered for evaluating the detection of individuals who are homozygous for deficient alleles of *TMPT*. When comparing genotyping to TPMT enzymatic testing as a reference standard, the sensitivity of genotyping for detecting TPMT-deficient individuals ranges from 55% to 100%, with a specificity of 95–100%. Alternatively, five of the six studies that used genotyping as the reference standard demonstrate a sensitivity of 100% for enzymatic testing. A lower specificity in the range of 86–98% is reported for these studies that is likely due to both unknown genetic factors contributing to TPMT deficiency and falsely low test results arising due to the known limitations of erythrocyte enzyme testing. In the context of the typical prevalence of TPMT deficiency in the mostly white European populations studied, the negative predictive value (NPV) of genetic testing for deficiency detection ranged from 82% to 100%. A NPV of less than 100% is expected, given the inability of a limited set of genetic factors to explain all causes of TPMT deficiency. The situation is further complicated by the generally underpowered studies, which fail to include many homozygous, severely deficient individuals. Thus, either test identifies mostly individuals with intermediate (heterozygous) deficiency. While toxicity from 6-mercaptopurine, such as leukopenia, is associated with intermediate enzyme activity, the frequency, severity and the clinical relevance of the toxicity is unclear. The package inserts for 6-mercaptopurine and azathioprine currently contain information for clinicians regarding TPMT deficiency. Few studies have attempted to evaluate the utility of genotypic or phenotypic testing in a randomized, prospective clinical trial.

Irinotecan

Irinotecan (IRN, CPT-11, Camptosar™ [Pfizer, New York]) is an integral component of chemotherapy regimens in patients with colorectal carcinoma. It is most commonly combined with either 5-fluorouracil and leucovorin (FOLFIRI regimen) or a platinum compound such as oxaliplatin (FOLFOX and IROX regimens). Early phase evaluation of irinotecan identified hematologic and gastrointestinal toxicity as the major dose-limiting adverse effects of this drug. Gastrointestinal toxicity and the combined occurrence of multiple toxicities have been associated with fatalities on an irinotecan-containing regimen, supporting the importance of early recognition and prevention of these adverse events [44]. While toxicity from irinotecan likely depends upon the regimen, with bolus 5-fluorouracil therapy exhibiting potentially greater toxicity compared with infusional regimens [45], hematologic and gastrointestinal toxicity occurs with all regimens. As with most drugs, irinotecan toxicity correlates with dose and likely exposure to the drug [44]. While pharmacokinetic assessment can sometimes aid in predicting toxicity, as in busulfan, the pharmacokinetic behavior of irinotecan, while variable [46, 47], is also rather complex. Irinotecan is primarily a pro-drug that is rapidly metabolized by ubiquitously expressed carboxylesterase to 7-ethyl-10-hydroxycamptothecin (also known as SN-38), which is a potently active metabolite; however, SN-38 is a lactone that isomerizes to its open carboxylate form in a pH-dependent manner with activity of only the lactone form. Given that pH may vary widely throughout tissues, the ability to predict active SN-38 at the site of action from blood concentrations is limited. Traditional concentration monitoring is therefore unlikely to be very helpful for this drug. SN-38 elimination occurs predominantly via UDP-glucuronosyltransferase 1A (UGT1A) mediated conjugation and hepatic elimination [48]. It was recognized early that glucuronidation correlated with the risk for irinotecan toxicity [49]. These findings led to investigation of UGT1A enzymes and irinotecan toxicity.

Case reports of individuals with Gilbert's syndrome and severe toxicity supported the association of irinotecan toxicity and UGT1A activity [50], and the activity of UGT1A1 as the principle enzyme responsible for irinotecan glucuronidation was subsequently confirmed [51]. The relatively common UGT1A1*28 allele associated with reduced activity in Gilbert's syndrome showed altered glucuronidation *in vivo*, setting the stage for several studies evaluating UGT1A1 genetics and irinotecan toxicity. Multiple studies over the past decade have clearly confirmed the association between homozygosity for the UGT1A1*28 allele and irinotecan-induced neutropenia. Hu *et al.* reviewed this important topic [52]. The association with gastrointestinal toxicity has been somewhat less clear, but a meta-analysis of 20 trials totaling 1760 patients demonstrated that the risk for severe diarrhea is significantly increased in patients who are homozygous for the UGT1A1*28 allele and receive a high-dose irinotecan regimen [53]. Based upon the data available, the FDA encouraged relabeling of irinotecan to include a warning regarding the administration of irinotecan at standard doses to patients with the UGT1A1*28 allele. Nevertheless, it remains unclear whether the association between UGT1A1*28 and toxicity applies to all treatment regimens. A recent study by McLeod *et al.* of 520 patients receiving the IFL (irinotecan + -fluorouracil), FOLFOX (fluorouracil + oxaliplatin) or IROX (irinotecan + oxaliplatin) regimens demonstrated a association between UGT1A1*28 homozygosity and toxicity; however, the association was only statistically significant in the IROX treatment group [54]. They also found lower overall treatment response for patients with the UGT1A1*28 allele on IROX, suggesting that UGT1A1*28/*28 patients may tend to be under-dosed on this regimen. This study and others also demonstrate that a number of polymorphisms in additional genes, such as GSTM1, GSTP1 (genes controlling activities of glutathione S transferases superfamily of dimeric Phase II metabolic enzymes that catalyze the conjugation of reduced glutathione with various electrophilic compounds) and CYP3A5 were associated with toxicity or efficacy of irinotecan-containing regimens for colorectal carcinoma, demonstrating the potential complexity of pharmacogenetics for this drug that is primarily used in combination [54, 55]. The UGT1A1*28 polymorphism also may not be useful in all populations, such as in Asian populations where it is rarely found. UGT1A1*6, defined by a separate non-synonymous SNP in exon 1 of UGT1A1, has been observed with a higher frequency in Asians, and this allele exhibits a similar association with irinotecan toxicity, illustrating the importance of population considerations in pharmacogenetics [56–58].

Finally, a challenge faced by most oncologists who might attempt to use UGT1A1 genetics to adjust irinotecan chemotherapy is determining the degree of dose reduction that is safe but will still be effective in an individual patient such as a homozygous UTG1A1*28 carrier. Innocenti et al. have recommended a reduction to 30% of the standard dose of irinotecan in patients bearing the UGT1A1*28/*28 genotype [55]. While this may produce less toxicity, it is unclear whether it may also result in more failed therapies since not every patient with the UGT1A1*28/*28 genotype exhibits severe toxicity. Two recent Phase I dose escalation studies driven by UGT1A1 genetics demonstrate that patients carrying the wild-type UGT1A1*1 allele (i.e., homozygotes and heterozygotes) can tolerate substantially higher doses of irinotecan that are well above the current standard doses established prior to consideration of genetic factors [59, 60]. Given the established relationship between exposure and efficacy, these pharmacogenetically guided approaches to dosing suggest that greater efficacy may be achievable with personalized dosing, but more studies with other regimens and randomization based upon genetics are sorely needed.

5-Fluorouracil

5-Fluorouracil exhibits limited effectiveness as a single agent anticancer drug, but it is the most widely use anticancer agent worldwide, with incorporation into combination therapies for a range of malignancies of the gastrointestinal tract, the breast and the head and neck. Following conversion to a pyrimidine nucleotide, 5-fluorouracil exerts its cytotoxic activity through several mechanisms, including inhibition of thymidylate synthase and incorporation into DNA and RNA. The effects of 5-fluorouracil can be further enhanced by administration of leucovorin, which also inhibits thymidylate synthase, and this combination is frequently used. Numerous administration schemes are currently employed for 5-fluorouracil and leucovorin with some variation in timing, but there are two general approaches: continuous intravenous infusion of 5-fluorouracil, or bolus administration performed over repeated treatment cycles spaced by 1 to several weeks apart. The optimal administration of 5-fluorouracil that maximizes efficacy with minimized toxicity appears to depend upon the cancer and the co-administered chemotherapeutic drugs. A thorough discussion of the various 5-fluorouracil regimens can be found in Chabner and Longo [30].

5-Fluorouracil has been shown to display significant pharmacokinetic variability (%CV of ~ 35% for clearance with 24-hour constant infusion) [61]. Based upon this PK variability, dose adaptation based upon concentration monitoring has been advocated. In a randomized concentration-controlled trial of 5-fluorouracil that compared fixed dose to concentration-adapted dosing, patients who underwent pharmacokinetic-guided (PK-guided) dose adjustment experienced a statistically significant improvement in their objective response rate (33.7% in the adjusted-dose group versus 18.3% in the fixed-dose control group). Although toxicity was primarily grade I/II diarrhea and hand—foot syndrome, there was also a significant reduction in overall adverse events in the dose-adjusted group [62]. This study suggests that many patients receiving 5-fluorouracil at tolerable dosing determined by population-level studies may be receiving too little or too much of the drug. Unfortunately, this trial used a somewhat unconventional 5-fluorouracil regimen, so the transferability of their results to other regimens is less clear. Nevertheless, it does support the notion that we may be able to do better with more individualized dosing of anticancer drugs, including a drug like 5-fluorouracil that has been in use for over 40 years.

While active concentration monitoring is one potential method of individualization of 5-fluorouracil therapy, understanding the factors that affect 5-fluorouracil metabolism may be useful in predicting 5-fluorouracil pharmacokinetic and pharmacodynamic behavior. More than 80% of a single 5-fluorouracil dose is metabolized rapidly to inactive metabolites, with only 1—3% converted to active, cytotoxic metabolites through the cells' normal nucleotide synthetic pathways (see Fig. 14.2). The rate-limiting enzyme in 5-fluorouracil metabolism is the enzyme dihydropyrimidine dehydrogenase. Several studies have demonstrated that dihydropyrimidine dehydrogenase activity is highly variable in the general population, and 3—5% of Caucasians exhibit low dihydropyrimidine dehydrogenase activity. A single nucleotide polymorphism (SNP) at the splice site between exons 13 and 14 that leads to skipping of the 14th exon and a non-functional enzyme (known as c.1905+G>A, IVS14+G>A or DPD*2A) has been consistently demonstrated to be associated with dihydropyrimidine dehydrogenase deficiency in Caucasians and severe 5-FU toxicity; however, dihydropyrimidine dehydrogenase is a large gene with 23 exons and over 7000 SNPs. An association between a number of additional SNPs (e.g., 1679T>9 and 2846A>T) and dihydropyrimidine dehydrogenase and/or 5-fluorouracil toxicity has been reported (extensively reviewed in [63]). Of course, additional polymorphisms in genes involved in 5-fluorouracil action have also been shown to impact 5-fluorouracil efficacy and toxicity, either directly (thymidylate synthase) or indirectly (methylene-tetrahydrofolate reductase) [64]. It is clear that an individual's genetics impacts 5-fluorouracil therapy. The challenge of using this genetic information prospectively in routine clinical care remains, especially for 5-fluorouracil with such varied dosing schemes and combinations with other chemotherapeutic agents.

Tamoxifen

The estrogen receptor (ER) antagonist tamoxifen (trade names include Nolvadex™, Istubal™, Valodex™), is widely used in the treatment of ER-positive breast cancer and breast cancer chemoprevention. Despite the success of tamoxifen in the treatment of ER-positive breast cancer, 30—50% of patients will fail tamoxifen therapy [65, 66]. Although tamoxifen exhibits direct anti-estrogenic activity, it is best thought of as a pro-drug. Metabolism by CYP enzymes generates several metabolites of tamoxifen (Fig. 14.3). Two of these metabolites, 4-hydroxy-tamoxifen and endoxifen, exhibit much greater anti-estrogenic effects compared with tamoxifen. These metabolites are believed to be the primary compounds mediating tamoxifen's clinical activity, with endoxifen probably playing the more important role due to its higher plasma concentration relative to 4-hydroxy-tamoxifen in patients taking tamoxifen [67]. Although several CYPs are capable of metabolizing tamoxifen, CYP3A4/5 and CYP2D6 are the principle CYPs involved in tamoxifen metabolism. The formation of

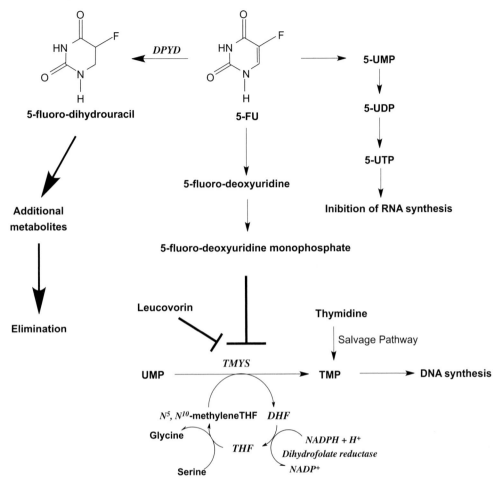

FIGURE 14.2 5-FU metabolism. 5-Fluorouracil enters the pathways of normal pyrimidine nucleotide synthesis leading to the formation of 5-fluoro-deoxyuridine monophosphate (5-dUMP), which is a potent inhibitor of thymidylate synthase (TYMS). The inhibition of *de novo* deoxythymidine monophosphate (dTMP) synthesis from deoxyuridine monophosphate (dUMP) by TYMS leads to cellular deficiency of dTTP affecting DNA synthesis. Incorporation of 5-fluoro-uridine triphosphate (5-FUTP) and 5-fluoro-deoxyuridine triphosphate (5-FdUTP) from 5-FU precursor further affects RNA and DNA synthesis. More than 80% of 5-FU is eliminated by dihydropyrimidine dehydrogenase (DPYD), which is the rate-limiting enzyme in the metabolism of 5-FU.

endoxifen appears to be highly dependent upon the presence of functional CYP2D6 alleles for its production [68].

The recognition of metabolism by CYP2D6 as a critical step in the biological activation of tamoxifen into endoxifen, and the recognition that CYP2D6 enzyme activity is highly variable in humans, led to clinical studies that evaluated the impact of CYP2D6 pharmacogenetics on tamoxifen efficacy (reviewed in [69]). The largest study performed, in a cohort of 1325 German and US women with early-stage (I–III) breast cancer, clearly demonstrated

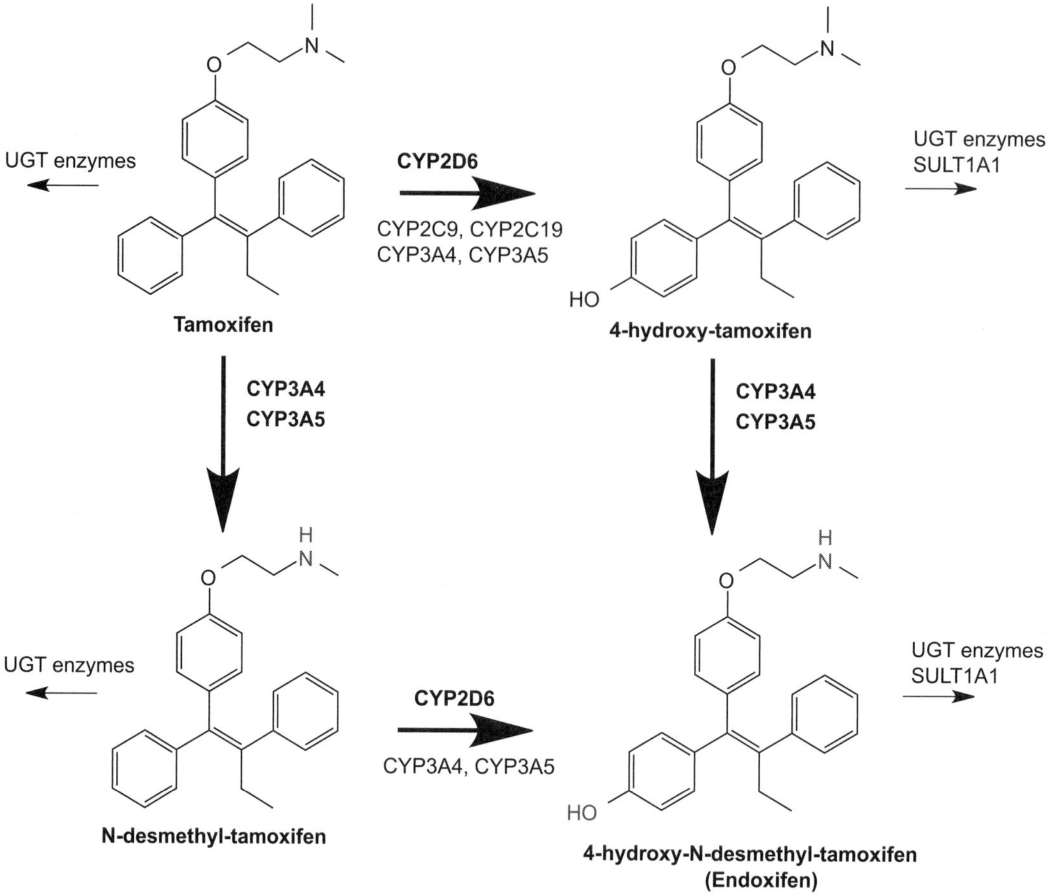

FIGURE 14.3 Tamoxifen metabolism. Tamoxifen undergoes metabolism via cytochrome P450 enzymes to form the active metabolites, 4-hydroxy-tamoxifen (4-OHT) and endoxifen. Both tamoxifen and its metabolites undergo further phase II conjugation via UDP-glucuronosyltransferase (UGT) and sulfotransferase (SULT1A1) enzymes.

an association between CYP2D6 alleles with reduce function and increased disease recurrence [70]. Compared with extensive metabolizers (extensive metabolizer, EM, defined by absence of CYP2D6*3, *4, *5, *10 or *41 alleles) comprising 46% of the population, poor metabolizers (poor metabolizers, PM, defined as homozygotes or compound heterozygotes for the CYP2D6*3, *4 or *5 alleles) that comprised 6% of women in the study exhibited an approximately two-fold increased risk of breast cancer recurrence (12.5% in EM versus 24.1% in PM after 9 years of follow-up). A statistically significant effect on overall survival (16.7% in EM versus 22.8% in PM) could not be demonstrated; however, the length of follow-up and the number of patients were probably insufficient to evaluate this endpoint. While an impact of CYP2D6 genetics on tamoxifen efficacy seems clear, additional genetic factors such as CYP2C19, CYP3A5 and ABCC2 (ATP-binding cassette, subfamily 2, member 2, also known as Mrp2) drug transporter polymorphisms may also influence the efficacy of tamoxifen

[71–73]. To further complicate matters, the association between CYP2D6 and perhaps other genetic factors and tamoxifen efficacy may be limited by the observation that patients bearing the highly active CYP2D6 alleles are also the patients most likely to discontinue therapy prematurely [74]. Thus, while there may be benefit in knowledge of CYP2D6 genotype prior to tamoxifen therapy, there are currently no prospective studies demonstrating a benefit to genotyping. It is therefore unclear how tamoxifen therapy ought to be modified (change in dose or timing), if it indeed should be, in order to improve outcome.

Given that CYP2D6 genetics may be primarily predicting the pharmacokinetics of tamoxifen and its metabolites, measurement of endoxifen and 4-hydroxy-tamoxifen may provide complementary and perhaps more useful information. This may be particular important as a number of prescription drugs such as selective serotonin inhibitors (SSRIs) and over-the-counter drugs such as antihistamines and alternative therapies (e.g., St John's Wort) inhibit CP2D6 activity [75]. At least two methods for quantitative measurement of both active metabolites have been described in the literature [76, 77]. Unfortunately, no commercial assays are currently available for tamoxifen or its metabolites, and no clinical data on the use of concentration monitoring have been reported.

Anti-Epidermal Growth Factor Receptor (EGFR) Antibodies

The EGFR (also known as ErbB1 or HER1) was recognized in the early 1980s as an important pathway contributing to the oncogenic phenotype in a range of epithelial cancers. This receptor provides survival and mitogenic signals to cells, and dysregulated EGFR activity has been described in tumors through both altered receptor expression and kinase activity [78–82]. The link between EGFR pathway activity and cancer led to a significant research effort aimed at disrupting this important signaling pathway with a series of anti-EGFR antibodies developed in the mid-1990s [83, 84]. One of these antibodies, cetuximab (mAb225, C225 or Erbitux™ [Bristol-Myers Squibb, New York, NY]) demonstrated potent anticancer activity *in vitro* and using preclinical tumor xenograft models in mice [85]. Directed against the extracellular domain of the EGFR, cetuximab mediates its effects through multiple mechanisms, including blockade of EGF binding [86], stimulation of EGFR internalization and degradation [87], and antibody-dependent cellular cytotoxicity [88]. Based upon highly promising Phase II and III studies of cetuximab in patients with metastatic colorectal carcinoma, Cetuximab received FDA approval in 2004 and has become an important component of the chemotherapeutic regimen for this disease [89–92]. Subsequent studies demonstrating efficacy in head and neck squamous cell carcinoma led to extended approval for patients with locally and regionally advanced tumors as an adjunct to radiotherapy [93–95]. Panitumumab (ABX-EGF [Amgen, Seattle, WA]) is a fully human EGFR-specific antibody that demonstrates similar efficacy in metastatic colorectal carcinoma [96, 97]. Similar to cetuximab, panitumumab received FDA approval in 2006 for EGFR-expressing tumors with progression on standard FOLFOX (5-fluorouracil/oxaliplatin) or FOLFIRI (5-fluorouracil/irinotecan) regimens [98].

Despite the significant success of these agents, the overall objective response rate for anti-EGFR therapy is still relatively low, with less than 25% of patients achieving a complete or partial response. Despite the highly targeted nature of these drugs, adverse events such as fatal infusion reactions (~2%) and sudden cardiac death (~3% of head and neck squamous cell carcinoma patients receiving concomitant radiotherapy) have been observed. Thus, optimal selection of patients who are most likely to achieve clinical benefit from these agents is warranted. Several laboratory-based biomarkers have been explored for patient selection, which are discussed further below.

EGFR Expression and Gene Copy Number

Clinical studies with cetuximab and panitumumab in metastatic colorectal carcinoma have generally restricted enrollment to patients with documented expression of EGFR by the primary or metastatic tumor by immunohistochemistry (IHC) due to an assumed relationship between expression and response [89–92, 96, 97]. Clinical trials with cetuximab in head and neck squamous cell carcinoma have included patients without detectable expression of EGFR by IHC, but these cases represent a very small percentage ($< 2\%$) of cases in this disease. The package inserts for both cetuximab and panitumumab currently list EGFR-expressing metastatic colorectal carcinoma as a primary indication for use of these drugs. Nonetheless, the relationship between EGFR expression and clinical response is far from clear. Unlike anti-HER2/neu therapy, where objective response rates exhibit a relationship with receptor expression on the tumor [99–101], the objective response rate for EGFR-targeted antibody therapy does not show a relationship to either the percentage or the intensity of EGFR-positive tumor cells as assessed by an IHC test [89]. Additional reports have further suggested clinical responses are possible in EGFR-negative metastatic colorectal carcinoma [102–105]. The detection of EGFR expression by IHC continues to be used for treatment decisions, as this biomarker served as a primary inclusion criterion in early trials that formed the basis for FDA approval of these drugs. Nevertheless, the sensitivity and specificity of this test for predicting response to anti-EGFR antibody therapy appears to be poor in metastatic colorectal carcinoma and head and neck squamous cell carcinoma.

Amplification of the EGFR gene has also been evaluated as a surrogate biomarker for expression based upon the assumption that high gene copy number might be a superior predictor of the tumor dependence on EGFR signaling and, in turn, clinical response (Fig. 14.4). Overall, the number of studies and evaluated patients is very small. Nevertheless, there is some evidence that higher EGFR gene copy number is associated with a greater likelihood of response. In a retrospective analysis of tumor specimens from 31 patients with metastatic colorectal carcinoma that were treated with either cetuximab or panitumumab, 8 out of 9 patients (89%) of patients with increased EGFR gene copy number determined by fluorescence *in situ* hybridization (FISH) achieved an objective response by response evaluation criteria in solid tumor (RECIST) compared with only 1 of 21 patients (5%) with normal EGFR gene copy number. A follow-up study by the same investigators using a different patient population less enriched for responders, as done in the prior study, confirmed the association between EGFR gene copy number and treatment response. These results suggest that EGFR gene copy number testing could be superior to EGFR expression analysis by IHC, and may be helpful in identifying patients who are most likely to benefit from anti-EGFR antibody therapy. Nevertheless, they also demonstrate that even in patients with an elevated EGFR gene copy number the objective response rate is ~30%, pointing to additional mechanisms for therapy resistance in most patients. The ability for EGFR gene copy number testing to distinguish responders from non-responders may also not be that straightforward. Studies by other investigators have either confirmed some of these findings [104, 106] or failed to

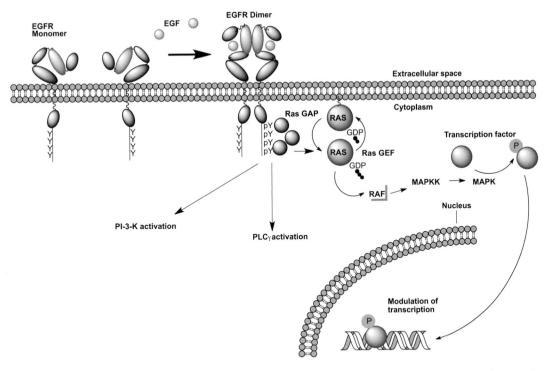

FIGURE 14.4　EGFR signal transduction. The EGFR, upon binding to receptor ligands, forms dimers that permit the kinase domain of the receptor to cross-phosphorylate the substrate domains within the EGFR cytoplasmic domain. The phosphorylated EGFR activates several downstream signal transduction pathways, including the Ras/ MAP kinase, phosphatidylinositol-3(OH)-kinase (PI3K) and phospholipase C gamma (PLCγ) pathways.

demonstrate a significant association between EGFR gene copy number and objective response [107]. Some of these discrepancies may be due to differences in the techniques used or selection of patients for inclusion in these retrospective studies.

EGFR Mutations

Several mutations within the EGFR kinase domain that lead to constitutive activation of the receptor have been described. While these mutations occur in cases of non-small cell lung cancer, they appear quite rare in metastatic colorectal carcinoma [105, 108]. Although their frequency is low, no significant correlation between the presence of these mutations and clinical response has been observed in patients with metastatic colorectal carcinoma treated with cetuximab or panitumumab [105]. Head and neck squamous cell carcinoma also shows a similarly low EGFR mutation frequency with no discernible relationship to clinical response [94]. An EGFR mutant termed EGFRvIII, bearing a large in-frame 801 base-pair (268 amino acid) deletion in exons 2–7 of the EGFR has been described. Expression studies demonstrate that this mutant EGFR is not expressed in normal tissues, but is present in a variety of tumors including ~27% of breast carcinomas, ~52% of malignant gliomas and ~45% of head and neck squamous cell carcinoma [109, 110]. In contrast, this variant is exceedingly rare in colorectal carcinoma [111, 112]. Studies with tumor models in culture and in animals suggested that tumors bearing the EGFRvIII may be resistant to anti-EGFR antibody therapy [109]. A recent study by Tinhofer *et al.* lends support to the negative prognostic outlook for EGFRvIII-positive tumors [113] but, given the small and retrospective nature of this study, further prospective evaluation is clearly required to determine the sensitivity and specificity of this biomarker for cetuximab and panitumumab therapy.

KRAS Mutation

The less than 25% objective response rates observed in clinical trials of cetuximab and panitumumab, despite expression of EGFR, suggested that other mechanisms beside loss of the receptor must be present. The EGFR stimulates several downstream signal transduction pathways with the cell (Fig. 14.3). The small plasma-membrane localized GTPase, Ras, represents one of the key pathways leading to MAP kinase (MAPK) activation, which is central to cell survival, proliferation and differentiation. The Ras (Rat sarcoma) proteins are encoded by a family of related genes, and mutated versions of HRAS (also known as transforming protein p21), NRAS (also known as Neuroblastoma Ras viral oncogene homolog) and KRAS (also known as v-ki-ras2 Kirsten rat sarcoma viral oncogene homolog) genes that lead to constitutive Ras activity are frequently found within a variety of human cancers [114]. Approximately 40% of colorectal carcinomas have a detectable mutation in KRAS [115, 116].

Over 150 studies evaluating the impact of KRAS mutations on the outcome of anti-EGFR antibody therapy have been published in the past decade. Two relatively recent systematic reviews and meta-analyses of the literature have attempted to summarize this large body of literature composed of mostly small, retrospective cohort studies with patient selection based upon convenience sampling rather than prospective recruitment using pre-specified inclusion criteria [117, 118]. Both analyses support the notion that KRAS mutations are associated with resistance to cetuximab and panitumumab therapy in metastatic colorectal carcinoma; however, they also acknowledge the limited ability to explore important effect modifiers such as concurrent therapy or other patient-specific characteristics that might modify the impact of KRAS mutation. The ability of KRAS mutation analysis to prospectively predict response to therapy is also difficult to ascertain, since the performance characteristics of a test are dependent upon the population to which the test is applied. Adelstein *et al.* focused their meta-analysis upon data from randomized controlled studies with prospective recruitment of patients, which may provide the best indication of test performance in a clinical setting [118]. While the overall anti-EGFR antibody response rate was not statistically different from the standard therapy to which it was compared in patient with tumors bearing mutated forms of KRAS, the response rate ranged from no improvement to a 25% improvement in response depending upon the study and the concurrent treatment partner (overall mean response improved by 11% with anti-EGFR therapy). Based upon the available data, the American Society of Clinical Oncology (ASCO) issued a provisional clinical opinion in 2009 recommending that all patients with metastatic colorectal carcinoma who are anti-EGFR treatment candidates should have their tumors tested for mutant KRAS prior to therapy, and patients with tumors bearing mutations at codons 12 or 13 should not receive anti-EGFR antibody therapy [119].

While the role of KRAS mutation in anti-EGFR therapy resistance appears clear, there are different mutations that occur in KRAS. Not all mutations may impact anti-EGFR therapy equally. De Roock *et al.* identified 32 patients out of 579 patients pooled from several single arm studies of cetuximab with tumors bearing a Glycine to Aspartatic acid change at codon 13 (G13D) [120]. Compared to patients bearing other forms of mutated KRAS (primarily codon 12 mutations), patients with the G13D mutations experienced a greater median overall survival (7.6 months [95% CI 5.7–20.5] versus 5.7 months [95% CI 4.9–6.8]) and progression-free survival (4.0 months [95% CI 1.9–6.2] versus 1.9 months [95% CI 1.8–2.8]), raising the question of whether the exclusion of tumors bearing all codon 12 and 13 mutations of KRAS is justified. Stratification of anti-EGFR antibody therapy is further complicated by the fact that most assays currently offered for KRAS mutations are restricted to only codon 12 and codon 13 mutations, but other mutations in KRAS (codons 61 and 146) that may confer resistance to anti-EGFR therapy have also been identified [121]. The impact of tumor composition (i.e. normal cells variably mixed with cancer cells) and testing methodologies also cannot be ignored, and may contribute to misclassification of KRAS status [122].

Other Potential Biomarkers

In addition to assessing EGFR gene copy number and KRAS mutational analysis, additional factors have been identified that might contribute to sensitivity to anti-EGFR antibody therapy. Naturally occurring polymorphisms in two Fc receptors for IgG (FcγRIIa and FcγRIIIa) have been identified with significant minor allele frequencies (15–30%) in Caucasians. These variant Fc receptors have been demonstrated to affect antibody-dependent cellular cytotoxicity, which may contribute to the mechanism of action for anti-EGFR antibody therapy. Two studies have evaluated the impact of these polymorphisms on cetuximab therapy in metastatic colorectal carcinoma patients, and both have demonstrated independent effects on progression-free survival (PFS). Studies further suggested that the hazard ratio for progression-free survival for homozygous carriers of the minor allele of both receptors was comparable in magnitude to the impact of KRAS mutation. In addition to KRAS, dysregulation of other signaling pathways downstream of the EGFR may also occur, contributing to an anti-EGFR antibody resistant tumor phenotype. Recently, two independent groups identified mutations in genes including BRAF (also known as v-Raf murine sarcoma viral oncogene homolog B1), NRAS and PIK3CA, the 110-kD catalytic subunit of phosphoinositide-3(OH)-kinase [122, 123]. De Roock *et al.* demonstrated that patients with metastatic colorectal carcinoma bearing these mutations are also unlikely to respond to cetuximab therapy [123].

In addition to tumor and constitutional genetics, other investigators have sought gene expression and protein biomarkers that might be predictive of anti-EGFR antibody therapeutic response. In a study of 110 patients with metastatic colorectal carcinoma that were enrolled in a cetuximab monotherapy trial, high levels of the EGFR ligands amphiregulin and epiregulin were identified as significant predictors of disease control [124]. The association of these expression biomarkers with response has been confirmed in at least two subsequent published studies from independent groups supporting the potential utility of this type of biomarker, especially in tumors with wild-type KRAS [125, 126].

ANTI-EGFR TYROSINE KINASE INHIBITORS

Simultaneously with the development of antibody-based therapeutics for EGFR, small molecule inhibitors of the EGFR cytoplasmic tyrosine kinase domain were sought as an alternative approach to blocking this important oncogenic signal transduction pathway. Gefitinib represented the first EGFR-specific tyrosine kinase inhibitor (TKI). Similar to antibody-based inhibitors, gefitinib (ZD1839, Iressa™ [AstraZeneca, London, UK]), erlotinib (OSI-774, Tarceva™ [Genentech, South San Francisco, CA]) and other EGFR TKIs have demonstrated robust inhibition of EGFR signaling and antitumor activity in both preclinical and clinical studies. As a result of very promising results from Phase II studies, gefitinib and erlotinib both received FDA approval for non-small cell lung cancer in 2003 and 2004, respectively, through a newly developed accelerated approval process. Somewhat surprisingly at the time, subsequent Phase III studies failed to demonstrate improved overall survival (OS) or time to tumor progression (TTP). These disappointing Phase III results combined with apparent responses in some patients led to exploration of factors that might distinguish responsive and non-responsive patients.

EGFR Mutation Status

Retrospective analysis of data from several early Phase II/III trials in non-small cell lung cancer demonstrated that response to TKIs was strongly associated with female gender, Asian ancestry and the absence of a smoking history. Further genetic analysis of tumors from responders (~10% of non-selected non-Asian patients) and non-responders to gefitinib demonstrated that response to TKIs was strongly associated with adenocarcinomas bearing certain mutations in the tyrosine kinase domain of EGFR [127, 128]. Mutations varied among small in-frame deletions (predominantly in exon 19) or missense mutations (predominantly L858R in exon 21) that were clustered around the ATP binding pocket of the EGFR kinase domain, which serves as the target of the TKIs. These mutations also occurred with higher frequency in females and in individuals from Japanese ancestry, perhaps explaining the association of these traits with response in the early clinical trials.

A meta-analysis of 38 separate published reports, mostly derived from retrospective cohort studies of EGFR-TKIs used as a single agent in non-small cell lung cancer, demonstrates that patients with an EGFR mutation have a 5.92-fold increase in probability of objective response compared with patients with non-small cell lung cancer bearing a wild-type EGFR. One important caveat of this pooled analysis is the relative over-representation of studies conducted solely with Asian patients. Only a handful of the 38 published studies included non-Asian patients. The largest, by Tsao et al., evaluated potential predictive markers in 731 patients from the BR.21 study of single agent erlotinib compared with placebo in patients who had progression following standard chemotherapy for non-small cell lung cancer [129]. Due to technical limitations and the failure to secure tissue of all patients, only 395 patients in the study had tumor material available, and EGFR mutational analysis could be attempted on only 195 patients. From this subset, 110 (56% of attempted samples) yielded sufficient DNA for analysis, with more than half requiring microdissection to yield material with sufficiently enriched tumor representation. Mutations in exon 19 or 21 of the EGFR were identified in 24 out of 107 (22%) tumors. Evaluation of patients with wild-type and mutated EGFR-bearing tumors failed to demonstrate a significant difference in overall survival between erlotinib- and placebo-treated patients, despite a difference between the treatments in the full study population. This finding was quite surprising, but perhaps relates to the relatively small subset (26%) of the original study population analyzed. Evaluation of data from the IDEAL (Iressa Dose Evaluation in Advanced Lung Cancer) and INTACT (Iressa NSCLC Trial Assessing Combination Treatment) studies of gefitinib in patients who previously demonstrated progression on chemotherapy also failed to identify an improved overall survival; however, this study did demonstrate a significant difference in the surrogate endpoint of progression-free survival, suggesting that the presence of a mutated form of EGFR has a potentially clinically relevant impact on TKI response [130]. The recently published IPASS (IRESSA Pan-Asia Study), a randomized controlled trial of gefitinib versus carboplatin/docetaxel chemotherapy as first-line therapy in 1217 patients with advanced lung cancer, further supports the predictive nature of EGFR mutation analysis prior to initiation of therapy with a TKI [131, 132]. The study population for IPASS was composed of East Asian patients who were either non-smokers or light smokers with adenocarcinoma, a population with significantly higher likelihood of harboring EGFR mutations. Patients with tumors bearing activating mutations of EGFR exhibited a 25% decreased rate of disease progression and death with gefitinib therapy compared with chemotherapy. More importantly, patients with wild-type EGFR-bearing tumors exhibited a 2.8-fold decreased rate of disease progression on gefitinib compared with chemotherapy. Similar to early studies, IPASS failed to demonstrate a difference in OS between patients with wild-type or mutated EGFR-expressing tumors treated with gefitinib; however, PFS was the primary endpoint of the study, and it was likely insufficiently powered to detect a small difference in OS. Similar results were obtained in the analysis of the INTEREST (IRESSA Non-Small Cell Lung Cancer Trial Evaluating Response and Survival against Taxotere) population [133]. While concerns regarding the use of a surrogate endpoint such as PFS have been raised, high rates of crossover to alternative treatments were not infrequent in most of these studies, and this has been proposed as a confounding variable for the analysis of OS. In addition to these retrospective cohort studies, two studies evaluated patients with non-small cell lung cancer bearing a mutated EGFR, who were prospectively randomized to gefitinib or conventional chemotherapy-based first-line therapy [134, 135]. Both studies, performed in Asian populations, demonstrated a substantially improved objective response rate and progression-free survival in the TKI treatment group compared with conventional chemotherapy, indicating that TKI therapy is the preferred therapy in this population.

Based upon the aggregated data, and especially the more recent clinical trial results that included EGFR mutation assessment *a priori* in their analysis, the American Society of Clinical Oncology (ASCO) issued a provisional opinion recommending EGFR mutational analysis prior to initiation of first-line TKI therapy in patients with advanced non-small cell lung cancer [136]. Nevertheless, they recognize the paucity of data in non-Asian populations and using erlotinib, which may differ due to unknown factors such as genetics. Supporting the role of EGFR mutations in non-Asian populations, the large Phase III Sequential Tarceva in Unresectable NSCLC (SATURN, B018192) study comparing erlotinib maintenance therapy to a placebo control in platinum chemotherapy-treated, advanced non-small cell lung cancer patients demonstrates that EGFR mutation is strongly correlated with PFS in non-Asian patients, with a 90% reduction in risk of progression or death with erlotinib [137].

Interestingly, this study further demonstrated a smaller but significant 22% reduction in risk in patients bearing a wild-type EGFR. These results suggest that TKI therapy may still be helpful in the absence of EGFR mutations, especially as second-line therapy.

EGFR Expression and Gene Copy Number

Similar to anti-EGFR antibody therapy, both EGFR protein expression assessed by IHC and EGFR gene copy number assessed by FISH or chromogenic *in situ* hybridization have been evaluated as potential predictive markers for TKI therapeutic response in patients with non-small cell lung cancer. Retrospective evaluation of EGFR gene copy number in relation to response rates, PFS and OS in several prospective TKI trials, including the ISEL (IRESSA Survival Evaluation in Lung Cancer) [138], BR.21 [129] and SWOG (South-West Oncology Group) [139] and Italian population [140] studies demonstrated a strong correlation of this marker to these clinically relevant endpoints. A recent meta-analysis of 22 different studies of TKIs in non-small cell lung cancer that included assessment of EGFR gene copy number confirms the predictive nature of EGFR gene copy number [141]. An interesting result of this analysis was the demonstration of EGFR gene copy number as a predictor of response and survival in non-East Asian populations, but the failure of this marker to predict response in the Asian population. These findings illustrate some of the challenges faced in biomarker studies, where the performance characteristics of a biomarker may differ depending upon the population being assessed. While EGFR gene copy number may be a useful marker for TKI therapy, it is also a far more technically challenging analysis compared with EGFR mutational analysis. The interpretation of EGFR gene copy number is also somewhat subjective, with varying thresholds for an increased gene copy number used in some studies; however, criteria developed by Cappuzzo *et al.* have helped to standardize this assay [140].

Prospective evaluation of EGFR gene copy number or of protein expression are not currently recommended tests prior to TKI treatment. The data demonstrating improvements in response rate and survival, particularly in non-East Asian populations, suggest that EGFR gene copy number may have some utility as a predictive biomarker for TKI therapy as well as a potential prognostic biomarker for non-small cell lung cancer. Nevertheless, larger prospective studies using validated and standardized methods are required. Along these lines, the recent data from the SATURN study performed in non-East Asians failed to demonstrate improved PFS with maintenance erlotinib therapy in patients with either EGFR gene copy number or protein, suggesting that these markers are much less useful than EGFR mutational status [137].

Other Potential Biomarkers

The significant number of patients who fail to respond to TKIs (~10–20%) led to a search for molecular markers that might predict responders, with the activating mutations of EGFR serving as very promising candidates. Markers that might help to identify patients who are unlikely to benefit from a therapy could also be useful by avoiding futile therapy with associated toxicity. KRAS mutations have been proposed as potential markers for both anti-EGFR antibodies (see discussion above) and EGF-targeted TKIs. At least 17 studies have attempted to explore KRAS mutations in the context of TKIs in non-small cell lung cancer. In a meta-analysis of these relatively small respective cohort studies comprising a total of 1008 patients, Linardou *et al.* demonstrated that KRAS mutations occur in ~16% of cases [142]. In this pooled cohort, KRAS mutations exhibited an overall sensitivity of 21% and a specificity of 94% for the detection of TKI non-responders, with no detectable differences in subsets of patients based upon TKI (erlotinib versus gefitinib), ethnicity (Asian versus white) or prior chemotherapy (naïve versus ≥ one line of chemotherapy). Thus, similar to the situation with anti-EGFR antibody therapy in metastatic colorectal carcinoma, KRAS mutation status appears to have a high positive predictive value for non-responsiveness to TKI therapy in patients with non-small cell lung cancer. In contrast, the absence of KRAS mutations is a poor predictor of response. It should also be noted that KRAS mutations and EGFR mutations rarely occur in the same tumor. These data suggest that prospective testing for KRAS mutations would be an efficient way to eliminate a portion of non-responders. Intriguingly, the recent data from the SATURN study that evaluated 889 prospectively recruited patients randomized to erlotinib or placebo as maintenance following platinum-based chemotherapy suggest that KRAS mutations may be more of a prognostic biomarker of non-small cell lung cancer natural history irrespective of therapy rather than a predictive biomarker for TKIs [137]. There are also some data suggesting that patients with non-small cell lung cancer bearing mutant KRAS can achieve long-term stable disease on TKIs [143, 144]. Thus, unlike the situation in metastatic colorectal carcinoma, it is still unclear whether KRAS testing should be used prospectively for decisions related to TKI therapy.

Concentration Monitoring

In addition to the pharmacodynamics variability that may arise from molecular changes within the target tumor, both erlotinib and gefitinib exhibit appreciable pharmacokinetic variability. Gefitinib and erlotinib AUC has been reported to vary significantly, with 36%−113% coefficients of variations (%CV). This may be due in part to interactions with other co-administered drugs such as phenytoin and azole antifungals [145]. Smoking may also contribute to appreciable variation in PK for these drugs [146]. The relationship between clinical response and drug exposure has not been rigorously investigated, but there is some evidence for a relationship between PK, toxicity and efficacy for erlotinib [147].

CONCLUSIONS

The oncologist who treats a patient with cancer has long attempted to choose the right therapy that best fits with a patient's cancer, overall health, personal values and expectations. The medical laboratory is an integral part of this individualization process, and its role is certainly destined to increase. Applied pharmacokinetics using drug concentration data and other clinical and laboratory data to adjust a drug's dosage continues to be important; however, applied pharmacokinetics is limited by its inability to account for pharmacodynamics differences between patients and their cancers. The genomics revolution of the past two decades brings us many steps closer to the ideally individualized therapeutic for cancer.

TABLE 14.1 Summary of Selected Biomarkers for Personalized Therapy with Anticancer Drugs

Drug(s)	Disease	Marker associations
Tamoxifen	Breast cancer	• CYP2D6 deficient or hypofunctioning alleles (CYP2D6*3, *4, *5, *10 or *41) are associated with an increased risk of disease recurrence and progression
Irinotecan	Colon cancer	• UGT1A1*28 homozygosity is associated with an increased risk of leukopenia and diarrhea
5-Fluorouracil	Colon cancer	• DPDY, TMYS polymorphisms are associated with an increased risk of severe toxicity
EGFR-specific TKIs Erlotinib Gefitinib	Non-small cell lung cancer	• EGFR mutations are strongly associated with improved efficacy • Increased EGFR gene copy number is associated with efficacy • KRAS mutations are associated with resistance to therapy and poor efficacy
EGFR-specific antibodies Cetuximab Panitumumab	Colon cancer Non-small cell lung cancer	• Increased EGFR gene copy number and protein expression is associated with increased efficacy • KRAS mutations are associated with resistance to therapy and poor efficacy
Thiopurine antimetabolites Azathioprine 6-Mercaptopurine	Acute lymphoblastic leukemia Inflammatory bowel disease	• Reduced TPMT enzymatic activity (RBC enzymatic assay or homozygous carrier of TPMT*2, *3A, *3B or *3C alleles) is associated with severe toxicity
Methotrexate + Leucovorin	High-dose therapy for lymphoma	• Plasma methotrexate concentration is associated with the risk for toxicity
Busulfan	Myeloablation for bone marrow transplantation in several malignant and non-malignant diseases	• Plasma busulfan C_{ss} or AUC is associated with the risk for toxicity (primarily veno-occlusive disease) and efficacy (bone marrow engraftment and disease relapse)

The technology to assess an individual's constitutional genetics and the genetic changes of a cancer are rapidly becoming routine within clinical laboratories. Table 14.1 summarizes the most well-established relationships between laboratory biomarkers and anticancer drug therapy results. The current challenge is determining how to effectively apply this wealth of genetic information to the individualization process. While biomarkers, including genetic biomarkers, are increasingly being included in early phase trials of new drugs, prospective studies that evaluate approaches to using genetic information to guide pharmacotherapy and improve meaningful clinical outcomes are generally lacking for existing drugs such as those in Table 14.1. This is also no trivial matter, particularly in cancer, where it may take a decade or longer to reach clinically relevant outcomes, especially translating findings of basic research into successful clinical application.

References

[1] Chabner B, Longo DL. Cancer Chemotherapy and Biotherapy: Principles and Practice. 4th ed. vol. XV. Philadelphia, PA: Lippincott Williams & Wilkins; 2006.

[2] Woods RL, Fox RM, Tattersall MH. Methotrexate treatment of squamous-cell head and neck cancers: dose—response evaluation. Br Med J (Clin Res Ed.) 1981;282:600—2.

[3] Delepine N, Delepine G, Cornille H, et al. Dose escalation with pharmacokinetics monitoring in methotrexate chemotherapy of osteosarcoma. Anticancer Res 1995;15(2):489—94.

[4] Delepine N, Delepine G, Jasmin C, et al. Importance of age and methotrexate dosage: prognosis in children and young adults with high-grade osteosarcomas. Biomed Pharmacother 1988;42(4):257—62.

[5] Evans WE, Crom WR, Abromowitch M, et al. Clinical pharmacodynamics of high-dose methotrexate in acute lymphocytic leukemia. Identification of a relation between concentration and effect. N Engl J Med 1986;314(8):471—7.

[6] Evans WE, Pratt CB, Taylor RH, et al. Pharmacokinetic monitoring of high-dose methotrexate. Early recognition of high-risk patients. Cancer Chemother Pharmacol 1979;3(3):161—6.

[7] Evans WE, Relling MV, Rodman JH, et al. Conventional compared with individualized chemotherapy for childhood acute lymphoblastic leukemia. N Engl J Med 1998;338(8):499—505.

[8] Isacoff WH, Morrison PF, Aroesty J, et al. Pharmacokinetics of high-dose methotrexate with citrovorum factor rescue. Cancer Treat Rep 1977;61(9):1665—74.

[9] Nirenberg A, Mosende C, Mehta BM, et al. High-dose methotrexate with citrovorum factor rescue: predictive value of serum methotrexate concentrations and corrective measures to avert toxicity. Cancer Treat Rep 1977;61(5):779—83.

[10] Stoller RG, Hande KR, Jacobs SA, et al. Use of plasma pharmacokinetics to predict and prevent methotrexate toxicity. N Engl J Med 1977;297(12):630—44.

[11] Gibbs JP, Gooley T, Corneau B, et al. The impact of obesity and disease on busulfan oral clearance in adults. Blood 1999;93(12):4436—40.

[12] Busulfex Product Information. Fremont, CA: PDL BioPharma; 2007.

[13] Slattery JT, Risler LJ. Therapeutic monitoring of busulfan in hematopoietic stem cell transplantation. Ther Drug Monit 1998;20(5):543—9.

[14] Vassal G, Fischer A, Challine D, I, et al. Busulfan disposition below the age of three: alteration in children with lysosomal storage disease. Blood 1993;82(3):1030—4.

[15] Dix SP, Wingard JR, Mullins RE, Jerkunica I, et al. Association of busulfan area under the curve with veno-occlusive disease following BMT. Bone Marrow Transpl 1996;17(2):225—30.

[16] Grochow LB. Busulfan disposition: the role of therapeutic monitoring in bone marrow transplantation induction regimens. Semin Oncol 1993;20(4 Suppl. 4):18—25. quiz 26.

[17] Grochow LB, Jones RJ, Brundrett RB, et al. Pharmacokinetics of busulfan: correlation with veno-occlusive disease in patients undergoing bone marrow transplantation. Cancer Chemother Pharmacol 1989;25(1):55—61.

[18] Slattery JT, Sanders JE, Buckner CD, et al. Graft-rejection and toxicity following bone marrow transplantation in relation to busulfan pharmacokinetics. Bone Marrow Transplant 1995;16(1):31—42.

[19] Slattery JT, Clift RA, Buckner CD, et al. Marrow transplantation for chronic myeloid leukemia: the influence of plasma busulfan levels on the outcome of transplantation. Blood 1997;89(8):3055—60.

[20] Bolinger AM, Zangwill AB, Slattery JT, et al. Target dose adjustment of busulfan in pediatric patients undergoing bone marrow transplantation. Bone Marrow Transplant 2001;28(11):1013—8.

[21] Eichelbaum M, Ingelman-Sundberg M, Evans WE. Pharmacogenomics and individualized drug therapy. Annu Rev Med 2006;57:119—37.

[22] Suhre K, Shin SY, Petersen AK, et al. Human metabolic individuality in biomedical and pharmaceutical research. Nature 2011;477(7362):54—60.

[23] Weinshilboum R. Inheritance and drug response. N Engl J Med 2003;348(6):529—37.

[24] Sissung TM, Baum CE, Kirkland CT, et al. Pharmacogenetics of membrane transporters: an update on current approaches. Mol Biotechnol 2010;44(2):152—67.

[25] Thummel KE, Wilkinson GR. In vitro and in vivo drug interactions involving human CYP3A. Annu Rev Pharmacol Toxicol 1998;38:389—430.

[26] Plant N. The human cytochrome P450 sub-family: transcriptional regulation, inter-individual variation and interaction networks. Biochim Biophys Acta 2007;1770(3):478—88.

[27] FDA. Table of Pharmacogenomic Biomarkers in Drug Labels [cited 7 November 2011]; Available at, http://www.fda.gov/drugs/scienceresearch/researchareas/pharmacogenetics/ucm083378.htm; 2011.

[28] Gomez-Roca C, Raynaud CM, Penault-Llorca F, et al. Differential expression of biomarkers in primary non-small cell lung cancer and metastatic sites. J Thorac Oncol 2009;4(10):1212—20.

[29] Marchetti A, Felicioni L, Buttitta F. Assessing EGFR mutations. N Engl J Med 2006;354(5):526—8. author reply 526—528.

[30] Chabner B, Longo DL. Cancer Chemotherapy and Biotherapy: Principles and Practice. 5th ed, vol. XV. Philadelphia PA: Wolters Kluwer Health/Lippincott Williams & Wilkins; 2011.

[31] Weinshilboum RM, Sladek SL. Mercaptopurine pharmacogenetics: monogenic inheritance of erythrocyte thiopurine methyltransferase activity. Am J Hum Genet 1980;32(5):651—62.

[32] Relling MV, Hancock ML, Rivera GK, et al. Mercaptopurine therapy intolerance and heterozygosity at the thiopurine S-methyltransferase gene locus. J Natl Cancer Inst 1999;91(23):2001—8.

[33] Evans WE, Hon YY, Bomgaars L, et al. Preponderance of thiopurine S-methyltransferase deficiency and heterozygosity among patients intolerant to mercaptopurine or azathioprine. J Clin Oncol 2001; 19(8):2293—301.

[34] McLeod HL, Siva C. The thiopurine S-methyltransferase gene locus — implications for clinical pharmaco-genomics. Pharmacogenomics 2002;3(1):89—98.

[35] Stocco G, Cheok MH, Crews KR, et al. Genetic polymorphism of inosine triphosphate pyrophosphatase is a determinant of mercaptopurine metabolism and toxicity during treatment for acute lymphoblastic leukemia. Clin Pharmacol Ther 2009;85(2):164—72.

[36] McBride KL, Gilchrist GS, Smithson WA, et al. Severe 6-thioguanine-induced marrow aplasia in a child with acute lymphoblastic leukemia and inherited thiopurine methyltransferase deficiency. J Pediatr Hematol Oncol 2000;22(5):441—5.

[37] Lennard L, Chew TS, Lilleyman JS. Human thiopurine methyltransferase activity varies with red blood cell age. Br J Clin Pharmacol 2001;52(5):539—46.

[38] Oliveira E, Quental S, Alves S, et al. Do the distribution patterns of polymorphisms at the thiopurine S-methyltransferase locus in sub-Saharan populations need revision? Hints from Cabinda and Mozambique. Eur J Clin Pharmacol 2007;63(7):703—6.

[39] Alves S, Rocha J, Amorim A, Prata MJ. Tracing the origin of the most common thiopurine methyltransferase (TPMT) variants: preliminary data from the patterns of haplotypic association with two CA repeats. Ann Hum Genet 2004;68(Pt. 4):313—23.

[40] Ando M, Ando Y, Hasegawa Y, et al. Genetic polymorphisms of thiopurine S-methyltransferase and 6-mercaptopurine toxicity in Japanese children with acute lymphoblastic leukaemia. Pharmacogenetics 2001;11(3):269—73.

[41] Jun JB, Cho DY, Kang C, et al. Thiopurine S-methyltransferase polymorphisms and the relationship between the mutant alleles and the adverse effects in systemic lupus erythematosus patients taking azathioprine. Clin Exp Rheumatol 2005;23(6):873—6.

[42] Schaeffeler E, Zanger UM, Eichelbaum M, et al. Highly multiplexed genotyping of thiopurine S-methyl-transferase variants using MALD-TOF mass spectrometry: reliable genotyping in different ethnic groups. Clin Chem 2008;54(10):1637—47.

[43] Donnan JR, Ungar WJ, Mathews M, et al. Systematic review of thiopurine methyltransferase genotype and enzymatic testing strategies. Ther Drug Monit 2011;33(2):192—9.

[44] Rothenberg ML, Meropol NJ, Poplin EA, et al. Mortality associated with irinotecan plus bolus fluorouracil/leucovorin: summary findings of an independent panel. J Clin Oncol 2001;19(18):3801—7.

[45] Van Cutsem E, Douillard JY, Kohne CH. Toxicity of irinotecan in patients with colorectal cancer. N Engl J Med 2001;345(18):1351—2.

[46] Mathijssen RH, Verweij J, de Jonge MJ, et al. Impact of body-size measures on irinotecan clearance: alternative dosing recommendations. J Clin Oncol 2002;20(1):81—7.

[47] Miya T, Goya T, Fujii H, et al. Factors affecting the pharmacokinetics of CPT-11: the body mass index, age and sex are independent predictors of pharmacokinetic parameters of CPT-11. Invest New Drugs 2001;19(1):61—7.

[48] Gupta E, Mick R, Ramirez J, et al. Pharmacokinetic and pharmacodynamic evaluation of the topoisomerase inhibitor irinotecan in cancer patients. J Clin Oncol 1997;15(4):1502–10.

[49] Gupta E, Lestingi TM, Mick R, et al. Metabolic fate of irinotecan in humans: correlation of glucuronidation with diarrhea. Cancer Res 1994;54(14):3723–5.

[50] Wasserman E, Myara A, Lokiec F, et al. Severe CPT-11 toxicity in patients with Gilbert's syndrome: two case reports. Ann Oncol 1997;8(10):1049–51.

[51] Iyer L, King CD, Whitington PF, et al. Genetic predisposition to the metabolism of irinotecan (CPT-11). Role of uridine diphosphate glucuronosyltransferase isoform 1A1 in the glucuronidation of its active metabolite (SN-38) in human liver microsomes. J Clin Invest 1998;101(4):847–54.

[52] Hu ZY, Yu Q, Pei Q, et al. Dose-dependent association between UGT1A1*28 genotype and irinotecan-induced neutropenia: low doses also increase risk. Clin Cancer Res 2010;16(15):3832–42.

[53] Hu ZY, Yu Q, Zhao YS. Dose-dependent association between UGT1A1*28 polymorphism and irinotecan-induced diarrhoea: a meta-analysis. Eur J Cancer 2010;46(10):1856–65.

[54] McLeod HL, Sargent DJ, Marsh S, et al. Pharmacogenetic predictors of adverse events and response to chemotherapy in metastatic colorectal cancer: results from North American Gastrointestinal Intergroup Trial N9741. J Clin Oncol 2010;28(20):3227–33.

[55] Innocenti F, Kroetz DL, Schuetz E, et al. Comprehensive pharmacogenetic analysis of irinotecan neutropenia and pharmacokinetics. J Clin Oncol 2009;27(16):2604–14.

[56] Han JY, Lim HS, Shin ES, et al. Comprehensive analysis of UGT1A polymorphisms predictive for pharmacokinetics and treatment outcome in patients with non-small-cell lung cancer treated with irinotecan and cisplatin. J Clin Oncol 2006;24(15):2237–44.

[57] Minami H, Sai K, Saeki M, et al. Irinotecan pharmacokinetics/pharmacodynamics and UGT1A genetic polymorphisms in Japanese: roles of UGT1A1*6 and *28. Pharmacogenet Genomics 2007;17(7):497–504.

[58] Onoue M, Terada T, Kobayashi M, et al. UGT1A1*6 polymorphism is most predictive of severe neutropenia induced by irinotecan in Japanese cancer patients. Intl J Clin Oncol 2009;14(2):136–42.

[59] Marcuello E, Paez D, Pare L, et al. A genotype-directed phase I–IV dose-finding study of irinotecan in combination with fluorouracil/leucovorin as first-line treatment in advanced colorectal cancer. Br J Cancer 2011;105(1):53–7.

[60] Toffoli G, Cecchin E, Gasparini G, et al. Genotype-driven phase I study of irinotecan administered in combination with fluorouracil/leucovorin in patients with metastatic colorectal cancer. J Clin Oncol 2010;28(5):866–71.

[61] Young AM, Daryanani S, Kerr DJ. Can pharmacokinetic monitoring improve clinical use of fluorouracil? Clin Pharmacokinet 1999;36(6):391–8.

[62] Gamelin E, Delva R, Jacob J, et al. Individual fluorouracil dose adjustment based on pharmacokinetic follow-up compared with conventional dosage: results of a multicenter randomized trial of patients with metastatic colorectal cancer. J Clin Oncol 2008;26(13):2099–105.

[63] Amstutz U, Froehlich TK, Largiader CR. Dihydropyrimidine dehydrogenase gene as a major predictor of severe 5-fluorouracil toxicity. Pharmacogenomics 2011;12(9):1321–36.

[64] Scartozzi M, Maccaroni E, Giampieri R, et al. 5-Fluorouracil pharmacogenomics: still rocking after all these years? Pharmacogenomics 2011;12(2):251–65.

[65] Abe O, Abe R, Enomoto K. Effects of chemotherapy and hormonal therapy for early breast cancer on recurrence and 15-year survival: an overview of the randomised trials. Lancet 2005;365(9472):1687–717.

[66] Early Breast Cancer Trialists' Collaborative Group. Tamoxifen for early breast cancer: an overview of the randomised trials. Lancet 1998;351(9114):1451–67.

[67] Stearns V, Johnson MD, Rae JM, Morocho A, et al. Active tamoxifen metabolite plasma concentrations after coadministration of tamoxifen and the selective serotonin reuptake inhibitor paroxetine. J Natl Cancer Inst 2003;95(23):1758–64.

[68] Borges S, Desta Z, Li L, et al. Quantitative effect of CYP2D6 genotype and inhibitors on tamoxifen metabolism: Implication for optimization of breast cancer treatment. Clin Pharmacol Ther 2006;80(1):61–74.

[69] Seruga B, Amir E. Cytochrome P450 2D6 and outcomes of adjuvant tamoxifen therapy: results of a meta-analysis. Breast Cancer Res Treat 2010;122(3):609–17.

[70] Schroth W, Goetz MP, Hamann U, et al. Association between CYP2D6 polymorphisms and outcomes among women with early stage breast cancer treated with tamoxifen. J Am Med Assoc 2009;302(13):1429–36.

[71] Kiyotani K, Mushiroda T, Imamura CK, et al. Significant effect of polymorphisms in CYP2D6 and ABCC2 on clinical outcomes of adjuvant tamoxifen therapy for breast cancer patients. J Clin Oncol 2010;28(8):1287—93.

[72] Schroth W, Antoniadou L, Fritz P, et al. Breast cancer treatment outcome with adjuvant tamoxifen relative to patient CYP2D6 and CYP2C19 genotypes. Journal of Clinical Oncology 2007;25(33):5187—93.

[73] Wegman P, Elingarami S, Carstensen J, et al. Genetic variants of CYP3A5, CYP2D6, SULT1A1, UGT2B15 and tamoxifen response in postmenopausal patients with breast cancer. Breast Cancer Res 2007;9(1):R7.

[74] Rae JM, Sikora MJ, Henry NL, et al. Cytochrome P450 2D6 activity predicts discontinuation of tamoxifen therapy in breast cancer patients. Pharmacogenomics Journal 2009;9(4):258—64.

[75] Flockhart DA. Drug Interactions: Cytochrome P450 Drug Interaction Table [cited 18 November 2011]; Available at, http://medicine.iupui.edu/clinpharm/ddis/table.aspx; 2007.

[76] Jaremko M, Kasai Y, Barginear MF, et al. Tamoxifen metabolite isomer separation and quantification by liquid chromatography-tandem mass spectrometry. Anal Chem 2010;82(24):10186—93.

[77] Dahmane E, Mercier T, Zanolari B, et al. An ultra performance liquid chromatography-tandem MS assay for tamoxifen metabolites profiling in plasma: first evidence of 4'-hydroxylated metabolites in breast cancer patients. J Chromatogr B Analyt Technol Biomed Life Sci 2010;878(32):3402—14.

[78] Veale D, Ashcroft T, Marsh C, et al. Epidermal growth factor receptors in non-small cell lung cancer. Br J Cancer 1987;55(5):513—6.

[79] Libermann TA, Razon N, Bartal AD, et al. Expression of epidermal growth factor receptors in human brain tumors. Cancer Res 1984;44(2):753—60.

[80] Weichselbaum RR, Dunphy EJ, Beckett MA, et al. Epidermal growth factor receptor gene amplification and expression in head and neck cancer cell lines. Head Neck 1989;11(5):437—42.

[81] Libermann TA, Nusbaum HR, Razon N, et al. Amplification, enhanced expression and possible rearrangement of EGF receptor gene in primary human brain tumours of glial origin. Nature 1985; 313(5998):144—7.

[82] Ullrich A, Coussens L, Hayflick JS, et al. Human epidermal growth factor receptor cDNA sequence and aberrant expression of the amplified gene in A431 epidermoid carcinoma cells. Nature 1984;309(5967): 418—25.

[83] Sato JD, Kawamoto T, Le AD, et al. Biological effects *in vitro* of monoclonal antibodies to human epidermal growth factor receptors. Mol Biol Med 1983;1(5):511—29.

[84] Kawamoto T, Sato JD, Le A, et al. Growth stimulation of A431 cells by epidermal growth factor: identification of high-affinity receptors for epidermal growth factor by an anti-receptor monoclonal antibody. Proc Natl Acad Sci USA 1983;80(5):1337—41.

[85] Masui H, Kawamoto T, Sato JD, et al. Growth inhibition of human tumor cells in athymic mice by anti-epidermal growth factor receptor monoclonal antibodies. Cancer Res 1984;44(3):1002—7.

[86] Li S, Schmitz KR, Jeffrey PD, et al. Structural basis for inhibition of the epidermal growth factor receptor by cetuximab. Cancer Cell 2005;7(4):301—11.

[87] Patel D, Lahiji A, Patel S, et al. Monoclonal antibody cetuximab binds to and down-regulates constitutively activated epidermal growth factor receptor vIII on the cell surface. Anticancer Res 2007;27(5A):3355—66.

[88] Kurai J, Chikumi H, Hashimoto K, et al. Antibody-dependent cellular cytotoxicity mediated by cetuximab against lung cancer cell lines. Clin Cancer Res 2007;13(5):1552—61.

[89] Cunningham D, Humblet Y, Siena S, et al. Cetuximab monotherapy and cetuximab plus irinotecan in irinotecan-refractory metastatic colorectal cancer. N Engl J Med 2004;351(4):337—45.

[90] Folprecht G, Lutz MP, Schöffski P, et al. Cetuximab and irinotecan/5-fluorouracil/folinic acid is a safe combination for the first-line treatment of patients with epidermal growth factor receptor expressing metastatic colorectal carcinoma. Ann Oncol 2006;17(3):450—6.

[91] Sobrero AF, Maurel J, Fehrenbacher L, et al. EPIC: Phase III trial of cetuximab plus irinotecan after fluoropyrimidine and oxaliplatin failure in patients with metastatic colorectal cancer. J Clin Oncol 2008;26(14):2311—9.

[92] Saltz LB, Meropol NJ, Loehrer Sr PJ, et al. Phase II trial of cetuximab in patients with refractory colorectal cancer that expresses the epidermal growth factor receptor. J Clin Oncol 2004;22(7):1201—8.

[93] Bonner JA, Harari PM, Giralt J, et al. Radiotherapy plus cetuximab for squamous-cell carcinoma of the head and neck. N Engl J Med 2006;354(6):567—78.

[94] Vermorken JB, Mesia R, Rivera F, et al. Platinum-based chemotherapy plus cetuximab in head and neck cancer. N Engl J Med 2008;359(11):1116–27.

[95] Burtness B, Goldwasser MA, Flood W, et al. Phase III randomized trial of cisplatin plus placebo compared with cisplatin plus cetuximab in metastatic/recurrent head and neck cancer: an Eastern Cooperative Oncology Group study. J Clin Oncol 2005;23(34):8646–54.

[96] Hecht JR, Mitchell E, Chidiac T, et al. A randomized phase IIIB trial of chemotherapy, bevacizumab, and panitumumab compared with chemotherapy and bevacizumab alone for metastatic colorectal cancer. J Clin Oncol 2009;27(5):672–80.

[97] Van Cutsem E, Peeters M, Siena S, et al. Open-label Phase III trial of panitumumab plus best supportive care compared with best supportive care alone in patients with chemotherapy-refractory metastatic colorectal cancer. J Clin Oncol 2007;25(13):1658–64.

[98] Giusti RM, Shastri K, Pilaro AM, et al. US Food and Drug Administration approval: panitumumab for epidermal growth factor receptor-expressing metastatic colorectal carcinoma with progression following fluoropyrimidine-, oxaliplatin-, and irinotecan-containing chemotherapy regimens. Clin Cancer Res 2008;14(5):1296–302.

[99] Cobleigh MA, Vogel CL, Tripathy D, et al. Multinational study of the efficacy and safety of humanized anti-HER2 monoclonal antibody in women who have HER2-overexpressing metastatic breast cancer that has progressed after chemotherapy for metastatic disease. J Clin Oncol 1999;17(9):2639–48.

[100] Mass RD, Press MF, Anderson S, et al. Evaluation of clinical outcomes according to HER2 detection by fluorescence in situ hybridization in women with metastatic breast cancer treated with trastuzumab. Clin Breast Cancer 2005;6(3):240–6.

[101] Slamon DJ, Leyland-Jones B, Shak S, et al. Use of chemotherapy plus a monoclonal antibody against HER2 for metastatic breast cancer that overexpresses HER2. N Engl J Med 2001;344(11):783–92.

[102] Hecht JR, Mitchell E, Neubauer MA, et al. Lack of correlation between epidermal growth factor receptor status and response to panitumumab monotherapy in metastatic colorectal cancer. Clin Cancer Res 2010;16(7):2205–13.

[103] Chung KY, Shia J, Kemeny NE, et al. Cetuximab shows activity in colorectal cancer patients with tumors that do not express the epidermal growth factor receptor by immunohistochemistry. J Clin Oncol 2005;23(9):1803–10.

[104] Cappuzzo F, Finocchiaro G, Rossi E, et al. EGFR FISH assay predicts for response to cetuximab in chemotherapy refractory colorectal cancer patients. Ann Oncol 2008;19(4):717–23.

[105] Moroni M, Veronese S, Benvenuti S, et al. Gene copy number for epidermal growth factor receptor (EGFR) and clinical response to antiEGFR treatment in colorectal cancer: a cohort study. Lancet Oncol 2005;6(5):279–86.

[106] Personeni N, Fieuws S, Piessevaux H, et al. Clinical usefulness of EGFR gene copy number as a predictive marker in colorectal cancer patients treated with cetuximab: a fluorescent in situ hybridization study. Clin Cancer Res 2008;14(18):5869–76.

[107] Italiano A, Follana P, Caroli FX, et al. Cetuximab shows activity in colorectal cancer patients with tumors for which FISH analysis does not detect an increase in EGFR gene copy number. Ann Surg Oncol 2008;15(2):649–54.

[108] Barber TD, Vogelstein B, Kinzler KW, Velculescu VE. Somatic mutations of EGFR in colorectal cancers and glioblastomas. N Engl J Med 2004;351(27):2883.

[109] Sok JC, Coppelli FM, Thomas SM, et al. Mutant epidermal growth factor receptor (EGFRvIII) contributes to head and neck cancer growth and resistance to EGFR targeting. Clin Cancer Res 2006;12(17):5064–73.

[110] Wikstrand CJ, Hale LP, Batra SK, et al. Monoclonal antibodies against EGFRvIII are tumor specific and react with breast and lung carcinomas and malignant gliomas. Cancer Res 1995;55(14):3140–8.

[111] Spindler KL, Olsen DA, Nielsen JN, et al. Lack of the type III epidermal growth factor receptor mutation in colorectal cancer. Anticancer Res 2006;26(6C):4889–93.

[112] Azuma M, Danenberg KD, Iqbal S, et al. Epidermal growth factor receptor and epidermal growth factor receptor variant III gene expression in metastatic colorectal cancer. Clin Colorectal Cancer 2006;6(3):214–8.

[113] Tinhofer I, Klinghammer K, Weichert W, et al. Expression of amphiregulin and EGFRvIII affect outcome of patients with squamous cell carcinoma of the head and neck receiving cetuximab-docetaxel treatment. Clin Cancer Res 2011;17(15):5197–204.

[114] Ellis CA, Clark G. The importance of being K-Ras. Cell Signal 2000;12(7):425−34.

[115] Bos JL, Fearon ER, Hamilton SR, et al. Prevalence of ras gene mutations in human colorectal cancers. Nature 1987;327(6120):293−7.

[116] Arber N, Shapira I, Ratan J, et al. Activation of c-K-ras mutations in human gastrointestinal tumors. Gastroenterology 2000;118(6):1045−50.

[117] Dahabreh IJ, Terasawa T, Castaldi PJ, et al. Systematic review: Anti-epidermal growth factor receptor treatment effect modification by KRAS mutations in advanced colorectal cancer. Ann Intern Med 2011;154(1):37−49.

[118] Adelstein BA, Dobbins TA, Harris CA, et al. A systematic review and meta-analysis of KRAS status as the determinant of response to anti-EGFR antibodies and the impact of partner chemotherapy in metastatic colorectal cancer. Eur J Cancer 2011;47(9):1343−54.

[119] Allegra CJ, Jessup JM, Somerfield MR, et al. American society of clinical oncology provisional clinical opinion: testing for KRAS gene mutations in patients with metastatic colorectal carcinoma to predict response to anti-epidermal growth factor receptor monoclonal antibody therapy. J Clin Oncol 2009;27(12):2091−6.

[120] De Roock W, Jonker DJ, Di Nicolantonio F, et al. Association of KRAS p.G13D mutation with outcome in patients with chemotherapy-refractory metastatic colorectal cancer treated with cetuximab. JAMA 2010;304(16):1812−20.

[121] Loupakis F, Ruzzo A, Cremolini C, et al. KRAS codon 61, 146 and BRAF mutations predict resistance to cetuximab plus irinotecan in KRAS codon 12 and 13 wild-type metastatic colorectal cancer. Br J Cancer 2009;101(4):715−21.

[122] Baldus SE, Schaefer KL, Engers R, et al. Prevalence and heterogeneity of KRAS, BRAF, and PIK3CA mutations in primary colorectal adenocarcinomas and their corresponding metastases. Clin Cancer Res 2010;16(3):790−9.

[123] De Roock W, Claes B, Bernasconi D, et al. Effects of KRAS, BRAF, NRAS, and PIK3CA mutations on the efficacy of cetuximab plus chemotherapy in chemotherapy-refractory metastatic colorectal cancer: A retrospective consortium analysis. Lancet Oncol 2010;11(8):753−62.

[124] Khambata-Ford S, Garrett CR, Meropol NJ, et al. Expression of epiregulin and amphiregulin and K-ras mutation status predict disease control in metastatic colorectal cancer patients treated with cetuximab. J Clin Oncol 2007;25(22):3230−7.

[125] Jacobs B, De Roock W, Piessevaux H, et al. Amphiregulin and epiregulin mRNA expression in primary tumors predicts outcome in metastatic colorectal cancer treated with cetuximab. J Clin Oncol 2009;27(30):5068−74.

[126] Saridaki Z, Tzardi M, Papadaki C, et al. Impact of KRAS, BRAF, PIK3CA mutations, PTEN, AREG, EREG expression and skin rash in ≥ 2nd line cetuximab-based therapy of colorectal cancer patients. PLoS ONE 2011;6(1):e15980.

[127] Paez JG, Jänne PA, Lee JC, et al. EGFR mutations in lung cancer: correlation with clinical response to gefitinib therapy. Science 2004;304(5676):1497−500.

[128] Lynch TJ, Bell DW, Sordella R, S, et al. Activating mutations in the epidermal growth factor receptor underlying responsiveness of non-small-cell lung cancer to gefitinib. N Engl J Med 2004;350(21):2129−39.

[129] Tsao MS, Sakurada A, Cutz JC, et al. Erlotinib in lung cancer − molecular and clinical predictors of outcome. N Engl J Med 2005;353(2):133−44.

[130] Bell DW, Lynch TJ, Haserlat SM, et al. Epidermal growth factor receptor mutations and gene amplification in non-small-cell lung cancer: molecular analysis of the IDEAL/INTACT gefitinib trials. J Clin Oncol 2005;23(31):8081−92.

[131] Mok TS, Wu YL, Thongprasert S, et al. Gefitinib or carboplatin-paclitaxel in pulmonary adenocarcinoma. N Engl J Med 2009;361(10):947−57.

[132] Fukuoka M, Wu YL, Thongprasert S, et al. Biomarker analyses and final overall survival results from a phase III, randomized, open-label, first-line study of gefitinib versus carboplatin/paclitaxel in clinically selected patients with advanced non-small-cell lung cancer in Asia (IPASS). J Clin Oncol 2011;29(21):2866−74.

[133] Douillard JY, Shepherd FA, Hirsh V, et al. Molecular predictors of outcome with gefitinib and docetaxel in previously treated non-small-cell lung cancer: data from the randomized phase III INTEREST trial. J Clin Oncol 2010;28(5):744−52.

[134] Mitsudomi T, Morita S, Yatabe Y, et al. Gefitinib versus cisplatin plus docetaxel in patients with non-small-cell lung cancer harbouring mutations of the epidermal growth factor receptor (WJTOG3405): an open label, randomised Phase 3 trial. Lancet Oncol 2010;11(2):121−8.

[135] Zhou C, Wu YL, Chen G, et al. Erlotinib versus chemotherapy as first-line treatment for patients with advanced EGFR mutation-positive non-small-cell lung cancer (OPTIMAL, CTONG-0802): a multicentre, open-label, randomised, Phase 3 study. Lancet Oncol 2011;12(8):735—42.

[136] Keedy VL, Temin S, Somerfield MR, et al. American Society of Clinical Oncology provisional clinical opinion: epidermal growth factor receptor (EGFR) mutation testing for patients with advanced non-small-cell lung cancer considering first-line EGFR tyrosine kinase inhibitor therapy. J Clin Oncol 2011;29(15):2121—7.

[137] Brugger W, Triller N, Blasinska-Morawiec M, et al. Prospective molecular marker analyses of EGFR and KRAS from a randomized, placebo-controlled study of erlotinib maintenance therapy in advanced non-small-cell lung cancer. J Clin Oncol 2011;29(31):4113—20.

[138] Hirsch FR, Varella-Garcia M, Bunn Jr PA, et al. Molecular predictors of outcome with gefitinib in a Phase III placebo-controlled study in advanced non-small-cell lung cancer. J Clin Oncol 2006;24(31):5034—42.

[139] Hirsch FR, Varella-Garcia M, McCoy J, et al. Increased epidermal growth factor receptor gene copy number detected by fluorescence *in situ* hybridization associates with increased sensitivity to gefitinib in patients with bronchioloalveolar carcinoma subtypes: a Southwest Oncology Group Study. J Clin Oncol 2005;23(28):6838—45.

[140] Cappuzzo F, Hirsch FR, Rossi E, et al. Epidermal growth factor receptor gene and protein and gefitinib sensitivity in non-small-cell lung cancer. J Natl Cancer Inst 2005;97(9):643—55.

[141] Dahabreh IJ, Linardou H, Kosmidis P, et al. EGFR gene copy number as a predictive biomarker for patients receiving tyrosine kinase inhibitor treatment: a systematic review and meta-analysis in non-small-cell lung cancer. Ann Oncol 2011;22(3):545—52.

[142] Linardou H, Dahabreh IJ, Kanaloupiti D, et al. Assessment of somatic k-RAS mutations as a mechanism associated with resistance to EGFR-targeted agents: a systematic review and meta-analysis of studies in advanced non-small-cell lung cancer and metastatic colorectal cancer. Lancet Oncol 2008;9(10):962—72.

[143] Zhu CQ, da Cunha Santos G, Ding K, et al. Role of KRAS and EGFR as biomarkers of response to erlotinib in National Cancer Institute of Canada Clinical Trials Group Study BR.21. J Clin Oncol 2008;26(26):4268—75.

[144] Schneider CP, Heigener D, Schott-von-Romer K, et al. Epidermal growth factor receptor-related tumor markers and clinical outcomes with erlotinib in non-small cell lung cancer: an analysis of patients from german centers in the TRUST study. J Thorac Oncol 2008;3(12):1446—53.

[145] Klumpen HJ, Samer CF, Mathijssen RH, et al. Moving towards dose individualization of tyrosine kinase inhibitors. Cancer Treat Rev 2011;37(4):251—60.

[146] Hamilton M, Wolf JL, Rusk J, et al. Effects of smoking on the pharmacokinetics of erlotinib. Clin Cancer Res 2006;12(7 Pt. 1):2166—71.

[147] Soulieres D, Senzer NN, Vokes EE, et al. Multicenter Phase II study of erlotinib, an oral epidermal growth factor receptor tyrosine kinase inhibitor, in patients with recurrent or metastatic squamous cell cancer of the head and neck. J Clin Oncol 2004;22(1):77—85.

[148] Gerlinger M, Rowan AJ, et al. Intratumor heterogeneity and branched evolution revealed by multiregion sequencing. N Engl J Med 2012;366:883—92.

CHAPTER

15

Immunosuppressive Drug Monitoring
Limitations of Immunoassays and the Application of Liquid Chromatography Mass Spectrometry

Kathleen A. Kelly, Anthony W. Butch

Department of Pathology and Laboratory Medicine, Geffen School of Medicine,
University of California at Los Angeles, Los Angeles, CA

OUTLINE

Therapeutic Drug Monitoring: Newer Drugs and Biomarkers
DOI: 10.1016/B978-0-12-385467-4.00015-4

INTRODUCTION

It has been more than a half-century since the first successful kidney transplant was performed between monozygotic twins [1]. Since then, vast improvements in organ transplantation have occurred despite the need for continuous immunosuppression to prevent graft rejection. In order to optimize and individualize immunosuppressive therapy, reliable and precise methods are required for drug monitoring. Not all immunosuppressive drugs are routinely monitored — for example, corticosteroids are dosed based on empirical guidelines. Several methods have been developed to measure azathioprine; however, this antiproliferative agent is seldom monitored in transplant patients [2–4]. The immunosuppressive drugs cyclosporine A (commonly refered to as cyclosporine), tacrolimus, sirolimus and mycophenolic acid, are routinely monitored for the following reasons: (1) there is a clear relationship between drug concentration and clinical response; (2) the drug has a narrow therapeutic index; (3) drug levels exhibit a high degree of inter- and intra-patient variability; (4) the pharmacological response is difficult to distinguish from unwanted side effects; (5) there is a risk of poor or non-compliance because the drug is administered for the lifetime of the graft or patient; and (6) there are significant drug–drug interactions. Therapeutic drug monitoring of everolimus is also warranted since the drug received United States Food and Drug Administration (FDA) approval in 2010 for use in adult kidney transplantation.

Combination immunosuppressive therapy is widely used today and drug interactions have been extensively documented. The most common combinations of immunosuppressive drugs used in solid organ transplant patients are tacrolimus and mycophenolic acid, followed by cyclosporine and mycophenolic acid [5]. Cyclosporine and sirolimus or tacrolimus and sirolimus are also used together. Corticosteroids are typically included in all drug regimens [6]. Cyclosporine inhibits transport of a mycophenolic acid metabolite from the liver into bile, which results in lower mycophenolic acid concentrations when the drugs are used in combination [6, 7]. The combination of cyclosporine and sirolimus or tacrolimus and sirolimus results in higher than expected blood concentrations of sirolimus [6, 8]. This can result in unpredictable drug concentrations, and emphasizes the need for therapeutic drug monitoring.

Until recently, most laboratories measured immunosuppressive drugs by semi-automated and automated immunoassays. The development of automated sample extraction systems and improvements in mass spectrometers have made liquid chromatography mass spectrometry (LC-MS) and liquid chromatography combined with tandem mass spectrometry (LC-MS/MS) systems more attractive to laboratories that monitor immunosuppressive drugs.

TABLE 15.1 Immunosuppressive Drugs Monitored in Solid Organ Transplantation

Drug class	Generic name	Brand names
Antimetabolites	Mycophenolate mofetil Mycophenolate sodium	CellCept Myfortic
Calcineurin Inhibitors	Cyclosporine A Tacrolimus (FK-506)	Sandimmune, Neoral, generic forms Prograf
mTOR Inhibitors	Sirolimus (Rapamycin) Everolimus	Rapamune Zortress, Certican

This chapter focuses on methods to measure FDA-approved immunosuppressive drugs (Table 15.1). Chemical structures of FDA-approved immunosuppressants are shown in Fig. 15.1. Analytical methods for drugs not commonly monitored, such as corticosteroids, azathioprine and cyclophosphamide, will not be discussed. We will also discuss the advantages and potential problems associated with immunoassays, LC-MS and LC-MS/MS methods, as they relate to specific drugs. We will use LC-MS and (/MS) throughout the chapter when referring to both LC-MS and LC-MS/MS methods.

APPLICATION OF IMMUNOASSAYS AND LC-MS TO IMMUNOSUPPRESSIVE DRUG MONITORING

There are a number of immunoassay technologies on the market that are considered either semi-automated or automated methods [9]. Since most of cyclosporine, tacrolimus, sirolimus and everolimus are found in red blood cells (RBCs), all testing methods require a processing step to extract the drug from RBCs. For these drugs semi-automated immunoassays dominate (five available) and require an off-line manual pretreatment step before analysis. There is currently one fully automated immunoassay (ACMIA) that does not require a manual pretreatment step. Assay formats and immunosuppressant drug (which are monitored in whole blood, except mycophenolic acid) applications are shown in Table 15.2.

The fully automated immunoassay uses antibody conjugate magnetic immunoassay (ACMIA) technology that is available on the Dimension® (Siemens Healthcare Diagnostics, Tarrytown, NY) series of instruments. The instrument mixes and sonicates an aliquot of whole blood followed by incubation with an anti-drug antibody conjugated to β-galactosidase. Drug-coated magnetic beads are used to remove unbound conjugate and the concentration of drug in the sample is measured spectrophotometrically after hydrolysis of substrate by β-galactosidase.

The chemiluminescent microparticle immunoassay (CMIA) uses an antibody that is attached to paramagnetic microparticles to capture drug from a pre-extracted sample hemolysate. After washing, acridinium-labeled drug is added and the amount of chemiluminescent light is monitored. The amount of light generated is inversely related to the drug concentration.

The cloned enzyme donor immunoassay (CEDIA) is a homogeneous assay (no wash step) that utilizes two inactive fragments of β-galactosidase (a drug conjugated enzyme donor and an unconjugated enzyme acceptor) that, when combined, have enzymatic activity. An antibody against the drug is added that interferes with the binding of drug–enzyme donor to enzyme acceptor and prevents enzymatic activity. As the concentration of drug in the sample increases, fewer antibodies are available to interfere with the formation of active enzyme. Hydrolysis of substrate by active enzyme is monitored and directly related to the amount of drug in the sample.

The enzyme multiplied immunoassay technique (EMIT) is a homogeneous assay that has the drug conjugated to the enzyme glucose-6-phosphate dehydrogenase. Drug in the sample competes with enzyme-labeled drug for binding to antibody. Unbound enzyme is active and converts NAD^+ (nicotinamide adenine dinucleotide) to NADH, which is monitored. There is a direct relationship between signal and drug concentration.

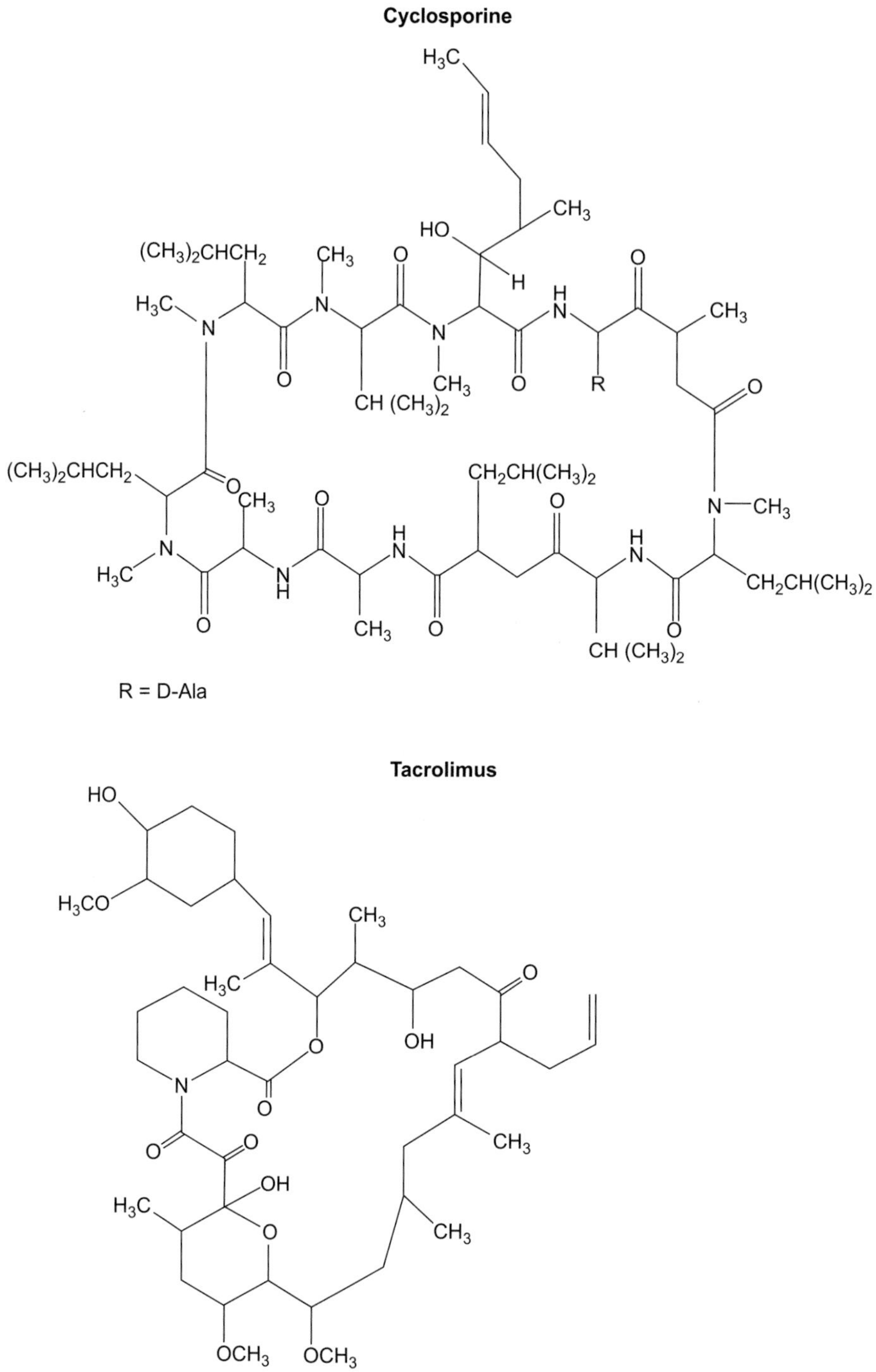

FIGURE 15.1   Chemical structures of FDA-approved immunosuppressants.

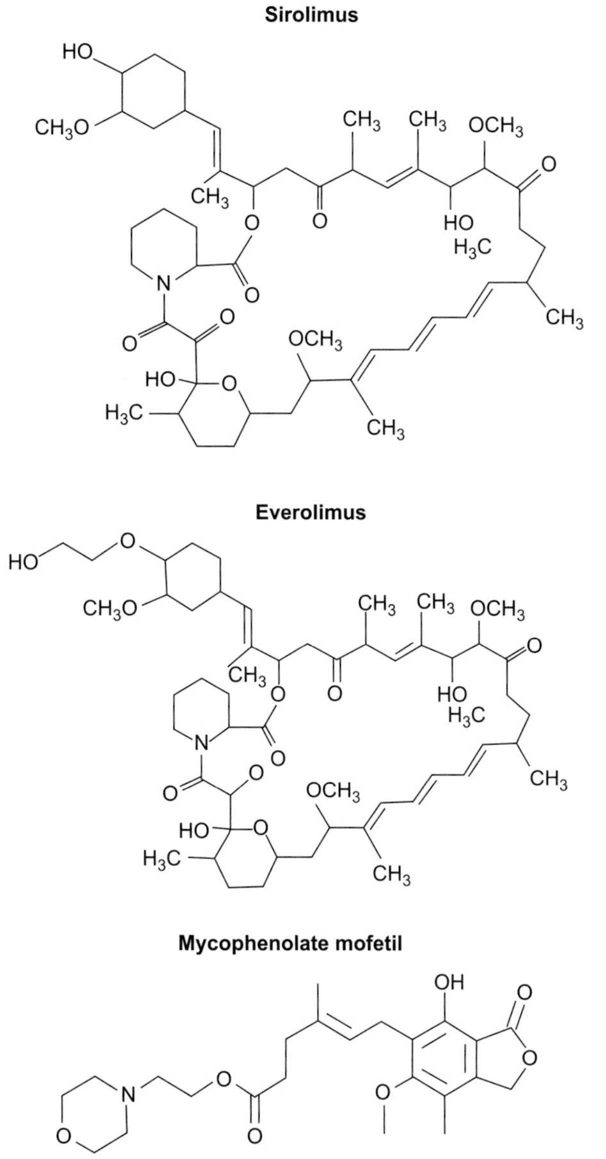

Sirolimus

Everolimus

Mycophenolate mofetil

FIGURE 15.1 (*Continued*).

The ADVIA Centaur® assay is a competitive assay that uses an antibody conjugated to biotin. Drug in the sample completes with acridinium-labeled drug for antibody binding. Streptavidin-coated magnetic particles are used to capture antibody–biotin complexes, and the amount of chemiluminescent signal is indirectly related to the drug concentration.

TABLE 15.2 Immunoassay Formats Used to Measure Whole Blood Immunosuppressants

Immunoassay*	Drug applications	Manufacturer
ACMIA	Cyclosporine, tacrolimus, sirolimus	Siemens Healthcare
CMIA	Cyclosporine, tacrolimus, sirolimus	Abbott Laboratories
CEDIA Plus	Cyclosporine, tacrolimus, sirolimus	Microgenics/Thermo Fisher
QMS	Everolimus	Microgenics/Thermo Fisher
Syva EMIT 2000	Cyclosporine, tacrolimus	Siemens Healthcare
ADVIA Centaur	Cyclosporine	Siemens Healthcare
FPIA	Cyclosporine	Abbott Laboratories

ACMIA, antibody conjugated magnetic immunoassay; CMIA, chemiluminescent microparticle immunoassay; CEDIA, cloned enzyme donor immunoassay; QMS, quantitative microsphere system; EMIT, enzyme-multiplied immunoassay technique; FPIA, fluorescence polarization immunoassay.

The fluorescence polarization immunoassay (FPIA) is a homogeneous assay that uses fluorescein-labeled drug that competes with the drug in the sample for antibody binding. When fluorescein-labeled drug is bound to antibody, the amount of polarized light is increased compared to unbound fluorescein-labeled drug. The concentration of drug in the sample is inversely proportional to the amount of polarized light.

In general, the advantages of immunoassays for measuring immunosuppressive drugs are the low start-up costs and ease of incorporation into the routine clinical laboratory, since the analytical methods and instruments do not require highly specialized training. The major limitation of immunoassays is cross-reactivity with drug metabolites, which is not always predictable and can vary significantly among patients.

Liquid chromatography (LC) separation with ultraviolet (UV), MS and tandem MS (MS/MS) detection methods have been available for many years for measuring immunosuppressive drug levels in blood. Before MS detection methods became widely available, LC-UV was considered the "gold standard" for measuring cyclosporine and was used to evaluate immunoassays. LC-UV methods to measure cyclosporine require extensive sample clean-up to minimize potential interfering substances, and have been largely replaced by LC-MS (/MS) methods [10]. The addition of MS/MS detection greatly increases specificity and can dramatically decrease run times, making this approach competitive with immunoassays from a throughput standpoint [11]. Despite the high cost of LC-MS (/MS) systems, numerous protocols have been developed and validated to measure immunosuppressive drugs and are routinely used by laboratories supporting large solid organ transplant programs [12, 13].

A critical component when monitoring immunosuppressive drugs by LC-MS (/MS) is the sample clean-up procedure. Blood contains large amounts of protein that can be absorbed onto chromatographic columns, which can reduce efficiency and increase column back-pressure, resulting in poor chromatographic separation [14]. Matrix components that are not removed during sample clean-up can also produce inaccurate measurements by either suppressing or enhancing ionization efficiency of the target compound or internal standard [15]. An extensive sample clean-up procedure can minimize matrix effects and ion suppression, but often requires additional time and labor that can impact the sample throughput.

Sample preparation can be performed manually (off-line) or can be automated and integrated into the front-end of the LC-MS (/MS) systems. Off-line techniques using solid phase extraction columns can be automated and have the advantage of concentrating the drug of interest. Liquid—liquid extraction methods are also used because they produce the cleanest extracts, but are highly labor-intensive and more time-consuming than other procedures. Because of these issues, off-line sample preparation is not amenable to testing large sample numbers.

LC-MS (/MS) systems with automated on-line solid phase sample preparation have the potential to greatly increase sample throughput and provide faster turnaround times. On-line sample preparation systems contain an additional column for sample clean-up that alternates between on-line and off-line by a series of automated switches. Since the same column is used to process many samples, there is the potential for column clogging and sample carryover. These concerns can be eliminated by using disposable single-use cartridges [16]. The other obstacle when using on-line solid phase sample preparation columns is introduction of internal standard prior to sample extraction to account for variable drug recovery between samples. Alnouti *et al.* developed a method for automated injection of internal standard into plasma samples prior to on-line sample clean-up. The accuracy, recovery and inter-assay precision of the method for propranolol and diclofenac were found to be comparable to those obtained using off-line sample preparation [17]. Koster *et al.* also reported favorable results when introducing an internal standard prior to on-line sample extraction [18]. Numerous on-line methods for LC-MS (/MS) have been reported with encouraging results, and have resulted in turnaround times that are competitive with immunoassays [14]. While encouraging, LC-MS (/MS) systems with on-line sample preparation are not widely used for monitoring immunosuppressive drugs despite having the potential for improving the specificity and dramatically reducing testing times.

Another important consideration using LC-MS (/MS) methods is the selection of internal standards. Ideally, the internal standard should have the same physiochemical properties as the immunosuppressive drug being monitored in order to correct for recovery and matrix effects that can reduce or enhance ionization efficiency. The internal standard can be a structurally unrelated compound, a structural analog, or a stable isotope-labeled compound. The preferred choice for an internal standard is the stable isotope-labeled immunosuppressive drug. When considering stable-isotope labeled internal standards it is important that the internal standard and analyte of interest co-elute, but do not have isotopic overlap. The internal standard should be used at a concentration above the limit of quantification that can be reliably measured, but not at a concentration that introduces ion suppression. The purity of stable isotope-labeled internal standards should also be established prior to use, since significant contamination with unlabeled compound can result in measurement bias.

Typically, sodium adducts are monitored when quantitating immunosuppressive drugs by LC-MS since they give the strongest signal in positive mode using electrospray ionization [19—21]. For LC-MS/MS methods, either ammonium acetate or ammonium formate is added to the mobile phase for monitoring ammonium adducts in positive mode using electrospray ionization [22—24]. A major advantage of LC-MS/MS is that selected product ions from specific precursor ions (transitions) can be monitored, which greatly improves the specificity of the method. The major disadvantage of LC-MS/MS detection is the increased cost over LC-MS systems.

THERAPEUTIC DRUG MONITORING OF CALCINEURIN INHIBITORS (CYCLOSPORINE AND TACROLIMUS)

Cyclosporine and tacrolimus are two calcineurin inhibitors commonly used for immunosuppression. They block activation and proliferation of $CD4^+$ and $CD8^+$ T lymphocytes by inhibiting interleukin-2 production [25, 26]. Under normal circumstances, binding of major histocompatibility complex—peptide conjugates to T lymphocytes results in activation of calcium/calmodulin-dependent serine/threonine phosphatase calcineurin. This produces dephosphorylation of the nuclear factor of activated T lymphocytes (NF-AT) and nuclear translocation of NF-AT. In the nucleus, NF-AT binds pro-inflammatory cytokine genes such as interleukin-2, resulting in upregulated gene transcription and proliferation of T lymphocytes [27]. Cyclosporine and tacrolimus freely cross lymphocyte membranes and form complexes with specific cytoplasmic binding proteins called immunophilins. Cyclosporine and tacrolimus bind the immunophilin cyclophilin and FK506-binding protein-12, respectively [28, 29]. Complexes of drug—immunophilin inhibit calcineurin activity and prevent nuclear translocation of NF-AT, which in turn downregulates cytokine gene transcription. The end result is a block in $CD4^+$ and $CD8^+$ lymphocyte activation [30—32].

Monitoring of Cyclosporine A

Cyclosporine is a small cyclic polypeptide originally isolated from fungal cultures of *Tolypocladium inflatum Gams* in 1970 [33]. Cyclosporine is approved in the United States to prolong organ and patient survival following kidney, liver, heart and bone marrow transplants. Cyclosporine is administered orally and intravenously (Sandimmune®). Neoral® is a microemulsion formulation of cyclosporine with more reproducible absorption characteristics following oral administration [34]. Numerous generic microemulsion formulations are also available [35, 36]. The majority of cyclosporine is found in RBCs and is bound to lipoproteins in plasma.

Immunoassays for Cyclosporine Monitoring

Improvements in immunosuppressive therapies and the demand for tighter control of immunosuppressive drug levels have made it critical for laboratories to provide rapid and precise drug concentrations. There are currently six different immunoassays for measuring whole blood cyclosporine in the United States (Table 15.2). Immunoassays are used by approximately 86% of all laboratories, according to the 2011 College of American Pathologists Immunosuppressive Drug Monitoring Survey, despite the fact that many of these immunoassays have significant cross-reactivity with cyclosporine metabolites (Table 15.3). Recommendations by numerous consensus panels specify that the analytical method for cyclosporine should be specific for parent compound [37—39]. Thus, other factors besides metabolite cross-reactivity are most likely being considered when selecting a suitable cyclosporine assay. These include instrumentation and reagent costs, technical skill requirements, testing volume, expected turnaround times, and familiarity of transplant physicians with specific immunoassays. All of the immunoassays, with the exception of the ACMIA, are semi-automated and require a whole blood pre-treatment step. This typically involves adding an extraction reagent such as methanol to an aliquot of whole blood. The hemolysate is

TABLE 15.3   Cyclosporine Immunoassay Metabolite Cross-Reactivity

Immunoassay	% Cyclosporine metabolite cross-reactivity*			
	AM1	AM4N	AM9	AM19
ACMIA	0	< 7	< 4	< 2
CMIA	0	< 4	< 3	< 2
CEDIA Plus	8	30	18	2
Syva EMIT 2000	≤ 5	8–13	≤ 4	0
FPIA	6–12	≤ 6	14–27	≤ 4

* Each metabolite was evaluated at 1000 μg/L except AM1, which was tested at 500 μg/L in the CEDIA Plus assay. Data are derived from references [45–49, 163].
ACMIA, antibody conjugated magnetic immunoassay; CMIA, chemiluminescent microparticle immunoassay; CEDIA, cloned enzyme donor immunoassay; EMIT, enzyme-multiplied immunoassay technique; FPIA, fluorescence polarization immunoassay.

then centrifuged and the supernatant is loaded onto the instrument for analysis. The CEDIA® Plus and the ADVIA Centaur methods do not require centrifugation after addition of the extraction reagent.

LC-MS (/MS) Methods for Cyclosporine

LC-UV is subject to interferences, requires laborious sample preparation and has largely been replaced by LC-MS (/MS) methods [40]. LC-MS (/MS) methods are specific for cyclosporine parent compound, and are now considered the reference method for validating immunoassays. Sample preparation usually involves a protein precipitation step followed by solid phase extraction using disposable columns containing C_{18} or another solid phase material. Sample extraction using disposable solid phase columns can be performed manually, or automated using liquid handling systems [16, 22]. Alternatively, liquid–liquid extraction can be performed manually or can be semi-automated [41]. Several methods using on-line solid phase extraction have also been described [21, 42]. Cyclosporine is a large neutral molecule that does not readily protonate under electrospray ionization but forms Na^+, K^+ and NH_4^+ adducts in the mobile phase. LC-MS methods mainly measure a sodium adduct (m/z 1224.6) since this produces the strongest signal [20, 21]. The majority of LC-MS/MS methods monitor an ammonium adduct transition (m/z 1220 → 1203), since ammonium adducts are relatively unstable and easy to fragment under the condition of tandem mass spectrometry and produce characteristic daughter ions [11, 43].

Analytical Issues

The major advantages of immunoassays are that the instruments are easy to operate and do not require the purchase of capital equipment. Immunoassays can also be performed by medical technologists without the need for specialized training. Another advantage of immunoassays is rapid turnaround times. Turnaround times can be a critical issue, especially in an outpatient setting where it is desirable for the drug concentration to be available when the patient is seen in clinic. This can require a 1- to 2-hour turnaround time for immunosuppressive drug testing.

The biggest drawback using cyclosporine immunoassays is metabolite cross-reactivity (Table 15.3). None of the immunoassays appears to be completely free from cross-reactivity with cyclosporine metabolites. The CEDIA Plus and FPIA have the highest overall metabolite cross-reactivity, and have significant cross-reactivity with AM1 and AM9 (Table 15.3) — metabolites that are typically present in the highest concentrations after transplantation [44]. As expected, the magnitude of metabolite cross-reactivity contributes to the positive bias when comparing immunoassays with LC methods. Mean concentrations of cyclosporine were shown to be approximately 12%, 13%, 17%, 22% and 40% higher than results obtained by LC-UV when measured by ACMIA, Syva EMIT, CEDIA Plus, FPIA on the TDx, and FPIA on the AxSYM, respectively [45–49]. Thus, it is important to consider metabolite cross-reactivity and the degree of positive bias when selecting an immunoassay for monitoring cyclosporine.

A potential problem with all cyclosporine immunoassays that require a manual extraction step is poor laboratory technique, which can significantly contribute to overall assay imprecision. Careful attention to detail and good technique can minimize variations at this critical pre-analytical step. This can be a problem with any of the whole blood immunosuppressive drug assays requiring a manual extraction step.

The advent of C2 monitoring for cyclosporine (cyclosporine levels 2 hours post-dosing) results in concentrations that range from 660 to 1700 µg/L (1700 ng/mL), depending on the type of graft and time after transplantation [50]. This can be a problem for some immunoassays with calibration curves that do not have sufficient analytical linearity to measure C2 concentrations without sample dilution. Sample dilution can lead to inaccuracies in quantitation since cyclosporine metabolites may not dilute in a linear fashion. Differences in the time needed for cyclosporine metabolites to re-equilibrate after dilution can vary depending on the immunoassay and dilution protocol [51, 52]. Some of the immunoassay manufacturers have eliminated the potential for dilution error by providing a separate calibration curve for C2 monitoring (ACIMA, CEDIA Plus and ADVIA Centaur).

Clearly, the major advantage of LC-MS (/MS) methods over immunoassays is their excellent specificity and lack of interference from cyclosporine metabolites. MS detection methods have excellent correlation with UV detection methods ($r = 0.998$) [53]. It is important that the linearity of the method is high enough to cover C2 monitoring of cyclosporine otherwise the method can produce dilution errors, as described above for immunoassays. Most methods are typically linear from 10 to 2000 µg/L (10–2000 ng/mL) [53]. Another advantage is that other immunosuppressive drugs can be measured in the same sample, which reduces labor costs, analysis time, and sample volume requirements [54]. Turnaround times can be a drawback for LC-MS (/MS) methods, especially when expedited test results are needed. Run time per sample can be long, ranging from 5 to 15 minutes, depending on the method [53]. Liquid handling systems and solid phase extraction in a 96-well plate format can help improve sample throughput and reduce turnaround times, especially at institutions that have large testing volumes. Other potential solutions to improve sample throughput include using LC-MS/MS systems equipped with on-line sample extraction and measuring multiple immunosuppressive drugs in the same sample [11, 43].

The selection of internal standard is critical and can potentially contribute to assay imprecision. Cyclosporine D, deuterium-labeled (d_{12}) cyclosporine and ascomycin are commonly used internal standards. Ascomycin is often used when monitoring cyclosporine and another immunosuppressive drug in the same sample. Some metabolites in blood can interfere with non-deuterated internal standards such as cyclosporine D by increasing peak areas for certain transitions [55, 56]. The use of cyclosporine D as an internal standard results in lower cyclosporine results compared with deuterium-labeled (d_{12}) cyclosporine as the internal standard. Ascomycin produces the highest imprecision when compared to cyclosporine D and deuterium-labeled cyclosporine as internal standard [55]. Thus, internal standards must be carefully selected and evaluated when developing LC-MS (/MS) methods to monitor cyclosporine either separately or simultaneously with other immuno-suppressive drugs [57].

Despite the specificity of LC-MS (/MS) methods for measuring cyclosporine, the majority of laboratories in the United States are still using immunoassays. The lack of widespread acceptance of LC-MS (/MS) methods for measuring cyclosporine clearly reflects the high initial equipment costs and the need for specialized training in chromatographic techniques and mass spectrometry detection methods. Unfortunately this type of specialized training is only available in a limited number of clinical laboratories, and is not part of many medical technology training programs. As newer LC-MS (/MS) systems emerge that are easier to operate and less expensive to purchase, more clinical laboratories may consider switching to these systems for measuring immunosuppressive drugs.

Monitoring of Tacrolimus

Tacrolimus (also known as FK-506) is a macrolide antibiotic, originally isolated from the fungus *Streptomyces tsukubaensis* [58]. In the United States, tacrolimus (brand name Prograf®) was approved for use in liver transplantation in 1994 and kidney transplantation in 1997. Tacrolimus is ~100-times more potent than cyclosporine, and is associated with less acute and chronic rejection and better long-term graft survival [59]. Tacrolimus monitoring is an integral part of any organ transplant program because of variable blood concentrations and a narrow therapeutic index. Tacrolimus is rapidly replacing cyclosporine. The majority of tacrolimus is found within RBCs and is bound in plasma to albumin, α_1-acid glycoprotein and lipoproteins [60].

Tacrolimus Immunoassays

Tacrolimus can be measured by ELISA and immunoassay. The ELISA takes ~4 hours to complete, requires numerous manual steps, and is used by only a few laboratories in the United States. More than 85% of laboratories measure tacrolimus by immunoassay. The ACMIA is fully automated, whereas the CMIA, CEDIA Plus and Syva EMIT 2000 are semi-automated methods requiring a separate whole blood pre-treatment step.

The CMIA is the most popular immunoassay (used by 49% of all laboratories in the United States) and is available on ARCHITECT *i* systems. The CMIA uses the same mouse mono-clonal anti-tacrolimus antibody that was used in the microparticle enzyme immunoassay, which is no longer commercially available. The fully automated ACMIA has been available since 2006 and is the second most popular tacrolimus immunoassay. The Syva EMIT 2000 has recently received FDA approval and is used by only 4% of laboratories. The Microgenics CEDIA for tacrolimus is also not widely used, despite being available for measuring tacroli-mus on several different instruments.

LC-MS (/MS) Methods for Tacrolimus

Tacrolimus cannot be measured by LC-UV because it does not possess a chromophore. LC-MS (/MS) methods are used by only 14% of laboratories in the United States, despite the fact that LC-MS (/MS) methods satisfy the recommendations in consensus documents regarding specificity for parent compound [39]. LC-MS/MS methods for tacrolimus have been shown to correlate better with biochemical data from transplant patients followed longitudinally than results by immunoassay [61]. Although the original LC-MS methods only measured tacrolimus, other immunosuppressive drugs such as cyclosporine, sirolimus and everolimus can be measured in the same sample because of similar solubility in alcohols, acetonitrile, ethers and halogenated hydrocarbons [62, 63]. There are numerous protocols to measure tacrolimus by LC-MS (/MS) with a lower limit of quantitation around 0.2 µg/L (0.2 ng/mL) [11, 18, 64–66]. LC-MS methods mainly monitor a sodium adduct (*m/z* 826) in positive ion mode while LC-MS/MS methods monitor an ammonium adduct transition (*m/z* 821 → 768) [11, 20, 43]. Kushnir *et al.* compared the specificity of LC-MS and LC-MS/MS for measuring tacrolimus and other immunosuppressive drugs and concluded, as expected, that LC-MS/MS is the superior method for verifying drug identity and avoiding interferences [67].

Analytical Issues

All of the immunoassays have significant cross-reactivity with tacrolimus metabolites. The ELISA, CMIA and EMIT cross-react with M-II (31-*O*-demethyl), M-III (15-*O*-demethyl) and M-V (15,13-di-*O*-demethyl) metabolites of tacrolimus [68, 69]. The CEDIA has significant cross-reactivity with M-I (13-*O*-demethyl), but does not cross-react with M-II or M-III. Cross-reactivity of the CEDIA with M-V has not been examined [70]. The ACMIA is expected to have metabolite cross-reactivity similar to the EMIT, since both assays use the same mono-clonal antibody. Metabolite cross-reactivity in patients with good liver function is typically not a problem because metabolite concentrations are relatively low compared to the parent drug [71]. However, metabolites tend to accumulate with reduced liver function and imme-diately after liver transplant, resulting in significant metabolite cross-reactivity and falsely elevated tacrolimus concentrations [72].

The ACMIA, CMIA and EMIT produce tacrolimus results that are 0.12 µg/L (0.12 ng/mL) lower, 0.92 µg/L (0.92 ng/mL) higher and 1.50 µg/L (1.50 ng/mL) higher than results obtained by LC-MS/MS, respectively [73]. The CMIA produces results that are 1.21 µg/L (1.21 ng/mL) higher and 0.47 µg/L (0.47 ng/mL) lower than results obtained by the ACMIA and EMIT, respectively. The ACMIA was shown to produce results that are 1.66 µg/L (1.66 ng/mL) lower than results by the EMIT, and produced a falsely high tacrolimus result for a patient not receiving tacrolimus [74]. A multi-site study found that the CMIA produces results similar to results by the ACMIA, and 0.51–1.63 µg/L (0.51 to 1.63 ng/mL) higher than results obtained by LC-MS/MS [75]. The CEDIA produces results that are 19–22% higher than results obtained by LC-MS/MS [70, 76]. Calibration error may contribute to some of the overall positive bias.

The recommended therapeutic range for whole blood tacrolimus concentrations after kidney and liver allograft transplants is 5.0–20 µg/L (5–20 ng/mL) by LC-MS [77]. When tacrolimus is used with other immunosuppressive agents such as sirolimus, the desired target tacrolimus concentration can be reduced to 2.0–4.0 µg/L (2.0–4.0 ng/mL). Because of this, the European Consensus Conference on Tacrolimus Optimization recommends a limit of quantitation of 1 µg/L (1.0 ng/mL) for tacrolimus in order to provide reliable concentrations during low-dose tacrolimus therapy [78]. Thus, it is important for laboratories to use a tacrolimus testing method that has acceptable performance at low concentrations and to make transplant services aware of the imprecision at the limit of quantitation. The limit of quantitation (between-day CV $< 20\%$) of the ACMIA was shown to range from 2.5 to 4.0 µg/L (2.5 to 4.0 ng/mL), whereas the CMIA ranged from 0.5 to 0.8 µg/L (0.5 to 0.8 ng/mL) [73, 75, 77]. The CEDIA and EMIT have a limit of quantitation of 3.6 µg/L (3.6 ng/mL) and 3.0 µg/L (3.0 ng/mL), respectively [76, 79]. These data indicate that only the CMIA meets the recommended limit of quantitation of 1 µg/L (1 ng/mL).

Assay standardization and reagent lot variations have been shown to be a major source of within-lab imprecision for tacrolimus immunoassays [80]. To minimize this type of variation it is recommended that laboratories sequester a large supply of a single lot of reagents, and carefully monitor new lots for bias and imprecision before beginning patient testing. The previously used MEIA produced falsely elevated tacrolimus concentrations with low hematocrit values, but the CMIA is not affected by changes in hematocrit [81, 82].

LC/MS (/MS) methods for measuring tacrolimus have the advantage of specificity (no metabolite cross-reactivity) and have limits of quantitation suitable for monitoring tacrolimus during low-dose treatment regiments. However, the initial introduction of LC-MS methods to clinical laboratories provided highly variable results [69]. The variability in tacrolimus testing was due to poor chromatography, variability in calibration curves, the absence of an isotope-labeled internal standard, and lack of experience with LC-MS testing methods. Unlike immunoassay kits that contain all the necessary reagents including calibrators and controls, LC-MS (/MS) methods typically require the in-house preparation of calibrators, controls and internal standards, which can contribute to variability. A commercially available kit containing freeze-dried calibrators and controls, and a solution of internal standard, is currently available (MassTrak™ Immunosuppressants Kit) but is not widely used due to cost. The kit performed well in a multi-center evaluation, and has the potential to help harmonize tacrolimus testing across laboratories [73]. Another potential source of variability is the use of ascomycin as the internal standard. Ascomycin is not structurally identical to tacrolimus (ethyl analog), and may behave differently and not completely compensate for variable recovery during sample extraction and matrix effects that produce ion suppression.

THERAPEUTIC DRUG MONITORING OF MAMMALIAN TARGET OF RAPAMYCIN (MTOR) INHIBITORS (SIROLIMUS AND EVEROLIMUS)

The mTOR inhibitors (also called proliferation signal inhibitors) sirolimus and everolimus are macrocyclic lactones. Sirolimus (also known as rapamycin) is a lipophilic molecule derived from *Streptomyces hygroscopicus*. This actinomycete fermentation product was identified in the early 1970s, and was approved by the FDA in 1999 for use with cyclosporine to reduce acute kidney rejection [83]. Sirolimus is available for both oral and intravenous administration. Everolimus is a chemically modified version of sirolimus (it contains a 2-hydroxyethyl group at position 46 of sirolimus) that is more hydrophilic and has improved pharmacokinetic characteristics and bioavailability [84]. Everolimus was approved by the FDA in April 2010 for oral use in adult kidney transplant patients.

The mTOR inhibitors readily cross the lymphocyte plasma membrane and bind the intracellular immunophilin, FK506 binding protein-12 [85]. Sirolimus and everolimus do not inhibit calcineurin activity after forming complexes with immunophilin. Instead, the complexes are highly specific inhibitors of the mammalian target of rapamycin (mTOR), a cell cycle serine/threonine kinase involved in the protein kinase B signaling pathway. This suppresses cytokine-induced T lymphocyte proliferation by blocking cell cycle progression into S phase [86]. The mTOR inhibitors can be used to minimize or allow complete withdrawal of calcineurin inhibitors in patients that experience declining renal allograph function. It was shown that kidney allograph patients at risk of renal dysfunction benefited from conversion from calcineurin inhibitors to mTOR inhibitors based on an improvement in renal glomerular filtration rate (mean increase of 38%) and serum creatinine (mean reduction of 17%) [87].

Monitoring of Sirolimus

Sirolimus synergizes with calcineurin inhibitors to produce profound immunosuppression of T lymphocytes. Sirolimus is primarily found in RBCs (96%), with a small amount in plasma and lymphocytes/granulocytes [88]. Almost all the sirolimus in plasma is bound to lipoproteins.

Sirolimus Immunoassays

Therapeutic monitoring of sirolimus is critical, because the administered dose is a poor predictor of total drug exposure due to patient variables. Because of the long drug half-life, daily monitoring of sirolimus is typically not necessary. Weekly monitoring may be needed shortly after transplantation, followed by monthly monitoring. Target concentrations for sirolimus range from 4.0 to 12.0 μg/L (4−12 ng/mL) when used with a calcineurin inhibitor [89]. Similar to tacrolimus, these relatively low whole blood concentrations can be a challenge analytically for some immunoassays. As combination immunosuppressant therapies continue to evolve, target concentrations for sirolimus may become even lower, further challenging the analytical performance of immunoassays.

According to the most recent College of American Pathologist Immunosuppressive Drug Monitoring Survey, there are 249 laboratories performing sirolimus testing. Approximately 55% of the laboratories in the United States measure whole blood sirolimus by CMIA (ARCHITECT *i* instruments) [90]. Another 14% of the laboratories use the ACMIA (Dimension instruments) and only a handful use the CEDIA.

LC-MS (/MS) Methods for Sirolimus

LC-UV methods for sirolimus suffer from the same drawbacks as described previously for cyclosporine. Approximately 28% of laboratories measure sirolimus using LC-MS (/MS) methods. LC-MS (/MS) methods typically have limits of quantitation below 0.3 μg/L (0.3 ng/mL) [16, 20, 21, 24, 91, 92]. LC-MS methods mainly monitor a sodium adduct (m/z 936.6) while LC-MS/MS methods monitor an ammonium adduct transition (m/z 931 → 864) in selected reaction monitoring mode [11, 20]. These assays have acceptable total imprecision that ranges from 0.96% to 10.8%, with a reported accuracy of 92–108% [11]. As indicated previously for calcineurin inhibitors, some of these methods use on-line extraction methods to improve turnaround times. A rapid LC-MS/MS method with turbulent flow technology has recently been introduced with markedly reduced run times of less than 20 minutes, compared with 2-hour run times for traditional LC-MS methods [93].

Analytical Issues

As with other immunoassays, the major problem with sirolimus immunoassays is metabolite cross-reactivity. The CMIA has 37% cross-reactivity with 11-hydroxy-sirolimus and 20% cross-reactivity with 41-O-demethyl-sirolimus [94]. The CEDIA has 44% cross-reactivity with 11-hydyroxy-sirolimus and 73% cross-reactivity with 41-O- and 32-O-demethyl-sirolimus [95]. However, immunoassay metabolite cross-reactivity may be less of an issue from a clinical standpoint since the distribution of metabolites in whole blood is similar among patients and relatively stable over long periods of time [96].

Sirolimus results using the ACMIA were shown to be 0.95 µg/L (0.95 ng/mL) higher than results obtained by LC/MS-MS [97]. At the authors' institution, sirolimus results obtained by CMIA are 0.74 µg/L (0.74 ng/mL) higher than results obtained by LC-MS. A multi-site evaluation found that the CMIA produced results that were 14–39% higher across three sites compared with results obtained by LC-MS/MS [94]. The CEDIA produces whole blood sirolimus results with a mean positive bias of 20.4%, compared with results obtained by LC-UV and LC-MS/MS methods [97].

The ACMIA, CMIA and CEDIA have limits of quantitation of 2.0, ≤ 1.5 and 3.0 µg/L (ng/mL), respectively [94, 97–99]. Although these limits of detection are adequate for monitoring sirolimus it is important that laboratories experimentally determine their own limit of quantitation (using whole blood samples) and do not rely on package insert information or published data. As noted above for the calcineurin inhibitors, a major advantage of LC-MS (/MS) sirolimus methods is increased sensitivity and specificity compared to immunoassays. A drawback is the longer turnaround times compared to immunoassay, but this problem can be partially addressed with on-line sample extraction. The use of in-house calibrators and controls, and different internal standards, can result in variable results across laboratories [100]. Hopefully, the variability across laboratories using LC-MS (/MS) methods can be reduced when kits containing all the critical reagents become commercially available.

Another potential problem with LC-MS (/MS) methods for sirolimus is the choice of internal standard. Many of the published methods currently use desmethoxy-rapamycin as the internal standard. A recent study compared sirolimus results by LC-MS/MS using deuterium-labeled-sirolimus and desmethoxy-rapamycin as internal standards, and experienced matrix effects that produced variable suppression/enhancement of the desmethoxy-rapamycin response [100]. This can result in a positive bias for sirolimus when compared with results obtained using a deuterium-labeled internal standard. The interpatient assay imprecision is also higher using desmethoxy-rapamycin as the internal standard. Thus, internal standards need to be carefully validated in LC-MS (/MS) methods when quantitating immunosuppressive drugs, and, whenever possible, deuterium-labeled internal standards should be used after verifying that they do not contain a significant amount of unlabeled drug.

Monitoring of Everolimus

Everolimus was recently approved for use in adult kidney transplant patients by the FDA, although it has been used for a number of years in European countries and other parts of the world. In a large international multicenter study called RECORD-1 (Renal Cell cancer treatment with Oral RaD001 given Daily), everolimus was found to prevent organ rejection and preserve kidney function using lower doses of cyclosporine [101]. Sirolimus partitions between RBCs and plasma, with approximately 75% of everolimus in RBCs [102]. Almost all of the everolimus in plasma is bound to proteins [102]. Everolimus metabolites are in relatively low concentrations when monitoring trough blood levels [103]. The recommendation is to monitor tough levels of everolimus, since they correlate well with the level of immunosuppression and rate of adverse effects [104].

Everolimus Immunoassays

The quantitative microsphere system (QMS®) everolimus immunoassay (Thermo Fisher Scientific) is the only FDA-approved immunoassay (approved in early 2011) for monitoring whole blood everolimus concentrations. The QMS everolimus assay is a particle-enhanced turbidimetric assay that uses a six-point calibration curve. The limit of quantitation was shown to be 1.3 µg/L (1.3 ng/mL), and the immunoassay produces everolimus results with a positive bias of 11% compared with LC-MS/MS [105]. Since everolimus trough concentrations are typically maintained at or above 3.0 µg/L (3.0 ng/mL) after kidney transplantation, this immunoassay has an adequate limit of quantitation [106, 107]. The immunoassay has 46% cross-reactivity with sirolimus, which is not surprising given the structural similarity between molecules. An FPIA (Seradyn, Inc.) to measure everolimus has been available outside the United States for many years and has a lower limit of detection of 2.0 µg/L (2.0 ng/mL) [108]. Metabolite cross-reactivity ranges from 5.0% to 72.0% [109]. When compared with LC-MS, the FPIA has a positive bias of 24.4% in renal transplant recipients [110].

LC-MS (/MS) Methods for Everolimus

LC-UV methods have been developed to measure everolimus, but they only have a limit of quantitation of 2.0 µg/L (2.0 ng/mL) [104]. At least nine LC-MS (/MS) methods have been developed to measure everolimus, with limits of quantitation around 0.25 µg/L (0.25 ng/mL) [104, 111, 112]. LC-MS methods monitor a sodium adduct (m/z 980.6) in positive ion mode. The LC-MS/MS methods monitor an ammonium adduct transition (m/z 975→908) in selected reaction monitoring mode. A deuterium-labeled everolimus is available and highly recommended, since ascomycin underestimates everolimus concentrations when used as internal standard [113–115].

THERAPEUTIC DRUG MONITORING OF MYCOPHENOLIC ACID

Mycophenolic acid is a fermentation product of *Penicillium* species that was originally shown to have antibacterial, antifungal and immunosuppressive properties [116, 117]. To improve bioavailability, the 2-morpholinoethyl ester of mycophenolic acid, mycophenolate mofetil (brand name CellCept®), was developed for oral and intravenous use [118]. Myco-phenolate mofetil received FDA approval in 1995. A sodium salt of mycophenolic acid, mycophenolate sodium (brand name Myfortic®), is also available as delayed-release (enteric-coated) tablets for oral use. Mycophenolic acid has largely replaced azathioprine in organ transplantation.

Mycophenolic acid non-competitively inhibits the enzymatic activity of inosine mono-phosphate dehydrogenase (IMPDH), the rate-limiting step in the production of guanosine nucleotides [119]. Guanosine nucleotides are needed for DNA synthesis and cellular prolif-eration, and are synthesized by the IMPDH pathway and an alternate salvage pathway. The salvage pathway is not present in lymphocytes, so mycophenolic acid selectively inhibits lymphocyte proliferation [120, 121]. Two isoforms of IMPDH exist, and mycophenolic acid selectively inhibits the one expressed predominantly by activated lymphocytes [122]. Almost all mycophenolic acid (> 99%) is located in plasma, so mycophenolic acid concentrations are measured in serum and plasma samples [123]. The use of plasma from EDTA-anticoagulated whole blood allows the same sample to be used to measure other immunosuppressive drugs using LC-MS/MS methods.

When mycophenolic acid was originally approved for use as mycophenolate mofetil, ther-apeutic drug monitoring was not considered necessary. However, studies have found wide variations in total drug exposure (as high as 10-fold) following a fixed dose, suggesting that individualized dosing may be beneficial [124, 125]. A round-table meeting recently rec-ommended therapeutic drug monitoring based on inter-patient variability and significant drug interactions during combination immunosuppressive therapy [126]. Trough levels of mycophenolic acid are a relatively good indicator of total drug exposure [127]. The generally accepted therapeutic range for mycophenolic acid is 1.0–3.5 mg/L (1.0–3.5 µg/mL), which can be easily measured by current analytical methods with good precision [128–130].

Circulating mycophenolic acid is mostly bound to albumin, and concentrations of free (unbound) mycophenolic acid range from 1.2% to 2.5% of total mycophenolic acid concentra-tions [123]. Free mycophenolic acid can be increased in certain clinical conditions, such as hypoalbuminemia, hyperbilirubinemia and uremia [131]. Several studies have shown that the immunosuppressive effects of mycophenolic acid and clinical toxicity correlate better with free mycophenolic acid rather than total mycophenolic acid concentrations [123]. This is especially true for children, because they have higher concentrations of mycophenolic acid that are more variable due to differences in glucuronosyltransferase activity [132]. In contrast, a few studies have found that free mycophenolic acid is not superior to total myco-phenolic acid in predicting clinical outcomes in transplant patients [133]. The most recent consensus report recommends measuring total mycophenolic acid, but does not recommend separate monitoring of free mycophenolic acid or mycophenolic acid metabolites [134].

Immunoassays for Mycophenolic Acid

Currently only 45 laboratories in the United States offer therapeutic drug monitoring of mycophenolic acid, which is only one-tenth the number of all laboratories that measure tacro-limus. Five laboratories use the EMIT and seven laboratories use the Roche enzymatic immu-noassay for measuring total mycophenolic acid. Even fewer laboratories use the CEDIA to measure mycophenolic acid. The Roche enzymatic immunoassay uses mycophenolic acid in the sample to inhibit IMPDH II, the enzyme that normally catalyzes the conversion of ino-sine monophosphate to xanthosine monophosphate. During this reaction, NAD^+ is converted to NADH, and the rate of NADH generation is monitored. The concentration of mycophenolic acid in the sample is inversely related to NADH.

LC-UV and LC-MS/MS Methods for Mycophenolic Acid

Most laboratories use LC-UV (25%) and LC-MS/MS (33%) methods to monitor mycophenolic acid. LC-MS methods are not commonly used to monitor mycophenolic acid. A LC-MS method that monitors the deprontonated molecular ion (*m/z* 319) of mycophenolic acid has been described that correlates well with LC-UV methods [135]. LC-UV and LC-MS/MS methods have excellent specificity and sensitivity for the parent compound [136–140]. The LC-UV methods differ from the LC-MS/MS methods primarily in sample extraction, analytical column, length of run, and limit of quantitation.

Free mycophenolic acid can be measured after removal of protein-bound mycophenolic acid by ultrafiltration or precipitation. However, free mycophenolic acid is typically in low concentration (~2% of total) and is more appropriately quantitated using LC-MS/MS methods [43]. Although LC-MS/MS methods have been described to measure multiple immunosuppressants in the same sample, mycophenolic acid is structurally different and requires separate calibrators and sample preparation techniques [136, 141–144]. LC-MS/MS methods for mycophenolic acid typically monitor a ammonium adduct transition (*m/z* 338→207) in selected reaction monitoring mode, utilizing positive electrospray ionization and mycophenolic acid carboxybutoxy ether as the internal standard.

Analytical Issues

As previously described for other immunosuppressive drugs, the major benefits of mycophenolic acid immunoassays are the simple testing format, rapid turnaround times, and minimal start-up costs. The major limitation is metabolite cross-reactivity, which can translate into significant assay bias. The two major metabolites are the 7-*O*-glucuronide and acyl glucuronide conjugates of mycophenolic acid. Mycophenolic acid glucuronide does not have immunosuppressive activity, whereas the acyl glucuronide metabolite of mycophenolic acid has anti-IMPDH activity [145, 146]. The EMIT, Roche enzymatic assay and CEDIA have 30%, < 5% and 158% cross-reactivity with the acyl glucuronide metabolite of mycophenolic acid, respectively [147–149]. Bias due to metabolite cross-reactivity for the EMIT and CEDIA can be further exaggerated in transplant patients with impaired renal function due to the accumulation of acyl glucuronide of mycophenolic acid [150, 151].

The EMIT has been shown to overestimate mycophenolic acid concentrations by 10–30% when compared with LC-UV methods [150, 152–154]. Other studies have shown that the positive bias of the EMIT ranges from 19–61% compared with LC-MS/MS methods, and is dependent on whether the patient is also receiving sirolimus or cyclosporine [151, 155]. The Roche enzymatic immunoassay produces results that are only 0.26–0.45 mg/L (0.26–0.45 μg/mL) lower than results obtained by LC-MS/MS [156]. Further studies across multiple testing centers have confirmed that the Roche enzymatic immunoassay produces mycophenolic acid results that are in close agreement with those produced by LC-UV and

LC-MS/MS [156, 157]. The CEDIA for mycophenolic acid has a mean positive bias of around 55% when compared with a LC-UV method [158].

LC-UV and LC-MS/MS methods for mycophenolic acid are specific for the parent compound and are used for validating immunoassays [138—140, 159]. LC-UV methods typically do not have a limit of quantitation suitable for monitoring free mycophenolic acid unless the sample is extensively concentrated before analysis [160]. When using a LC-MS/MS method to measure mycophenolic acid in conjunction with other immunosuppressive drugs, it is important to carefully validate the method for drug recovery and eliminate any assay bias. Another concern when monitoring mycophenolic acid by LC-MS/MS is the selection of the internal standard. Due to structural similarity, the carboxybutoxy ether of mycophenolic acid is typically used as the internal standard. However, there are reports that mycophenolic acid carboxybutoxy ether is subject to in-source ion fragmentation to mycophenolic acid, which may result in significant bias when measuring free mycophenolic acid concentrations [161, 162].

CONCLUSIONS

Therapeutic monitoring of immunosuppressive drugs is essential for optimizing therapeutic effectiveness and minimizing unwanted adverse effects following organ transplantation. Although it has been firmly established that immunoassays suffer from significant metabolite cross-reactivity, the majority of laboratories in the United States still use immunoassays to measure most immunosuppressive drugs. The exception is mycophenolic acid, which is commonly monitored by LC-UV and LC-MS/MS, given the limited availability of immunoassay applications. Immunoassays have gained widespread use, and will continue to dominant the market because they are simple to operate, have fast turnaround times and low start-up costs, and do not require specialized training. These considerations overshadow the excellent sensitivity, specificity and versatility of LC-MS (/MS) methods for immunosuppressive drug monitoring. The high cost of LC-MS (/MS) systems is a major obstacle, especially for hospitals with limited capital equipment budgets. Furthermore, it is difficult to recruit testing personnel with experience in chromatographic separation techniques and mass spectrometry, and even more difficult to train a novice.

References

[1] Merrill JP, Murray JE, Harrison JH, Guild WR. Successful homotransplantation of the human kidney between identical twins. J Am Med Assoc 1956;160:277—82.

[2] Bruunshuus I, Schmiegelow K. Analysis of 6-mercaptopurine, 6-thioguanine nucleotides and 6-thiuric acid in biological fluids by high-performance liquid chromatography. Scand J Clin Invest 1989;49:799—784.

[3] Kreuzenkamp-Jansen CW, De Abreu RA, Bokkerink JPM, Trijbels JMF. Determination of extracellular and intracellular thiopurines and methylthiopurines with HPLC. J Chromatogr 1995;672:53—61.

[4] Rabel SR, Stobaugh JF, Trueworthy R. Determination of intracellular levels of 6-mercaptopurine metabolites in erythrocytes utilizing capillary electrophoresis with laser-induced fluorescence detection. Anal Biochem 1995;224:315—22.

[5] Wolfe RA, Roys EC, Merion RM. Trends in organ donation and transplantation in the United States, 1999—2008. Am J Transpl 2010;10(4 Part 2):961—72.

[6] Filler G, Lepage N, Delisle B, Mai I. Effect of cyclosporine on mycophenolic acid area under the concentration–time curve in pediatric kidney transplant recipients. Ther Drug Monit 2001;23:514–9.

[7] van Gelder T, Klupp J, Barten MJ, et al. Comparison of the effects of tacrolimus and cyclosporine on the pharmacokinetics of mycophenolic acid. Ther Drug Monit 2001;23:119–28.

[8] Undre NA. Pharmacokinetics of tacrolimus based combination therapies. Nephrol Dial Transpl. 2003;18:i12–5.

[9] Wild DG, editor. The Immunoassay Handbook. 3rd edn. North Holland: Elsevier B V; 2006.

[10] Napoli KL, Kahan BD. Sample clean-up and high-performance liquid chromatographic techniques for measurement of whole blood rapamycin concentrations. J Chromatogr B Biomed Appl. 1994;654:111–20.

[11] Korecka MSL. Review of the newest HPLC methods with mass spectrometry detection for determination of immunosuppressive drugs in clinical practice. Ann Transplant 2009;14:61–72.

[12] Whitman DA, Abbott V, Fregien K, Bowers LD. Recent advances in high-performance liquid chromatography/mass spectrometry and high-performance liquid chromatography/tandem mass spectrometry: detection of cyclosporine and metabolites in kidney and liver tissue. Ther Drug Monit 1993;15:552–6.

[13] Zhou L, Tan D, Theng J, et al. Optimized analytical method for cyclosporine A by high-performance liquid chromatography-electrospray ionization mass spectrometry. J Chromatogr B Biomed Sci Appl 2001;754:201–7.

[14] Mullett WM. Determination of drugs in biological fluids by direct injection of samples for liquid-chromatographic analysis. J Biochem Biophys Methods 2007;70:263–73.

[15] Taylor PJ. Matrix effects: the Achilles heel of quantitative high-performance liquid chromatography-electrospray-tandem mass spectrometry. Clin Biochem 2005;38:328–34.

[16] Koal T, Deters M, Casetta B, Kaever V. Simultaneous determination of four immunosuppressants by means of high speed and robust on-line solid phase extraction-high performance liquid chromatography-tandem mass spectrometry. J Chromatogr B 2004;805:215–22.

[17] Alnouti Y, Li M, Kavetskaia O, et al. Method for internal standard introduction for quantitative analysis using on-line solid-phase extraction LC-MS/MS. Anal Chem 2006;78:1331–6.

[18] Koster RA, Dijkers ECF. Robust, high-throughput LC-MS/MS method for therapeutic drug monitoring of cyclosporine, tacrolimus, everolimus, and sirolimus in whole blood. Ther Drug Monit 2009;31:116–25.

[19] Kirchner GI, Vidal C, Jacobsen W, et al. Simultaneous on-line extraction and analysis of sirolimus (rapamycin) and ciclosporin in blood by liquid chromatography-electrospray mass spectrometry. J Chromatogr B: Biomed Sci Appl 1999;721:285–94.

[20] Deters M, Kirchner G, Resch K, Kaever V. Simultaneous quantification of sirolimus, everolimus, tacrolimus and cyclosporine by liquid chromatography-mass spectrometry (LC-MS). Clin Chem Lab Med 2002;40:285–92.

[21] Vidal C, Kirchner GI, Wunsch G, Sewing K-F. Automated simultaneous quantification of the immunosuppressants 40-O-(2-hydroxyethyl)rapamycin and cyclosporine in blood with electrospray-mass spectrometric detection. Clin Chem 1998;44:1275–82.

[22] Annesley TM, Clayton L. Simple extraction protocol for analysis of immunosuppressant drugs in whole blood. Clin Chem 2004;50:1845–8.

[23] Taylor PJ, Salm P, Lynch SV, Pillans PI. Simultaneous quantification of tacrolimus and sirolimus, in human blood, by high-performance liquid chromatography-tandem mass spectrometry. Ther Drug Monit 2000;22:608–12.

[24] Holt DW, Lee T, Jones K, Johnston A. Validation of an assay for routine monitoring of sirolimus using HPLC with mass spectrometric detection. Clin Chem 2000;46:1179–83.

[25] Shibasaki F, Hallin U, Uchino H. Calcineurin as a multifunctional regulator. J Biochem 2002;131:1–15.

[26] Siekierka JJ, Hung SHY, Poe M, et al. A cytosolic binding protein for the immunosuppressant FK506 has peptidyl-prolyl isomerase activity but is distinct from cyclophilin. Nature 1989;341:755–7.

[27] Schreiber SL, Crabtree GR. The mechanism of action of cyclosporin A and FK-506. Immunol Today 1992;13:136–42.

[28] Flanagan WM, Corthesy B, Bram RJ, Crabtree GR. Nuclear association of a T-cell transcription factor blocked by FK-506 and cyclosporin A. Nature 1991;352:803–7.

[29] Clipstone NA, Crabtree GR. Identification of calcineurin as a key signalling enzyme in T-lymphocyte activation. Nature 1992;357:695–7.

[30] Schreiber SL. Chemistry and biology of immunophilins and their immunosuppressive ligands. Science 1991;251:283–7.

[31] Gummert JF, Ikonen T, Morris R. Newer immunosuppressive drugs: A Review. J Am Soc Nephrol 1999;10:1366—80.

[32] Jørgensen KA, Koefoed-Nielsen PB, Karamperis N. Calcineurin phosphatase activity and immunosuppression. A review on the role of calcineurin phosphatase activity and the immunosuppressive effect of cyclosporin A and tacrolimus. Scand J Immunol 2003;57:93—8.

[33] Borel JF, Feurer C, Gubler HU, Stahelin H. Biological effects on cyclosporin A: A new antilymphocytic agent. Agents and Actions 1976;6:468—75.

[34] Vonderscher J, Meinzer A. Rationale for the development of Sandimmune Neoral. Transplant Proc 1994;26:2925—7.

[35] Bartucci MR. Issues in cyclosporine drug substitution: implications for patient management. J Transpl Coord 1999;9:137—42.

[36] Alloway RR. Generic immunosuppressant use in solid organ transplantation. Transplant Proc 1999;31:2S—5S.

[37] Kahan B, Shaw L, Holt D, et al. Consensus document: Hawk's Cay meeting on therapeutic drug monitoring of cyclosporine. Clin Chem 1990;36:1510—6.

[38] Shaw L, Yatscoff R, Bowers L, et al. Canadian Consensus Meeting on cyclosporine monitoring: report of the consensus panel. Clin Chem 1990;36:1841—6.

[39] Ollerich M, Armstrong VW, Kahan B, et al. Lake Louise consensus conference on cyclosporin monitoring in organ transplantation: report of the consensus panel. Ther Drug Monit 1995;17:642—54.

[40] Ansermot N, Fathi M, Veuthey J-L, et al. Simultaneous quantification of cyclosporine, tacrolimus, sirolimus and everolimus in whole blood by liquid chromatography-electrospray mass spectrometry. Clin Biochem 2008;41:728—35.

[41] Brignol N, McMahon LM, Luo S, Tse FLS. High-throughput semi-automated 96-well liquid/liquid extraction and liquid chromatography/mass spectrometric analysis of everolimus (RAD 001) and cyclosporin A (Cyclosporine) in whole blood. Rapid Commun Mass Spectrom 2001;15:898—907.

[42] Jemal M. High-throughput quantitative bioanalysis by LC/MS/MS. Biomed Chromatogr 2000;14:422—9.

[43] Sallustio BC. LC-MS/MS for immunosuppressant therapeutic drug monitoring. Bioanalysis 2010;2:1141—53.

[44] Ryffel B, Foxwell BM, Mihatsch MJ, et al. Biologic significance of cyclosporine metabolites. Transplant Proc 1988;20:575—84.

[45] Steimer W. Performance and specificity of monoclonal immunoassays for cyclosporine monitoring: How specific is specific? Clin Chem 1999;45:371—81.

[46] Schutz E, Svinarov D, Shipkova M, et al. Cyclosporin whole blood immunoassays (AxSYM, CEDIA, and Emit): A critical overview of performance characteristics and comparison with HPLC. Clin Chem 1998;44:2158—64.

[47] Hamwi A, Veitl M, Manner G, et al. Evaluation of four automated methods for determination of whole blood cyclosporine concentrations. Am J Clin Pathol 1999;112:358—65.

[48] Terrell AR, Daly TM, Hock KG, et al. Evaluation of a no-pretreatment cyclosporin A assay on the Dade Behring Dimension RxL clinical chemistry analyzer. Clin Chem 2002;48:1059—65.

[49] Butch AW, Fukuchi AM. Analytical performance of the CEDIA cyclosporine PLUS whole blood immunoassay. J Anal Toxicol 2004;28:204—10.

[50] Oellerick M, Armstrong VW. Two-hour cyclosporine concentration determinations: an appropriate tool to monitor neoral therapy? Ther Drug Monit 2022;24:40-46

[51] Morris RG, Holt DW, Armstrong VW, et al. Analytic aspects of cyclosporine monitoring, on behalf of the IFCC/IATDMCT Joint Working Group. Ther Drug Monit 2004;26:227—30.

[52] Holt DW, Johnston A, Kahan BD, et al. New approaches to cyclosporine monitoring raise further concerns about analytical techniques. Clin Chem 2000;46:872—4.

[53] Salm P, Taylor PJ, Lynch SV, et al. A rapid HPLC-mass spectrometry cyclosporin method suitable for current monitoring practices. Clin Biochem 2005;38:667—73.

[54] Taylor PJ. Therapeutic drug monitoring of immunosuppressant drugs by high-performance liquid chromatography-mass spectrometry. The Drug Monit 2004;26:215—9.

[55] Taylor PJ, Brown SR, Cooper DP, et al. Evaluation of 3 internal standards for the measurement of cyclosporin by HPLC-mass spectrometry. Clin Chem 2005;51:1890—3.

[56] Vogeser M, Spöhrer U. Pitfall in the high-throughput quantification of whole blood cyclosporin A using liquid chromatography-tandem mass spectrometry. Clin Chem Lab Med 2005;43:400—2.

[57] Taylor PJ. Internal standard selection for immunosuppressant drugs measured by high-performance liquid chromatography tandem mass spectrometry. Ther Drug Monit 2007;29:131–2.

[58] Goto T, Kino T, Hatanaka H, et al. Discovery of FK-506, a novel immunosuppressant isolated from *Streptomyces tsukubaensis*. Transplant Proc 1987;19:4–8.

[59] First MR. Tacrolimus based immunosuppression. J Nephrol 2004;17:25–31.

[60] Zahir H, Nand RA, Brown KF, et al. Validation of methods to study the distribution and protein binding of tacrolimus in human blood. J Pharmacol Toxicol Methods 2001;46:27–35.

[61] Napoli KL. Is microparticle enzyme-linked immunoassay (MEIA) reliable for use in tacrolimus TDM? Comparison of MEIA to liquid chromatography with mass spectrometric detection using longitudinal trough samples from transplant recipients. Ther Drug Monit 2006;28:491–504.

[62] Alak AM. Measurement of tacrolimus (FK506) and its metabolites: a review of assay development and application in therapeutic drug monitoring and pharmacokinetic studies. Ther Drug Monit 1997;19:338–51.

[63] Christians U, Jacobsen W, Serkova N, et al. Automated, fast and sensitive quantification of drugs in blood by liquid chromatography-mass spectrometry with on-line extraction: immunosuppressants. J Chromatogr B Biomed Sci Appl 2000;748:41–53.

[64] Wang S, Magill JE, Vicente FB. A fast and simple high-performance liquid chromatography/mass spectrometry method for simultaneous measurement of whole blood tacrolimus and sirolimus. Arch Pathol Lab Med 2005;129:661–5.

[65] Lensmeyer GL, Poquette MA. Therapeutic monitoring of tacrolimus concentrations in blood: semi-automated extraction and liquid chromatography-electrospray ionization mass spectrometry. The Drug Monit 2001;23:239–49.

[66] Keevil B, McCann S, Cooper D, Morris M. Evaluation of a rapid micro-scale assay for tacrolimus by liquid chromatography-tandem mass spectrometry. Ann Clin Biochem 2002;39:487–92.

[67] Kushnir MM, Rockwood AL, Nelson GJ, et al. Assessing analytical specificity in quantitative analysis using tandem mass spectrometry. Clin Biochem 2005;38:319–27.

[68] Iwasaki K, Shiraga T, Matsuda H, et al. Further metabolism of FK506 (tacrolimus). Identification and biological activities of the metabolites oxidized at multiple sites of FK506. Drug Metab Dispos 1995;23:28–34.

[69] Wallemacq P, Armstrong VW, Brunet M, et al. Opportunities to optimize tacrolimus therapy in solid organ transplantation: Report of the European Consensus Conference. Ther Drug Monit 2009;31:139–52.

[70] CEDIA® Tacrolimus Assay (package insert). Fremont, CA: Microgenics Corporation; 2005.

[71] Staatz CE, Taylor PJ, Tett SE. Comparison of an ELISA and an LC/MS/MS method for measuring tacrolimus concentrations and making dosage decisions in transplant recipients. Ther Drug Monit 2002;24:607–15.

[72] Gonschior A, Christians U, Winkler M, et al. Tacrolimus (FK506) metabolite patterns in blood from liver and kidney transplant patients. Clin Chem 1996;42:1426–32.

[73] Napoli KL, Hammett-Stabler C, Taylor PJ, et al. Multi-center evaluation of a commercial kit for tacrolimus determination by LC/MS/MS. Clin Biochem 2010;43:910–20.

[74] Bazin C, Guinedor A, Barau C, et al. Evaluation of the ARCHITECT tacrolimus assay in kidney, liver, and heart transplant recipients. J Pharm Biomed Anal 2010;53:997–1002.

[75] Wallemacq P, Goffinet J-S, O'Morchoe S, et al. Multi-site analytical evaluation of the Abbott ARCHITECT tacrolimus assay. Ther Drug Monit 2009;31:198–204.

[76] Westley IS, Taylor PJ, Salm P, Morris RG. Cloned enzyme donor immunoassay tacrolimus assay compared with high-performance liquid chromatography-tandem mass spectrometry and microparticle enzyme immunoassay in liver and renal transplant recipients. Ther Drug Monit 2007;29:584–91.

[77] Busuttil RW, Klintmalm GBG, Lake JR, et al. General guidelines for the use of tacrolimus in adult liver transplant patients. Transplantation 1996;61:845–7.

[78] Amann S, Parker TS, Levine DM. Evaluation of 2 immunoassays for monitoring low blood levels of tacrolimus. Ther Drug Monit 2009;31:273–6.

[79] LeGatt DF, Shalapay CE, Cheng SB. The EMIT 2000 tacrolimus assay: an application protocol for the Beckman Synchron LX20 PRO analyzer. Clin Biochem 2004;37:1022–30.

[80] Steele BW, Wang E, Soldin SJ, et al. A longitudinal replicate study of immunosuppressive drugs. Arch Pathol Lab Med 2003;127:283–8.

[81] Marubashi S, Nagano H, Kobayashi S, et al. Evaluation of a new immunoassay for therapeutic drug monitoring of tacrolimus in adult liver transplant recipients. J Clin Pharmacol 2010;50:705–9.

[82] Akbas SH, Ozdem S, Caglar S, et al. Effects of some hematological parameters on whole blood tacrolimus concentration measured by two immunoassay-based analytical methods. Clin Biochem 2005;38: 552–7.

[83] Miller JL. Sirolimus approved with renal transplant indication. Am J Health Syst Pharm 1999;56:2177–8.

[84] Sedrani R, Cottens S, Kallen J, Schuler W. Chemical modification of rapamycin: the discovery of SDZ RAD. Transplant Proc 1998;30:2192–4.

[85] Abraham RT, Wiederrecht GJ. Immunopharmacology of rapamycin. Annu Rev Immunol 1996;14:483–510.

[86] Kimball PM, Derman RK, Van Buren CT, et al. Cyclosporine and rapamycin affect protein kinase C induction of intracellular activation signal, activator of DNA replication. Transplantation 1993;55:1128–32.

[87] Sahin S, Gürkan A, Uyar M, et al. Conversion to proliferation signal inhibitors-based immunosuppressive regimen in kidney transplantation: to whom and when? Transplan Proc 2011;43:837–40.

[88] Yatscoff R, LeGatt D, Keenan R, Chackowsky P. Blood distribution of rapamycin. Transplantation 1993;56:1202–6.

[89] Holt DW, Denny K, Lee TD, Johnston A. Therapeutic monitoring of sirolimus: its contribution to optimal prescription. Transplant Proc 2003;35:S157–61.

[90] Kahn SE, Vazquez D, Meyer P, et al. Analytical evaluation of the Abbott ARCHITECT sirolimus assay. Clin Chem 2008;54:A14 (abstr).

[91] Poquette MA, Lensmeyer GL, Doran TC. Effective use of liquid chromatography-mass spectrometry (LC/MS) in the routine clinical laboratory for monitoring sirolimus, tacrolimus, and cyclosporine. Ther Drug Monit 2005;27:144–50.

[92] Streit F, Armstrong VW, Oellerich M. Rapid liquid chromatography-tandem mass spectrometry routine method for simultaneous determination of sirolimus, everolimus, tacrolimus, and cyclosporin A in whole blood. Clin Chem 2002;48:955–8.

[93] Wang S, Miller A. A rapid liquid chromatography-tandem mass spectrometry analysis of whole blood sirolimus using turbulent flow technology for online extraction. Clin Chem Lab Med 2008;46:1631–4.

[94] Schmid RW, Lotz J, Schweigert R, et al. Multi-site analytical evaluation of a chemiluminescent magnetic microparticle immunoassay (CMIA) for sirolimus on the Abbott ARCHITECT analyzer. Clin Biochem 2009;42:1543–8.

[95] Wilson D, Johnston F, Holt D, et al. Multi-center evaluation of analytical performance of the microparticle enzyme immunoassay for sirolimus. Clin Biochem 2006;39:378–86.

[96] Holt DW, McKeown DA, Lee TD, et al. The relative proportions of sirolimus metabolites in blood using HPLC with mass-spectrometric detection. Transplant Proc 2004;36:3223–5.

[97] Westley IS, Morris RG, Taylor PJ, et al. CEDIA(R) Sirolimus assay compared with HPLC-MS/MS and HPLC-UV in transplant recipient specimens. Ther Drug Monit 2005;27:309–14.

[98] Mahalati K, Kahan BD. Clinical pharmacokinetics of sirolimus. Clin Pharmacokinet 2001;40:573–85.

[99] Cervinski MA, Duh S-H, Hock KG, et al. Performance characteristics of a no-pretreatment, random access sirolimus assay for the Dimension® RxL clinical chemistry system. Clin Biochem 2009;42:1123–7.

[100] O'Halloran S, Ilett KF. Evaluation of a deuterium-labeled internal standard for the measurement of sirolimus by high-throughput HPLC electrospray ionization tandem mass spectrometry. Clin Chem 2008;54:1386–9.

[101] Motzer RJ, Escudier B, Oudard S, et al. Phase 3 trial of everolimus for metastatic renal cell carcinoma. Cancer 2010;116:4256–65.

[102] Kovarik JM, Kahan BD, Kaplan B, et al. Longitudinal assessment of everolimus in de novo renal transplant recipients over the first post-transplant year: pharmacokinetics, exposure–response relationships, and influence on cyclosporine. Clin Pharmacol Ther 2001;69:48–56.

[103] Kirchner GI, Winkler M, Mueller L, et al. Pharmacokinetics of SDZ RAD and cyclosporin including their metabolites in seven kidney graft patients after the first dose of SDZ RAD. Br J Clin Pharmacol 2000;50:449–54.

[104] Kirchner GI, Meier-Wiedenbach I, Manns MP. Clinical pharmacokinetics of everolimus. Clin Pharmacokinet 2004;43:83–95.

[105] Dasgupta A, Davis B, Chow L. Evaluation of QMS everolimus assay using Hitachi 917 analyzer: comparison with liquid chromatography/mass spectrometry. Ther Drug Monit 2011;33:149–54.

[106] Kovarik JM, Kaplan B, Tedesco Silva H, et al. Exposure–response relationships for everolimus in de novo kidney transplantation: defining a therapeutic range. Transplantation 2002;73:920–5.

[107] Lehmkuhl H, Ross H, Eisen H, Valantine H. Everolimus (Certican) in heart transplantation: optimizing renal function through minimizing cyclosporine exposure. Transplant Proc 2005;37:4145–9.

[108] Innofluor Certican Assay System (package insert). Indianapolis, IN: Seradyn Inc; 2003.

[109] Nashan B. Review of the proliferation inhibitor everolimus. Expert Opin Investig Drug 2002;11:1841–50.

[110] Salm P, Warnholtz C, Boyd J, et al. Evaluation of a fluorescent polarization immunoassay for whole blood everolimus determination using samples from renal transplant recipients. Clin Biochem 2006;39:732–8.

[111] Baldelli S, Murgia S, Merlini S, et al. High-performance liquid chromatography with ultraviolet detection for therapeutic drug monitoring of everolimus. J Chromatogr B 2005;816:99–105.

[112] Salm P, Taylor PJ, Lynch SV, Pillans PI. Quantification and stability of everolimus (SDZ RAD) in human blood by high-performance liquid chromatography-electrospray tandem mass spectrometry. J Chromatogr B Analyt Technol Biomed Life Sci 2002;772:283–90.

[113] Taylor PJ, Franklin ME, Graham KS, Pillans PI. A HPLC-mass spectrometric method suitable for the therapeutic drug monitoring of everolimus. J Chromatogr B 2007;848:208–14.

[114] Boernsen KO, Egge-Jacobsen W, Inverardi B, et al. Assessment and validation of the MS/MS fragmentation patterns of the macrolide immunosuppressant everolimus. J Mass Spectrom 2007;42:793–802.

[115] Hoogtanders K, van der Heijden J, Stolk LM, et al. Internal standard selection for the high-performance liquid chromatography tandem mass spectroscopy assay of everolimus in blood. Ther Drug Moni 2007;29:673–4.

[116] Sollinger HW. From mice to man: the preclinical history of mycophenolate mofetil. Clin Transplant 1996; 10: 85–92.

[117] Quinn CM, Bugeja VC, Gallagher JA, Whittaker PA. The effect of mycophenolic acid on the cell cycle of *Candida abicans*. Mycopathologia 1990;111:165–8.

[118] Lee WA, Gu L, Miksztal AR, et al. Bioavailability improvement of mycophenolic acid through amino ester derivatization. Pharm Res 1990;7:161–6.

[119] Franklin TJ, Cook JM. The inhibition of nucleic acid synthesis by mycophenolic acid. Biochem J 1969; 113:185–204.

[120] Wu JC. Mycophenolate mofetil: molecular mechanisms of action. Perspect Drug Discov Design 1994; 2:185–204.

[121] Eugui EM, Allison AC. Immunosuppressive activity of mycophenolate mofetil. Ann NY Acad Sci 1993;685:309–29.

[122] Allison AC, Eugui EM. Purine metabolism and immunosuppressive effects of mycophenolate mofetil (MMF). Clin Transplant 1996;10:77–84.

[123] Nowak I, Shaw L. Mycophenolic acid binding to human serum albumin: characterization and relation to pharmacodynamics. Clin Chem 1995;41:1011–7.

[124] van Gleder T, Shaw LM. The rationale for and limitations of therapeutic drug monitoring for mycophenolate mofetil in transplantation. Transplantation 2005;80:S244–53.

[125] Brunet M, Cirera I, Martorell J, et al. Sequential determination of pharmacokinetics and pharmacodynamics of mycophenolic acid in liver transplant patients treated with mycophenolate mofetil. Transplantation 2006;81:541–6.

[126] van Gelder T, Meur YL, Shaw LM, et al. Therapeutic drug monitoring of mycophenolate mofetil in transplantation. Ther Drug Monit 2006;28:145–54.

[127] Mahalati KKB. Pharmacological surrogates of allograft outcome. Ann Transplant 2000;5:14–23.

[128] Shaw LM, Holt DW, Oellerich M, et al. Current issues in therapeutic drug monitoring of mycophenolic acid: report of a roundtable discussion. Ther Drug Monit 2001;23:305–15.

[129] Oellerich M, Shipkova M, Schütz E, et al. Pharmacokinetic and metabolic investigations of mycophenolic acid in pediatric patients after renal transplantation: implications for therapeutic drug monitoring. Ther Drug Monit 2000;22:20–6.

[130] Shaw L, Korecka M, Aradhye S, et al. Mycophenolic acid area under the curve values in African American and Caucasian renal transplant patients are comparable. J Clin Pharmacol 2000;40:624–33.

[131] Kaplan B, Meier-Kriesche H, Friedman G, et al. The effect of renal insufficiency on mycophenolic acid protein binding. J Clin Pharmacol 1999;39:715–20.

[132] Filler G, Bendrick-Peart J, Christians U. Pharmacokinetics of mycophenolate mofetil and sirolimus in children. Ther Drug Monit 2008;30:138–42.

[133] Weber LT, Shipkova M, Armstrong VW, et al. The pharmacokinetic–pharmacodynamic relationship for total and free mycophenolic acid in pediatric renal transplant recipients: a report of the German Study Group on mycophenolate mofetil therapy. J Am Soc Nephrol 2002;13:759–68.

[134] Kuypers DRJ, Meur YL, Cantarovich M, et al. Consensus report on therapeutic drug monitoring of myco-phenolic acid in solid organ transplantation. Clin J Am Soc Nephrol 2010;5:341–58.

[135] Shaw LM, Korecka M, Van Breeman R, et al. Analysis, pharmacokinetics and therapeutic drug monitoring of mycophenolic acid. Clin Biochem 1998;31:323–8.

[136] Streit F, Shipkova M, Armstrong VW, Oellerich M. Validation of a rapid and sensitive liquid chromatography-tandem mass spectrometry method for free and total mycophenolic acid. Clin Chem 2004;50:152–9.

[137] Saunders DA. Simple method for the quantitation of mycophenolic acid in human plasma. J Chromatogr B Biomed Sci Appl 1997;704:379–82.

[138] Teshima D, Kitagawa N, Otsubo K, et al. Simple determination of mycophenolic acid in human serum by column-switching high-performance liquid chromatography. J Chromatogr B Analyt Technol Biomed Life Sci 2002;780:21–6.

[139] Sparidans RW, Hoetelmans RM, Beijnen JH. Liquid chromatographic assay for simultaneous determination of abacavir and mycophenolic acid in human plasma using dual spectrophotometric detection. J Chromatogr B Biomed Sci Appl 2001;750:155–61.

[140] Renner UD, Thiede C, Bornhauser M, et al. Determination of mycophenolic acid and mycophenolate mofetil by high-performance liquid chromatography using postcolumn derivatization. Anal Chem 2001;73:41–6.

[141] Ceglarek U, Casetta B, Lembcke J, et al. Inclusion of MPA and in a rapid multi-drug LC-tandem mass spectrometric method for simultaneous determination of immunosuppressants. Clinica Chimica Acta 2006;373:168–71.

[142] Kuhn J, Prante C, Kleesiek K, Götting C. Measurement of mycophenolic acid and its glucuronide using a novel rapid liquid chromatography-electrospray ionization tandem mass spectrometry assay. Clin Biochem 2009;42:83–90.

[143] Brandhorst G, Streit F, Goetze S, et al. Quantification by liquid chromatography tandem mass spectrometry of mycophenolic acid and its phenol and acyl glucuronide metabolites. Clin Chem 2006;52:1962–4.

[144] Annesley TM, Clayton LT. Quantification of mycophenolic acid and glucuronide metabolite in human serum by HPLC-tandem mass spectrometry. Clin Chem 2005;51:872–7.

[145] van Gleder T, Shaw LM. The rationale for and limitations of therapeutic drug monitoring for mycophenolate mofetil in transplantation. Transplantation 2005;80:S244–53.

[146] Schutz E, Shipkova M, Armstrong VW, et al. Identification of a pharmacologically active metabolite of mycophenolic acid in plasma of transplant recipients treated with mycophenolate mofetil. Clin Chem 1999;45:419–22.

[147] Shipkova M, Schutz E, Armstrong VW, et al. Overestimation of mycophenolic acid by EMIT correlates with MPA metabolite. Transplant Proc 1999;31:1135–7.

[148] Brandhorst G, Marquet P, Shaw LM, et al. Multicenter evaluation of a new inosine monophosphate dehydrogenase inhibition assay for quantification of total mycophenolic acid in plasma. Ther Drug Monit 2008;30:428–33.

[149] CEDIA® Mycophenolic Acid Immunoassay (MDA) package insert (n.d.), Fremont, CA: Thermo Scientific.

[150] Weber LT, Shipkova M, Armstrong VW, et al. Comparison of the EMIT immunoassay with HPLC for ther-apeutic drug monitoring of mycophenolic acid in pediatric renal-transplant recipients on mycophenolate mofetil therapy. Clin Chem 2002;48:517–25.

[151] Prémaud A, Rousseau A, Le Meur Y, et al. Comparison of liquid chromatography-tandem mass spectrometry with a commercial enzyme-multiplied immunoassay for the determination of plasma MPA in renal transplant recipients and consequences for therapeutic drug monitoring. Ther Drug Monit 2004;26:609–19.

[152] Beal JL, Jones CE, Taylor PJ, Tett SE. Evaluation of an immunoassay (EMIT) for mycophenolic acid in plasma from renal transplant recipients compared with a high-performance liquid chromatography assay. Ther Drug Monit 1998;20:685–90.

[153] Schütz E, Shipkova M, Armstrong VW, et al. Therapeutic drug monitoring of mycophenolic acid: comparison of HPLC and immunoassay reveals new MPA metabolites. Transplant Proc 1998;30:1185–7.

[154] Westley IS, Sallustio BC, Morris RG. Validation of a high-performance liquid chromatography method for the measurement of mycophenolic acid and its glucuronide metabolites in plasma. Clin Biochem 2005;38:824–9.

[155] Prémaud A, Rousseau A, Picard N, Marquet P. Determination of mycophenolic acid plasma levels in immuno-assay technique (EMIT) and liquid chromotagraphy-tandem mass spectrometry. The Drug Monit 2005;27:354–61.

[156] Decavele AS, Favoreel N, Heyden FV, Verstraete AG. Performance of the Roche Total Mycophenolic Acid® assay on the Cobas Integra 400®, Cobas 6000® and comparison to LC-MS/MS in liver transplant patients. Clin Chem Lab Med 2011;49:1159–65.

[157] van Gelder T, Domke I, Engelmayer J, et al. Clinical utility of a new enzymatic assay for determination of mycophenolic acid in comparison with an optimized LC-MS/MS method. Ther Drug Monit 2009;31:218—23.

[158] Westley IS, Ray JE, Morris RG. CEDIA® mycophenolic acid assay compared with HPLC-UV in specimens from transplant recipients. Ther Drug Monit 2006;28:632—6.

[159] Tsina I, Kaloostian M, Lee R, et al. High-performance liquid chromatographic method for the determination of mycophenolate mofetil in human plasma. J Chromatogr B Biomed Appl 1996;681:347—53.

[160] Mandla R, Line P-D, Midtvedt K, Bergan S. Automated determination of free mycophenolic acid and its glucuronide in plasma from renal allograft recipients. Ther Drug Monit 2003;25:407—14.

[161] Patel CG, Mendonza AE, Akhlaghi F, et al. Determination of total mycophenolic acid and its glucuronide metabolite using liquid chromatography with ultraviolet detection and unbound mycophenolic acid using tandem mass spectrometry. J Chromatogr B 2004;813:287—94.

[162] Atchison CR, West AB, Balakumaran A, et al. Drug enterocyte adducts: possible causal factor for diclofenac enteropathy in rats. Gastroenterology 2000;119:1537—47.

[163] Wallemacq P, Maine GT, Berg K, et al. Multisite analytical evaluation of the Abbott ARCHITECT cyclosporine assay. Ther Drug Monit 2010;32:145—51.

CHAPTER

16

Biomarkers: The Link between Therapeutic Drug Monitoring and Pharmacodynamics of Immunosuppressants

Michael Oellerich[1], Gunnar Brandhorst[1], Maria Shipkova[2], Eberhard Wieland[2]

[1]Department of Clinical Chemistry, George-August University, Goettingen, Germany
[2]Central Institute for Clinical Chemistry and Laboratory Medicine, Klinikum Stuttgart, Stuttgart, Germany

Therapeutic Drug Monitoring: Newer Drugs and Biomarkers
DOI: 10.1016/B978-0-12-385467-4.00016-6

INTRODUCTION

In the traditional therapeutic drug monitoring (TDM) approach it is assumed that for certain drugs like immunosuppressants, blood levels reflect the pharmacodynamic effect better than the dose [1]. However, it has been shown that immunosuppressants can have different effects in different patients even when drug levels and dosages are the same. Therefore, the question arises as to whether TDM really sufficiently reflects pharmacodynamics. Measuring appropriate biomarkers in addition to immunosuppressive drug levels may be useful to predict the actual pharmacodynamic effect in an individual patient in order to achieve personalized immunosuppression [2].

Individually tailored immunosuppression is indeed a critical issue. TDM does not precisely predict the effects of immunosuppressive drugs on immune cells. The primary value of TDM is to prevent toxicity. Inter-subject variability may occur in the sensitivity to suppression of immune function. Furthermore, there is an inter-individual variability in intra-lymphocyte immunosuppressive drug levels which is not reflected by whole blood drug concentrations [3]. It could be demonstrated that the *ABCB1* genotype has an influence on intra-lymphocyte cyclosporin concentrations [4]. The assessment of immunological risk prior to transplantation could be useful to identify patients who would benefit from a more potent immunosuppression. The optimization of immuno-suppressive multi-drug regimens is difficult with drug levels alone. Combinations of immunosuppressive drugs may be associated with synergistic and antagonistic effects. Chronic over- and under-immunosuppression occurs and needs to be avoided.

TABLE 16.1　Proposed Peripheral Blood Biomarkers in Solid Organ Transplantation

DRUG TARGET ENZYMES
IMPDH (Inosine monophosphate dehydrogenase)   CN (Calcineurin phosphatase)   P70S6K phosphorylation
CYTOKINES
IL-2, IFN-γ expression
NFAT REGULATED GENES
IL-2, IFN-γ, GM-CSF
MARKER OF IMMUNE CELL RESPONSE
PHA-stimulated ATP production (Immuknow® Cylex®)
MARKER OF LYMPHOCYTE PROLIFERATION AND LYMPHOCYTE ACTIVATION
PCNA, CD25, sCD30, CD71
POTENTIAL PREDICTORS OF TOLERANCE
Natural regulatory T-cells (CD4$^+$CD25^{high}FOXP3$^+$)   Signature of B-cell differentiation genes (*IGKV4-1, IGLLA, IGKV1D-13*)

Furthermore, there is a lack of biomarkers capable of identifying tolerant recipients before undergoing drug weaning. It has been argued that the inability to measure effects of immunosuppressive drugs on immune cells *in vivo* has severely limited the pre-clinical drug development, design and interpretation of clinical trials and optimal clinical use in transplantation [5].

There are two major factors limiting long-term outcome in transplantation, namely irreversible chronic rejection and the side effects of standard immunosuppression, which include nephrotoxicity, cardiovascular disease, opportunistic infection and malignancy. Therefore, numerous attempts have been made to develop biomarkers that would complement therapeutic drug monitoring. Drug target enzymes, cytokine expression and production by T cells, IL-2 receptor expression, proliferating cell nuclear antigen and global markers of immune cell response have been proposed as peripheral blood biomarkers (Table 16.1), all of which address key functions in T cell activation and proliferation. Furthermore, potential predictors of tolerance have been described [6–8].

SPECIFIC PHARMACODYNAMIC MARKERS

There are specific pharmacodynamic markers for immunosuppressants, including drug target enzymes, interleukin-2 in $CD8^+$ T cells, and nuclear factor of activated T lymphocytes (NFAT)-regulated gene expression. This section will address these specific pharmacodynamic markers.

Drug Target Enzymes

A pharmacodynamic assay for cyclosporine and tacrolimus is the measurement of inhibition of calcineurin phosphatase. Halloran *et al.* [9] related calcineurin activity to cyclosporine A blood levels in humans. Cyclosporine induces partial calcineurin inhibition, and there is a close temporal relationship between cyclosporine concentration and calcineurin inhibition. The greatest calcineurin inhibition ($> 50\%$) was found to correlate with the highest cyclosporine blood concentrations at 1 and 2 hours after dosing. This assay is, however, technically demanding, and its usefulness for routine pharmacodynamic monitoring has been questioned [10].

P70 S6 kinase phosphorylation is a marker of mTOR inhibition by sirolimus and everolimus [2]. Hartmann *et al.* [11] reported, in a small study with 24 kidney transplant patients receiving sirolimus in combination with either calcineurin inhibitors (CNIs) or mycophenolate mofetil (MMF), on 70S6 kinase phosphorylation, which was assessed by Western Blot technique. There was no correlation between p70S6 kinase activity and sirolimus trough concentrations. However, p70S6 kinase activity was significantly inhibited when sirolimus trough concentrations were > 6 ng/mL. A high degree of phosphorylation was observed in five patients who experienced a rejection event independently of the sirolimus trough concentrations. In contrast, non-rejectors showed significant inhibition of phosphorylation [11]. Although these results suggest that the phosphorylation status of the p70S6 kinase is a suitable indicator of the pharmacodynamic effect of sirolimus, the use of this assay is hampered by its laborious assay procedure and the semi-quantitative read out. Whether this disadvantage can be overcome by recently commercially available ELISA methods remains to be demonstrated [12].

Inosine monophosphate dehydrogenase (IMPDH) Type I and II is inhibited in peripheral blood mononuclear cells by mycophenolic acid. Glander *et al.* [13] studied the predictive value of pre-transplant IMPDH activity for MMF dosing. IMPDH activity was determined in isolated peripheral mononuclear cells from 79 dialysis patients prior to renal transplantation, and showed a substantial inter-individual variability. Patients with high IMPDH activity above a certain cut-off point and a dose reduction in the post-transplant period had the highest incidence of acute rejection. These preliminary data suggest that pre-transplant IMPDH activity may perhaps influence outcome.

Pharmacokinetic/pharmacodynamic relationships of MMF have been studied in pediatric and adult kidney transplant recipients. It has been shown that IMPDH activity is inversely related to mycophenolic acid (MPA) plasma concentration, with the highest level of inhibition associated with the highest concentration after which activity returned to near pre-dose values [14, 15]. Fukuda *et al.* observed that over time the overall IMPDH inhibition curve in pediatric patients shifted downward as a result of increasing MPA exposure. It was concluded in this study that there may be a potential utility of combining PK and IMPDH biomarker data to optimize MMF therapy [14]. Baseline IMPDH activity in children may serve as a potential clinical marker to guide the level of required MPA exposure. Furthermore, IMPDH variability was studied in renal transplant patients on long-term mycophenolate mofetil therapy [16]. In contrast to the study by Fukuda [14], pre-dose IMPDH activity in peripheral blood mononuclear cells from transplant recipients increased from 5.9 nmol/h·mg to 9.0 nmol/h·mg with an intra- and inter-patient variability of 28% and 48.2%, respectively [16]. Increases in pre-dose IMPDH activity were consistent in patients on MMF for 20–50 months. Pre-dose IMPDH activity was increased during rejection versus non-rejection.

In an outcome study, IMPDH activity was measured as the area under the enzyme curve over the first 4 hours after dose administration in renal transplant recipients treated with enteric coated mycophenolate sodium (EC-MPS) [17]. It was demonstrated that IMPDH inhibition was significantly lower in patients with rejection compared to patients with no rejection during the first and second weeks after transplantation. The test may be useful for the early identification of patients at risk for rejection.

In a recent study [18], *IMPDH1* and *IMPDH2* were resequenced using DNA from 288 individuals from three ethnic groups. In *IMPDH1*, 73 SNPs (59 novel) were identified; in *IMPDH2*, 25 SNPs (24 novel) were identified. Two alloenzymes, IMPDH1 Leu275 and IMPDH2 Phe263, displayed a strong decrease in cytosolic IMPDH activity. The novel IMPDH1 alloenzyme (Leu275) had only 10% of the wild-type activity. Variation in MPA response may result, in part, from genetic variation in *IMPDH1* and *IMPDH2*.

The polymorphisms in Type I and II *IMPDH* genes and association with clinical outcome were investigated in renal transplant patients on mycophenolate mofetil [19]. DNA and clinical data of 456 patients from clinical trials (Apomygre, FDCC) were evaluated. It was demonstrated that an *IMPDH* I SNP was associated with lower risk of biopsy proven acute rejection and higher risk of leukopenia over the first year post-transplantation. *IMPDH II* genotyping seems not to improve MPA treatment outcome, in contrast to MPA and calcineurin inhibitor therapeutic drug monitoring and *IMPDH I* genotyping.

Interleukin-2 in CD8$^+$ T cells

Interleukin-2 (IL-2) is a 15-kDa cytokine predominantly secreted by activated T cells and represents a key player in the cell-mediated immune response in allograft rejection. After binding to the IL-2-receptor on lymphocytes, IL-2 triggers a complex intracellular signaling involving several protein kinase pathways such as JAK-STAT (Janus kinase signal transduction and activation of transcription) and Ras-MAPK (ras-mitogen activated protein kinase) resulting in the clonal expansion of the target cell. Immunosuppressive therapy by calcineurin inhibitors (CNI) such as cyclosporine A and tacrolimus attenuates IL-2 response, leading to an inhibition of lymphocyte activation and proliferation, thereby mediating an immunosuppressive effect in patients after, for example, solid organ transplantation. The percentage of IL-2-producing CD8$^+$ T cells among total CD8$^+$ T cells has been proposed to be a non-invasive pharmacodynamic biomarker of T cell activation, and was demonstrated to be associated with the incidence of acute rejection in liver transplant recipients [20].

For the quantification of IL-2 expressing T cells in peripheral blood mononuclear cells (PBMC), flow cytometric assays are widely used. Briefly, in these assays heparinized whole blood is stimulated *ex vivo* for 4 hours with phorbol myristate acetate (PMA) and the calcium ionophore ionomycin (ION) while secretion of IL-2 is inhibited by brefeldin A. CD3 and CD8 as surface markers and intracellular IL-2 (after permeabilization) are stained simultaneously by fluorescent antibodies, and events are detected by a flow cytometer. After cell-counting, the number of IL-2 positive cells is expressed as a percentage of total CD8$^+$ T cells. The intra- and inter-assay imprecision of this procedure appears to be acceptable (CV $<$ 15% as stated by different authors [20, 21]). However, as in other flow cytometric assays, standardization remains a critical issue since, for example, different conditions for mitogenic stimulation lead to a high inter-laboratory variation [22].

In early studies it could be demonstrated that the percentage of IL-2-producing CD8$^+$ T cells was associated with an inhibition of IL-2 secretion during treatment with cyclosporine A [23]. Also, an association between the percentage of IL-2-producing CD8$^+$ T cells and graft stability in liver or kidney transplant recipients was proposed [24]. In a more recent approach by Boleslawski *et al.*, in 21 patients following liver transplantation the percentage of IL-2-producing CD8$^+$ T cells was found to be predictive for acute rejection [20]. Five patients in this study developed an acute rejection and tended to have higher numbers of IL-2-producing CD8$^+$ T cells as compared to the patients without acute rejection. Most interestingly, an increased number of IL-2-producing CD8$^+$ T cells in these patients could already be demonstrated before transplantation. Therefore, this assay might be useful to identify patients who require a more robust immunosuppression before transplantation. The results from Boleslaswki *et al.* were confirmed in two recent studies. Akoglu and coworkers demonstrated an association between IL-2-producing CD8$^+$ T cells and the histological Banff score in 66 patients after liver transplantation [22]. Furthermore, Millán *et al.*, who investigated the numbers of IL-2-producing CD8$^+$ T cells in stable liver transplant recipients undergoing weaning of immunosuppressive therapy during the withdrawal protocol, found that the percentage of IL-2-producing CD8$^+$ T cells was significantly higher in patients who rejected, compared to those who did not reject [25]. Stable liver transplant recipients that are candidates for immunosuppressive minimization appear to be at high risk of rejection if a high percentage of IL-2-producing CD8$^+$ T cells is detected. In conclusion, the percentage of

IL-2-producing $CD8^+$ T cells is a promising biomarker for a personalized immunosuppressive therapy when using calcineurin inhibitors with regards to the identification of patients at risk for acute rejection.

NFAT-Regulated Gene Expression

Cyclosporine A and tacrolimus work through inhibition of the calcium-dependent phosphatase calcineurin. This results in inhibition of the dephosphorylation of nuclear factor of activated T lymphocytes (NFAT), its nuclear translocation and subsequent transcriptional activation of NFAT-regulated expression of a variety of genes required for T cell activation.

During recent years the group of Zeier *et al.* [26] has extensively investigated the determination of residual expression of the NFAT-regulated genes interleukin-2 (*IL-2*), interferon-γ (*INF*-γ) and granulocyte macrophage colony-stimulating factor (*GM-CSF*) as a tool for pharmacodynamic monitoring of treatment with cyclosporine and tacrolimus. The combination of three genes aimed to adjust for random variations in expression of individual genes. To improve selectivity toward calcineurin inhibition, the gene expression is determined before (T_0) and 2 h (T_2, cyclosporine A) or 1.5 h ($T_{1.5}$, tacrolimus) after drug intake, and the % residual expression at the second time point is reported in relation to the expression at T_0. The method relies on *ex vivo* stimulation of whole blood by PMA and ION (3 h, 37 °C), avoiding artefacts associated with cell isolation [26]. Gene expression is quantified using an RT-PCR technique on a LightCycler® instrument (Roche Diagnostics, Mannheim, Germany) using a commercially available LightCycler "Cyclosporine Monitoring" amplification kit, and can be performed semi-automatically. These characteristics seem to be a promising basis for method standardization.

Most clinical evidence with this procedure has been generated with stable kidney transplant recipients. With this population on similar co-medication, Sommerer *et al.* [27] demonstrated that the intra-individual variability of the expression of NFAT-regulated genes was less than 10% if the cyclosporine A dose remained constant. In contrast, the inter-individual variability reached up to 50%, suggesting an individually varying degree of immunosuppression despite similar cyclosporine A or tacrolimus doses [27, 28]. The reduction of gene transcripts was found to be inversely correlated with the individual cyclosporine A or tacrolimus concentration. Low residual expression ($< 15\%$) of the three genes was associated with signs of probable over-immunosuppression, such as increased frequency of recurrent infections and malignancies (e.g., non-melanoma skin carcinoma) in stable patients treated with cyclosporine [27].

In a small biopsy-controlled pilot study the utility of the pharmacodynamic approach to monitor cyclosporine A tapering was investigated [29]. The dose reduction was accompanied by an increase in gene expression and was free from adverse events such as acute rejections, so long as the residual expression remained below 30%. Therefore, a range between 20% and 30% has been proposed as optimal in long-term stable renal transplant recipients [2]. These results have in general been confirmed in single studies with pediatric and elderly kidney transplanted patients, as well in pilot studies with stable liver and heart recipients [30–33].

The results suggest that the residual expression of NFAT-related genes might be a promising tool, complementary to therapeutic drug monitoring, to optimize immunosuppression with cyclosporine A in long-term stable transplant recipients. Now, as a next step, confirmation of the results in larger randomized prospective and multicentre studies is required to validate the appropriateness of this approach for clinical routine. Of particular importance is that the benefit of its introduction must be proven in controlled interventional trials.

Finally, the investigations on the applicability of the residual NFAT-regulated gene expression to monitor therapy with tacrolimus as well as to manage therapy with both cyclosporine and tacrolimus during the early post-transplant phase are very limited as yet, and open questions have to be addressed in additional studies. The first results demonstrated some difficulties. For example, with regard to tacrolimus therapy, a considerably higher residual activity compared to cyclosporine therapy has been found [28, 34] that suggested a need for different optimal target ranges for the two drugs. In addition, the time to reach adequate levels of suppression after drug intake seems to be more variable with tacrolimus than with cyclosporine A. In the early post-transplantation period a very high inhibition in nearly all patients complicates the use of the biomarker [35].

GLOBAL MARKERS OF RESPONSE TO IMMUNOSUPPRESSANTS

In addition to specific pharmacodynamic markers to assess response to an immunosuppressant drug, there are also global markers for investigating response to such drugs. In this section, various such markers are discussed.

ATP Concentration in $CD4^+$ T Lymphocytes

The commercial ImmuKnow® Cylex® assay (Cylex Inc., Columbia, MD) is designed to assess immune function based on the intracellular increase of adenosine triphosphate (ATP) in $CD4^+$ cells following activation by mitogenic stimulation. After overnight incubation (15—18 hours) of the patient blood sample with phytohemagglutinin (PHA), $CD4^+$ cells are selected by magnetic separation. After cell lysis, intercellular ATP is released and detected with luciferin/luciferase reagents using a luminometer [36]. The test works only with sodium heparinate as an anticoagulant. Sample integrity was shown to be maintained through 30 hours post-draw at room temperature [37].

The assay is carried out by use of microtiter plates. Each patient is run in quadruplicates without and with stimulation. For quality control purposes, a fresh blood specimen from an apparently healthy individual should to be used, which has to meet certain specifications for the iATP (intracellular ATP) result. The coefficient of variation (CV) of sample quadruplicates for stimulated wells should be < 20%. At an iATP concentration of 652 ng/ml, a CV of 6.1% is achieved (according to these authors' observations). The ImmuKnow Cylex assay has the advantage that it is standardized and a quality control system is available. The assay has been cleared by the Federal Drug Administration (FDA) for detection of immunity in an immunosuppressed patient population. There is no significant correlation between the absolute CD4 number and the iATP levels ($r^2 = 0.24$). Therefore, CD4 cell numbers and their functional activity as measured by ATP production are independent variables [38].

A comparison of ATP production in mitogen-stimulated CD4 cells and immunosuppressive drug concentrations before and 2 hours post-dose showed that the ImmuKnow test results are independent of the blood or plasma concentration of an immunosuppressive agent [39]. The ImmuKnow test therefore seems to be a marker for the overall level of immune function, and not a pharmacodynamic marker of any particular immunosuppressive agent [39]. In line with these data, there was also no significant correlation between tacrolimus or cyclosporine trough concentrations and iATP concentrations in pediatric stable transplant recipients [40]. Earlier studies by Kowalski [36] compared the ImmuKnow Cylex cell response between patients receiving different calcineurin inhibitors and apparently healthy individuals. As to be expected, the median values were lower in patients under immunosuppressive therapy; however, there was a substantial overlap between the different groups. Normal subjects showed a range of iATP values between about 200 and 1000 ng/mL. The trough calcineurin inhibitor (CNI; cyclosporine and tacrolimus) drug levels and immune cell response showed no correlation. These data further indicate that immunosuppressive drug level monitoring has limitations regarding the pharmacodynamic assessment of immunosuppression.

In a meta-analysis including 10 US transplant centers, the combined immune response of solid organ transplant recipients during periods of rejection, infection and stability was investigated [37]. It was demonstrated that during periods of clinical stability the median ATP release was lower than in patients with confirmed rejections and higher than in patients with documented infections. A putative zone of minimal risk was proposed; however, this would have to be confirmed in prospective outcome studies.

In a recent study, the association between pre-transplant iATP levels as determined by the ImmuKnow assay with kidney graft outcome has been investigated in a prospective multi-center clinical trial [41]. It was demonstrated that increased pre-transplant iATP levels were significantly associated with biopsy proven acute rejection (Banff grade 2 or greater). Those recipients who had negative biopsies had an intermediate mean value. Recipients with antibody-mediated acute rejection had pre-transplant iATP values comparable with those of recipients who did not have a biopsy. The results showed that recipients with pre-transplant iATP values > 375 ng/mL had a significantly higher risk of experiencing acute rejection. In contrast to these results, in a more recent study [42] on renal transplant recipients with opportunistic infections or rejection no association between single time-point ImmuKnow test results and adverse effects was observed in the subsequent 90 days. This was a retrospective analysis of 1330 ImmuKnow assay values evaluated in 583 renal transplant recipients with respect to infection or rejection. The authors of this study conclude that the optimal use of the ImmuKnow assay in kidney transplantation has yet to be determined.

Further studies have been published on the use of the ImmuKnow Cylex test in heart transplant patients with infection and rejection [43, 44]. It was demonstrated that patients with infection had significantly lower iATP values and patients with rejection significantly higher iATP values compared to stable heart transplant recipients [43]. CNI levels did not reflect the state of under-immunosuppression, as 64% of the CNI levels were within or above target. Serial longitudinal monitoring of the cellular immune function in heart transplant recipients may be useful to maintain an optimal personalized immunosuppression. In heart transplantation in particular it is essential to maintain tight monitoring of the patient to predict and prevent states of under- or over-immunosuppression in order to avoid infection or rejection. One patient in this study [43] demonstrated a unique immune function profile where immunologic stability was achieved at ImmuKnow levels that were lower than the defined moderate zone. In this case, an increase of iATP levels into the "moderate" zone brought about a rejection episode. It appears that this specific patient's immune function was in a state of under-immunosuppression already in the moderate response zone, and that the patient needed a more robust immunosuppression. Therefore, individual baseline values may be important for a personalized longitudinal follow-up. Snapshot ImmuKnow measurements seem not to be useful.

In a further study [44] with 296 adult heart transplant recipients, the average iATP values were significantly lower during infection than compared to stable patients. The average iATP concentrations, however, were not significantly different during rejection when compared to stable patients. It was concluded that the test appears to be useful to predict infection risk. The association between high iATP values and rejection risk was inconclusive, presumably due to the small number ($n = 8$) of rejection episodes.

The immune cell response was also studied in lung transplant recipients with infections (bacterial pneumonia, cytomegalovirus, fungal pneumonia). Again, patients with infection had significantly lower immune cell response values compared to the non-infected patients [45]. The improved immune response was in part related to decreasing immunosuppression in the majority of these cases. Functional immunity as measured by the ImmuKnow Cylex assay increased as infection resolved. The ImmuKnow assay seems to be particularly useful in lung transplant recipients, as those patients require higher levels of immunosuppression to avoid acute allograft rejection. On the other hand, however, these patients have a higher risk for infections. In an additional study [46], immune monitoring was carried out in lung transplant recipients with a stable course and in those with infections compared to stable patients. The median ImmuKnow values in cytomegalovirus disease (CMV), viral diseases and bacterial pneumonia were significantly lower. The median values of patients with fungal disease and tracheobronchitis had a tendency to be lower than the stable state, whereas patients with fungal colonization had comparable ImmuKnow values. The data from the Cylex assay may be useful in identifying patients with fungal colonization who are at risk for a progression to fungal disease and might benefit from antifungal prophylaxis and minimization of immunosuppression.

Various studies have been conducted with the Cylex assay in adult and pediatric liver transplant patients [40, 47, 48]. Again, it could be demonstrated that iATP concentrations were significantly lower in patients with infection compared to stable transplant recipients and healthy controls. In a retrospective study, the usefulness of the ImmuKnow test was examined in aiding in the distinction between adult liver transplant recipients with acute rejection and those with recurrent HCV [48]. The mean iATP level of recipients with recurrent HCV was significantly lower than in those with acute rejection, and also lower when compared to that with a normal biopsy. In contrast, the iATP level with acute rejection was significantly higher than that with a normal biopsy. The group with overlapping features was not significantly different from the remaining groups. The study revealed that the iATP values were related to the biopsy findings and that the test could be useful to identify patients with over-immunosuppression, who are at risk for recurrent HCV. The Cylex assay may also be useful to detect non-compliance and irregular drug intake, as the observed immune cell response is not determined by the actual immunosuppressant drug level alone rather than the exposure over a certain period of time. This phenomenon would have to be studied, however, in more detail.

In a further study, immune profiles obtained by the ImmuKnow Cylex assay were investigated in 10 liver transplant recipients in whom immunosuppressive treatment was gradually reduced until complete withdrawal at 6 months from the start of the protocol [49]. Two patterns of immune cell response were observed in these patients. As to be expected, iATP levels increased during immunosuppressive drug withdrawal in a subgroup of six patients as a consequence of recovery of the immune response, especially when the patients were free of immunosuppression. In a second subgroup, however, iATP levels were decreased, and these patients were free of immunosuppressive treatment. Although some of the iATP values were in the strong immune response zone, none of these patients developed rejection. On the other hand, iATP levels were investigated in 8/22 liver transplant recipients who developed rejection when immunosuppressive treatment was gradually reduced. Surprisingly, none of these patients showed iATP values in the strong immune response zone. Individual baselines, however, were not obtained in these patients. The data show that single time-points obtained with this assay may not reliably predict rejection.

Table 16.2 summarizes studies that have shown the presence or absence of a significant relationship between the immune cell response as determined by ImmuKnow Cylex and acute rejection. As can be seen, in renal and cardiac transplantation an equal number of studies have shown either the presence or absence of a significant relationship. In hepatic transplantation, the majority of studies showed a relationship. It seems that at least single time-point measurements may perhaps not be sufficient to detect acute rejection, and individual baseline values may perhaps be required. On the other hand, in the vast majority of studies a significant relationship with all listed allograft types was obtained between immune response and infection (Table 16.3). Based on this information, it seems that the Cylex assay is useful to detect over-immunosuppression.

In a more recent study, the association between immune response and short-term mortality risk was investigated [56]. In this study 1031 ImmuKnow assays in 362 patients with different allograft types were evaluated. It could be demonstrated that 14.4 % of patients with at least one ImmuKnow assay value below 175 ng/mL died, compared to 5.2 % of

TABLE 16.2 Relationship between Immune Cell Response (Cylex®) and Acute Rejection (AR)

Significant results ($P < 0.05$)	Authors and references
Renal transplantation	
⇑ AR risk with higher iATP levels	Kowalski *et al.* [37], Reinsmoen *et al.* [41]
No significant relationship	Huskey *et al.* [42], Serban *et al.* [50]
Cardiac transplantation	
⇑ AR risk with higher iATP levels	Israeli *et al.* [43], Kowalski *et al.* [37]
No significant relationship	Gupta *et al.* [51], Kobashigawa *et al.* [44]
Hepatic transplantation	
⇑ AR risk with higher iATP levels	Kowalski *et al.* [37], Cabrera *et al.* [52] Shulz-Juergensen *et al.* [40] Hashimoto *et al.* [48]
No significant relationship	Millán *et al.* [49]

TABLE 16.3 Relationship between Immune Cell Response (Cylex®) and Infection

Significant results (P < 0.05)	Authors and references
Renal transplantation	
⇑ Incidence of infection with lower iATP levels	Kowalski *et al.* [37]; Serban *et al.* [50] Cadillo-Chivez *et al.* [53]; De Paolis *et al.* [54]
No significant relationship	Huskey *et al.* [42]
Cardiac transplantation	
⇑ Incidence of infection with lower iATP levels	Israeli *et al.* [43], Kowalski *et al.* [37], Kobashigawa *et al.* [44]
No significant relationship	Gupta *et al.* [51]
Hepatic transplantation	
⇑ Incidence of infection with lower iATP levels	Xue *et al.* [47], Hashimoto *et al.* [48], Kowalski *et al.* [37], Cabrera *et al.* [52], Lee *et al.* [55]
No significant relationship	—
Lung transplantation	
⇑ Incidence of infection with lower iATP levels	Bhorade *et al.* [45], Husain *et al.* [46]
No significant relationship	—

patients with all ImmuKnow assays above 175 ng/mL. It was concluded that Cylex assays may have the potential to identify patients with increased risk of short-term mortality.

Immunosuppressant drug weaning is a further area of interest. In a retrospective analysis, it was demonstrated in stable small bowel transplant recipients that sequential Cylex ImmuKnow assay results may be useful to guide immunosuppressant weaning [57]. It was shown that histologically confirmed immune activation was associated with a corresponding increase in immune function.

Interferon-γ in Alloreactive T cells

T cells are the initiators and mediators of the alloimmune response elicited by organ transplantation. Activated recipient T cells synthesize cytokines and differentiate into subtypes with typical cytokine profiles. Th1 (type 1 helper) cells have been associated with the cellular immune response, whereas Th2 cells drive the humoral immune response. Th1 cells produce IL-2, IFN-γ, and TNF-α. Typical Th2 cytokines are IL-4, IL-5, IL-6 and IL-10 [58].

A very elegant method to monitor the frequency of cytokine-producing alloreactive T cells is the enzyme linked immunosorbent spot (ELISPOT) assay. In this assay, cytokine secreting T cells are counted after *in vitro* stimulation of recipient peripheral blood mononuclear cells (PBMCs) by donor specific or non-specific antigens for 18–48 hours. The secreted cytokine is detected by a specific monoclonal antibody, and the cells producing the product become visible as discrete spots. The assay is commercially available as a ready-to-use kit, and the read-out can be automated by video imaging. The assay has been used for detecting T cells secreting IL-2, IFN-γ, IL-10 or gramzyme B [59]. Like the ImmuKnow assay, the ELISPOT test is a general indicator of T cell activation rather than a specific pharmacodynamic marker.

By using the ELISPOT assay, Heeger and colleagues have reported that allogen-induced IFN-γ production before transplantation was associated with post-transplant outcome in kidney transplant recipients. African-American patients with a higher number of IFN-γ producing lymphocytes before kidney transplantation experienced significantly more acute rejection episodes [60]. Hricik *et al.* described post-transplantation correlations of both donor reactive and third party responses and the glomerular filtration rate at 6 and 12 months [61].

In order to better predict the immunological risk before transplantation in cases when no donor cells are available, a modification of the test was developed independently by Andree *et al.* [62] and Poggio *et al.* [63] using a panel of stimulator cells possessing the most important human leukocyte antigens (HLA). Using this approach, it was confirmed that pre-transplant ELISPOT results were associated with post-transplant acute rejection and renal function [64]. However, in living-donor kidney transplantation the finding that a higher frequency of IFN-γ producing T cells was associated with acute rejection could only be confirmed with donor-specific lymphocytes but not with third party cells [65]. T cell depletion and maintenance immunosuppression with sirolimus and MMF has been suggested to favor induction of tolerance. Hyporesponsesiveness of T cells associated with a better graft function has been demonstrated using the IFN-γ ELISPOT in patients treated with such a regime [66, 67].

Using a defined virus antigen, it has been shown that the IFN-γ ELISPOT assay generates reproducible results for T cell immune monitoring among different laboratories when it is performed according to a standardized protocol [68]. In addition, the ELISPOT assay is suitable for multicenter trials since it can be performed with cryopreserved PBMCs, which also makes it possible to generate reference cells that can be used as a control and proficiency testing. When it comes to transplantation medicine, the comparability of results between different laboratories has to be shown with a defined alloantigen or a mitogen as a T cell stimulus. Standardization of results with donor-specific lymphocytes can be expected to be very difficult.

Although there is some potential for the ELISPOT assay for pharmacodynamic monitoring, no data have been published so far indicating that the immunosuppressive therapy can be tailored based on T cell reactivity assessed by this method. Currently a trial is underway to assess if low pretransplantation donor specific T-cell reactive patients measured by the ELISPOT assay can be safely managed with calcineurin inhibitor-free sirolimus-based immunosuppression [69]. A drawback of the ELISPOT assay is the need for *ex vivo* incubation of isolated PBMCs and the long incubation time of about 24 hours.

T Cell Activation Surface Markers

Activated T cells express molecules on their cell surfaces, which clearly distinguishes them from naïve T cells. These molecules include receptor proteins, co-stimulatory molecules, adhesion molecules, chemokine receptors and major histocompatibility complex (MHC) class II molecules. Examples of receptor proteins are CD25 (the interleukin-2 receptor) and CD71 (the transferrin receptor) [70]. Members of co-stimulatory molecules include CD26, CD28, CD30 and CD154 [2, 70]. Examples of adhesion molecules on activated T cells include members of the integrin family, such as LFA-1 (lymphocyte function associated antigen 1) or

VLA-4 (very late antigen 4) and ICAM-1 (intercellular adhesion molecule 1 or CD54), as well as CD2 (LFA-2), which belong to the immunoglobulin superfamily [71]. Chemokine receptors, such as CXCR3 and CCR5, are also strongly upregulated in activated T cells and are involved in transplant rejection [72]. MHC Class II molecules expressed on activated T cells encompass all isotypes [73]. Data on transplant patients have been mainly generated with cell surface receptors and co-stimulatory molecules.

T cell surface activation markers can be easily detected on the cells by flow cytometry after staining with fluorescence-labeled monoclonal antibodies. Most of the published data are derived from using *in vitro* models in which diluted whole blood was non-specifically stimulated *ex vivo* by mitogens such as PMA, PHA or concanvalin A (CON A) in the presence of various immunosuppressants at different concentrations.

Böhler *et al.* have shown that CD25 and CD71 expression on CD3$^+$ cells (T cells) in stimulated whole blood (72 h) was dose-dependently inhibited by cyclosporine A, tacrolimus, sirolimus, mycophenolic acid and methylprednisolone with an acceptable intra-assay (CV < 10%) and intra-individual variability (CV < 21%) [74]. Expression of CD25 and CD71 has been shown to be lower in immunosuppressed patients when compared to healthy volunteers and dialysis patients [75, 76].

As reported by Premaud *et al.*, a transient mycophenolic acid concentration-dependent decrease in T cell expression of CD25 and CD71 was observed after a single dose of mycophenolic acid mofetil in liver transplant candidates on the waiting list [77]. In addition, Kamar *et al.* demonstrated that both markers dramatically declined in parallel to IMPDH activity during the first hour after mycophenolic acid mofetil intake in kidney transplant patients [78]. A reduced expression of CD28, CD54 and CD154 has been reported by Weimer *et al.* following conversion from cyclosporine A to tacrolimus, which may reflect differences in the effect of the two calcineurin inhibitors [79].

These results suggest that cell surface marker expression has the potential to serve as a pharmacodynamic measure to reflect immunmodulatory effects. However, there are only very limited data concerning an association between surface marker expression, immunosuppression and clinical events. CD25 and CD71 expression on CD3$^+$ and CD4$^+$ cells distinguished allograft dysfunction from rejection in heart graft recipients receiving a CNI-based therapy [80, 81]. Decreased CD25 and CD71 expression probably indicated over-immunosuppression in patients with allograft dysfunction [80].

In kidney transplant recipients, CD25 expression was helpful to distinguish patients with cyclosporine A nephrotoxicity from patients with rejection or infection [82]. The results from our group suggest that kidney transplant patients with a spontaneously low level of CD26 expression on CD3$^+$ cells within the first week after transplantation are less prone to rejection, whereas a low level of CD71 expression was associated with more infections, probably indicating over-immunosuppression [83].

Boleslawski *et al.* reported an association between a decreased level of CD28 expression on CD8$^+$ cells and malignancies in long-term liver transplant patients, as well as an association between increased expression and rejection [84, 85]. So far, no standardization of assay protocols has been achieved and no sound data from larger clinical trials have been published. This suggests that the demanding assay procedures have so far precluded the dissemination of T cell activation surface markers as a complementary tool to conventional therapeutic drug monitoring.

Soluble CD30 in Serum

Soluble CD 30 in serum (sCD30) is the soluble form of CD30, a member of the tumor necrosis factor (TNF) receptor family that was originally identified as a marker for Reed-Sternberg cells in Hodgkin's disease [86]. CD30 is expressed on CD4$^+$ and CD8$^+$ T lymphocytes, B and NK cells, as well as some non-lymphoid cells, and represents a co-stimulatory molecule with an important role in T and B cell growth, differentiation and function [87–89]. The soluble form, sCD30 with a molecular mass of about 85 kDa, is released after activation from the cell surface into the bloodstream by proteolytic cleavage [90]. In most healthy individuals sCD30 is present in only low concentrations [91]. There is age-dependency, with children and young people having higher concentrations than adults [92]. A clear gender dependency could not be demonstrated until now.

Over recent years a considerable number of studies on the utility of sCD30 as a new tool for immunologic testing in transplantation have been published. Particularly in kidney transplantation, results of large outcome studies with hundreds to thousands of patients have been reported [93–96] that provide a significantly greater body of clinical evidence compared to other biomarkers. An important reason for this is the availability of commercial assays based on enzyme linked immunosorbent assay (ELISA) technology, which can be easily performed, do not require *ex vivo* stimulation of immune cells, and offer a certain level of standardization and comparability of the results. In addition, the development and validation of a fluorescent microsphere immunoassay (Luminex® technology) has been more recently described which allows multiplex determination of sCD30 along with other molecules in the same sample and opens new analytical perspectives [97].

The diagnostic role of sCD30 has been studied in a variety of diseases, such as viral infections, autoimmune and allergic disorders, etc., and more recently in transplantation medicine. Numerous studies, primarily in kidney transplantation, have demonstrated an association between high sCD30 concentrations in serum and impaired graft outcome. High pre-transplant concentrations (> 100 U/mL) were significantly related to the incidence of acute allograft rejection and the need for anti-rejection treatment in the first year post-transplantation, as well as the risk of graft loss during a 5-year follow-up [93]. Plasma sCD30 concentrations remaining high early after transplantation (3–5 days) were identified as an additional prognostic marker for the development of acute rejection [98]. sCD30 was able to discriminate, with a specificity of 100% and a sensitivity of 88%, patients with an uncomplicated course or rejection, as well as, with a specificity of 91% and a sensitivity of 72%, those with acute tubular necrosis or rejection.

Moreover, a recent multicenter study which included over 2000 kidney transplant recipients investigated the time course of sCD30 after transplantation, and showed that a nadir of the concentration was reached at day 30 and that values over 40 U/mL were associated with a significantly lower 3-year graft survival rate, irrespective of whether the sCD30 concentration before transplantation was high or low [95].

Finally, results of a separate study by the same group suggested that 1-year sCD30 concentrations can differentiate graft deterioration from chronic allograft nephropathy [99]. In addition, high sCD30 concentrations, both pre- and post-transplantation, were shown to be a risk factor for low graft survival independent of antibody sensitization and HLA mismatch [93, 95], with a particularly poor prognosis for patients with simultaneously high levels of the markers.

There have been some studies in kidney transplantation which failed to find the associations described above, and it can be speculated that possible reasons for the discrepancies are the lower number of patients included or a short follow-up period. As shown by Altermann et al. [96], there is considerable intra-individual variation of the sCD30 concentrations in about 20% patients on the waiting list; thus, sequential monitoring (e.g., quarterly) might be advantageous. Furthermore, as reported by López-Hoyos et al. [100] and Spiridon et al. [101], there is a correlation between higher sCD30 concentrations and increased serum creatinine concentrations that may complicate interpretation of results, particularly those close to the cut-offs.

In addition to the association between sCD30 and graft outcome in kidney transplantation, some research groups have evaluated the relation between this marker and the occurrence of infections [101, 102] as well as its utility as a predictor of outcome of non-renal transplantation (e.g., lung, heart, islet cells and liver) [103–106]. However, these studies were smaller and their results often discrepant. Particularly important questions, such as the optimal time-points for sCD30 determination as well as cut-offs, are still open and more research is needed to clarify the diagnostic value of sCD30 for these applications. Moreover, studies investigating the effects of different immunosuppressive drugs or drug combinations on sCD30 are unfortunately lacking. This very important issue must be addressed in the future.

Lymphocyte Proliferation

Lymphocyte proliferation can be assessed by flow cytometry by using monoclonal antibodies binding to proliferating cell nuclear antigen (PCNA) and propidium iodide-labeled DNA [107]. An alternative approach is to determine PCNA mRNA expression by real-time polymerase chain reaction (PCR) [108]. Whereas PCNA protein expression requires approximately 72 hours to become reliably measurable, PCNA mRNA expression can be assessed 24 hours after the onset of stimulation.

In addition, a number of other methods exist to follow cell proliferation in various cell populations. If labeled DNA precursors, such as radioactive thymidine (^{3}H-thymidine) or the thymidine analog BrdU (bromoedoxyuridine), are added to the cells, then they are incorporated into the newly synthesized DNA. Levels of ^{3}H-thymidine can be detected by a scintillation counter, while BrdU can be detected by a quantitative cellular enzyme immunoassay using monoclonal antibodies [109, 110]. The succinimidyl ester of carboxyfluorescein diacetate (CFSE) can also be utilized to assess cell proliferation [111].

Clinical data linked to cell proliferation have been published using such assays as PCNA protein and mRNA expression, BrdU incorporation, and CFSE dilution [108, 25, 83, 112]. Millán et al. reported, in a study of stable liver transplant recipients undergoing weaning of immunosuppressive therapy, increased cell proliferation in CD8$^+$ cells in patients with rejections, using flow cytometry and PCNA/DNA expression [25]. In a small study with 55 renal transplant patients, reduced PCNA mRNA expression was associated with the risk of virus infections and reactivation whereas increased expression was observed in 3 out of 4 patients with rejection [108]. Using the CFSE dilution assay increased cell proliferation, indicating under-immunosuppression was associated with risk of rejection in 28 pediatric patients with small bowel transplantation [112]. BrdU incorporation was reduced in kidney transplant recipients who had an increased risk for developing leukopenia [83].

Cell proliferation has been assessed in parallel with T cell activation in many published reports, and the results are in most cases comparable. The assays require *ex vivo* lymphocyte stimulation by mitogens, and in general need 3 days for completion. The variability of the flow cytometric determination of PCNA/DNA seems to be greater than that of cell surface marker expression [74]. Although cell proliferation can principally be used to assess non-specific effects of immunosuppressants on lymphocytes, it is very unlikely that it will become a helpful pharmacodynamic marker to complement therapeutic drug monitoring. The assay procedure is laborious, difficult to standardize and time-consuming.

BIOMARKER SIGNATURES RELATED TO TOLERANCE

Schröppel *et al.* [113] recently pointed to the fact that more than 50% of transplanted kidneys from deceased donors fail within 10 years. Therefore, there is a need to better understand the mechanisms underlying rejection and tolerance. Biomarkers could be helpful in identifying tolerant liver or kidney transplant recipients who would benefit from immunosuppression withdrawal or minimization. Spontaneous operational tolerance is defined as the long-term maintenance of stable graft function without a clinically significant detrimental immune response or immune deficit following discontinuation of conventional immunosuppression [114].

Preliminary clinical studies indicate that the numbers of circulating regulatory T cells (Tregs) may contribute to determining the long-term fate of renal transplants [115]. It was demonstrated that the number of $CD4^+CD25^{high}FOXP3^+$ cells as determined by flow cytometry was significantly decreased in patients with chronic rejection compared to healthy volunteers and operationally-tolerant patients, as well as patients with stable graft function. Immune profiling of operational tolerance was performed in liver transplant recipients [116]. The study included 16 operationally-tolerant adult recipients with successful immunosuppression discontinuation and 16 immunosuppression-dependent recipients as well as 10 age-matched healthy controls. Tolerant recipients displayed a significantly greater proportion of $CD4^+CD25^{high}FOXP3^+$ T cells than immunosuppression-dependent patients. On the other hand, no significant differences in the percentages were observed between operationally-tolerant patients and healthy controls. So far, however, these studies cannot answer the question as to whether a normal or even enhanced number of $CD4^+CD25^{high}FOXP3^+$ T cells is a robust marker for drug weaning.

Experimental evidence exists that Tregs expand after lymphopenia induced by T cell depleting agents (such as the humanized anti-CD52 mAb Campath-1H). $CD3^+CD4^+$ cells that were isolated 24 months after transplantation from sirolimus-treated patients had significantly higher *FOXP3* (fork head box protein P3) expression compared with $CD3^+CD4^+$ cells from the same patients' baseline or from healthy individuals [117]. In CsA-treated patients, *FOXP3* expression in $CD3^+CD4^+$ cells was much lower than in the sirolimus group. These results indicate that, after lymphocyte depletion, sirolimus but not CsA increased the pool of *FOXP3* expression in $CD4^+CD25^{high}$ cells. It seems that CNI may inhibit *FOXP3* gene transcription in contrast to sirolimus and thereby the development of tolerance.

In a further study, immune monitoring was performed in liver transplant recipients with renal dysfunction treated either with a combination of mycophenolic acid mofetil (MMF) and minimal dose CNI or with a reduced CNI regimen [118]. After 12 months' treatment, $CD3^+CD8^+$ cytotoxic T lymphocytes and $CD3^+CD4^+$ T helper cells significantly declined in the MMF group but not in the control group, with only reduced CNI immunosuppression. Despite a general decline in circulating lymphocytes in the MMF group after 12 months, the absolute numbers of $CD4^+CD25^{high}FOXP3^+$ T cells were preserved during the whole study period. On the contrary, in the control group there was a significant decrease in the absolute number of Tregs in peripheral blood. This indicates that CNI treatment reduces the numbers of circulating Tregs. This report suggests that MMF combined with only minimal CNI exposure may potentially promote allograft tolerance.

FOXP3 mRNA expression was investigated during immunosuppression withdrawal in liver transplant recipients [119]. The *FOXP3* mRNA levels increased significantly in the operationally-tolerant group. Patients with rejections showed no increase in FOXP3 messenger RNA. All these preliminary findings may be regarded as a first step towards developing "tolerance permissive" immunosuppressive regimens in the clinical setting.

Various methods have been described for the determination of regulatory T cells. Flow cytometric assays and *FOXP3* mRNA expression are widely used methods which have, however, the disadvantage that they are not able to differentiate between Tregs and activated effector T cells, which transiently express *FOXP3*. A new assay has been developed, which is based on Treg-specific DNA demethylation within the *FOXP3* locus [120, 121]. *FOXP3* TSDR demethylation occurs only in natural Tregs. This assay may be useful for fast and reliable screening of Tregs.

Although it is unlikely that a single biomarker may be sufficient for identifying tolerance, because of the complexicity of the involved mechanisms, the number of regulatory T cells ($CD4^+CD25^{high}FOXP3^+$) may be one potential biomarker candidate. To use this parameter for guiding drug weaning, however, appropriate cut-off levels would have to be defined [122].

Presumably, a set of biomarkers would be necessary to predict tolerance [6, 122]. Recently, a tolerance-specific signature of 49 genes was identified in kidney transplant recipients, which suggests that TGF-β might contribute to this process by regulating specific phenotypes of Tregs or altering the threshold for T cell activation [123].

Newell and colleagues [8] conducted a study on the identification of a B cell signature associated with renal transplant tolerance in humans. A cohort of 25 tolerant transplant recipients, as defined by stable graft function and receiving no immunosuppression for more than 1 year, was included in this study. Gene expression profiles and peripheral blood lymphocytes subsets observed in tolerant transplant recipients were compared with those of subjects with stable graft function receiving immunosuppressive drugs and those of healthy controls. Tolerant patients exhibited increased numbers of total and naïve B cells, and showed increased expression of multiple B cell differentiation genes. A signature of three genes (*IGKV4-1, IGLLA, IGKV1D-13*) was highly predictive of tolerance, and a simple PCR assay may be used for screening purposes. It was concluded that transitioning or maturing B cells may be involved in tolerance induction and/or maintenance. Such approaches could be used to screen stable patients under conventional immunosuppression and identify those that could undergo a controlled reduction in immunosuppression.

Sagoo *et al.* [7] developed a cross-platform biomarker signature to detect renal transplant tolerance in humans (Table 16.4). Operationally-tolerant recipients were defined as stable

TABLE 16.4 Biomarker Signature to Detect Renal Transplant Tolerance

Tolerance signature comprising:

- a set of 10 genes with significantly altered expressions
- elevated numbers of peripheral blood B and NK cell
- diminished numbers of recently activated CD4$^+$ T cells
- donor-specific hyporesponsiveness of CD4$^+$ T cells (IFN-γ ELISpot)
- high ratio of *FoxP3*/α-1,2-mannosidase (*MAN1A2*) gene expression in peripheral blood

Data from Sagoo et al. [7].

renal transplant recipients without immunosuppression for more than 1 year with an increase in serum creatinine < 10%. In this study, biomarkers and bioassays were screened on a training set of 11 operationally-tolerant renal transplant recipients. Predictive assays were repeated on an independent test set of 24 tolerant recipients. It was found that tolerant patients displayed an expansion of peripheral blood B and NK lymphocytes, fewer activated CD4$^+$ T cells, a lack of donor-specific antibodies, donor-specific hyporesponsiveness of CD4$^+$ T cells and a high ratio of *FOXP3* to α-1,2-mannosidase (*MAN1A2*) gene expression.

Biomarkers of tolerance [124] are currently being validated in a prospective withdrawal study supported through the European Union RISET consortium (www.risetfp6.org).

CONCLUSIONS

In conclusion, the discussed biomarkers are potential complementary tools in addition to TDM. Such biomarkers may be useful to identify patients who are candidates for a minimization of immunosuppressive therapy, may identify patients at risk for acute rejection or infection, and may be useful to manage the timing and rate of immunosuppressant weaning. Serial longitudinal immune monitoring may allow maintenance of an individualized immunosuppressive regimen.

Pharmacodynamic monitoring using biomarkers is, however, still in its early stages. Optimal combinations of biomarkers seem to be necessary. Promising biomarkers of immune function are the CD4$^+$ cellular response measured by iATP synthesis reflecting mitochondrial metabolic competence, primarily as a marker of over-immunosuppression, and altered IL-2 expression by CD8$^+$ T-lymphocytes to assess cytotoxic properties as a marker of increased rejection risk. The assessment of T cell activation by the determination of iATP, sCD30, IFN-γ producing T cells by ELISPOT, and NFAT-regulated gene expression have a potential to be used more broadly in clinical trials since for these markers assay kits are in the meantime commercially available, thus facilitating their use in less experienced laboratories under routine conditions.

The number and function of regulatory T cells and the increased expression of B cell differentiation genes are potential predictors of tolerance. Before combinations of such molecular and functional biomarkers can be used as a decisional tool in the clinical setting, careful validation in appropriately designed prospective studies is necessary. Therapeutic drug monitoring in combination with such biomarkers seems to be a promising approach to improve the outcome in organ transplantation.

References

[1] Koch-Weser J. Drug therapy. Serum drug concentrations as therapeutic guides. N Engl J Med 1972;287:227—31.

[2] Wieland E, Olbricht CJ, Süsal C, et al. Biomarkers as a tool for management of immunosuppression in transplant patients. Ther Drug Monit 2010;32:560—72.

[3] Falck P, Asberg A, Guldseth H, et al. Declining intracellular T-lymphocyte concentration of cyclosporine A precedes acute rejection in kidney transplant recipients. Transplantation 2008;85:179—84.

[4] Crettol S, Venetz JP, Fontana M, et al. Influence of ABCB1 genetic polymorphisms on cyclosporine intracellular concentration in transplant recipients. Pharmacogenet Genomics 2008;18:307—15.

[5] Dambrin C, Klupp J, Morris RE. Pharmacodynamics of immunosuppressive drugs. Curr Opin Immunol 2000;12:557—62.

[6] Castellaneta A, Thomson AW, Nayyar N, et al. Monitoring the operationally tolerant liver allograft recipient. Curr Opin Organ Transplant 2010;15:28—34.

[7] Sagoo P, Perucha E, Sawitzki B, et al. Development of a cross-platform biomarker signature to detect renal transplant tolerance in humans. J Clin Invest 2010;120:1848—61.

[8] Newell KA, Asare A, Kirk AD, et al. Identification of a B cell signature associated with renal transplant tolerance in humans. J Clin Invest 2010;120:1836—47.

[9] Halloran PF, Helms LM, Kung L, Noujaim J. The temporal profile of calcineurin inhibition by cyclosporine *in vivo*. Transplantation 1999;68:1356—61.

[10] Marquet P. Is pharmacokinetic or pharmacodynamic monitoring of calcineurin inhibition therapy necessary? Clin Chem 2010;56:736—9.

[11] Hartmann B, Schmid G, Graeb C, et al. Biochemical monitoring of mTOR inhibitor-based immunosuppression following kidney transplantation: a novel approach for tailored immunosuppressive therapy. Kidney Intl 2005;68:2593—8.

[12] Dekter HE, Romijn FP, Temmink WP, et al. A spectrophotometric assay for routine measurement of mammalian target of rapamycin activity in cell lysate. Anal Biochem 2010;403:79—87.

[13] Glander P, Hambach P, Braun KP, et al. Pre-transplant inosine monophosphate dehydrogenase activity is associated with clinical outcome after renal transplantation. Am J Transplant 2004;4:2045—51.

[14] Fukuda T, Goebel J, Thøgersen H, et al. Inosine monophosphate dehydrogenase (IMPDH) activity as a pharmacodynamic biomarker of mycophenolic acid effects in pediatric kidney transplant recipients. J Clin Pharmacol 2011;51:309—20.

[15] Vethe NT, Mandla R, Line PD, et al. Inosine monophosphate dehydrogenase activity in renal allograft recipients during mycophenolate treatment. Scand J Clin Lab Invest 2006;66:31—44.

[16] Chiarelli LR, Molinaro M, Libetta C, et al. Inosine monophosphate dehydrogenase variability in renal transplant patients on long-term mycophenolate mofetil therapy. Br J Clin Pharmacol 2010;69:38—50.

[17] Raggi MC, Siebert SB, Steimer W, et al. Customized mycophenolate dosing based on measuring inosine-monophosphate dehydrogenase activity significantly improves patients' outcomes after renal transplantation. Transplantation 2010;90:1536—41.

[18] Wu TY, Peng Y, Pelleymounter LL, et al. Pharmacogenetics of the mycophenolic acid targets inosine monophosphate dehydrogenases IMPDH1 and IMPDH2: gene sequence variation and functional genomics. Br J Pharmacol 2010;161:1584—98.

[19] Gensburger O, van Schaik RHN, Picard N, et al. Polymorphisms in type I and II inosine monophosphate dehydrogenase genes and association with clinical outcome in patients on mycophenolate mofetil. Pharmacogenetics and Genomics 2010;20:537—43.

[20] Boleslawski E, Conti F, Sanquer S, et al. Defective inhibition of peripheral CD8+ T cell IL-2 production by anti-calcineurin drugs during acute liver allograft rejection. Transplantation 2004;77:1815—20.

[21] Brandt C, Liman P, Bendfeldt H, et al. Whole blood flow cytometric measurement of NFATc1 and IL-2 expression to analyze cyclosporine A-mediated effects in T cells. Cytometry A 2010;77:607—13.

[22] Akoglu B, Kriener S, Martens S, et al. Interleukin-2 in CD8+ T cells correlates with Banff score during organ rejection in liver transplant recipients. Clin Exp Med 2009;9:259—62.

[23] van den Berg AP, Twilhaar WN, Mesander G, et al. Quantitation of immunosuppression by flow cytometric measurement of the capacity of T cells for interleukin-2 production. Transplantation 1998;65:1066—71.

[24] Chen Y, McKenna GJ, Yoshida EM, et al. Assessment of immunologic status of liver transplant recipients by peripheral blood mononuclear cells in response to stimulation by donor alloantigen. Ann Surg 1999;230:242—50.

[25] Millán O, Benitez C, Guillén D, et al. Biomarkers of immunoregulatory status in stable liver transplant recipients undergoing weaning of immunosuppressive therapy. Clin Immunol 2010;137:337—46.

[26] Giese T, Zeier M, Schemmer P, et al. Monitoring of NFAT-regulated gene expression in the peripheral blood of allograft recipients: a novel perspective toward individually optimized drug doses of cyclosporine A. Transplantation 2004;77:339—44.

[27] Sommerer C, Konstandin M, Dengler T, et al. Pharmacodynamic monitoring of cyclosporine A in renal allograft recipients shows a quantitative relationship between immunosuppression and the occurrence of recurrent infections and malignancies. Transplantation 2006;82:1280—5.

[28] Sommerer C, Zeier M, Czock D, et al. Pharmacodynamic disparities in tacrolimus-treated patients developing cytomegalus virus viremia. Ther Drug Monit. 2011;33:373—9.

[29] Sommerer C, Giese T, Schmidt J, et al. Ciclosporin A tapering monitored by NFAT-regulated gene expression: a new concept of individual immunosuppression. Transplantation 2008;85:15—21.

[30] Zahn A, Schott N, Hinz U, et al. Immunomonitoring of nuclear factor of activated T cells-regulated gene expression: the first clinical trial in liver allograft recipients. Liver Transpl 2011;17:466—73.

[31] Billing H, Giese T, Sommerer C, et al. Pharmacodynamic monitoring of cyclosporine A by NFAT-regulated gene expression and the relationship with infectious complications in pediatric renal transplant recipients. Pediatr Transplant 2010;14:844—51.

[32] Konstandin MH, Sommerer C, Doesch A, et al. Pharmacodynamic cyclosporine A-monitoring: relation of gene expression in lymphocytes to cyclosporine blood levels in cardiac allograft recipients. Transpl Int 2007;20:1036—43.

[33] Sommerer C, Zeier M, Schnitzler P, et al. Pharmacodynamic monitoring of ciclosporin A reveals risk of opportunistic infections and malignancies in renal transplant recipients 65 years and older. Ther Drug Monit 2011;33:694—8.

[34] Sommerer C, Zeier M, Meuer S, Giese T. Individualized monitoring of nuclear factor of activated T cells-regulated gene expression in FK506-treated kidney transplant recipients. Transplantation 2010;89:1417—23.

[35] Sommerer C, Zeier M, Meurer S, Giese T. Pharmacodynamic monitoring of CsA therapy in the early post-transplant period. Kidney Intl 2011;(Suppl.):1000. Abstract #M0518.

[36] Kowalski R, Post D, Schneider MC, et al. Immune cell function testing: an adjunct to therapeutic drug monitoring in transplant patient management. Clin Transplant 2003;17:77—88.

[37] Kowalski RJ, Post DR, Mannon RB, et al. Assessing relative risks of infection and rejection: a meta-analysis using an immune function assay. Transplantation 2006;82:663—8.

[38] Kowalski RJ, Zeevi A, Mannon RB, et al. Immunodiagnostics: evaluation of functional T-cell immunocompetence in whole blood independent of circulating cell numbers. J Immunotoxicol 2007;4:225—32.

[39] Akhlaghi F, Gohh RY. The level of ATP production in mitogen-stimulated $CD4^+$ lymphocytes is independent of the time of ingestion of immunosuppressive agents. Ther Drug Monit 2010;32:116—7.

[40] Schulz-Juergensen S, Burdelski M, Oellerich M, Brandhorst G. Intracellular ATP production in $CD4^+$ T cells as a predictor for infection and allograft rejection in trough-level guided pediatric liver transplant recipients under calcineurin-inhibitor therapy. The Drug Monit 2012;34:4—10.

[41] Reinsmoen NL, Cornett KM, Kloehn R, et al. Pretransplant donor-specific and non-specific immune parameters associated with early acute rejection. Transplantation 2008;85:462—70.

[42] Huskey J, Gralla J, Wiseman AC. Single time point immune function assay (ImmuKnowTM) testing does not aid in the prediction of future opportunistic infections or acute rejection. Clin J Am Soc Nephrol 2011;6:423—9.

[43] Israeli M, Ben-Gal T, Yaari V, et al. Individualized immune monitoring of cardiac transplant recipients by noninvasive longitudinal cellular immunity tests. Transplantation 2010;89:968—76.

[44] Kobashigawa JA, Kiyosaki KK, Patel JK, et al. Benefit of immune monitoring in heart transplant patients using ATP production in activated lymphocytes. J Heart Lung Transplant 2010;29:504—8.

[45] Bhorade SM, Janata K, Vigneswaran WT, et al. Cylex ImmuKnow assay levels are lower in lung transplant recipients with infection. J Heart Lung Transplant 2008;27:990—4.

[46] Husain S, Raza K, Pilewski JM, et al. Experience with immune monitoring in lung transplant recipients: correlation of low immune function with infection. Transplantation 2009;87:1852—7.

[47] Xue F, Zhang J, Han L, et al. Immune cell functional assay in monitoring of adult liver transplantation recipients with infection. Transplantation 2010;89:620–6.

[48] Hashimoto K, Miller C, Horose K, et al. Measurement of CD4$^+$ T-cell function in predicting allograft rejection and recurrent hepatitis C after liver transplantation. Clin Transplant 2010;24:701–8.

[49] Millán O, Sánchez-Fueyo A, Rimola A, et al. Is the intracellular ATP concentration of CD4$^+$ T-cells a predictive biomarker of immune status in stable transplant recipients? Transplantation 2009;88(Suppl.):S78–84.

[50] Serban G, Whittaker V, Fan J, et al. Significance of immune cell function monitoring in renal transplantation after thymoglobulin induction therapy. Hum Immunol 2009;70:882–92.

[51] Gupta S, Mitchell JD, Markham DW, et al. Utility of the Cylex assay in cardiac transplant patients. J Heart Lung Transplant 2008;27:817–22.

[52] Cabrera R, Ararat M, Soldevila-Pico C, et al. Using an immune functional assay to differentiate acute cellular rejection from recurrent hepatitis C in liver transplant patients. Liver Transpl 2009;15:216–22.

[53] Cadillo-Chávez R, de Echegaray S, Santiago-Delpín EA, et al. Assessing the risk of infection and rejection in Hispanic renal transplant recipients by means of an adenosine triphosphate release assay. Transplant Proc 2006;38:918–20.

[54] De Paolis P, Favarò A, Piola A, et al. "ImmuKnow" to measurement of cell-mediated immunity in renal transplant recipients undergoing short-term evaluation. Transplant Proc 2011;43:1013–6.

[55] Lee TC, Goss JA, Roonex CM, et al. Quantification of a low cellular immune response to aid in identification of pediatric liver transplant recipients at high-risk for EBV infection. Clin Transplant 2006;20:689–94.

[56] Berglund D, Bengtsson M, Biglarnia A, et al. Screening of mortality in transplant patients using an assay for immune function. Transpl Immunol 2011;24:246–50.

[57] Zeevi A, Britz JA, Bentlejewski CA, et al. Monitoring immune function during tacrolimus tapering in small bowel transplant recipients. Transpl Immunol 2005;15:17–24.

[58] Nankivell B, Alexander SI. Rejection of the kidney allograft. N Engl J Med 2010;363:1451–62.

[59] Nickel P, Bestard O, Volk HD, Reinke P. Diagnostic value of T-cell monitoring assays in kidney transplantation. Curr Opin Organ Transplant 2009;14:426–31.

[60] Augustine JJ, Siu DS, Clemente MJ, et al. Pre-transplant IFN-gamma ELISPOTs are associated with post-transplant renal function in African American renal transplant recipients. Am J Transplant 2005;5:1971–5.

[61] Hricik DE, Rodriguez V, Riley J, et al. Enzyme linked immunosorbent spot (ELISPOT) assay for interferon-gamma independently predicts renal function in kidney transplant recipients. Am J Transplant 2003;3:878–84.

[62] Andree H, Nickel P, Nasiadko C, et al. Identification of dialysis patients with panel-reactive memory T cells before kidney transplantation using an allogeneic cell bank. J Am Soc Nephrol 2006;17:573–80.

[63] Poggio ED, Clemente M, Hricik DE, Heeger PS. Panel of reactive T cells as a measurement of primed cellular alloimmunity in kidney transplant candidates. J Am Soc Nephrol 2006;17:564–72.

[64] Poggio ED, Augustine JJ, Clemente M, et al. Pretransplant cellular alloimmunity as assessed by a panel of reactive T cells assay correlates with acute renal graft rejection. Transplantation 2007;83:847–52.

[65] Kim SH, Oh EJ, Kim MJ, et al. Pretransplant donor-specific interferon-gamma ELISPOT assay predicts acute rejection episodes in renal transplant recipients. Transplant Proc 2007;39:3057–60.

[66] Bestard O, Cruzado JM, Mestre M, et al. Achieving donor-specific hyporesponsiveness is associated with FOXP3$^+$ regulatory T cell recruitment in human renal allograft infiltrates. J Immunol 2007;179:4901–9.

[67] Noris M, Casiraghi F, Todeschini M, et al. Regulatory T cells and T cell depletion: role of immunosuppressive drugs. J Am Soc Nephrol 2007;18:1007–18.

[68] Zhang W, Caspell R, Karulin AY, et al. ELISPOT assays provide reproducible results among different laboratories for T-cell immune monitoring—even in hands of ELISPOT-inexperienced investigators. J Immunotoxicol 2009;6:227–34.

[69] US National Institutes of Health (n.d.). Clinical Trials. Available at, http://clinicaltrials.gov/ct2/show/. NCT01195194.

[70] Barraclough KA, Staatz CE, Isbel NM, McTaggart SJ. Review: pharmacodynamic monitoring of immunosuppression in kidney transplantation. Nephrology 2010;15:522–32.

[71] Heemann UW, Tullius SG, Azuma H, et al. Adhesion molecules and transplantation. Ann Surg 1994;219:4–12.

[72] Tan J, Zhou G. Chemokine receptors and transplantation. Cell Mol Immunol 2005;2:343–9.

[73] Holling TM, Schooten E, van Den Elsen PJ. Function and regulation of MHC class II molecules in T-lymphocytes: of mice and men. Hum Immunol 2004;65:282–90.

[74] Böhler T, Nolting J, Kamar N, et al. Validation of immunological biomarkers for the pharmacodynamic monitoring of immunosuppressive drugs in humans. Ther Drug Monit 2007;29:77–86.

[75] Stalder M, Bîrsan T, Holm B, et al. Quantification of immunosuppression by flow cytometry in stable renal transplant recipients. Ther Drug Monit 2003;25:22–7.

[76] Böhler T, Canivet C, Nguyen PN, et al. Cytokines correlate with age in healthy volunteers, dialysis patients and kidney-transplant patients. Cytokine 2009;45:169–73.

[77] Prémaud A, Rousseau A, Johnson G, et al. Inhibition of T-cell activation and proliferation by mycophenolic acid in patients awaiting liver transplantation: PK/PD relationships. Pharmacol Res 2011;63:432–8.

[78] Kamar N, Glander P, Nolting J, et al. Pharmacodynamic evaluation of the first dose of mycophenolate mofetil before kidney transplantation. Clin J Am Soc Nephrol 2009;4:936–42.

[79] Weimer R, Zipperle S, Daniel V, et al. Pretransplant CD4 helper function and interleukin 10 response predict risk of acute kidney graft rejection. Transplantation 1996;62:1606–14.

[80] Deng MC, Erren M, Roeder N, et al. T-cell and monocyte subsets, inflammatory molecules, rejection, and hemodynamics early after cardiac transplantation. Transplantation 1998;65:1255–61.

[81] Chang DM, Ding YA, Kuo SY, et al. Cytokines and cell surface markers in prediction of cardiac allograft rejection. Immunol Invest 1996;25:13–21.

[82] Beik AI, Morris AG, Higgins RM, Lam FT. Serial flow cytometric analysis of T-cell surface markers can be useful in differential diagnosis of renal allograft dysfunction. Clin Transplant 1998;12:24–9.

[83] Wieland E, Shipkova M, Martius Y, et al. Association between pharmacodynamic biomarkers and clinical events in the early phase after kidney transplantation: a single-center pilot study. Ther Drug Monit 2011;33:341–9.

[84] Boleslawski E, BenOthman S, Grabar S, et al. CD25, CD28 and CD38 expression in peripheral blood lymphocytes as a tool to predict acute rejection after liver transplantation. Clin Transplant 2008;22: 494–501.

[85] Boleslawski E, Othman SB, Aoudjehane L, et al. CD28 expression by peripheral blood lymphocytes as a potential predictor of the development of *de novo* malignancies in long-term survivors after liver transplantation. Liver Transpl 2011;17:299–305.

[86] Schwab U, Stein H, Gerdes J, et al. Production of a monoclonal antibody specific for Hodgkin and Sternberg-Reed cells of Hodgkin's disease and a subset of normal lymphoid cells. Nature 1982;299:65–7.

[87] Pellegrini P, Berghella AM, Contasta I, Adorno D. CD30 antigen: not a physiological marker for TH2 cells but an important costimulator molecule in the regulation of the balance between TH1/TH2 response. Transpl Immunol 2003;12:49–61.

[88] Okamoto A, Yamamura M, Iwahashi M, et al. Pathophysiological functions of CD30$^+$ CD4$^+$ T cells in rheumatoid arthritis. Acta Med Okayama 2003;57:267–77.

[89] Dai Z, Li Q, Wang Y, et al. CD4$^+$CD25$^+$ regulatory T cells suppress allograft rejection mediated by memory CD8$^+$ T cells via a CD30-dependent mechanism. J Clin Invest 2004;113:310–7.

[90] Josimovic-Alasevic O, Dürkop H, Schwarting R, et al. Ki-1 (CD30) antigen is released by Ki-1-positive tumor cells *in vitro* and *in vivo*. I. Partial characterization of soluble Ki-1 antigen and detection of the antigen in cell culture supernatants and in serum by an enzyme-linked immunosorbent assay. Eur J Immunol 1989;19:157–62.

[91] Bauwens AM, van de Graaf EA, van Ginkel WG, et al. Pre-transplant soluble CD30 is associated with bronchiolitis obliterans syndrome after lung transplantation. J Heart Lung Transplant 2006;25:416–9.

[92] Chrul S, Polakowska E. Age-dependent changes of serum soluble CD30 concentration in children. Pediatr Transplant 2011;15:515–8.

[93] Süsal C, Pelzl S, Döhler B, Opelz G. Identification of highly responsive kidney transplant recipients using pretransplant soluble CD30. J Am Soc Nephrol 2002;13:1650–6.

[94] Pelzl S, Opelz G, Wiesel M, et al. Soluble CD30 as a predictor of kidney graft outcome. Transplantation 2002;73:3–6.

[95] Süsal C, Döhler B, Sadeghi M, et al. Posttransplant sCD30 as a predictor of kidney graft outcome. Transplantation 2011;91:1364–9.

[96] Altermann W, Schlaf G, Rothhoff A, Seliger B. High variation of individual soluble serum CD30 levels of pre-transplantation patients: sCD30 a feasible marker for prediction of kidney allograft rejection? Nephrol Dial Transplant 2007;22:2795–9.

[97] Pavlov I, Martins TB, Delgado JC. Development and validation of a fluorescent microsphere immunoassay for soluble CD30 testing. Clin Vaccine Immunol 2009;16:1327—31.

[98] Pelzl S, Opelz G, Daniel V, et al. Evaluation of posttransplantation soluble CD30 for diagnosis of acute renal allograft rejection. Transplantation 2003;75:421—3.

[99] Weimer R, Süsal C, Yildiz S, et al. Post-transplant sCD30 and neopterin as predictors of chronic allograft nephropathy: impact of different immunosuppressive regimens. Am J Transplant 2006;6:1865—74.

[100] López-Hoyos M, San Segundo D, Benito MJ, et al. Association between serum soluble CD30 and serum creatinine before and after renal transplantation. Transplant Proc 2008;40:2903—5.

[101] Spiridon C, Nikaein A, Lerman M, et al. CD30, a marker to detect the high-risk kidney transplant recipients. Clin Transplant 2008;22:765—9.

[102] Nikaein A, Spiridon C, Hunt J, et al. Pre-transplant level of soluble CD30 is associated with infection after heart transplantation. Clin Transplant 2007;21:744—7.

[103] Shah AS, Leffell MS, Lucas D, Zachary AA. Elevated pretransplantation soluble CD30 is associated with decreased early allograft function after human lung transplantation. Hum Immunol 2009;70:101—3.

[104] Ypsilantis E, Key T, Bradley JA, et al. Soluble CD30 levels in recipients undergoing heart transplantation do not predict post-transplant outcome. J Heart Lung Transplant 2009;28:1206—10.

[105] Hire K, Hering B, Bansal-Pakala P, et al. Relative reductions in soluble CD30 levels post-transplant predict acute graft function in islet allograft recipients receiving three different immunosuppression protocols. Transpl Immunol 2010;23:209—14.

[106] Kim KH, Oh EJ, Jung ES, et al. Evaluation of pre- and posttransplantation serum interferon-gamma and soluble CD30 for predicting liver allograft rejection. Transplant Proc 2006;38:1429—31.

[107] Böhler T, Waiser J, Budde K, et al. The in vivo effect of rapamycin derivative SDZ RAD on lymphocyte proliferation. Transplant Proc 1998;30:2195—7.

[108] Niwa M, Miwa Y, Kuzuya T, et al. Stimulation index for PCNA mRNA in peripheral blood as immune function monitoring after renal transplantation. Transplantation 2009;87:1411—4.

[109] Wu J, Palladino MA, Figari IS, Morris RE. Comparative immunoregulatory effects of rapamycin, FK 506 and cyclosporine on mitogen-induced cytokine production and lymphoproliferation. Transplant Proc 1991;23:238—40.

[110] Shipkova M, Wieland E, Schütz E, et al. The acyl glucuronide metabolite of mycophenolic acid inhibits the proliferation of human mononuclear leukocytes. Transplant Proc 2001;33:1080—1.

[111] Lyons AB, Parish CR. Determination of lymphocyte division by flow cytometry. J Immunol Methods 1994;71:131—7.

[112] Ashokkumar C, Bentlejewski C, Sun Q, et al. Allospecific CD154+ B cells associate with intestine allograft rejection in children. Transplantation 2010;90:1226—31.

[113] Schröppel B, Heeger PS. Gazing into a crystal ball to predict kidney transplant outcome. J Clin Invest 2010;120:1803—6.

[114] Sánchez-Fueyo A, Strom TB. Immunologic basis of graft rejection and tolerance following transplantation of liver or other solid organs. Gastroenterology 2011;140:51—64.

[115] Braudeau C, Racape M, Giral M, et al. Variation in numbers of CD4+CD25highFOXP3+ T cells with normal immuno-regulatory properties in long-term graft outcome. Transpl Intl 2007;20:845—55.

[116] Martínez-Llordella M, Puig-Pey I, Orlando G, et al. Mulitparameter immune profiling of operational tolerance in liver transplantation. Am J Transplant 2007;7:309—19.

[117] Noris M, Casiraghi F, Todeschini M, et al. Regulatory T cells and T cell depletion: role of immunosuppressive drugs. J Am Soc Nephrol 2007;18:1007—18.

[118] Cicinnati VR, Yu Z, Klein CG, et al. Clinical Trial: switch to combined mycophenolate mofetil and minimal dose calcineurin inhibitor in stable liver transplant patients—assessment of renal and allograft function, cardiovascular risk factors and immune monitoring. Aliment Pharmacol Ther 2007;26:1195—208.

[119] Pons JA, Revilla-Nuin B, Baroja-Mazo A, et al. FoxP3 in peripheral blood is associated with operational tolerance in liver transplant patients during immunosuppression withdrawal. Transplantation 2008;86:1370—8.

[120] Baron U, Floess S, Wieczorek G, et al. DNA demethylation in the human FOXP3 locus discriminates regulatory T cells from activated FOXP3(+) conventional T cells. Eur J Immunol 2007;37:2378—89.

[121] Wieczorek G, Asemissen A, Model F, et al. Quantitative DNA methylation analysis of FOXP3 as a new method for counting regulatory T cells in peripheral blood and solid tissue. Cancer Res 2009;69:599—608.

[122] Volk HD. Predicting tolerance by counting natural regulatory T cells (CD4$^+$CD25^{++}FoxP$^+$)? Transpl Intl 2007;20:842–4.

[123] Brouard S, Mansfield E, Braud C, et al. Identification of a peripheral blood transcriptional biomarker panel associated with operational renal allograft tolerance. Proc Natl Acad Sci USA 2007;104:15448–53.

[124] Sarwal MM, Benjamin J, Butte AJ, et al. Transplantomics and biomarkers in organ transplantation: a report from the first international conference. Transplantation 2011;91:379–82.

CHAPTER

17

Therapeutic Drug Monitoring of Antiretroviral Drugs in the Management of Human Immunodeficiency Virus Infection

Natella Y. Rakhmanina[1], Charles J.L. la Porte[2]

[1]The George Washington University School of Medicine,
and the Children's National Medical Center, Washington, DC

[2]The Ottawa Hospital Research Institute and University of Ottawa, Ottawa, ON, Canada

OUTLINE

DOI: 10.1016/B978-0-12-385467-4.00017-8

INTRODUCTION

Human immunodeficiency virus (HIV) causes human disease by infecting and subsequently depleting T lymphocytes with CD4 cell receptor. The depletion of CD4 T cells creates an immunodeficiency state, and renders the host susceptible to infections and malignancies. HIV can also induce serious co-morbidities such as HIV-associated nephropathy, encephalopathy and other conditions leading to multiple organ damage. HIV infection is a highly dynamic process capable of creating well-hidden and preserved latent viral reservoirs. Moreover, HIV is prone to multiple genetic mutations leading to changes in viral RNA and high genetic diversity. Together, these characteristics make the virus an evasive target for the development of vaccine and drug therapy. As of today, no cure exists to permanently eliminate the virus from the human body.

Antiretroviral therapy (ART) is designed to maximally suppress the replication of HIV in the infected patient and to decrease and/or prevent systemic acute and chronic inflammation associated with the virus. Currently available antiretroviral (ARV) drugs are comprised of five classes, each with a unique mechanism of ARV action, capable of complementing each other.

Nucleoside/nucleotide reverse transcriptase inhibitors (NRTIs) and non-nucleoside reverse transcriptase inhibitors (NNRTIs) both inhibit the virally encoded reverse transcriptase enzyme in the host cell cytoplasm. NRTIs mimic viral nucleoside bases and act as DNA chain terminators, while NNRTIs bind the reverse transcriptase adjacent to the active site, causing structural change that prevents further elongation of the DNA chain [1]. Protease inhibitors (PIs) block the HIV core maturation process by binding to HIV-1 protease and blocking protease cleavage of newly formed HIV virions [2]. Entry and fusion inhibitors prevent HIV from entering the cells by binding HIV envelope protein (fusion inhibitor) and chemokine type 5 receptor (CCR5) (entry inhibitors) [3, 4]. Finally, integrase inhibitors inhibit the viral enzyme integrase and block the insertion of the HIV proviral DNA into the host cell's DNA [5].

In order to achieve maximal viral suppression and prevent the development of resistance, three or more ARV drugs are administered concomitantly as combination ART. The current US and European guidelines recommend the combination of two NRTIs (emtricitabine/tenofovir) with the NNRTIs (efavirenz) or PI (ritonavir) boosted atazanavir, or darunavir or integrase inhibitor (raltegravir), as a starting regimen for treatment-naïve patients [6, 7]. Such a wide choice of PIs is not practical in resource-limited settings where the regimen has to depend on cost and availability, or in treatment of co-morbidities such as tuberculosis, where there is the potential for significant drug–drug interactions. The World Health Organization (WHO) recommends the combination of two NRTIs (zidovudine/lamivudine, tenofovir/lamivudine, tenofovir/emtricitabine) plus NNRTI (efavirenz or nevirapine) as the preferred starting regimen [8]. Several important factors, such as ARV-associated toxicity, pill burden and dosing frequency, drug–drug and drug–food interactions, concomitant therapies and co-morbidities with hepatitis and tuberculosis affect the selection of the first and subsequent ART regimens. For selecting the second- and third-line regimens, virologic efficacy in the presence of ARV drug resistance frequently becomes the most significant factor.

Multiple studies have demonstrated that combination ART reduces HIV-associated morbidity and mortality and prevents development of acquired immunodeficiency syndrome (AIDS), as well as AIDS- and non-AIDS-related complications, in HIV-infected children and adults. ART has also been proven significant in the prevention of vertical (mother-to-child) and horizontal (through sex, injection drug use, blood products, etc.) transmission of HIV. Recently, the accumulated evidence that uncontrolled HIV infection has long-term negative consequences on health, and the improved toxicity profile of newer ARV drugs, has suggested the initiation of ART with higher baseline CD4 cell counts. Early initiation of ART in HIV-infected patients has also been shown to diminish the spread of HIV and decrease the rates of epidemic worldwide [9]. As the result of these findings, the current HIV treatment guidelines emphasize the need to initiate ART at early stages of the disease [6].

The response to ART is primarily measured through the qualitative evaluation of clinical symptoms (such as concomitant and opportunistic infections, nutritional status, development of neoplasms and other HIV-related co-morbidities) and quantitative laboratory parameters (primarily CD4 T cell count and HIV RNA viral load). Therapeutic drug monitoring (TDM) of ARV drugs is a laboratory tool for monitoring the efficacy and toxicity of ART. Current US and European ART guidelines recommend the use of ART TDM for the evaluation of non-adherence, multiple drug—food and drug—drug interactions, and treatment failure in the absence of viral resistance and non-adherence to medications [6, 10]. By identifying and adjusting ARV suboptimal exposures, TDM can help prevent the development of viral resistance. TDM could be instrumental in overcoming moderately decreased viral susceptibilities by allowing controlled increase of the ARV drugs' exposure [11]. Moreover, TDM may prevent suboptimal ARV drug concentrations which limit the response to ART even in the absence of HIV resistance [12].

TDM has been shown to be helpful in the management of drug—drug interactions among different ARV drugs, and between ARV drugs and other drug classes [13]. TDM is the only direct measurement of patient adherence to ART, which is a major challenge to the successful treatment of HIV disease [14, 15]. Finally, by identifying and reducing high ARV concentrations, TDM helps to prevent ART-related toxicities and toxicity-triggered non-adherence [16, 17]. It must be recognized, however, that TDM of ART has been investigated and applied primarily in the settings of developed countries, and significantly fewer data and a smaller number of clinical centers practicing TDM of ART exist in resource-limited settings.

THERAPEUTIC TARGETS OF THERAPEUTIC DRUG MONITORING (TDM) IN HIV-INFECTED PATIENTS

The goal of achieving the maximal suppression of viral replication and HIV-induced inflammation can be expressed as reaching maximal efficacy (EC) concentrations sufficient to reduce viral replication of the wild-type virus by at least 50% (EC_{50}) and up to 90% (EC_{90}) [18, 19]. Different pharmacokinetic (PK) targets, such as area under the concentration—time curve (AUC), peak plasma concentration (C_{max}) and trough plasma concentration (C_{min}), have been evaluated in relationship to the efficacy concentrations and toxicity of ARV drugs. As with many other pharmacologic agents, particularly antibacterial and antiviral drugs, the AUC plus C_{max} are mostly associated with the drug exposure/toxicity relationship, while AUC plus C_{min} are mostly linked to drug exposure/efficacy and sustained virologic suppression. Target concentrations for the exposure/effect relationship have been suggested for many ARV drugs, but targets for exposure/toxicity relationships have been established for only two drugs.

Failure to achieve and maintain inhibitory concentrations of ARV drugs may lead to continued replication of HIV and generation of ARV-resistant viral populations. Resistance to the NNRTIs has been shown to have a low plasma concentration threshold and is preventable by maintaining therapeutic concentrations of these drugs. Resistance to efavirenz and nevirapine is usually irreversible, regardless of drug exposure. The second-generation NNRTI etravirine has a different mechanism of developing viral resistance. However, no data have been published to date evaluating the dose adjustment in case of etravirine resistance. It is well recognized that PIs have higher plasma concentration threshold for the development of resistance than NNRTIs. In patients who develop resistance to PIs, increasing plasma PI concentrations has been shown to overcome resistance and improve virologic outcome [18, 20]. Therefore, combining the use of a virologic resistance test with TDM provides a mechanism for individualizing and optimizing the pharmacodynamics (PD) of PIs [21].

Currently, phenotypic viral resistance tests are used to calculate phenotypic inhibitory quotient (pIQ), virtual inhibitory quotient (vIQ) or normalized inhibitory quotient (nIQ), whereas genotypic tests are used to calculate a genotypic inhibitory quotient (gIQ) [22, 23]. In each instance the inhibitory quotient (IQ) represents the ratio of real time plasma trough concentration (C_{min}) to the various parameters of viral resistance or susceptibility to ARV drugs. For pIQ, the divisor in the ratio represents plasma concentration required to achieve 50% inhibition of HIV replication *in vitro* (IC_{50}). In case of vIQ, the C_{min} is divided by fold change in virtual IC_{50} derived from genotype and multiplied by the matched reference wild-type protein adjusted IC_{50}. The nIQ is calculated as a ratio of patient-specific IQ divided by a reference IQ calculated as the ratio of typical C_{min} for a given dose and wild-type viral IC_{50}, which normalizes the IQ target across ARV to the ratio of > 1. In addition to considering IC_{50} for the divisor, the target of IC_{90} has also been proposed for the pIQ, vIQ and nIQ estimates. Finally, gIQ is the ratio of the C_{min} to the number of ARV-specific resistance-associated mutations. Various IQ targets have been proposed for the majority of PIs [18, 22]. Pursuing IQ for a particular virus isolate based on genotypic and phenotypic sensitivity, however, is expensive, and requires highly specialized virologic and pharmacological expertise. To date, this practice has largely been reserved to the setting of developed countries.

Studies Conducted to Evaluate the Role of TDM in HIV-infected Patients

Over the past 10 years, several studies have examined the application of ARV TDM in the treatment of HIV. The 2003 Dutch ATHENA study included two clinical trials of TDM in treatment-naïve patients who started indinavir- or nelfinavir-based regimens. With only 20% of physicians responding to the dose adjustment recommendations by the study team, TDM of nelfinavir improved virologic suppression but did not significantly reduce toxicity, while dose adjustment for indinavir reduced toxicity but did not improve virologic suppression [24, 25]. TDM did prevent virologic failure and ART discontinuation due to ARV concentration-related toxicities.

Following the ATHENA study, the same group of investigators recently evaluated the adherence of Dutch medical providers to the national TDM guidelines [26]. Adherence to the 2005

TDM guidelines was 46.7% for the ART with lopinavir/ritonavir plus efavirenz or nevirapine; 9.5% for ART with efavirenz; and 58.5% for the use of nelfinavir during pregnancy. Clinics where an ARV assay was available locally and academic clinics were most likely to implement TDM. A higher baseline HIV viral load was also a significant predictor for performing TDM [26].

A Spanish study supporting the usefulness of TDM analyzed 3 years of clinical TDM requests in outpatient settings [27]. The most common reason for a TDM request was ARV drug toxicity (59%), followed by virologic failure (39%) and suspected drug interactions (2%). In 36% of drug-related toxicity cases TDM confirmed elevated ARV drug concentrations, whereas in 37% of patients with virologic failure TDM detected subtherapeutic concentrations of an ARV drug. Most importantly, TDM-based dose modification was done for 37% of the patients, resulting in 80% corrections of toxicities and virologic failure altogether [27].

In the Pharmacologic Optimizations of PIs and NNRTIs (POPIN) study conducted in England, a significant proportion of patients had ARV drug concentrations outside the therapeutic range [28]. No difference, however, was observed between study arms in the risk of reaching a study end-point, or between groups of patients with abnormal versus "therapeutic" ARV drug concentrations [28]. This finding was supported by a prospective randomized TDM study conducted in France (PharmAdapt), which failed to find a significant benefit of TDM versus standard care [29]. It is important to note that the study did not include a power analysis, and the concentrations obtained at Week 4 were used to adjust the dosage at Week 8, which may have been too late to prevent genotypic evaluation of the virus.

Another short-term (24-week) French study, GENOPHAR, also did not find a statistically significant benefit from routine TDM in patients who appeared to be adherent, but supported the incorporation of genetic susceptibility and expert advice as useful tools in the management of ART [30]. Integration of viral genotypic resistance and expert advice to optimize therapy based on the combination of the TDM and genotypic viral resistance was shown to be associated with higher antiviral efficacy [30, 31].

A randomized controlled trial of TDM in treatment-naïve and treatment-experienced patients in the US has demonstrated a significant proportion (39%) of patients with Week-2 ARV drugs concentrations outside the target range [32]. Most importantly, this proportion rose significantly over time, with the majority of patients (64%) having non-target exposure to ARV drugs at least once over 48 weeks. In this large multi-center open-label trial, TDM recommendations were well accepted and improved ARV drug exposure. Patients with ARV concentrations below TDM targets showed a trend toward worse virologic outcome [32]. In a smaller US trial of nIQ-guided TDM of PIs in treatment-experienced patients, no overall benefit of TDM was demonstrated [33]. TDM did, however, appear to be beneficial in Black and Hispanic patients, and in patients whose virus retained some susceptibility to the PIs. Finally, the use of a TDM-guided ART strategy in pregnancy and pediatrics demonstrated benefits in clinical reports and study protocols which incorporated the ARV dose adjustment into the study design when evaluating PK and PD of ART in children and pregnant women [34–41].

Overall, the inclusion of TDM into the ART studies has been limited by a lack of guaranteed access to laboratories with validated ARV drug measurement capabilities. The need for rapid adjustments in ARV dosage based on early clinical response and TDM is another significant barrier to inclusion of this approach into study design. Moreover, the limited PK and toxicity information at adjusted ARV doses and the high inter-subject variability of many ARV drugs limit the application of TDM in research and clinical practice [13, 18, 42]. Creation of a large TDM database may facilitate the establishment of expected concentration ranges for a variety of ARV drugs, including newer, more potent and less toxic agents. One example of such a database, the AIDS Clinical Trials Group (ACTG) Study 5145 (A5146), provided a valuable summary of specific issues in the TDM process that could be improved in the multicenter clinical trial [43]. These include collecting samples within the targeted sampling window, decreasing the time of sample shipment, increasing the number of patients in adherence counseling, and decreasing the time to the TDM-based dose adjustment.

CURRENT APPROACH TO TDM IN THE MANAGEMENT OF THERAPY IN HIV-INFECTED PATIENTS

A decade of experience with TDM management of HIV infection [44] has created a good sense of "dos and don'ts" in applying it as a clinical tool. TDM is incorporated in a number of HIV treatment guidelines, including Department of Health and Human Services (DHHS), British HIV Association (BHIVA), European AIDS Clinical Society (EACS) and other national guidelines [6, 10, 45, 46]. Furthermore, a specific guideline on performing TDM in the management of HIV was published in 2006, bringing together experience and advice from a number of expert clinical HIV pharmacologists involved in TDM of ARV drugs [47].

TDM in the management of ART is mostly utilized for PI and NNRTI classes of ARV drugs. For most of these drugs therapeutic ranges have been established, which is a key prerequisite for success when performing TDM [48]. TDM is not considered helpful for the NRTIs, since these ARV drugs undergo intracellular metabolism into active triphosphates. Assessment of intracellular triphosphate concentrations is extremely complicated, and is only used in research applications [49]. As new drugs from the new classes emerge, TDM may prove more useful, pending the results from ongoing studies.

The interpretation of laboratory results is paramount in TDM in HIV management. A TDM specialist with experience in HIV clinical pharmacology should be involved in the interpretation of pharmacokinetic results, clinical decision-making and follow-up TDM to investigate whether an intervention had the desired effect on drug levels. There are a number of specific recommendations to consider when planning TDM in the management of HIV [47]. A specimen submitted for TDM to the laboratory should be accompanied by a form with all the necessary information. At a minimum, the form should provide: the information linking the specimen to the patient; the indication for TDM; drug-specific information, including drug names, doses and frequency of administration; resistance mutation information in case of virologic failure; time of last intake of drugs; information on co-medications; and the exact date and time the sample was obtained.

TDM in Special Populations

TDM is frequently considered in special patient populations, including pregnant women, children, geriatric patients, and patients with abnormal body weight or hepatic impairment.

Clinical indications include drug–drug interactions, unconventional dosing options, side effects, virologic failure and non-adherence to the treatment regimen.

Pregnancy

Prevention of mother-to-child transmission of HIV during pregnancy is crucial, and requires efficient and timely establishment and/or maintenance of an undetectable viral load. Changes in PK parameters of ARV have been reported during pregnancy and may be due to physiological and metabolic changes, which are usually most evident during the third trimester [50]. These changes include, among others, longer gastric and intestinal transit time, decreased gastric secretions, nausea, and increased volume of distribution as a result of increased body water and fat. In addition, plasma protein concentrations may be decreased, resulting in increased amount of free (unbound) drug, although this ratio may be compensated by changes in drug metabolism. A recent report on a group of pregnant women using lopinavir called for the use of TDM during pregnancy [51]. In addition, PK studies during pregnancy have shown modest decreases in drug concentrations for lopinavir and nelfinavir [52, 53], while atazanavir and saquinavir [54–56] exposures remained at a stable level.

Pediatric and Adolescent Patients

HIV-infected pediatric and adolescent patients face a multitude of dose changes over the years of ART, but only limited dosing guidelines exist for pediatric use of many ARV drugs. Due to developmental differences in drug metabolism and disposition, PKs of ARV drugs are highly variable in younger children, which creates a risk of subtherapeutic ARV exposure. TDM is a useful tool in managing pediatric ART for establishing and guiding ARV drug dosing, and addressing adherence and abnormal drug concentrations [57, 58]. Unfortunately, due to the invasive nature of TDM and difficulties in conducting pediatric PK studies, there is a lack of specific TDM studies to confirm the role of HIV TDM in the management of HIV in the pediatric population. This complicates incorporation of ARV TDM into clinical practice and pediatric research.

Geriatric Patients

The impressive success of HIV treatment has allowed the HIV-infected population to grow older over the years, and geriatric patients present one of the next challenges for ART. Geriatric patients in general, and geriatric patients with HIV infection in particular, use multiple drugs, which results in polypharmacy and multiple drug–drug interactions. Furthermore, physiological and metabolic changes of aging may affect the PK of ARV drugs. Most of these effects are understudied and are not clear at this point. For these reasons, TDM of ART in the elderly may serve as a tool to support interventions based on the toxicity of drug–drug interactions. Unfortunately, even more than in pediatrics, data are missing both on PK differences and on the use of TDM in this population.

Patients with Hepatitis

Hepatic impairment, commonly observed among HIV-infected patients, is mainly caused by hepatitis B virus (HBV) and hepatitis C virus (HCV) infections, but can also be the result of alcohol abuse. Damage to the liver may result in changed hepatic architecture, reduced

CYP450 metabolism, changed blood flow (e.g., shunting) and changes in protein binding, all resulting in increased ARV drug levels, primarily for the PIs and NNRTIs [59]. Although not always clinically relevant on a population basis, these changes may result in significant ARV-associated toxicity that could be managed by reducing the drug dosage, based on the results of TDM.

Drug Interactions

Drug–drug interactions and unconventional drug dosages can occasionally be managed without evaluating drug exposure, if there is enough information about specific clinical situation and changes in management (e.g., substitution for another agent without interaction) provide the solution. Nevertheless, there are many cases when this information is missing or incomplete. In such cases, TDM makes it possible to evaluate the severity of the interactions in a specific patient. For instance, a recent case report included a previously unknown complex drug interaction involving darunavir/ritonavir administered concomitantly with etravirine and voriconazole [60]. This report described bidirectional interactions involving CYP enzymes (cytochrome P450 family of drug-metabolizing enzymes) and resulting in decreased darunavir exposure with increased etravirine and voriconazole exposure [60]. This case illustrates how TDM can be extremely useful in cases of drug interactions, both in patient management, and for the generation of new knowledge in the field.

Avoiding Drug Toxicity

In the case of ARV-associated toxicity and side effects, TDM may help to eliminate or decrease toxicity by reducing the drug dose in a controlled manner. An example is TDM-guided dose reduction of efavirenz to prevent toxicity-induced discontinuation [61]. For ritonavir-boosted atazanavir, a TDM-guided approach was reported to be successful in un-boosting patients to atazanavir alone, resulting in lower atazanavir exposure and reduced drug-associated toxicity, while preserving the therapeutic use of the drug [62].

Virologic Failure

In a situation of virologic failure without resistance and/or adherence barriers, TDM may help to explain a failure to achieve the anticipated therapeutic response. If detectable ARV drug concentrations are below the target value, this may allow ongoing viral replication. In this case an increase in the ARV drug dose is likely to resolve the problem, although it will be important to investigate the reason for the low drug exposure, such as high metabolizing capacity (e.g., pharmacogenetic cause) and/or absorption problems, or unknown/ unreported/unnoticed drug–drug or drug–food interaction. In cases of combinations of "no detectable" ARV drug and a high viral load, the most likely reason is an adherence issue. It should be remembered, however, that detectable ARV drug concentrations do not always reflect long-term adherence to ART outside of medical settings, and that adherence can be overestimated by TDM as a result of "white coat compliance" − that is, a patient taking the drug prior to a medical visit [63].

As new ARV drugs are developed and newer techniques become more widely available, the approach to TDM in the management of HIV is constantly changing [22, 64]. TDM of ART requires a multidisciplinary approach, including an infectious disease specialist, a clinical pharmacist, a TDM specialist, a virologist and in the future perhaps a geneticist, to fully integrate TDM into optimal clinical management of the individual HIV-infected patient. For successful application of TDM, sustained access to a laboratory capable of analyzing concentrations of ARV drugs is crucially important.

CURRENT METHODOLOGIES IN TDM OF ANTIRETROVIRAL DRUGS

A variety of methods can be used for the analysis of ARV drug concentrations, but to date no immunoassay is commercially available. As a result, laboratories usually develop their own assays. Published methods of measuring ARV drug concentrations include high-performance liquid chromatography (HPLC) coupled to ultraviolet (UV) detection [65–67], photo diode array (PDA) detection [68, 69] and mass spectrometry (MS) [70–72]. For the preparation of plasma samples for analysis, liquid–liquid extraction [65, 67], solid phase extraction [66, 68, 69] and protein precipitation [70–72] have been used successfully. Furthermore, techniques involving thin layer chromatography (TLC) [73] and enzyme immunoassays [74–76] including immuno-chromatographic strips [77] are used. These techniques have the advantage of using small sample aliquots and provide ease of use and low cost of operation (specifically for TLC). Nevertheless, these techniques are not widely available, and the gold standard of ARV drug measurement is HPLC coupled to tandem MS. Although this equipment is highly versatile and capable of simultaneously analyzing a wide range of different compounds, it is expensive. The alternative of HPLC coupled with single MS or UV detection can give equally good results at a considerably lower equipment cost.

Independently of the assay techniques used in the laboratory, it is imperative that personnel are highly trained and capable of developing the right assay within the limitations of the equipment and compounds analyzed. Furthermore, proper internal and external quality control measures must be developed. Internal quality controls must be used in each analytical batch to ensure that conditions are within normal ranges to avoid errors. External quality controls, or inter-laboratory quality control, can help to ensure that results from different laboratories are interchangeable. Programs such as the International Inter-Laboratory Quality Control Program for Measurement of Antiretroviral Drugs in Plasma (www.kkgt.nl) typically include one or more rounds of controls per year [44]. The samples include a range of HIV drugs for which TDM is routinely performed. The concentrations of the samples are blinded to avoid bias.

Different sample matrixes have been evaluated for the TDM of ARV drugs. Blood, however, is the most commonly used specimen, since it is routinely and frequently taken for monitoring therapeutic response with evaluations of CD4 lymphocytes and HIV RNA viral load. In general, blood for ARV TDM can be collected in different types of tubes containing an anticoagulant such as ethylene-diamine tetraacetic acid (EDTA) or lithium-heparin. It is important to recognize that most ARV assays are designed for use with a specific collection tube, and the choice of tube for TDM sample collection must be confirmed with the laboratory. In general, 5 mL blood samples will yield enough plasma to analyze all ARV drugs, even when sample work-up needs to be repeated for individual drugs. In specific cases, particularly involving infants and young children, where the quantity of blood drawn needs to be limited, the amount of the smallest sample collection needs to be established and verified with the laboratory performing the assay. The blood needs to be centrifuged at 3000 g for 5 minutes, allowing the plasma to be separated from the cells. Plasma must be separated and stored in a freezer. For storage of up to 1 month, maintaining the temperature at −20°C is usually sufficient [45, 78]. However, if longer storage is needed, information on the specific stability for the ARV drug of interest is required. Samples are usually shipped to the laboratory on dry ice to ensure that they remain frozen. Some laboratories, however, will allow shipment of ARV TDM samples at ambient temperature, as long as they arrive at the laboratory in less than 2 days [45]. The process of TDM sample collection, storage and shipment requires personnel, equipment and space, and can be relatively costly. For that reason, efforts have been made to look at other options of sample matrix and processing, including dried blood spots, saliva, and hair samples. All of these present challenges, but they share good economics and ease of use, and are suitable candidates for expanding TDM of ART to resource-limited settings.

Hair samples are inexpensive, easy and painless to obtain. Storage and shipment of hair samples is simple, as hairs are stable and lightweight. Analysis of ARV drugs (indinavir) in hair samples was first reported in 1998 [79], and later it was shown that indinavir hair concentrations were associated with virologic suppression [80]. Indinavir concentrations in hair also showed an association with virologic outcome, while plasma concentrations did not [81]. The difference in correlation with outcome between blood and hair samples for indinavir is most likely due to the high intra-individual variation in plasma concentrations of this PI. More recent studies in other PIs have shown an association between hair concentrations of atazanavir and lopinavir and virologic outcome [82–84]. This evidence suggests that concentrations of ARV drugs in hair may measure ARV drug exposure over time, and therefore may incorporate some measure of lasting adherence to ART. Hair analysis could have potential to develop into an ART adherence monitoring tool in HIV, in the same manner as hemoglobin A1C concentrations are used to assess adherence with insulin therapy in diabetes. However, due to the concomitant use of several ARV drugs and a high potential for drug–drug interactions, it is unclear if hair samples will play a reliable role in HIV TDM for timely dosage adjustments. Furthermore, the use of hair analysis in TDM may be limited, as no ARV target concentrations have been derived to date.

The advantages of saliva samples include cost-effectiveness, as well as an easy and non-invasive methodology which allows patients to collect samples. Eliminating the need for medical personnel makes it possible to use this method in remote areas. A special tube (Salivette® by Sartedt, Nümbrecht, Germany; available at www.sarstedt.com) has been used successfully to obtain reliable saliva samples. This tube contains a saliva collector impregnated with citric acid to stimulate saliva production, which some patients may find unpleasant to chew on for several minutes. Alternatively non-stimulated saliva can be used for ARV drug analysis [85]. A saliva sample needs to be stored and shipped in a similar fashion as a blood plasma sample. While believed to be related, ARV drug concentrations in blood plasma and saliva are not equivalent. Studies with nevirapine found that nevirapine saliva concentrations are about half of the concentration in blood plasma [73]. To date, reports are available for the salivary ARV concentrations of efavirenz [86], nevirapine [73, 85], indinavir [87, 88], saquinavir [89], lopinavir [90] and maraviroc [91]. Expanding the use of saliva specimens for TDM requires more specific studies and validation for specific ARV drugs.

In contrast to hair and saliva samples, dried blood spots (DBS) involve an invasive sampling technique. The amount of blood, however, is smaller than with a standard blood sample, and sample processing is significantly simpler, making it a feasible option for resource-limited settings. For these reasons, DBS are also currently being considered for HIV RNA viral load and HIV resistance testing [92]. Furthermore, the small amount of blood collected for DBS makes it a potentially more suitable sampling strategy for children [93, 94]. Drug stability in the DBS is generally good and allows for shipping at ambient temperatures. The fact that no shipment of fluids is involved significantly facilitates the shipping process. Current studies of DBS in TDM of ART include development of the assays for most PIs and other frequently used ARV drugs [94–97]. Although most DBS methods use HPLC tandem MS, other mass spectrometry techniques are used as well, including matrix-assisted laser desorption/ionization-triple quadrupole tandem mass spectrometry (MALDI-MS/MS) [94]. As with saliva samples, more studies are needed to establish the ratio of drug concentrations found in DBS compared to regular plasma samples before they can become part of routine TDM work.

Other studies of ARV drugs' PK include the analysis of seminal plasma in men [91, 98], cervicovaginal fluid [99, 100] and breast milk in women [101, 102], and cerebrospinal fluid in both [103–105]. These TDM evaluations are primarily used to evaluate the distribution of ARV drugs into sanctuary sites in clinical studies aimed at the prevention of HIV transmission, and are not currently used for TDM of ART in clinical settings.

TDM OF ANTIRETROVIRAL DRUGS BY CLASSES

Synergy and antagonism between different ARV drugs may affect concentrations of each and alter the desirable exposure. Ideally, the TDM of ART should involve monitoring of all ARV drugs simultaneously. The rationale for and feasibility of measuring concentrations of ARV drugs depend on the drug class.

Nucleoside Reverse Transcriptase Inhibitors

While several studies have established relationships between plasma concentrations of NRTIs and virologic and immunologic outcomes, it is not clear whether plasma concentrations of NRTIs reflect real-time NRTIs exposure, because these drugs are metabolized inside the cell to active triphosphate metabolites [106, 107]. A study by Fletcher *et al.* in adults has shown significant correlation between target zidovudine plasma average steady-state concentrations and improved and sustained virologic suppression [39, 106]. These findings were supported by a study in infants showing zidovudine plasma exposure correlation with virologic outcome [108]. In a later study by Fletcher *et al.*, however, zidovudine and lamivudine plasma concentrations were not correlated with outcome parameters. On the contrary, the relationship between higher intracellular drug levels and improved virologic and immunologic outcome for zidovudine and lamivudine has been shown to be significant, though this correlation was relatively weak [107]. Decreased plasma concentrations of emtricitabine and lamivudine in younger pediatric patients did not seem to affect the virologic outcome, though the long-term effects of subtherapeutic exposure on the development of emtricitabine/lamivudine resistance are unknown [109, 110]. Another pediatric study indicated a possible relationship between plasma tenofovir exposure (single dose and steady-state tenofovir AUC) and virologic outcome [111]. Because of insufficient evidence, currently the monitoring of the NRTIs plasma concentrations is considered to be of use in only a few scenarios for the evaluation and management of rare drug–drug interactions that affect plasma concentrations of NRTIs, and only in certain cases of adherence assessment [112]. The detection of intracellular triphosphate NRTIs metabolites is expensive and labor-intensive; therefore, it is limited to a few highly specialized centers for research purposes only.

Non-Nucleoside Reverse Transcriptase Inhibitors

For the NNRTIs, the relationship between plasma drug concentrations, efficacy and toxicity has been well established for the first-generation drugs efavirenz and nevirapine [113, 114]. Patients taking nevirapine and efavirenz are at a greater risk for developing resistance due to the low-threshold to high-level virologic resistance requiring single codon mutation (K103N, Y188L or V106M) in HIV than patients receiving the second-generation NNRTI etravirine, which requires multiple mutations. Long-term virologic suppression of HIV has been associated with maintenance of efficacy plasma trough concentrations above 1000 ng/mL for efavirenz (C_{24h}) and 3000 ng/mL for nevirapine (C_{12h}) in adult and pediatric patients with HIV infection [112, 113, 115]. For efavirenz samples obtained at 12 hours postdose the cut-off value of efficacy concentration of 3000 ng/mL has been suggested [116], but the plasma concentration of 1000 ng/mL between 8–20 hours post-dose is considered to be a target in the clinical studies [17].

Higher nevirapine plasma trough concentrations (> 4300 ng/mL) have been reported to be associated with reduced nevirapine resistance compared to the range of 3000–4300 ng/mL concentrations in adults [117], but the recommended target remains at 3000 ng/mL for nevirapine due to the concern for potential toxicity and sustained virologic suppression at a lower target in other studies. Toxicity studies for nevirapine have not shown a significant association between elevated liver enzymes and plasma concentrations of nevirapine, except for a single study suggesting an association of nevirapine C_{min} with maximal-fold increase in alanine aminotransferase (ALT) and gamma-glutamyl transpeptidase (GGT). No toxicity concentration threshold has been established for nevirapine [118–120]. For efavirenz-associated central nervous system toxicity (dizziness, insomnia, agitation, hallucinations and other symptoms) a relationship between efavirenz clinical symptoms and higher plasma concentrations (> 4000 ng/mL) has been established in adult and pediatric patients [17, 35, 121, 122]. No strong correlation has been identified between plasma concentrations of etravirine, the second-generation NNRTI, and efficacy and toxicity [123]. A median (range) plasma trough concentration of 275 ng/mL (81–2980 ng/mL) in adults has been reported in clinical trials by the manufacturer, but has not been set as a target concentration [123].

With a well-defined efficacy and toxicity range for the first-generation NNRTIs, TDM of NNRTIs has earned recognition in multiple clinical settings, both in adult and in pediatric practice. TDM for NNRTIs is most commonly used in the evaluation of adherence due to the long half-life ($t_{1/2}$) of nevirapine and efavirenz, and for the evaluation of treatment failure in the presence of adherence [116]. Moreover, the contribution of a patient's pharmacogenetic background to the efavirenz and nevirapine exposure makes TDM of these drugs highly relevant to clinical practice. Both drugs are metabolized by the cytochrome (CYP) 450 enzyme CYP2B6 with the known polymorphism in allele 516G > T affecting clearance of efavirenz and nevirapine [124, 125]. This polymorphism is highly prevalent in patients of African descent, who comprise the majority of HIV-infected patients worldwide [126, 127]. Several studies have reported an association between increased plasma efavirenz and nevirapine concentration and a related increase in virologic suppression and toxicity, as well as CYP2B6 polymorphism. A few studies have reported successful TDM-based efavirenz dose reduction in adult and pediatric patients with CYP2B6 G516T polymorphism [34, 40, 128–130]. Consideration is being given to the selective genotyping of populations with high prevalence of CYP2B6 polymorphism [131], and future studies need to be conducted to evaluate the validity of CYP2B6 genotype/TDM-based efavirenz dose adjustment.

Protease Inhibitors

In clinical practice, TDM is most widely used for PIs. An important aspect of measuring the concentrations of PIs in patients with HIV infection is related to multiple documented drug–drug and drug–food interactions of these ARV drugs. Because all PIs are substrate/inducers/inhibitors of multiple isoenzymes (CYP3A4, CYP1A2, CYP2C9 and CYP2C19), they have complex interactions with CYP450 enzymes. This may lead to drug–drug interactions with multiple agents used to treat complications of HIV and other significant co-morbidities/co-infections, such as tuberculosis, fungal infections, hyperlipidemia, etc. In addition to identifying the drug–drug interactions, and evaluation of adherence and treatment failure, TDM of PIs has also been used for dose optimization in cases of mild to moderate virologic resistance.

While the relationship between efficacy and plasma concentrations has been established for the majority of PIs, there are limited data on the exposure/toxicity relationship. Indinavir is the single PI with a well-defined therapeutic window. A high frequency of nephrolithiasis is associated with an indinavir $C_{max} > 10\,000$ ng/mL and $C_{min} > 500$ ng/mL in adults [132, 133]. Atazanavir-induced hyperbilirubinemia has been associated with increased atazanavir plasma trough concentrations in adults, but no concentration threshold for the development of this drug-induced toxicity has been established [134, 135].

Efficacy plasma trough concentrations for atazanavir, fosamprenavir, indinavir, lopinavir, nelfinavir, ritonavir and saquinavir have been reported in treatment-naïve adults in combination with low-dose boosting ritonavir. The exception is atazanavir, where the C_{min} values for both un-boosted and ritonavir-boosted atazanavir have been described [112] (Table 17.1). The efficacy target C_{min} for nelfinavir represents the concentration of its active metabolite M8 nelfinavir with antiviral capacity at an estimated 25% of circulating plasma concentrations of the drug [24, 136, 137]. The efficacy concentration for tipranavir has been derived in treatment-experienced patients with documented HIV resistance [138]. The data on the efficacy/exposure relationship for the newer PI darunavir are limited, and currently exist in the form of the median plasma C_{min} of 3300 ng/mL (range: 1255–7368 ng/mL) reported in clinical trials [139, 140] and the suggested efficacy target C_{min} of 2200 ng/mL [141].

TABLE 17.1 Concentration and GIQ-Based Cut-Off Values for Performing TDM of Antiretroviral Agents

Drug	Efficacy (C_{trough}) mg/L	Toxicity (mg/L)	GIQ (mg/L/mutation)	Mutations used in calculation of GIQ
Efavirenz	1.0 [17]	C_{trough} 4.0 [17]	N/A	N/A
Nevirapine	3.0 [114]	N/A	N/A	N/A
(Fos)amprenavir	0.40 [149]	N/A	0.30 [150]	L10I/R/V/F, L33F, M36I, 46I/L, I54M/L/T/V, I62V, L63P, A71I/L/V/T, G73A/C/F/T, V82A/F/S/T, I84V, L90M [150]
Atazanavir	0.15 [151]	N/A	0.10 [151]	K20M/R, L24I, D30N, V32I, L33F, M36I, M46I/L, I47V/A, G48V, I50V, I50L, F53L, I54V/L/A/M/T/S, L63P, A71V/T, G73S, V77I, V82A/F/T, I84/V, N88D/S, L90M [151]
Darunavir*	2.2 [141]	N/A	2.15 [142]	11I, 32I, 33F, 47V, 50V, 54L/M, 73S, 76V, 84V, 89V [142]
Indinavir	0.10 [152]	C_{max} 10.0 [132]	N/A	N/A
Lopinavir	1.0 [153]	N/A	0.90 [154]	10, 20, 24, 30, 32, 33, 36, 46, 47, 48, 50, 53, 54, 63, 71, 73, 77, 82, 84, 88, 90 [154]
Nelfinavir	0.80 [24]	N/A	N/A	N/A
Saquinavir	0.10 [155, 156]	N/A	0.04 [156]	10, 20, 24, 30, 32, 33, 36, 46, 47, 48, 50, 53, 54, 63, 71, 73, 77, 82, 84, 88, 90 [156]
Tipranavir	20.5 [157]	N/A	4.7 [157]	D30, V32, M36, M46, I47, G48, I50, I54, F53, V82, I84, N88 and L90 [157]

*For experienced patients.
N/A, not applicable/no data.

In addition to plasma efficacy concentrations, pIQ and gIQ have been generated for the majority of the PIs, except for indinavir, nelfinavir and ritonavir, (used solely as a boosting drug in PI-based therapy) [116, 142, 143] (Table 17.1). Because all PIs are strongly protein bound, the pIQ and vIQ have to use reference wild-type IC_{50} corrected for protein binding to account for the concentration/effect of the free (unbound) fraction of the PIs [18]. The interest in IQ-guided TDM of the PIs is primarily based on the mechanism of resistance development for this class of ARV drugs. Unlike the first-generation NNRTIs, which require a single codon mutation for a high level of virologic resistance, the large majority of the PIs (except for nelfinavir, and un-boosted atazanavir, amprenavir and saquinavir) require stepwise development of several mutations, usually four or more, for the emergence of HIV resistance. The PIs also have higher biological (*in vitro*) and clinical (*in vivo*) cut-offs for the IC_{50} concentrations than other ARV drugs. It is therefore feasible to potentially overcome *"partial"* resistance to the PIs by increasing the concentrations of the drugs to the higher range in relationship to viral resistance threshold. Several studies have addressed the issue of IQ TDM-guided increased dose therapy in PI-experienced patients [116, 142, 143]. Emergence of newer, more potent ARV in recent years has decreased the need for this intervention in developed countries.

However, it could be applied in resource-limited settings as the delivery of the ART scales up and resistance of HIV to ARV drugs increases worldwide. It is important, however, to recognize that while various IQs have been shown to correlate with virologic outcome, very few prospective studies have been conducted for the validation of cut-off values for the many commonly used PIs, and data on the strategy of IQ-based TDM remain limited.

Other Antiretroviral Drug Classes

TDM in HIV for other drug classes, including integrase inhibitors and entry inhibitors, is not well developed at this point. Recently published bioanalytical assays for use in HIV TDM include the integrase inhibitor raltegravir [144] and the CCR5 entry inhibitor maraviroc [78, 144], but no recommendation on target concentrations of these agents have been developed.

Raltegravir is the first, and so far the only, licensed integrase inhibitor, although more compounds in this drug class are in development [145]. The PK of raltegravir are highly variable both within and between patients [146]. With regards to a concentration–effect relationship, C_{min} has not been related to virologic outcome. However, when the average throughout the dosing interval was studied, a weak but positive relationship was found with antiviral effect. At this time it seems that the (partial) AUC may be useful for TDM of this drug, although no target value has been set [146]. Future research may elucidate the role TDM can play in HIV treatment with raltegravir.

Maraviroc is the only CCR5 antagonist currently on the market, and it has been not been included in TDM-driven research. The target value for TDM based on clinical results is not established. The current DHHS guidelines have a target value of 50 ng/mL, although this value was not obtained through a clinical TDM study [6]. Research is needed to define the clinical cut-off value before TDM can be meaningfully applied to maraviroc treatment in terms of virologic effect.

Pending the availability of target values for new ARV drugs for TDM for the purpose of viral efficacy or toxicity, TDM is useful in the scenarios of drug–drug interactions and adherence, and in special populations. In these cases, the individual TDM result can be compared to available population average values to estimate the case-attributable effects. Performing TDM in these cases will generate more knowledge about the new drug and its use, and may reveal important information possibly leading to case reports.

CHALLENGES IN PRACTICAL APPLICATION OF TDM IN MANAGING PATIENTS WITH HIV

The use of TDM in the management of HIV continues to face a number of challenges, mostly related to location-specific practical issues. Challenges include the cost of analysis and shipping, availability of HIV TDM laboratories, availability of expert interpretation, and multidisciplinary uptake of HIV TDM in clinical care.

The cost of analysis for a TDM sample ranges from around US$25–75 (www. hivpharmacology.com), and averages around US$50. This may involve measurement of one or more drugs, although some laboratories will impose an extra charge for each additional drug. Some TDM labs are government funded, such as in The Netherlands and the province of Quebec in Canada. Other programs receive funding from the pharmaceutical industry or the hospital where they are located, or a combination of these [45]. If a laboratory is successful in securing third-party funding it can offer TDM free of charge to the end-user, while laboratories without such funding will have to directly charge the end-user the TDM fee. In addition to the cost of analysis, the fact that the number of laboratories that provide HIV TDM is limited necessitates shipping costs. As discussed previously, shipments of TDM samples regularly involve dry ice and courier costs, which may add up to a significant amount. Although many hospitals have arrangements in place for shipment of clinical samples, there may be additional costs for small and private clinics. In order to minimize shipping costs, it is worthwhile to combine several samples in a single shipment, as well as to investigate options such as shipping at ambient temperature.

A recent report from the largest inter-laboratory HIV TDM quality control program listed 56 HIV TDM laboratories worldwide as of 2009 [44], which is probably the best estimate to date. In practice, this means that on a worldwide scale only a few HIV clinics have direct access to TDM of ART. According to the report, the majority of laboratories (44) are located in Europe, with a much smaller representation in North America (8) and just 4 in the rest of the world [44]. These differences may be due to the stronger uptake of TDM in national treatment guidelines in Europe as opposed to other parts of the world. Moreover, government-supported funding for TDM of ARV drugs is more readily available in European countries. The costs for set-up and operation of a HIV TDM program are significant, as can be illustrated by the establishment of the Quebec Antiretroviral Therapeutic Drug Monitoring Program. Start-up costs for equipment were around 500 000 CAD, while annual operating costs are around 350 000 CAD [45]. Setting up an HIV TDM service without an extensive financial investment may not be feasible, although it may be cheaper for an existing TDM laboratory to move into the field of HIV TDM.

Interpretation of results from the laboratory sample analysis is an integral part of the TDM service, and requires expertise in the field of HIV pharmacology and TDM. An HIV TDM specialist must be able to communicate with the multidisciplinary team that works with an HIV-infected patient. As the field of HIV therapeutics continues to develop rapidly, the HIV TDM specialist should constantly keep up to date with the new data. The HIV TDM specialist needs to become a part of routine clinical HIV patient care, most likely in the capacity of a clinical pharmacist specializing in HIV. However, currently there are no training programs on the TDM of ART. The best way to acquire such expertise is to work at an established ART TDM laboratory and clinical program, following baseline training in pharmacology and medicine.

A recent study looked at the adherence of clinicians to treatment guidelines involving TDM in The Netherlands [147]. Three clinical scenarios in which TDM was recommended in the Dutch HIV treatment guideline for 2005 were studied. TDM was recommended at the start of lopinavir/ritonavir in combination with efavirenz or nevirapine, at the start of efavirenz, and when using nelfinavir during pregnancy. The study reported that TDM was performed in 46.7%, 9.5% and 58.5% of the three scenarios, respectively. It found that patients in clinics with access to TDM and patients with a higher baseline viral load were more likely to receive TDM [147]. The study also indicated that clinicians are more likely to use TDM in the case of a drug–drug interaction (scenario one) or during pregnancy (scenario three) rather than a check-up (scenario two) without specific indication. Across the three scenarios, uptake of

TDM was less than half ($< 50\%$), which is relatively low considering that HIV TDM is reimbursed in The Netherlands and multiple HIV TDM laboratories are available [147].

Other studies investigated the adherence of clinicians to TDM recommendations — for example, changing the dosage of an ARV drug based on the TDM results. In the POPIN study [28] the adherence rate was 35%, and the percentage was even lower in the RADAR [148] and ATHENA [25] studies. The low adherence rates reflect the continued imbalance between the suggestions of a TDM specialist and their acceptance by an HIV clinician. Achievement of a consensus on the target therapeutic values and clinical interventions, and the development of the algorithms for their implementation, would increase the clinicians' adherence to ART TDM. For the successful application of ART TDM, the dose adjustment advice must be accepted and supported by all members of the clinical care team, including medical, nursing and other support staff. Improved patient education regarding the significance and potential benefits of TDM of ART drugs is an equally important prerequisite for the successful implementation of this tool in the clinical practice of ART.

CONCLUSION

Understanding the relationship between systemic exposure and drug responses is crucial for dose selection and design of strategies to optimize response to and tolerability of ART in HIV-infected patients. While large prospective studies on the effect of TDM on clinical and virologic outcomes are yet to be conducted, several smaller studies have suggested its usefulness in an array of clinical scenarios, including unexplained virologic failure, exposure-related toxicity, and management of treatment-experienced patients and special populations such as pregnant women, children and patients with impaired drug-absorbing and -metabolizing capacity. For the organic incorporation of TDM into clinical practice of ART, further development of the new and established therapeutic ranges of concentrations (including intracellular exposure) for all ARV drugs, and incorporation of the pharmacogenetic, pharmacokinetic and virologic profiles in the modeling of the therapeutic response to the ARV drugs, are necessary. Training of clinical HIV specialists with pharmacologic expertise, development of web-based resources to assist with interpretation of ARV concentrations, and guidance on dosing regimens are important components of expanding the use of TDM of ARV drugs worldwide. Finally, provision of funds supporting new ARV TDM technologies and laboratory access in resource-limited settings is required to allow for optimization of the individual outcome of ART in areas with availability of ARV drugs.

References

[1] Squires KE. An introduction to nucleoside and nucleotide analogues. Antivir Ther 2001;6(Suppl.3):1–14.

[2] Flexner C. HIV-protease inhibitors. N Engl J Med 1998;338(18):1281–92.

[3] Eggink D, Berkhout B, Sanders RW. Inhibition of HIV-1 by fusion inhibitors. Curr Pharm Des 2010;16(33):3716–28.

[4] Gulick RM, Lalezari J, Goodrich J, et al. Maraviroc for previously treated patients with R5 HIV-1 infection. N Engl J Med 2008;359(14):1429–41.

[5] Pendri A, Meanwell NA, Peese KM, Walker MA. New first and second generation inhibitors of human immunodeficiency virus-1 integrase. Expert Opin Ther Pat 2011;21(8):1173–89.

[6] Department of Health and Human Services. Guidelines for the Use of Antiretroviral Agents in HIV-Infected Adults and Adolescents. Available at, http://www.aidsinfor.nih.gov; 2010 (accessed 25 April 2011).

[7] Clumeck N, Pozniak A, Raffi F. European AIDS Clinical Society (EACS) guidelines for the clinical management and treatment of HIV-infected adults. HIV Med 2008;9(2):65–71.

[8] World Health Organization. AntiretroviralTtherapy for HIV Infection in Adults and Adolescents: Recommendations for a Public Health Approach. Geneva: WHO. Available at, http://whqlibdoc.who.int/publications; 2010 (accessed 1 May 2011).

[9] Cohen MS, Chen YQ, McCauley M, et al. Prevention of HIV-1 infection with early antiretroviral therapy. N Engl J Med 2011;365(6):493–505.

[10] European AIDS Clinical Society (EACS). Guidelines for the Clinical Management and Treatment of HIV-Infected Adults in Europe. Available at, http://www.eacs.eu/guide/index.htm; 2007 (accessed 25 May 2011).

[11] Haas DW. Can responses to antiretroviral therapy be improved by therapeutic drug monitoring? Clin Infect Dis 2006;42(8):1197–9.

[12] Hoefnagel JG, Koopmans PP, Burger DM, et al. Role of the inhibitory quotient in HIV therapy. Antivir Ther 2005;10(8):879–92.

[13] Boffito M, Acosta E, Burger D, et al. Therapeutic drug monitoring and drug–drug interactions involving antiretroviral drugs. Antivir Ther 2005;10(4):469–77.

[14] Gerber JG, Acosta EP. Therapeutic drug monitoring in the treatment of HIV-infection. J Clin Virol 2003;27(2):117–28.

[15] Hugen PW, Burger DM, Aarnoutse RE, et al. Therapeutic drug monitoring of HIV-protease inhibitors to assess noncompliance. Ther Drug Monit 2002;24(5):579–87.

[16] Kappelhoff BS, Crommentuyn KM, de Maat MM, et al. Practical guidelines to interpret plasma concentrations of antiretroviral drugs. Clin Pharmacokinet 2004;43(13):845–53.

[17] Marzolini C, Telenti A, Decosterd LA, et al. Efavirenz plasma levels can predict treatment failure and central nervous system side effects in HIV-1-infected patients. AIDS 2001;15(1):71–5.

[18] Acosta EP, Gerber JG. Position paper on therapeutic drug monitoring of antiretroviral agents. AIDS Res Hum Retroviruses 2002;18(12):825–34.

[19] Back DJ, Khoo SH, Gibbons SE, et al. Therapeutic drug monitoring of antiretrovirals in human immunodeficiency virus infection. Ther Drug Monit 2000;22(1):122–6.

[20] Boffito M, Acosta E, Burger D, et al. Current status and future prospects of therapeutic drug monitoring and applied clinical pharmacology in antiretroviral therapy. Antivir Ther 2005;10(3):375–92.

[21] Morse GD, Catanzaro LM, Acosta EP. Clinical pharmacodynamics of HIV-1 protease inhibitors: use of inhibitory quotients to optimise pharmacotherapy. Lancet Infect Dis 2006;6(4):215–25.

[22] la Porte C. Inhibitory quotient in HIV pharmacology. Curr Opin HIV AIDS 2008;3(3):283–7.

[23] Winston A, Hales G, Amin J, et al. The normalized inhibitory quotient of boosted protease inhibitors is predictive of viral load response in treatment-experienced HIV-1-infected individuals. AIDS 2005;19(13):1393–9.

[24] Burger DM, Hugen PW, Aarnoutse RE, et al. Treatment failure of nelfinavir-containing triple therapy can largely be explained by low nelfinavir plasma concentrations. Ther Drug Monit 2003;25(1):73–80.

[25] Burger D, Hugen P, Reiss P, et al. Therapeutic drug monitoring of nelfinavir and indinavir in treatment-naive HIV-1-infected individuals. AIDS 2003;17(8):1157–65.

[26] van Luin M, Wit FW, Smit C, et al. Adherence to HIV therapeutic drug monitoring guidelines in The Netherlands. Ther Drug Monit 33(1):32–39.

[27] Rendon A, Nunez M, Jimenez-Nacher I, et al. Clinical benefit of interventions driven by therapeutic drug monitoring. HIV Med 2005;6(5):360–5.

[28] Khoo SH, Lloyd J, Dalton M, et al. Pharmacologic optimization of protease inhibitors and nonnucleoside reverse transcriptase inhibitors (POPIN) – a randomized controlled trial of therapeutic drug monitoring and adherence support. J Acquir Immune Defic Syndr 2006;41(4):461–7.

[29] Clevenbergh P, Garraffo R, Durant J, Dellamonica P. PharmAdapt: a randomized prospective study to evaluate the benefit of therapeutic monitoring of protease inhibitors: 12 week results. AIDS 2002;16(17):2311–5.

[30] Bossi P, Peytavin G, Ait-Mohand H, et al. GENOPHAR: a randomized study of plasma drug measurements in association with genotypic resistance testing and expert advice to optimize therapy in patients failing antiretroviral therapy. HIV Med 2004;5(5):352–9.

[31] Acosta EP, King JR. Methods for integration of pharmacokinetic and phenotypic information in the treatment of infection with human immunodeficiency virus. Clin Infect Dis 2003;36(3):373–7.

[32] Best BM, Goicoechea M, Witt MD, et al. A randomized controlled trial of therapeutic drug monitoring in treatment-naive and -experienced HIV-1-infected patients. J Acquir Immune Defic Syndr 2007;46(4):433–42.

[33] Demeter LM, Jiang H, Mukherjee AL, et al. A randomized trial of therapeutic drug monitoring of protease inhibitors in antiretroviral-experienced, HIV-1-infected patients. AIDS 2009;23(3):357–68.

[34] Neely M, Jelliffe R. Practical therapeutic drug management in HIV-infected patients: use of population pharmacokinetic models supplemented by individualized Bayesian dose optimization. J Clin Pharmacol 2008;48(9):1081–91.

[35] Fletcher CV, Brundage RC, Fenton T, et al. Pharmacokinetics and pharmacodynamics of efavirenz and nelfinavir in HIV-infected children participating in an area-under-the-curve controlled trial. Clin Pharmacol Ther 2008;83(2):300–6.

[36] Rakhmanina NY, Capparelli EV, van den Anker JN. Personalized therapeutics: HIV treatment in adolescents. Clin Pharmacol Ther 2008;84(6):734–40.

[37] Panel on Antiretroviral Therapy and Medical Management of HIV-Infected Children. Guidelines for the Use of Antiretroviral Agents in Pediatric HIV Infection, pp. 1–219. Available at, http://aidsinfo.nih.gov/contentfiles/PediatricGuidelines.pdf; 2010 (accessed 1 May 2011).

[38] Rakhmanina N, van den Anker J, Baghdassarian A, et al. Population pharmacokinetics of lopinavir predict suboptimal therapeutic concentrations in treatment-experienced human immunodeficiency virus-infected children. Antimicrob Agents Chemother 2009;53(6):2532–8.

[39] Fletcher CV, Anderson PL, Kakuda TN, et al. Concentration-controlled compared with conventional antiretroviral therapy for HIV infection. AIDS 2002;16(4):551–60.

[40] Rakhmanina NY, van den Anker JN, Soldin SJ, et al. Can therapeutic drug monitoring improve pharmacotherapy of HIV infection in adolescents? Ther Drug Monit 2011;32(3):273–81.

[41] Caswell RJ, Phillips D, Chaponda M, et al. Utility of therapeutic drug monitoring in the management of HIV-infected pregnant women in receipt of lopinavir. Int J STD AIDS 2011;22(1):11–4.

[42] Nettles RE, Kieffer TL, Parsons T, et al. Marked intraindividual variability in antiretroviral concentrations may limit the utility of therapeutic drug monitoring. Clin Infect Dis 2006;42(8):1189–96.

[43] DiFrancesco R, Rosenkranz S, Mukherjee AL, et al. Quality assessment for therapeutic drug monitoring in AIDS Clinical Trials Group (ACTG 5146): a multicenter clinical trial. Ther Drug Monit 2010;32(4):458–66.

[44] Burger D, Teulen M, Eerland J, et al. The International Interlaboratory Quality Control Program for Measurement of Antiretroviral Drugs in Plasma: a global proficiency testing program. Ther Drug Monit 2011;33(2):239–43.

[45] Higgings N, Tseng A, Sheehan N, la Porte C. Antiretroviral therapeutic drug monitoring in Canada: Current status and recommendations for clinical practice. Can J Hosp Pharm 2009;62(6):500–9.

[46] British HIV Association. British HIV Association guidelines for the treatment of HIV-1-infected adults with antiretroviral therapy 2008. HIV Med 2008;9:563–608.

[47] la Porte CJL, Back DJ, Blaschke T, et al. Updated guidelines to perform therapeutic drug monitoring for antiretroviral agents. Rev Antivir Ther 2006;3:4–14.

[48] van Luin M, Kuks PF, Burger DM. Use of therapeutic drug monitoring in HIV disease. Curr Opin HIV AIDS 2008;3(3):266–71.

[49] Bazzoli C, Jullien V, Le Tiec C, et al. Intracellular pharmacokinetics of antiretroviral drugs in HIV-Infected patients, and their correlation with drug action. Clin Pharmacokinet 2010;49(1):17–45.

[50] van der Lugt J, Colbers A, Burger D. Clinical pharmacology of HIV protease inhibitors in pregnancy. Curr Opin HIV AIDS 2008;3(6):620–6.

[51] Lambert JS, Else LJ, Jackson V, et al. Therapeutic drug monitoring of lopinavir/ritonavir in pregnancy. HIV Med 2011;12(3):166–73.

[52] Stek AM, Mirochnick M, Capparelli E, et al. Reduced lopinavir exposure during pregnancy. AIDS 2006;20(15):1931–9.

[53] Read JS, Best BM, Stek AM, et al. Pharmacokinetics of new 625-mg nelfinavir formulation during pregnancy and postpartum. HIV Med 2008;9(10):875–82.

[54] Conradie F, Zorrilla C, Josipovic D, et al. Safety and exposure of once-daily ritonavir-boosted atazanavir in HIV-infected pregnant women. HIV Med 2011;12(9):570–9.

[55] Ripamonti D, Cattaneo D, Maggiolo F, et al. Atazanavir plus low-dose ritonavir in pregnancy: pharmacokinetics and placental transfer. AIDS 2007;21(18):2409—15.

[56] van der Lugt J, Colbers A, Molto J, et al. The pharmacokinetics, safety and efficacy of boosted saquinavir tablets in HIV type-1-infected pregnant women. Antivir Ther 2009;14(3):443—50.

[57] Burger DM. The role of therapeutic drug monitoring in pediatric HIV/AIDS. Ther Drug Monit 2010;32(3):269—72.

[58] Rakhmanina NY, van den Anker JN, Soldin SJ, et al. Can therapeutic drug monitoring improve pharmacotherapy of HIV infection in adolescents? Ther Drug Monit 2010;32(3):273—81.

[59] McCabe SM, Ma Q, Slish JC, et al. Antiretroviral therapy: pharmacokinetic considerations in patients with renal or hepatic impairment. Clin Pharmacokinet 2008;47(3):153—72.

[60] Toy J, Giguere P, Kravcik S, la Porte CJ. Drug interactions between voriconazole, darunavir/ritonavir and etravirine in an HIV-infected patient with Aspergillus pneumonia. AIDS 2011;25(4):541—2.

[61] van Luin M, Gras L, Richter C, et al. Efavirenz dose reduction is safe in patients with high plasma concentrations and may prevent efavirenz discontinuations. J Acquir Immune Defic Syndr 2009;52(2):240—5.

[62] Rodriguez-Novoa S, Morello J, Barreiro P, et al. Switch from ritonavir-boosted to unboosted atazanavir guided by therapeutic drug monitoring. AIDS Res Hum Retrovir 2008;24(6):821—5.

[63] Podsadecki TJ, Vrijens BC, Tousset EP, et al. "White coat compliance" limits the reliability of therapeutic drug monitoring in HIV-1-infected patients. HIV Clin Trials 2008;9(4):238—46.

[64] Figueroa SC, de Gatta MF, Garcia LH, et al. The convergence of therapeutic drug monitoring and pharmacogenetic testing to optimize efavirenz therapy. Ther Drug Monit 2010;32(5):579—85.

[65] Choi SO, Rezk NL, Kashuba AD. High-performance liquid chromatography assay for the determination of the HIV-protease inhibitor tipranavir in human plasma in combination with nine other antiretroviral medications. J Pharm Biomed Anal 2007;43(4):1562—7.

[66] Notari S, Bocedi A, Ippolito G, et al. Simultaneous determination of 16 anti-HIV drugs in human plasma by high-performance liquid chromatography. J Chromatogr B Analyt Technol Biomed Life Sci 2006;831(1—2):258—566.

[67] Weller DR, Brundage RC, Balfour Jr HH, Vezina HE. An isocratic liquid chromatography method for determining HIV non-nucleoside reverse transcriptase inhibitor and protease inhibitor concentrations in human plasma. J Chromatogr B Analyt Technol Biomed Life Sci 2007;848(2):369—73.

[68] D'Avolio A, Baietto L, Siccardi M, et al. An HPLC-PDA method for the simultaneous quantification of the HIV integrase inhibitor raltegravir, the new nonnucleoside reverse transcriptase inhibitor etravirine, and 11 other antiretroviral agents in the plasma of HIV-infected patients. Ther Drug Monit 2008;30(6):662—9.

[69] Elens L, Veriter S, Di Fazio V, et al. Quantification of 8 HIV-protease inhibitors and 2 nonnucleoside reverse transcriptase inhibitors by ultra-performance liquid chromatography with diode array detection. Clin Chem 2009;55(1):170—4.

[70] D'Avolio A, Siccardi M, Sciandra M, et al. HPLC-MS method for the simultaneous quantification of the new HIV protease inhibitor darunavir, and 11 other antiretroviral agents in plasma of HIV-infected patients. J Chromatogr B Analyt Technol Biomed Life Sci 2007;859(2):234—40.

[71] Dickinson L, Robinson L, Tjia J, et al. Simultaneous determination of HIV protease inhibitors amprenavir, atazanavir, indinavir, lopinavir, nelfinavir, ritonavir and saquinavir in human plasma by high-performance liquid chromatography-tandem mass spectrometry. J Chromatogr B Analyt Technol Biomed Life Sci 2005;829(1—2):82—90.

[72] ter Heine R, Alderden-Los CG, Rosing H, et al. Fast and simultaneous determination of darunavir and eleven other antiretroviral drugs for therapeutic drug monitoring: method development and validation for the determination of all currently approved HIV protease inhibitors and non-nucleoside reverse transcriptase inhibitors in human plasma by liquid chromatography coupled with electrospray ionization tandem mass spectrometry. Rapid Commun Mass Spectrom 2007;21(15):2505—14.

[73] L'Homme RF, Muro EP, Droste JA, et al. Therapeutic drug monitoring of nevirapine in resource-limited settings. Clin Infect Dis 2008;47(10):1339—44.

[74] Bastiani E, Benedetti F, Berti F, et al. Development and evaluation of an immunoassay for the monitoring of the anti-HIV drug amprenavir. J Immunol Methods 2007;325(1—2):35—41.

[75] Roucairol C, Azoulay S, Nevers MC, et al. Development of a competitive immunoassay for efavirenz: hapten design and validation studies. Anal Chim Acta 2007;589(1):142—9.

[76] Uglietti A, Ravasi G, Meroni V, et al. Nelfinavir + M8 plasma levels determined with an ELISA test in HIV infected patients with or without HCV and/or HBV coinfection: the VIRAKINETICS II study. Curr HIV Res 2009;7(3):293−301.

[77] Cressey TR, Nangola S, Tawon Y, et al. Immunochromatographic strip test for rapid detection of nevirapine in plasma samples from human immunodeficiency virus-infected patients. Antimicrob Agents Chemother 2007;51(9):3361−3.

[78] Else L, Watson V, Tjia J, et al. Validation of a rapid and sensitive high-performance liquid chromatography-tandem mass spectrometry (HPLC-MS/MS) assay for the simultaneous determination of existing and new antiretroviral compounds. J Chromatogr B Analyt Technol Biomed Life Sci 2010;878(19):1455−65.

[79] Bernard L, Peytavin G, Vuagnat A, et al. Indinavir concentrations in hair from patients receiving highly active antiretroviral therapy. Lancet 1998;352(9142):1757−8.

[80] Bernard L, Vuagnat A, Peytavin G, et al. Relationship between levels of indinavir in hair and virologic response to highly active antiretroviral therapy. Ann Intern Med 2002;137(8):656−9.

[81] Duval X, Peytavin G, Breton G, et al. Hair versus plasma concentrations as indicator of indinavir exposure in HIV-1-infected patients treated with indinavir/ritonavir combination. AIDS 2007;21(1):106−8.

[82] Gandhi M, Ameli N, Bacchetti P, et al. Atazanavir concentration in hair is the strongest predictor of outcomes on antiretroviral therapy. Clin Infect Dis 2011;52(10):1267−75.

[83] Gandhi M, Ameli N, Bacchetti P, et al. Protease inhibitor levels in hair strongly predict virologic response to treatment. AIDS 2009;23(4):471−8.

[84] van Zyl GU, van Mens TE, McIlleron H, et al. Low lopinavir plasma or hair concentrations explain second-line protease inhibitor failures in a resource-limited setting. J Acquir Immune Defic Syndr 2011;56(4):333−9.

[85] Rakhmanina NY, Capparelli EV, van den Anker JN, et al. Nevirapine concentration in nonstimulated saliva: an alternative to plasma sampling in children with human immunodeficiency virus infection. Ther Drug Monit 2007;29(1):110−7.

[86] Theron A, Cromarty D, Rheeders M, Viljoen M. Determination of salivary efavirenz by liquid chromatography coupled with tandem mass spectrometry. J Chromatogr B Analyt Technol Biomed Life Sci 2010;878(28):2886−90.

[87] Hugen PW, Burger DM, de Graaff M, et al. Saliva as a specimen for monitoring compliance but not for predicting plasma concentrations in patients with HIV treated with indinavir. Ther Drug Monit 2000;22(4):437−45.

[88] Wintergerst U, Kurowski M, Rolinski B, et al. Use of saliva specimens for monitoring indinavir therapy in human immunodeficiency virus-infected patients. Antimicrob Agents Chemother 2000;44(9):2572−4.

[89] Hoetelmans RM, van Essenberg M, Meenhorst PL, et al. Determination of saquinavir in human plasma, saliva, and cerebrospinal fluid by ion-pair high-performance liquid chromatography with ultraviolet detection. J Chromatogr B Biomed Sci Appl 1997;698(1−2):235−41.

[90] Estrela RC, Ribeiro FS, Seixas BV, Suarez-Kurtz G. Determination of lopinavir and ritonavir in blood plasma, seminal plasma, saliva and plasma ultra-filtrate by liquid chromatography/tandem mass spectrometry detection. Rapid Commun Mass Spectrom 2008;22(5):657−64.

[91] Brown KC, Patterson KB, Malone SA, et al. Single and multiple dose pharmacokinetics of maraviroc in saliva, semen, and rectal tissue of healthy HIV-negative men. J Infect Dis 2011;203(10):1484−90.

[92] Johannessen A. Dried blood spots in HIV monitoring: applications in resource-limited settings. Bioanalysis 2010;2(11):1893−908.

[93] Pandya HC, Spooner N, Mulla H. Dried blood spots, pharmacokinetic studies and better medicines for children. Bioanalysis 2011;3(7):779−86.

[94] Meesters RJ, van Kampen JJ, Reedijk ML, et al. Ultrafast and high-throughput mass spectrometric assay for therapeutic drug monitoring of antiretroviral drugs in pediatric HIV-1 infection applying dried blood spots. Anal Bioanal Chem 2010;398(1):319−28.

[95] Ter Heine R, Mulder JW, van Gorp EC, et al. Clinical evaluation of the determination of plasma concentrations of darunavir, etravirine, raltegravir and ritonavir in dried blood spot samples. Bioanalysis 2011;3(10):1093−7.

[96] Koal T, Burhenne H, Romling R, et al. Quantification of antiretroviral drugs in dried blood spot samples by means of liquid chromatography/tandem mass spectrometry. Rapid Commun Mass Spectrom 2005;19(21):2995−3001.

[97] Van Schooneveld T, Swindells S, Nelson SR, et al. Clinical evaluation of a dried blood spot assay for atazanavir. Antimicrob Agents Chemother 2010;54(10):4124−8.

[98] Lorello G, la Porte C, Pilon R, et al. Discordance in HIV-1 viral loads and antiretroviral drug concentrations comparing semen and blood plasma. HIV Med 2009;10:548–54.

[99] Dumond JB, Patterson KB, Pecha AL, et al. Maraviroc concentrates in the cervicovaginal fluid and vaginal tissue of HIV-negative women. J Acquir Immune Defic Syndr 2009;51(5):546–53.

[100] Talameh JA, Rezk NL, Kashuba AD. Quantifying the HIV-1 integrase inhibitor raltegravir in female genital tract secretions using high-performance liquid chromatography with ultraviolet detection. J Chromatogr B Analyt Technol Biomed Life Sci 2010;878(1):92–6.

[101] Rezk NL, White N, Bridges AS, et al. Studies on antiretroviral drug concentrations in breast milk: validation of a liquid chromatography-tandem mass spectrometric method for the determination of 7 anti-human immunodeficiency virus medications. Ther Drug Monit 2008;30(5):611–9.

[102] Mirochnick M, Thomas T, Capparelli E, et al. Antiretroviral concentrations in breast-feeding infants of mothers receiving highly active antiretroviral therapy. Antimicrob Agents Chemother 2009;53(3):1170–6.

[103] DiCenzo R, DiFrancesco R, Cruttenden K, et al. Lopinavir cerebrospinal fluid steady-state trough concentrations in HIV-infected adults. Ann Pharmacother 2009;43(12):1972–7.

[104] Yilmaz A, Gisslen M, Spudich S, et al. Raltegravir cerebrospinal fluid concentrations in HIV-1 infection. PLoS One 2009;4(9):e6877.

[105] Best BM, Koopmans PP, Letendre SL, et al. Efavirenz concentrations in CSF exceed IC50 for wild-type HIV. J Antimicrob Chemother 2011;66(2):354–7.

[106] Fletcher CV, Acosta EP, Henry K, et al. Concentration-controlled zidovudine therapy. Clin Pharmacol Ther 1998;64(3):331–8.

[107] Fletcher CV, Kawle SP, Kakuda TN, et al. Zidovudine triphosphate and lamivudine triphosphate concentration–response relationships in HIV-infected persons. AIDS 2000;14(14):2137–44.

[108] Capparelli EV, Englund JA, Connor JD, et al. Population pharmacokinetics and pharmacodynamics of zidovudine in HIV-infected infants and children. J Clin Pharmacol 2003;43(2):133–40.

[109] Burger DM, Verweel G, Rakhmanina N, et al. Age-dependent pharmacokinetics of lamivudine in HIV-infected children. Clin Pharmacol Ther 2007;81(4):517–20.

[110] Saez-Llorens X, Violari A, Ndiweni D, et al. Long-term safety and efficacy results of once-daily emtricitabine-based highly active antiretroviral therapy regimens in human immunodeficiency virus-infected pediatric subjects. Pediatrics 2008;121(4):e827–835.

[111] Hazra R, Gafni RI, Maldarelli F, et al. Tenofovir disoproxil fumarate and an optimized background regimen of antiretroviral agents as salvage therapy for pediatric HIV infection. Pediatrics 2005;116(6):e846–854.

[112] Back D, Gibbons S, Khoo S. An update on therapeutic drug monitoring for antiretroviral drugs. Ther Drug Monit 2006;28(3):468–73.

[113] Leth FV, Kappelhoff BS, Johnson D, et al. Pharmacokinetic parameters of nevirapine and efavirenz in relation to antiretroviral efficacy. AIDS Res Hum Retroviruses 2006;22(3):232–9.

[114] Duong M, Buisson M, Peytavin G, et al. Low trough plasma concentrations of nevirapine associated with virologic rebounds in HIV-infected patients who switched from protease inhibitors. Ann Pharmacother 2005;39(4):603–9.

[115] Gonzalez de Requena D, Gallego O, Corral A, et al. Higher efavirenz concentrations determine the response to viruses carrying non-nucleoside reverse transcriptase resistance mutations. AIDS 2004;18(15):2091–4.

[116] la Porte CJL, Back DJ, Blaschke T, et al. Updated guideline to perform therapeutic drug monitoring for antiretroviral agents. Rev Antivir Ther 2006;3:4–14.

[117] Gonzalez de Requena D, Bonora S, Garazzino S, et al. Nevirapine plasma exposure affects both durability of viral suppression and selection of nevirapine primary resistance mutations in a clinical setting. Antimicrob Agents Chemother 2005;49(9):3966–9.

[118] Almond LM, Boffito M, Hoggard PG, et al. The relationship between nevirapine plasma concentrations and abnormal liver function tests. AIDS Res Hum Retrovir 2004;20(7):716–22.

[119] De Requena DG, Jimenez-Nacher I, Soriano V. Changes in nevirapine plasma concentrations over time and its relationship with liver enzyme elevations. AIDS Res Hum Retrovir 2005;21(6):555–9.

[120] Kappelhoff BS, van Leth F, Robinson PA, et al. Are adverse events of nevirapine and efavirenz related to plasma concentrations? Antivir Ther 2005;10(4):489–98.

[121] Wintergerst U, Hoffmann F, Jansson A, et al. Antiviral efficacy, tolerability and pharmacokinetics of efavirenz in an unselected cohort of HIV-infected children. J Antimicrob Chemother 2008;61(6):1336–9.

[122] Ren Y, Nuttall JJ, Egbers C, et al. High prevalence of subtherapeutic plasma concentrations of efavirenz in children. J Acquir Immune Defic Syndr 2007;45(2):133—6.

[123] Kakuda TN, Wade JR, Snoeck E, et al. Pharmacokinetics and pharmacodynamics of the non-nucleoside reverse-transcriptase inhibitor etravirine in treatment-experienced HIV-1-infected patients. Clin Pharmacol Ther 88(5):695-703.

[124] Mahungu T, Smith C, Turner F, et al. Cytochrome P450 2B6 516G→T is associated with plasma concentrations of nevirapine at both 200 mg twice daily and 400 mg once daily in an ethnically diverse population. HIV Med 2009;10(5):310—7.

[125] Rotger M, Tegude H, Colombo S, et al. Predictive value of known and novel alleles of CYP2B6 for efavirenz plasma concentrations in HIV-infected individuals. Clin Pharmacol Ther 2007;81(4):557—66.

[126] Klein K, Lang T, Saussele T, et al. Genetic variability of CYP2B6 in populations of African and Asian origin: allele frequencies, novel functional variants, and possible implications for anti-HIV therapy with efavirenz. Pharmacogenet Genomics 2005;15(12):861—73.

[127] Nyakutira C, Roshammar D, Chigutsa E, et al. High prevalence of the CYP2B6 516G→T(*6) variant and effect on the population pharmacokinetics of efavirenz in HIV/AIDS outpatients in Zimbabwe. Eur J Clin Pharmacol 2008;64(4):357—65.

[128] Gatanaga H, Hayashida T, Tsuchiya K, et al. Successful efavirenz dose reduction in HIV type 1-infected individuals with cytochrome P450 2B6 *6 and *26. Clin Infect Dis 2007;45(9):1230—7.

[129] Mello AF, Buclin T, Decosterd LA, et al. Successful efavirenz dose reduction guided by therapeutic drug monitoring. Antivir Ther 16(2):189-197.

[130] Ribaudo HJ, Liu H, Schwab M, et al. Effect of CYP2B6, ABCB1, and CYP3A5 polymorphisms on efavirenz pharmacokinetics and treatment response: an AIDS Clinical Trials Group study. J Infect Dis 202(5):717—22.

[131] Rotger M, Telenti A. Optimizing efavirenz treatment: CYP2B6 genotyping or therapeutic drug monitoring? Eur J Clin Pharmacol 2008;64(4):335—6.

[132] Dieleman JP, Gyssens IC, van der Ende ME, et al. Urological complaints in relation to indinavir plasma concentrations in HIV-infected patients. AIDS 1999;13(4):473—8.

[133] Solas C, Basso S, Poizot-Martin I, et al. High indinavir C_{min} is associated with higher toxicity in patients on indinavir-ritonavir 800/100-mg twice-daily regimen. J Acquir Immune Defic Syndr 2002;29(4):374—7.

[134] Rodriguez Novoa S, Barreiro P, Rendon A, et al. Plasma levels of atazanavir and the risk of hyperbilirubinemia are predicted by the 3435C→T polymorphism at the multidrug resistance gene 1. Clin Infect Dis 2006;42(2):291—5.

[135] Molto J, Santos JR, Valle M, et al. Monitoring atazanavir concentrations with boosted or unboosted regimens in HIV-infected patients in routine clinical practice. Ther Drug Monit 2007;29(5):648—51.

[136] Crommentuyn KM, Scherpbier HJ, Kuijpers TW, et al. Population pharmacokinetics and pharmacodynamics of nelfinavir and its active metabolite M8 in HIV-1-infected children. Pediatr Infect Dis J 2006;25(6):538—43.

[137] Droste JA, Verweij-Van Wissen CP, Burger DM. Simultaneous determination of the HIV drugs indinavir, amprenavir, saquinavir, ritonavir, lopinavir, nelfinavir, the nelfinavir hydroxymetabolite M8, and nevirapine in human plasma by reversed-phase high-performance liquid chromatography. Ther Drug Monit 2003;25(3):393—9.

[138] Morello J, Gasco PG, Rodriguez-Novoa S, et al. Association between tipranavir plasma levels and virological response in HIV-infected patients. AIDS Res Hum Retrovir 2008;24(3):389—91.

[139] Back D, Sekar V, Hoetelmans RM. Darunavir: pharmacokinetics and drug interactions. Antivir Ther 2008;13(1):1—13.

[140] Sekar V, DeMeyer S, Vangeneugden T, et al. Pharmacokinetic/pharmacodynamic (PK/PD) analyses of TMC114 in the POWER 1 and POWER 2 trials in treatment-experienced HIV-infected patients. Paper presented at 13th Conference on Retroviruses and Opportunistic Infections; 5 February 2006, Denver, CO. Abstract J-121.

[141] Sekar V, Vanden Abeele C, Van Baelen B, et al. Pharmacokinetic/pharmacodynamic analyses of once-daily Darunavir in the ARTEMIS study. In: 9th International Workshop on Clinical Pharmacology of HIV Therapy. New Orleans, LA 2008.

[142] Gonzalez de Requena D, Bonora S, Cometto C, et al. Effect of Darunavir (DRV) genotypic inhibitory quotient (gIQ) on the virological response to DRV-containing salvage regimens at 24 weeks. In: 9th International Workshop on Clinical Pharmacology of HIV Therapy. New Orleans, LA 2008.

[143] Gonzalez de Requena D, Bonora S, Vigano O, et al. Comparative evaluation of seven resistance interpretation algorithms and their derived genotypic inhibitory quotients for the prediction of 48 week virological response to darunavir-based salvage regimens. J Antimicrob Chemother 66(1):192—200.

[144] Fayet A, Beguin A, Zanolari B, et al. A LC-tandem MS assay for the simultaneous measurement of new antiretroviral agents: raltegravir, maraviroc, darunavir, and etravirine. J Chromatogr B Analyt Technol Biomed Life Sci 2009;877(1—2):1057—69.

[145] Prada N, Markowitz M. Novel integrase inhibitors for HIV. Expert Opin Investig Drugs 2010;19(9):1087—98.

[146] Burger DM. Raltegravir: a review of its pharmacokinetics, pharmacology and clinical studies. Expert Opin Drug Metab Toxicol 2010;6(9):1151—60.

[147] van Luin M, Wit FW, Smit C, et al. Adherence to HIV therapeutic drug monitoring guidelines in The Netherlands. Ther Drug Monit 2011;33(1):32—9.

[148] Torti C, Quiros-Roldan E, Regazzi M, et al. A randomized controlled trial to evaluate antiretroviral salvage therapy guided by rules-based or phenotype-driven HIV-1 genotypic drug-resistance interpretation with or without concentration-controlled intervention: the Resistance and Dosage Adapted Regimens (RADAR) study. Clin Infect Dis 2005;40(12):1828—36.

[149] Sadler BM, Gillotin C, Lou Y, Stein DS. Pharmacokinetic and pharmacodynamic study of the human immunodeficiency virus protease inhibitor amprenavir after multiple oral dosing. Antimicrob Agents Chemother 2001;45(1):30—7.

[150] Pellegrin I, Coureau G, Morlat P, et al. Clinically relevant interpretation of genotype and pharmacokinetics parameters for resistance to fosamprenavir/ritonavir-based regimens in ART-experienced patients: Zephir Study. In: 13th Conference on Retroviruses and Opportunistic Infections, Denver, CO 2006.

[151] Gonzalez de Requena D, Bonora S, Cavechia I, et al. Atazanavir C_{trough} is associated with efficacy and safety at 24 weeks: definition of therapeutic range. In: 6th International Workshop on Clinical Pharmacology of HIV Therapy. Quebec, QC 2005.

[152] Burger DM, van Rossum AM, Hugen PW, et al. Pharmacokinetics of the protease inhibitor indinavir in human immunodeficiency virus type 1-infected children. Antimicrob Agents Chemother 2001;45(3):701—5.

[153] Ananworanich J, Kosalaraksa P, Hill A, et al. Pharmacokinetics and 24-week efficacy/safety of dual boosted saquinavir/lopinavir/ritonavir in nucleoside-pretreated children. Pediatr Infect Dis J 2005;24(10):874—9.

[154] Hoefnagel JG, van der Lee MJ, Koopmans PP, et al. The genotypic inhibitory quotient and the (cumulative) number of mutations predict the response to lopinavir therapy. AIDS 2006;20(7):1069—71.

[155] Fletcher CV, Jiang H, Brundage RC, et al. Sex-based differences in saquinavir pharmacology and virologic response in AIDS Clinical Trials Group Study 359. J Infect Dis 2004;189(7):1176—84.

[156] Valer L, de Mendoza C, Soriano V. Predictive value of drug levels, HIV genotyping, and the genotypic inhibitory quotient (GIQ) on response to saquinavir/ritonavir in antiretroviral-experienced HIV-infected patients. J Med Virol 2005;77(4):460—4.

[157] Naeger L, Zheng J and Struble K. (2006). Virologic response to tipranavir based on plasma concentration and baseline resistance parameters. In: 13th Conference on Retroviruses and Opportunistic Infections Denver, CO.

Drug Testing in Pain Management

Roger L. Bertholf[1], Gary M. Reisfield[2]

[1]Department of Pathology, University of Florida College of Medicine, Jacksonville, FL

[2]Department of Psychiatry, University of Florida College of Medicine, Gainesville, FL

INTRODUCTION

Urine drug testing (UDT) has a history that now spans nearly half a century, and has evolved from its primitive beginnings during the Vietnam War era to the multibillion dollar industry it is today. Widespread drug use by troops deployed during the late 1960s to Southeast Asia, where marijuana (and its more concentrated form, hashish) and heroin were widely available, was an affront to President Richard Nixon, whose platform for his 1972 campaign included, prominently, the "War on Drugs". Nixon ordered that military personnel would be subject to drug testing, the technology for which had been recently developed but was crude by contemporary standards. Nixon's order, however, created the first systematic program of UDT, and out of that initiative grew the subsequent programs for testing all federal employees in safety-sensitive positions, anyone working in safety-sensitive positions

Therapeutic Drug Monitoring: Newer Drugs and Biomarkers
DOI: 10.1016/B978-0-12-385467-4.00018-X

regulated by a federal agency, and workplace drug testing programs instituted by state governments and private employers.

Along the evolution toward widespread use of UDT were seminal events that accelerated its adoption. In 1981, the crash of a Marine EA-6B Prowler attempting to land on the flight deck of the USS Nimitz claimed the lives of 14 seamen and left 45 others with serious injuries, along with an estimated US$150 million of damage to aircraft and their carrier. The subsequent investigation of the incident revealed marijuana in urine, using autopsy specimens collected from several members of the flight deck crew, prompting President Reagan to issue a "Zero Tolerance" policy for drug use in the US military, with mandated urine drug testing of all service personnel. The program would soon be expanded to include non-military federal employees in safety-sensitive positions. The National Institute on Drug Abuse (NIDA), an agency of the National Institutes of Health (NIH), was given responsibility for oversight of the federal drug-free workplace program, and the Research Triangle Institute (RTI) in North Carolina was awarded a grant to develop a protocol for UDT of federal employees. The RTI recommendations were codified into federal law in 1987, when Public Law 100-71 established the specifications for laboratories performing UDT for federal employees. Included in the specifications was a program to certify laboratories that met the standards established in PL 100-71; it became known as "NIDA certification", and clinical laboratories had to meet NIDA standards, and be certified, before they could compete for contracts to perform UDT for federal employees.

The NIDA drug testing program established specifications for UDT of federal employees. These specifications included which drugs or metabolites would be included in the test panel (opiates, amphetamines, cocaine, marijuana and phencyclidine), the analytical methods that would be used for screening and confirmation (immunoassay and gas chromatography/ mass spectrometry, respectively), and the concentration thresholds that would be used for determining whether a result was positive or negative for a particular drug or metabolite. In addition, requirements were set for documenting the collection, custody and control, and storage of specimens, along with security precautions for laboratories performing UDT analysis. For the first time laboratories had a common set of specifications for UDT, which were quickly adopted by other agencies, both public and private, that sought to institute drug testing programs. The drug testing program of the federal government is currently regulated by the Substance Abuse and Mental Health Services Administration, SAMHSA, which was established in 1992 under the auspices of NIDA. One important division within SAMHSA is the Center for Behavioral Health Statistics and Quality (formerly the Office of Applied Statistics), which gathers data on the prevalence and patterns of drug use. SAMHSA has rule-making authority to codify the specifications for the federal drug-free workplace program.

The NIDA program was limited to federal employees until 1987, when a horrific accident occurred that prompted President Reagan to expand the drug-free workplace program to include anyone working in a job that is regulated by a federal agency. On 4 January 1987, Amtrak train 94 (the "Colonial"), en route from Washington's Union Station to Boston South Station, collided with a Conrail three-locomotive tandem being moved from Bayview Yard east of Baltimore, MD, to Enola Yard near Harrisburg, PA. The Conrail tandem, operated by an engineer and brakeman, crossed into the path of Amtrak 94, which was traveling at 120 miles per hour; when the Amtrak engineer saw the Conrail locomotives, he could only slow his train to what was estimated to be 108 mph before impact with the third locomotive in the Conrail tandem. Fourteen of the Amtrak passengers were killed, along with the engineer and a lounge car attendant.

The National Transportation Safety Board investigation of the accident found that several safety protocols had not been observed by the Conrail engineer prior to departure, and electronic warnings *en route* were ignored (some safety features had been disabled prior to departure). More significantly, the Conrail brakeman turned state's evidence and testified that he and the engineer had smoked marijuana together prior to their departure; urine drug tests after the accident confirmed that fact. Summarily, the federal Drug Free Workplace Program was expanded to include employees in positions involving public safety that are regulated by federal agencies, and the Department of Transportation was the principal focus.

There was another influence on the development of UDT. Testing Olympic athletes for use of performance enhancing drugs (PEDs) began in the 1960s, and has evolved into a sophisticated program that includes laboratory certification, precise analytical specifications, and innovative approaches to detecting subtle changes that occur in urinary excretion of hormones and their metabolites when an athlete uses exogenous anabolic compounds in an effort to enhance strength, speed and endurance. The list of substances banned by the International Olympic Committee (IOC) is extensive, and the laboratory requirements for UDT in sports are correspondingly demanding. Some of the IOC specifications for testing athletes have been adopted by college and professional sports, and many laboratories have tailored UDT services to that market. There are considerable differences, however, between UDT for detecting illicit drug use by employees, and testing athletes for use of PEDs. Drug-free workplace UDT programs are limited in scope, and observe standardized protocols with regard to screening, confirmation, and quantitative thresholds. Sports testing, on the other hand, has a nearly limitless scope and continually has to adapt to changes in the pattern of PED use by athletes, as well as the emergence of new PEDs.

As technology has advanced, making available increasingly sophisticated analytical instruments for detecting and measuring drugs and metabolites in urine, sports and forensic drug testing have rapidly diverged. Sports testing laboratories face the continually changing requirements for detecting PEDs, whereas forensic drug testing laboratories only have to comply with a relatively narrow set of standards that are infrequently modified. In that regard, UDT in sports provides a much better model for the application of these laboratory methods to monitoring patients in pain management or substance abuse recovery programs than does UDT in workplace drug monitoring, because the focus of clinical UDT varies widely depending on the circumstances that prompt its use. In clinical settings, UDT is used both for verification of proper use of prescribed drugs and for detection of unauthorized drug use.

USE OF OPIOIDS IN PAIN MANAGEMENT

Chronic pain is the most common reason for seeking medical care in the United States; it is estimated that one-third of the population is affected [1]. Among the many therapeutic options for managing chronic pain, opioid analgesics are a frequent choice due to their effectiveness, relatively low cost, and comparatively low incidence of serious side effects. Opiates are isolated from the latex encased in the seed pods of the opium poppy, and include morphine and codeine, along with several non-analgesic alkaloids. Semi-synthetic pharmaceutical derivatives of the opium alkaloids ("opioids") include buprenorphine, hydromorphone, hydrocodone, oxymorphone and oxycodone. Heroin is a derivative of morphine (diacetylmorphine) that is used therapeutically in some countries, but is illegal in the US. Although opioids comprise the most effective analgesics available for pain management they also have a high potential for abuse, and recent data indicate that opioids now rival marijuana as the drug of choice for first time illegal drug users [2]. The prevalence of opioid-use disorders in chronic pain patients receiving opioid therapy is difficult to determine. In several recent studies, 25–50% of chronic pain patients exhibited aberrant drug-related behaviors [3–7]. The proportion with diagnosable addiction has been estimated to be between 3% and 19% [8].

Reflecting the movement toward more aggressive management of chronic pain, the prescribing of opioid analgesics has increased exponentially in recent years. Between 1997 and 2006, a decade during which the US population increased by 12%, retail sales of methadone, oxycodone, fentanyl, hydromorphone and hydrocodone increased by 1177%, 732%, 479%, 274% and 244%, respectively [9]. The liberalization of opioid prescribing as been associated with devastating unintended consequences. For example:

- In 2008, 2.2 million Americans initiated non-medical use of prescription opioids, equaling the number of those initiating use of cannabis and exceeding the numbers of those initiating use of any other class of illicit or prescription drug [2].
- In 2008, 1.24 million Americans met DSM-IV criteria for dependence (addiction) to prescription opioids, eclipsing the numbers of those addicted to heroin (253 000) and cocaine (959 000) combined [2]. Moreover, opioid-related admissions to drug treatment centers more than quadrupled – from 16 605 to 74 750 – during the decade from 1996 to 2006, while admissions for alcohol and cocaine dropped, and admissions for heroin remained flat [10].
- Emergency room visits related to the non-medical use of prescription opioids more than doubled – from 144 600 to 305 900 – during the 5-year period from 2004 to 2008 [11].
- Unintentional overdose deaths involving prescription opioids have increased dramatically in recent years. In Florida, from 2008 to 2009, deaths attributed to oxycodone, fentanyl and methadone increased by 26%, 17% and 5%, respectively, while deaths due to heroin and cocaine decreased by 16% and 18%, respectively [12].
- The societal cost of prescription opioid abuse and addiction is enormous, and was recently estimated at US$54.5 billion annually [13].

The sources of opioids destined for non-medical use are informative. According to SAMHSA's National Survey on Drug Use and Health (NSDUH), 56% of those endorsing non-medical use of opioids indicated that they obtained their most recent opioids from a friend or relative for free; 9% stated that they purchased the medication from a friend or relative; 5% stated that they stole the medication from a friend or relative; and 18% stated that they procured a prescription from one physician. Of those respondents who obtained opioids from a friend or relative for free, 82% indicated that the friend or relative obtained the prescription from a single physician [2]. Thus, according to this government data source, most opioids destined for non-medical use originate from valid prescriptions from physicians. Physicians thus face the often difficult task of distinguishing between the (non-mutually exclusive) groups of patients who have a legitimate need for opioid analgesia, and those who are seeking opioids for non-medical abuse purposes. Since it has been clearly demonstrated that self-reported drug use and behavioral observations are unreliable indicators of drug abuse, clinicians have increasingly used UDT to verify adherence to prescription instructions, detect unauthorized use of other prescription medications and reveal use of illegal drugs. There is encouraging evidence that UDT in pain management decreases illicit drug use by patients [14]; however, at the same time, the number of deaths from opioid overdose has nearly quadrupled over the past decade, despite greater surveillance by UDT [15]. Opioid abuse has increased by a similar proportion [16].

Although UDT is now widely used in monitoring patients being treated for chronic pain, as well in substance abuse recovery programs, questions have been raised over whether the UDT is being ordered appropriately and the results interpreted correctly. Surveys of family physicians participating in pain management symposia revealed a troubling lack of knowledge about drug testing sensitivity and specificity, drug metabolism, and passive exposure [17]. For example, only 29% of the physicians surveyed were aware that codeine is metabolized to morphine, 22% knew that eating poppy seeds can produce sufficient urinary morphine concentrations to result in a positive drug test, and 10% would taper or discontinue opioid therapy in a patient who tested negative for the prescribed drug, without verifying that the assay being used in the laboratory (or at the point-of-care) was capable of detecting that specific opioid. Disturbingly, 10% of physicians responding to the survey reported that they would notify law enforcement in the latter scenario.

ANALYTICAL METHODS FOR DRUG TESTING

Laboratory methods for detecting drug use include immunoassays, which are designed to have high sensitivity but may cross-react with structurally similar (and, occasionally, structurally dissimilar) compounds, and confirmatory methods that are highly specific but, in general, more expensive and technically demanding. Among the immunoassays available for UDT are methods adapted for rapid, on-site (point of care) use, and assays designed for use on automated chemistry analyzers. Most confirmatory methods involve mass spectrometry, but there are several permutations of inlet and mass filter options. Historically gas chromatography was most often used to separate drugs prior to mass spectrometric identification, but often required the synthesis of volatile derivatives to produce satisfactory chromatographic results. The development of thermospray and electrospray techniques for interfacing non-volatile chromatographic methods, such as liquid–liquid chromatography, enhanced the popularity of LC/MS methods, which often could be applied to specimens with minimal pre-analytical manipulation. The relative merits and limitations of measuring drugs in different body fluids — blood, urine, breath, saliva (or "oral fluid") — nails and hair are beyond the scope of this chapter, and have been reviewed elsewhere [18].

General Considerations in Immunoassays

The basic design of the competitive, heterogeneous immunoassay was described by Rosalind Yalow and Solomon Bersen in a landmark paper published in 1960 [19] in which they relate a method for measuring insulin in blood using radioisotopically-labeled bovine insulin and polyclonal anti-insulin antibodies generated in guinea pigs. The vast potential for radioimmunoassay (RIA) was immediately apparent, and the technique was applied to many hormones, vitamins and enzymes previously too difficult to detect at their low concentrations in blood. Yalow was awarded the 1977 Nobel Prize in Physiology and Medicine for the discovery of RIA, but Bersen died in 1972 and therefore could not share the award, since the Nobel Prize is not awarded posthumously.

Although immunochemical methods all share a common denominator — use of an antibody to recognize and bond with a specific analyte — there are several analytical strategies that have evolved from this approach. Some immunoassays rely on a ligand modified with a label to measure its concentration in the antibody-bound or free fraction. Radioactive labels gave rise to RIA, and radioisotopes are easily attached to organic molecules, preserve the structural integrity of proteins, and can be detected at very low concentrations. However, the instability of radioisotopes — shelf-life is limited — and the health risks of exposure to radioactivity have made radioisotopes an unpopular choice for detection labels, and they have been mostly replaced by enzymes and chemiluminescent probes in label-based immunoassays. In label-based methods, either the ligand or the antibody may carry the label. Other immunoassays do not involve a label, but instead depend on the formation of large cross-linked antibody—antigen complexes that alter the light-scattering properties of the solution.

Immunoassays are classified as competitive or non-competitive, depending on whether the antigen or antibody, respectively, is present in excess. In addition, immunoassays are heterogeneous if their design requires separation of the bound and free antigen fractions before measurement of the incorporated label, or homogeneous if separation is not required for distinguishing between bound and free antigen fractions. Heterogeneous immunoassays can be either competitive or non-competitive, whereas virtually all homogeneous immunoassays are competitive. Homogeneous immunoassays are more easily adapted to automated chemistry analyzers because the physical separation of the bound and free fractions is not required. Homogeneous methods typically involve an antigen labeled with a probe that has a unique physical or chemical property that changes when the antigen is bound to antibody. A generic scheme for a homogeneous immunoassay is illustrated in Fig. 18.1, and this is the most common configuration of automated methods for detecting drugs. Point-of-care assays ordinarily are heterogeneous, and may be classified as competitive or non-competitive, depending on the design; some have features of both. Finally, immunoassays may be one-site, which involves a single antigenic site against which a mixture of polyclonal antibodies or a monoclonal antibody is directed, or two-site, where the analyte has two distinct antigenic sites with antibodies directed at each. Immunoassays for detecting drugs typically are one-site, since drug (and drug metabolite) molecules ordinarily are too small to accommodate two antibodies. Two-site methods are often called "sandwich" methods, since the analyte is sandwiched between two antibodies.

A vast array of immunoassays has been developed around these basic principles — competitive versus non-competitive, homogeneous versus heterogeneous, one-site versus two-site — but for practical reasons only a few have been applied to detecting drugs or drug metabolites.

Immunoassays used in Point-of-Care Drug Testing

The technology for most point-of-care drug immunoassays is called lateral flow immunoassay or immuno-chromatographic assay. Although both terms appear in the literature, they

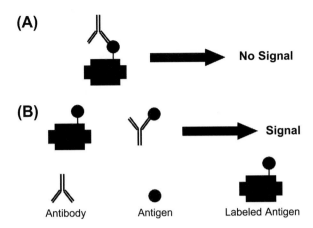

FIGURE 18.1 A general scheme for homogeneous immunoassay. The antigen is covalently attached to a label (or signal molecule), the properties of which are altered when an antibody is bound to the labeled antigen (A). Free antigen displaces the labeled antigen from the antibody (B). Typically, displacement of the labeled antigen results in a detectable signal that is proportional to free antigen concentration, but in some homogeneous immunoassays, the signal is inversely proportional to free antigen concentration. *From [34]: Reisfield, G. M., Salazar, E., and Bertholf, R. L. (2007). Rational use and interpretation of urine drug testing in chronic opioid therapy. Annals of Clinical and Laboratory Science 37(4), 301–314. Reprinted with permission.*

refer to the same basic approach, which is the capture of labeled antigens or antibodies moving across a solid support to which antibodies or antigens have been covalently linked. In one scheme, labeled antibodies bind to immobilized antigen as they pass across the test region unless they have been saturated with free antigens in the specimen applied to the sample pad that promotes capillary flow along the device membrane (Fig. 18.2). Another approach uses immobilized antibodies to capture labeled antigens that have been displaced from soluble antibodies by endogenous unlabeled antigens in the specimen (Fig. 18.3). A third strategy involves antigens covalently bound to gold particles, mixed with the specimen and free antibodies [20]. In the absence of free antigen, the antigens bound to the gold particles are obscured by antibodies, and cannot be captured by antibodies immobilized in the detection regions of the membrane (Fig. 18.4).

Lateral flow immunoassays are difficult to classify precisely. They incorporate elements of competitive immunoassays, in that the antigen usually is present in excess, but only when the free antigen exceeds a threshold concentration. They are mostly heterogeneous, since bound and free fractions are separated, but the separation step is subtle and integral to the lateral flow design. Both one-site and two-site lateral flow immunoassay designs have been developed.

Point-of-care drug testing devices are attractive to clinicians because they offer rapid results and allow contemporaneous discussion with patients with regard to unexpected test results. Many clinicians will recognize that unexpected positive or negative results, particularly when they conflict with a patient's self-reported drug use, should be confirmed by a more specific laboratory method, but some may not. Several thousand commercially available point-of-care urine drug testing devices have been granted a waiver from CLIA requirements by the FDA [21]. One of the conditions under which the FDA grants a waiver to an *in vitro* diagnostic test is that the manufacturer's instructions for its use must be

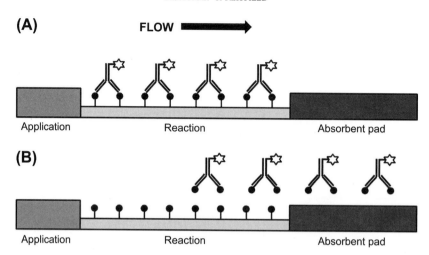

FIGURE 18.2   One design of a lateral flow immunoassay involves the flow of reagent across a reaction bed that can capture labeled antibodies on immobilized antigen (A). In the presence of free antigen, binding sites on the labeled antibodies are saturated and do not react with the immobilized antigen; the label ends up in the absorbent pad at the end of the device (B). The positive or negative result is determined by whether there is signal in the reaction region; the presence of signal is a negative result, whereas the absence of signal is a positive result.

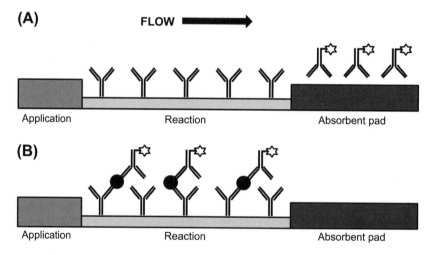

FIGURE 18.3   A two-site, non-competitive approach to lateral flow immunoassay involves an immobilized antibody and a soluble labeled antibody. In the absence of antigen to bridge the two antibodies, the label does not appear in the reaction region (A). When antigen is present, the antibodies can form a link with antigen, and signal appears in the reaction region (B). In this scheme, a signal is associated with a positive result.

followed, and product inserts for waived UDT devices usually include a statement variously recommending or requiring confirmation of positive results. In the context of pain management, however, a negative result may be as potentially important as a positive result if it is interpreted to mean that a patient has been non-adherent and may be misusing or diverting

(A)

FLOW ➡

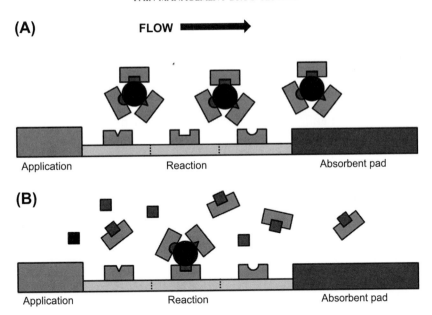

Application   Reaction   Absorbent pad

(B)

Application   Reaction   Absorbent pad

FIGURE 18.4 In the Ascend™ multi-analyte immunoassay technique (Triage™, Biosite Diagnostics, Roselle, CA), the specimen, antibodies, and colloidal gold-drug conjugates are applied to the lateral flow device. In the absence of free drug in the specimen, the antibodies react with the gold-conjugated drugs, preventing their reaction with the immobilized antibodies in the reaction region (A). In the presence of a free drug in the specimen, the antibodies against that drug are saturated, exposing the conjugated drug, which therefore is captured in the reaction region (B). A positive result is indicated by the presence of a red bar in the reaction region for a specific drug.

prescribed opioids. As noted in an earlier section of this chapter, clinicians' understanding of the sensitivities and specificities of immunoassays often is limited.

Homogeneous Immunoassays

The most popular methods for automated UDT are homogeneous immunoassays, several of which are adaptable to a variety of commercially available chemistry analyzers. Homogeneous immunoassays are relatively simple to automate, since separation of the bound and free fractions is not required. Depending on the type of label used, the detection system may involve spectrophotometry, turbidimetry, or fluorescence polarization (FPIA). With the exception of FPIA, which was a popular technology throughout the 1980s and 1990s but is no longer available, automated UDT screening methods are mostly enzyme immunoassays. Three homogeneous immunoassays dominate the market for automated UDT: enzyme-multiplied immunoassay (EMIT; Siemens Healthcare, Deerfield, IL), cloned enzyme donor immunoassay (CEDIA; Thermo Scientific, Waltham, MA), and kinetic interaction of microparticles in solution (KIMS; Roche Diagnostics, Indianapolis, IN).

ENZYME-MULTIPLIED IMMUNOASSAY TECHNIQUE (EMIT)

The patent for the EMIT homogeneous immunoassay was granted to Syva Corporation, a joint venture between Varian Associates and Syntex Corporation (Palo Alto, CA), in 1971.

In 1995, Behring Diagnostics, a newly spun subsidiary of Dade International, purchased Syva Corporation, and marketed the EMIT products under that corporate name until 1997, when the corporations merged to become Dade Behring. Recently, Siemens acquired Dade Behring and now it is a part of Siemens Diagnostics. In the design of an EMIT for detecting a drug or metabolite, the antigen is covalently attached to an enzyme, glucose-6-phosphate dehydrogenase (G-6-PD), in a position near the substrate binding site. When antibodies against the drug bind to the enzyme-linked antigen, the active site is sterically hindered by the antibody, and enzyme activity is inhibited. However, if free antigens are present in the specimen they will compete for the antibody, displacing the enzyme-linked antigen and restoring enzyme activity. Therefore, the enzyme activity is directly proportional to the amount of free antigen (drug or metabolite) in the specimen. The EMIT is an extraordinarily versatile assay because it only requires spectrophotometric measurement of the G-6-PD cofactor nicotinamide adenine dinucleotide phosphate ($NADP^+$), which can be distinguished from its reduced form (NADPH) by its UV absorption at 340 nm. Hence, an increase in absorption at 340 nm occurs as $NADP^+$ is reduced when glucose-6-phosphate is enzymatically oxidized to 6-phosphogluconate.

CLONED ENZYME DONOR IMMUNOASSAY (CEDIA)

Like the Syva Corporation, Microgenics Corporation (Concord, CA) was founded in 1981 in the biotechnology seedbed that evolved in northern California throughout the 1970s and 1980s. Microgenics used recombinant DNA technology to develop a homogeneous immunoassay based on cloned fragments of the β-galactosidase enzyme that spontaneously associated in solution to reconstitute the active enzyme. The CEDIA method was patented in 1985. CEDIA reagents currently are marketed through a partnership with Thermo Fisher Scientific. In the CEDIA method, the β-galactosidase enzyme is cloned in two sections, a smaller fragment (the "donor") and a larger fragment ("acceptor"). In solution, the donor and acceptor fragments spontaneously associate to form a monomer, and four monomeric units aggregate to form the active tetrameric enzyme. The antigen is covalently attached to the acceptor fragment such that when antibody is attached to the bound antigen, association with the donor fragment is sterically hindered. Free antigens in the specimen compete with the acceptor-labeled antigen for antibodies, releasing the acceptor fragments for association with donor fragments and resulting in reconstitution of enzyme activity. Therefore, β-galactosidase activity is proportional to free antigen (drug or metabolite) concentration, and is measured spectrophotometrically by enzymatic conversion of dye-labeled substrate. The CEDIA technology has the same attractive feature as the EMIT, which is portability to any clinical analyzer that has the capability of spectrophotometric measurements.

KINETIC INTERACTION OF MICROPARTICLES IN SOLUTION (KIMS)

A non-enzymatic homogeneous immunoassay for detecting drugs in urine was developed by Roche Diagnostics, one of two principal divisions of F. Hoffman-La Roche Ltd., a healthcare conglomerate headquartered in Basel, Switzerland. The other division develops and markets pharmaceuticals. The KIMS method (Fig. 18.5) borrowed the approach of earlier latex agglutination assays designed to measure antibodies. For UDT, a drug or metabolite is covalently bound to a latex microparticle, and, in the absence of free drug, antibodies crosslink the microparticles to form large complexes that scatter light, measured turbidimetrically.

FIGURE 18.5 In the KIMS method, antigens are attached to a microparticle. Antibodies cross-link the antigen-bound microparticles, forming large cross-linked complexes that result in turbidity (A). In the presence of free antigen, the microparticles are displaced from the antibody and do not form large complexes, reducing the turbidity (B). In the KIMS method, the signal (turbidity) is inversely proportional to the free antigen concentration. *From [34]: Reisfield, G. M., Salazar, E., and Bertholf, R. L. (2007). Rational use and interpretation of urine drug testing in chronic opioid therapy.* Annals of Clinical and Laboratory Science *37(4), 301–314. Reprinted with permission.*

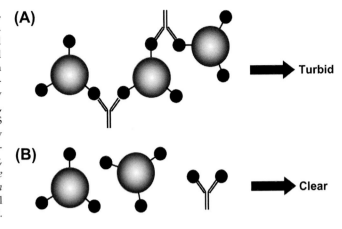

Free antigens occupy binding sites on the antibodies, inhibiting the formation of crosslinked complexes, thereby decreasing the turbidity of the mixture. The scheme is often called "immunoturbidimetric assay". There is no enzyme involved, so the KIMS assays are not susceptible to potential chemical interferences from enzyme inhibitors. On the other hand, turbidimetry is a less specific analytical method because it only detects particles capable of scattering light, as opposed to spectrophotometric measurements that detect specific compounds based on their absorption of UV or visible light. Turbidimetric methods are susceptible to interference from non-specific aggregates in solution that scatter light. The analytical performance of immunoturbidimetric methods for UDT is, however, substantially equivalent to that of enzyme immunoassays.

Confirmatory Methods

Mass spectrometry (MS) has been the standard for identifying and measuring organic compounds since a method for detecting methylated derivatives of amino acids was described over half a century ago by Carl-Ove Andersson, an analytical biochemist at the University of Uppsala in Sweden [22]. Mass filters used in MS applications include magnets, quadrupole radio frequency sectors, and time-of-flight (TOF) instruments. The fundamental design of a mass spectrometer involves an ion source, where a compound is subjected to a high-energy flux of electrons (electron ionization) or unstable ionization products (chemical ionization). Exposure to excess energy results in fragmentation of the molecule; charged fragments can be separated and quantified when they pass through the mass filter, and detected when they collide with the charged collecting plates in an electron multiplier. The fragmentation pattern of every molecule is unique, because it is related to the stability of individual bonds within the molecule, and even small biomolecules have many intramolecular bonds that contribute to the fragmentation pattern and resulting mass spectrum, which can be considered a "fingerprint" of the molecule. Gas chromatography (GC) was the first chromatographic method widely adapted to MS detectors. Capillary GC columns used in most gas chromatography-mass spectrometry are much longer than traditional glass columns, improving the chromatographic resolution by a factor of 10 to 100, and they do not require an interface to reduce pressure, so the GC effluent can be delivered directly to the ion source. Liquid chromatography (LC) is an attractive alternative to GC for coupling with an MS detector because it does not require volatile analytes. However, unlike capillary GC, LC involves a large volume of solvent (mobile phase) that must be removed before the column effluent can be introduced into the ion source. Several LC/MS interfaces have been devised. Early attempts to interface an LC to an MS involved a heated conveyer on which the volatile solvent was evaporated before introduction of the column effluent into the ion source. However, the introduction of thermospray and electrospray technologies revolutionized LC/MS applications. These interfaces involve atomizing the LC column effluent into small droplets from which the solvent can be rapidly evaporated (thermospray), abandoning the analyte in the vapor phase, or charging the droplets in an electrical field so their contents can be accelerated by a focusing lens into the ion source. Thermospray and electrospray interfaces are common in LC/MS and LC/MS-MS instruments available for drug testing. See Chapter 3 for more discussion on mass spectrometry.

LC/MS-MS methods are particularly well-suited to UDT in pain management, and have become common in laboratories offering those services. One reason for the unique adaptability of this analytical method is that it can detect and quantify multiple drugs and metabolites in small volumes without concern for volatility or GC chromatographic properties. The method is less susceptible to interferences from co-migrating compounds, due to the greater specificity of parent/daughter ion selectivity of tandem MS. Conjugated metabolites, such as ethyl glucuronide and ethyl sulfate, can be measured without extensive chemical manipulation. In unregulated UDT confirmatory methods have to be adapted to specific clinical needs, which typically involves confirming adherence to prescribed medications.

SPECIMEN TAMPERING

In forensic UDT, guidelines have been established for detecting tampering with a urine specimen. Acceptable ranges for temperature (immediately post-collection), pH (within certain time limits), creatinine concentration and specific gravity are intended to reveal specimens that have been substituted (temperature), adulterated (pH, and other specific adulterants such as nitrite) or diluted (creatinine and specific gravity). Substitution with a pet's urine is also encountered in unobserved collections, and may result in abnormal indices. Chemical warmers are sometimes used to warm a substituted specimen to a temperature within an acceptable range. In general, these specimen integrity checks are appropriate for non-forensic UDT, such as monitoring patients who are prescribed chronic opioid therapy, particularly when the screening is performed for the purpose of ensuring that the patient is not taking non-prescribed drugs.

However, UDT in pain management often serves the additional purpose of verifying adherence to prescribed opioid regimens; a negative screen for a prescribed drug may indicate that the drug has been used up early in the month and hence not administered in the days prior to the test, or that the drug has not been taken but instead has been diverted. Ironically, a non-adherent patient who is tested for a prescribed drug has an incentive to ensure the UDT is positive rather than negative (in contrast to drug abusers, whose incentive is to produce a negative specimen). Two potential approaches to gaining a positive result are substitution of a urine specimen from someone who is taking the drug, or addition of the drug to the negative urine specimen. The latter approach is more difficult to apply effectively, for two reasons:

1. Concentrations of drugs in the urine typically fall within predictable limits, although extremes are sometimes encountered. Addition of a few milligrams of drug to a 50-mL urine specimen can produce a urinary drug concentration of more than 100 000 ng/mL, which is unusually high for most opioid dosage ranges.

2. Drugs (particularly opioids) are rarely eliminated exclusively as the parent drug. Most opioids undergo some type of oxidative metabolism, as well as conjugation. Therefore, the presence of solely the parent drug in a urine specimen would be suspicious, and metabolites are prohibitively difficult to obtain by patients trying to wangle appropriate UDT results. While critical examination of the UDT results for a typical drug/metabolite combination would often reveal a specimen to which drug has been added, there are no widely-adopted protocols for this type of assessment, and it is unlikely that most physicians ordering UDT for their patients would scrutinize screening results if they appeared consistent with patient adherence.

There is precedent in forensic drug testing programs for follow-up of positive results with specific tests to look for additional drugs or metabolites. Methamphetamine, for example, is demethylated to produce amphetamine, but only the d-stereoisomer is significantly metabolized by that pathway. Desoxyephedrine (levmetam fetamine on vicks® nasal spray package), the l-isomer of methamphetamine, which is not a controlled drug and is a constituent of over-the-counter products, produces a mass spectrum nearly identical to methamphetamine, but is not significantly demethylated to amphetamine. Therefore, one protocol for confirmation of methamphetamine-positive specimens requires the presence of amphetamine. In addition, the dextrorotatory (d) stereoisomer of methamphetamine can also be distinguished from the l-isomer by using chiral derivatizing reagents, or on a chromatographic column with a chiral stationary phase. Some non-chiral chromatographic methods with sufficient resolution are capable of separating the stereoisomers.

Heroin is rapidly metabolized to morphine, so the presence of morphine in the urine is consistent with administration of morphine or codeine (of which several legal but controlled pharmaceutical preparations exist) or heroin, which is not approved in the US for pharmaceutical use and which is illegal to possess. In some cases heroin use can be confirmed by the presence of an intermediate metabolite, 6-acetylmorphine (or a contaminant, 6-acetylcodeine), and protocols exist for detecting this metabolite at very low concentrations in urine specimens that have morphine concentrations above the positive threshold.

METABOLISM OF OPIOID ANALGESICS

Opioid analgesics are widely prescribed for the treatment of acute and chronic pain of moderate to severe intensity. To wit, hydrocodone currently is by far the single most prescribed drug of any class in the United States. Knowledge of opioid metabolism is critical in clinical urine drug testing because several commercially available opioids are metabolized to other commercially available opioids or are present as process impurities in the manufacture of other commercially available opioids. Failure to recognize these facts can result in false conclusions that patients are using non-prescribed opioids.

Opioid metabolism occurs chiefly in the liver by Phase I and/or Phase II reactions. Phase I reactions are non-synthetic reactions (e.g., oxidation, reduction), and occur chiefly by means of the cytochrome P450 (CYP) superfamily of enzymes. Fig. 18.6 shows the principal Phase I metabolic pathways for several opioids. Phase II metabolism typically involves conjugation of the drug or metabolite to a moiety that may render it inactive or improve its excretion. In the case of opioids, glucuronic acid is the major conjugate.

The most important oxidative enzymes are CYP2D6 and CYP3A4, which constitute 2–4% and 30%, respectively, of hepatic CYPs, but are responsible for the oxidative metabolism of 25% and 50%, respectively, of commercially available drugs, including most opioids [23]. CYP enzymes are variously inducible (e.g., CYP3A4) and suppressible (e.g., CYP2D6, CYP3A4) by other drugs, and display a high degree of genetic polymorphism that imbues them with a wide spectrum of activity. CYP2D6 phenotypes comprise poor metabolizers (PMs), intermediate metabolizers (IMs), extensive metabolizers (EM) and ultra-rapid metabolizers (UMs), which account for 5–10%, 10–17%, 70–80% and 3–5%, respectively, of the Caucasian population [23]. In contrast, approximately 1% of the Chinese population are PMs and 29% of Ethiopians are UMs [24].

CYP2D6 metabolizes three pharmaceutically used opioids to other commercially available opioids. The most clinically significant example is the conversion of codeine to morphine. Codeine is metabolized primarily by glucuronidation to codeine-6-glucuronide, and secondarily by CYP3A4 to nor-codeine. However, approximately 10% of an administered dose is O-demethylated by CYP2D6 to morphine, the metabolite chiefly responsible for codeine's analgesic effects. Two other opioids undergo conversions that, while clinically minor, are toxicologically noteworthy. Oxycodone is a potent opioid analgesic of which approximately 10% is O-demethylated to the more potent oxymorphone [25]. Likewise, some individuals O-demethylate a small percentage of hydrocodone to the more potent hydromorphone. This conversion has been found in 6.6% of hydrocodone-positive postmortem cases [26].

Other toxicologically significant opioid metabolic conversions exist, although the responsible enzymatic pathways have not yet been identified. Several case reports have described the metabolism of morphine to hydromorphone. In each of these cases, the urinary hydromorphone concentration comprised less than 5% of the urinary morphine concentration. A minor pathway exists for the metabolism of codeine to hydrocodone. Hydrocodone can sometimes metabolize to dihydrocodeine, with the latter found in approximately 10% of hydrocodone-positive postmortem cases [26]. It is important to recognize that most commercially available opioids do not metabolize to other opioids. Thus, buprenorphine, fentanyl, levorphanol, meperidine, methadone, propoxyphene and tramadol are neither metabolized to, nor metabolites of, other commercially available opioids.

During the manufacture of several opioid products, other opioid(s) may appear as "process impurities", possibly confounding urine drug test interpretation. As can be seen in Table 18.1, allowable limits of these impurities do not exceed 0.5%. This has become an issue in recent years because of the increasing prescribing of opioids — particularly high-dose opioids — for the treatment of non-cancer pain, together with the increasing use of clinical urine drug testing, an expanded test menu for opioids, and use of lower analyte cut-off

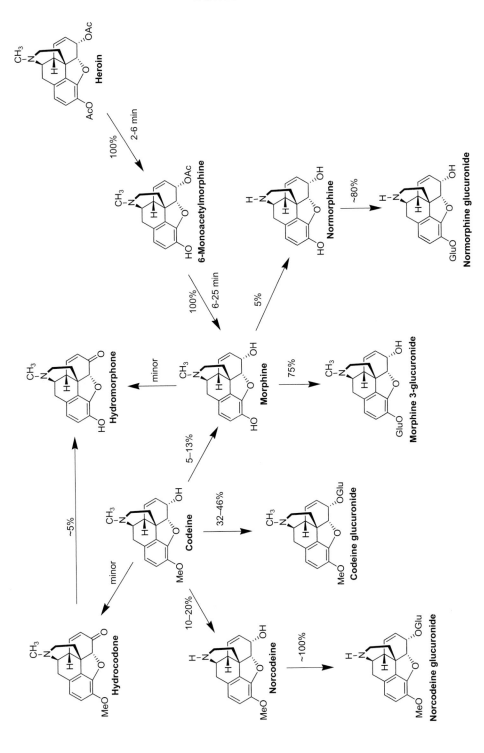

FIGURE 18.6 Metabolism of opioids. *Fom [34]: Reisfield, G. M., Salazar, E., and Bertholf, R. L. (2007). Rational use and interpretation of urine drug testing in chronic opioid therapy. Annals of Clinical and Laboratory Science 37(4), 301–314. Reprinted with permission.*

TABLE 18.1   Acceptable Impurities Present in Commercial Opioid Drugs[a]

Opioid drug	Impurity present	Allowable limit	Comments[b]
Codeine	Morphine	0.15%	Morphine impurity < 1%
Morphine	Codeine	0.5%	Codeine impurity < 1%
	6-Monoacetyl morphine	Not established	
Hydrocodone	Codeine	0.15%	Newer preparations may not contain any impurity
Oxycodone	Hydrocodone	1%	Hydrocodone < 0.2%
Oxymorphone	Hydromorphone	0.15%	Hydromorphone up to 1%
	Oxycodone		Oxycodone up to 0.5%
Hydromorphone	Hydrocodone	0.1%	Newer preparation may not contain any impurity
	Morphine		0.15%

[a]Source: Medical Review Officer Alter, April 2010; Volume 21, No. 3, Quadrangle Research, LLC, Research Triangle Park, NC.
[b]Manufacturer's certificate of analysis of products.

levels. Recently the heroin metabolite 6-acetylmorphine has been reported as a process impurity in the manufacture of morphine, but allowable limits have not yet been established and typically observed percentages have not been reported [27]. 6-Acetylmorphine also has been detected at concentrations above 20 ng/mL in specimens with morphine concentrations below the customary positive threshold of 300 ng/mL [28]. Table 18.1 lists the allowable limits for process impurities in the manufacture of several opioids.

Patients prescribed chronic opioid therapy often use benzodiazepines for various indications [29], including treatment of muscle spasm (diazepam), neuropathic pain (clonazepam), insomnia (temazepam; triazolam) and co-occurring anxiety disorders (e.g., alprazolam, diazepam, lorazepam, oxazepam). Benzodiazepines, like opioids, are also common drugs of abuse, and data indicate that individuals using both opioids and benzodiazepines are more likely to be diagnosed with an opioid use disorder [30]. Furthermore, unintentional drug overdose deaths often involve a combination of opioids and benzodiazepines [31]. Several benzodiazepines, like several opioids, are subject to bioconversion to other commercially available benzodiazepines. For example, temazepam is metabolized to oxazepam (via CYP2C19), diazepam is metabolized to temazepam (via CYP3A4) and thence to oxazepam [32], and chlordiazepoxide is metabolized to nor-diazepam and oxazepam [33]. Alprazolam, clonazepam, flunitrazepam, lorazepam, midazolam and triazolam are neither metabolites of, nor metabolized to, other commercially available benzodiazepines.

CHALLENGES IN DRUG TESTING IN PAIN MANAGEMENT

The principal focus of clinical laboratories has always been to provide analytical data that support and promote accurate medical diagnosis and treatment. The benefits of measuring plasma concentrations of drugs were immediately apparent, and clinical laboratories adapted to the emerging need for TDM by offering it, typically, within their "toxicology" services. It was a logical designation, since many of the analytical methods for measuring therapeutic drugs were the same as those used for detecting toxins. The advent of homogeneous immunoassays for therapeutic drugs, however, and the application of that same technology for detecting drugs of abuse in urine, blurred the distinction between toxicology and clinical chemistry. Most contemporary UDT assays have been adapted to routine chemistry analyzers.

There was diagnostic value to UDT in the evaluation and treatment of patients presenting to the emergency department, where drug overdose was an urgent diagnostic and therapeutic consideration that could often only be resolved by laboratory support. The division between medical and forensic UDT, however, was very clear: screening by immunochemical UDT assays was sufficient for urgent medical evaluation, but forensic UDT had to conform to statutory guidelines that specified concentration thresholds for positive results, confirmatory analyses for positive results, review of UDT results by a medical review officer, and restrictions with regard to collection and documentation of the specimen chain of custody. Laboratories offering forensic UDT services had to conform to state or federal regulations, which were rigorous.

Medical and forensic UDT diverged into two distinct disciplines. Urine toxicology for sports medicine became a third discipline, regulated by its own set of guidelines and regulatory agencies that exceeded the resources of most clinical and forensic drug testing laboratories. For hospital-based clinical laboratories, the division between medical and forensic UDT was clearly apparent; hospitals provided medical UDT, which rarely included confirmatory analyses, and referral laboratories with the resources to comply with NIDA and SAMSHA requirements sought certification to offer forensic UDT under federal contracts.

Drug testing in pain management straddles the divide between medical and forensic UDT. In some respects it is part of medical evaluation, but in other respects it is used to determine consequences in a manner similar to forensic UDT. To a patient prescribed opioid therapy for chronic pain, denial of treatment is a consequence tantamount to termination as an employee or removal of privileges to participate in sports activity. Patients face the stigma of being considered a drug abuser or, perhaps worse, a drug dealer, based on the results of UDT. As noted earlier in the discussion of physicians' lack of interpretive knowledge, some physicians may even report the patient to law enforcement authorities based on a UDT result. The severity of these consequences demands that utmost care must be taken to avoid the possibility of misinterpretation of UDT results, but currently there are no safeguards in place to ensure that this does not occur. Laboratories that offer UDT services to pain management practices typically have a toxicologist or medical director qualified to correctly interpret UDT results and perhaps recommend follow-up tests to clarify unexpected or ambiguous results of screening tests. However, effective use of such a resource requires the exchange of information between the clinician and laboratory that is often missing from UDT orders. Other laboratories may request no information about what drug(s) the patient is taking, or what result the clinician expects to confirm patient adherence. Without this information, the laboratory cannot recognize circumstances that require additional testing. This is a serious deficiency in current practices for using UDT to monitor patients on opioid therapy.

A critical and mandatory feature of forensic UDT is the review of all positive results by a medical review officer certified to interpret UDT. The same approach would be prohibitively expensive and time-consuming for UDT in pain management. In forensic UDT only positive results have adverse consequences, whereas in pain management positive or negative UDT results can have adverse consequences, so equal attention must be paid to unexpected negative results. Laboratory tests for drugs and their metabolites in urine have many limitations, and the proper interpretation of positive or negative results requires consideration of several factors, including the specific drug and dose that was administered, the recent administration pattern, metabolic factors that influence the urinary products characteristic of that drug or metabolite, the presence of other drugs that may influence metabolism, and the sensitivity and specificity of the analytical method used to detect the drug and its metabolites. Clinicians ordinarily do not receive the type of training necessary to resolve these various factors, and therefore the potential for misinterpretation of positive or negative UDT results is disturbingly high.

There is an unaddressed need for standardization, and perhaps regulation, of UDT services applied to patients on monitored opioid therapy, as well as enrollees in substance abuse recovery programs. Analytical methods exist for sensitive and specific detection of drugs in urine and other biological matrices, and many laboratories offer these services to pain management practices. Used correctly, UDT is an invaluable component of the responsible application of chronic opioid analgesic therapy. However, without precautions against the misinterpretation of results, UDT has the potential to cause harm to individuals who may be responsibly adherent to prescribed and essential medication regimens.

CONCLUSIONS

UDT in pain management has been widely adopted by clinicians to assist in determining whether patients are adherent with medical therapy, as patient records are unreliable. Despite available analytical methods, including confirmation of the presence of the intended drug in the urine, there are ethical and medical issues regarding the practice of drug monitoring in pain management.

References

[1] Starrels JL, Becker WC, Alford DP, et al. Systematic review: treatment agreements and urine drug testing to reduce opioid misuse in patients with chronic pain. Ann Intern Med 2010;152:712–20.
[2] The Substance Abuse and Mental Health Services Administration, Office of Applied Studies. National Survey on Drugs Use and Health. Rockville, MD: SAMHSA. Available at, http://www.oas.samhsa.gov/NSDUH/2k9NSDUH/2k9ResultsP.pdf; 2009.
[3] Reid MC, Engles-Horton LL, Weber MB, et al. Use of opioid medications for chronic noncancer pain syndromes in primary care. J Gen Intern Med 2002;17:173–9.
[4] Katz NP, Sherburne S, Beach M, et al. Behavioral monitoring and urine toxicology testing in patients receiving long-term opioid therapy. Anesth Analg 2003;97:1097–102.
[5] Passik SD, Kirsh KL. Opioid therapy in patients with a history of substance abuse. CNS Drugs 2004;18:13–25.

[6] Ives TJ, Chelminski PR, Hammett-Stabler CA, et al. Predictors of opioid misuse in patients with chronic pain: a prospective cohort study. BMC Health Serv Res 2006;6:46.

[7] Wiedemer NL, Harden PS, Arndt IO, Gallagher RM. The opioid renewal clinic: a primary care, managed approach to opioid therapy in chronic pain patients at risk for substance abuse. Pain Med 2007;8:573—84.

[8] Fishbain DA, Rosomoff HL, Rosomoff RS. Drug abuse, dependence, and addiction in chronic pain patients. Clin J Pain 1992;8:77—85.

[9] Trescot AM, Helm S, Hansen H, et al. Opioids in the management of chronic non-cancer pain: an update of American Society of the Interventional Pain Physicians' (ASIPP) Guidelines. Pain Physician 2008;11:S5—S62.

[10] The Substance Abuse and Mental Health Services Administration, Office of Applied Studies. Treatment Episode Data Set. Rockville, MD: SAMHSA. Available at, http://oas.samhsa.gov/2k2/TEDS/TEDS.pdf; 2009. 2008.

[11] Centers for Disease Control and Prevention (CDC). Atlanta, GA: Press release. Available at, http://www.cdc.gov/media/pressrel/2010/r100617.htm; 2010.

[12] Florida Department of Law Enforcement. Interim Report by Florida Medical Examiners Commission on Drugs Identified in Deceased Persons Report. Tallahassee, FL: FDLA. Available at, http://www.fdle.state.fl.us/Content/News/November-2009/2009-Interim-Report-by-Florida-Medical-Examiners-C.aspx; 2009.

[13] Katz NP, Birnbaum HG, Castor A. Volume of prescription opioids used nonmedically in the United States. J Pain Palliat Care Pharmacother 2010;24:141—4.

[14] Pesce A, West C, Rosenthal M, et al. Illicit drug use in the pain patient population decreases with continued drug testing. Pain Physician 2011;14:189—93.

[15] Okie S. A flood of opioids, a rising tide of deaths. N Engl J Med 2010;363:1981—5.

[16] Compton WM, Volkow ND. Major increases in opioid analgesic abuse in the United States: concerns and strategies. Drug Alcohol Depend 2006;81:103—7.

[17] Reisfield GM, Bertholf R, Barkin RL, et al. Urine drug test interpretation: what do physicians know? J Opioid Manag 2007;3:80—6.

[18] Ropero-Miller JD, Goldberger BA. Handbook of Workplace Drug Testing. 2nd ed. Washington, DC: AACC Press; 2008.

[19] Yalow RS, Berson SA. Immunoassay of endogenous plasma insulin in man. J Clin Invest 1960;39:1157—75.

[20] Buechler KF, Moi S, Noar B, et al. Simultaneous detection of seven drugs of abuse by the Triage panel for drugs of abuse. Clin Chem 1992;38:1678—84.

[21] Watson ID, Bertholf RL, Hammett-Stabler CA. Drugs and ethanol testing at the point of care. Point of Care 2007;6:227—30.

[22] Andersson BA. Mass spectrometric and gas chromatographic studies of n-heptafluorobutyryl derivatives of peptide methyl esters. Acta Chem Scand 1967;21:2906—8.

[23] Zhou SF, Liu JP, Chowbay B. Polymorphism of human cytochrome P450 enzymes and its clinical impact. Drug Metab Rev 2009;41:89—295.

[24] Aklillu E, Persson I, Bertilsson L, et al. Frequent distribution of ultrarapid metabolizers of debrisoquine in an ethiopian population carrying duplicated and multiduplicated functional CYP2D6 alleles. J Pharmacol Exp Ther 1996;278:441—6.

[25] Heiskanen T, Olkkola KT, Kalso E. Effects of blocking CYP2D6 on the pharmacokinetics and pharmacodynamics of oxycodone. Clin Pharmacol Ther 1998;64:603—11.

[26] Baker DD, Jenkins AJ. A comparison of methadone, oxycodone, and hydrocodone related deaths in Northeast Ohio. J Anal Toxicol 2008;32:165—71.

[27] American Association of Medical Review Officers. AAMRO news. Available at, http://www.aamro.com/docs/news/27.pdf; 2011.

[28] Crews B, Mikel C, Latyshev S, et al. 6-Acetylmorphine detected in the absence of morphine in pain management patients. Ther Drug Monit 2009;31:749—452.

[29] Cone EJ, Caplan YH, Black DL, et al. Urine drug testing of chronic pain patients: licit and illicit drug patterns. J Anal Toxicol 2008;32:530—43.

[30] Hojsted J, Nielsen PR, Guldstrand SK, et al. Classification and identification of opioid addiction in chronic pain patients. Eur J Pain 2010;14:1014—20.

[31] Toblin RL, Paulozzi LJ, Logan JE, et al. Mental illness and psychotropic drug use among prescription drug overdose deaths: a medical examiner chart review. J Clin Psychiatry 2010;71:491—6.

[32] Mandrioli R, Mercolini L, Raggi MA. Benzodiazepine metabolism: an analytical perspective. Curr Drug Metab 2008;9:827—44.

[33] Baselt RC. Disposition of Toxic Drugs and Chemicals in Man. 7th ed. Foster City, CA: Biomedical Publications; 2004.

[34] Reisfield GM, Salazar E, Bertholf RL. Rational use and interpretation of urine drug testing in chronic opioid therapy. Annals of Clinical and Laboratory Science 2007;37:301—14.

CHAPTER

19

Effect of Herbal Supplement–Drug Interactions on Therapeutic Drug Monitoring

Alex C. Chin, Leland B. Baskin

Calgary Laboratory Services, Calgary, AB, Canada

OUTLINE

Therapeutic Drug Monitoring: Newer Drugs and Biomarkers
DOI: 10.1016/B978-0-12-385467-4.00019-1

INTRODUCTION

Therapeutic drug monitoring (TDM) usually consists of measuring blood concentrations of a drug or metabolite in the body, or measuring an intended or unintended effect of the drug. Physicians and other medical practitioners must increase their awareness of herbal supplements for a variety of reasons. According to past polls, the use of herbal supplements in the United States has increased from 2.5% to 12% from 1990 to 1997 [1, 2]. Although there was an increase from 11% to 18% during this timeframe in patients informing their physicians that they were taking herbal supplements [1, 2], the figure remains alarmingly low and indicates the potential risks posed to both the patient and physician in regard to herbal–drug interactions. Standardization of the active ingredients in herbal supplements is almost non-existent, and many have been shown to contain contaminants or adulterants of various kinds. According to American Association of Poison Control Centers data, in 2009 there was a total of 1 564 773 adverse exposures to pharmaceuticals, including 7395 major outcomes and 497 deaths [3]. Of these adverse exposures, 29 417 (1.9% of all pharmaceutical exposures) were due to dietary herbal supplements, with 24 major outcomes (0.3% of all major outcomes) and 1 death (0.2% of all deaths) [3]. Despite the rarity of serious adverse effects and death from herbal products, direct interference by these agents on laboratory analysis can lead to unnecessary confusion and a drain on resources for both the laboratory and the clinical team. Furthermore, extra vigilance is recommended, given that research in herbal–drug interactions is very limited and the potential for harm still exists.

HERBAL SUPPLEMENTS AND PHARMACOKINETICS

In order to predict the effects of supplements on therapeutic drug monitoring, it is necessary to possess an understanding of the pharmacological actions which may affect diagnostic testing. These pre-analytical variables influence pharmacokinetic mechanisms such as absorption, distribution, metabolism and excretion. More specifically, herbal supplements may cause direct unintended pharmacological effects such as alteration of drug absorption, protein binding, enzyme induction or inhibition, synergy, and toxicity. Furthermore, the presence of contaminants from the environment or the manufacturing process, deliberate adulteration with other pharmaceutical substances, and misidentification of the active herbal ingredient can also interfere with drug therapy.

Drug Absorption

When taken orally, drug absorption is usually mediated by transport proteins at the apical brush border of intestinal epithelial cells. Conversely, efflux transporters assist in detoxification by expelling agents from the enterocytes. These transport proteins are specialized according to the transport of drugs as well as various compounds such as peptides and amino acids, nucleosides, anions and cations [4]. Drugs that are transported by these transporters are listed in Table 19.1 and depicted in Fig. 19.1.

Effect on Uptake Transporting Proteins

Most herbal supplements have been shown to affect the function of the organic anion transporting polypeptide (OATP) family of proteins. Common drugs taken up by OATP include 3-hydroxy-3-methyl-glutaryl (HMG)-CoA-reductase inhibitors (statins), antibiotics, anticancer agents and cardiac glycosides. Since OATPs are expressed in a variety of different tissues, including brain, intestine, liver and kidney [5, 6], they play a key role not only in drug absorption, but also in facilitating downstream pharmacokinetic mechanisms such as distribution, metabolism and excretion.

Effect on Efflux Transporters

While OATP mediates the uptake of drugs, P-glycoprotein (P-gp) is a member of the ATP-binding cassette (ABC) family of transporters. Formerly known as multidrug resistance gene (MDR1) due to overexpression in tumor cells conferring multi-drug resistance against certain antineoplastic agents, P-gp mediates the transport of a wide variety of

TABLE 19.1 Example of Drugs that are Substrates for Cellular Transports

Cellular transporter	Representative drug
P-Glycoprotein	Actinomycin D, amitriptyline, amoxicillin, atorvastatin, carbamazepine, chlorpromazine, cimetidine, ciprofloxacin, corticosteroids, cyclosporine, daunorubicin, dexamethasone digoxin, diltiazem, dipyridamole, doxepin, doxorubicin, doxycycline, erythromycin, fexofenadine, glyburide, gramicidin D, hydrocortisone, imatinib, irinotecan, itraconazole, ivermectin, ketoconazole, loperamide, losartan, lovastatin, methylprednisolone, mitomycin C, mitoxantrone, nifedipine, olanzapine, paclitaxel, paroxetine, prednisolone, quetiapine, quinidine, ranitidine, rifampin, risperidone, ritonavir, saquinavir, sertraline, sirolimus, tacrolimus, talinolol, tamoxifen, tetracycline, topiramate, verapamil, vinblastine, vincristine
OATP*-A (Brain capillary endothelial cells)	N-methyl-quinidine, exofenadine, D-penicillamine, enkephalin
OATP-C (liver)	Pravastatin, rifampin, thyroid hormones
OATP-8 (liver)	Dehydroepiandrosterone sulfate, estrone-3-sulfate, cholecystokinin, digoxin, D-penicillamine, enkephalin (DPDPE), rifampin

*Organic anion transporting polypeptide.
Adapted from: http://www.genemedrx.com/PGPtable.php.

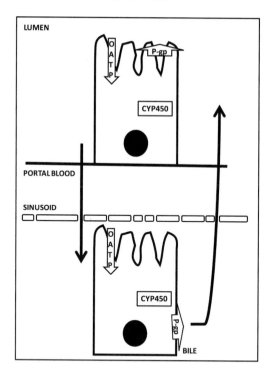

FIGURE 19.1   **First-pass metabolism.** Drugs are transported into the enterocyte via OATP or pumped back into the lumen via P-gp, which decreases drug levels. Drugs are metabolized by intestinal CYP450 and are transported to the hepatocytes through the portal blood into the sinusoids, where they are taken up through similar OATP mechanisms. Hepatic CYP450 further metabolize the drugs which then reenter the intestinal lumen for excretion by the action of the P-glycoprotein pump.

drugs and is distributed in the intestine, liver, blood–brain barrier, and kidney [7]. P-gp is one of the best-characterized efflux transporters, and studies have shown that herbal supplements can inhibit its function. Inhibition of P-gp leads to increased bioavailability or blood levels of co-administered drugs by preventing their efflux from the intestine.

Protein Binding

Once absorbed through the intestinal mucosa, drugs are carried in the blood to the liver for first-pass metabolism. Various plasma carrier proteins have the ability to bind drugs and their metabolites. Most acidic drugs are carried by albumin while basic drugs are carried by α1-acid glycoprotein (orosomucoid) and lipoproteins. By displacing drugs bound to protein carriers, the fraction of unbound "free" drug is increased, yielding increased apparent drug activity for a given drug concentration. Therefore, it is clear that herbal drugs which compete for plasma binding proteins can alter the equilibrium exhibited between bound and free co-administered drug concentrations.

Microsomal Enzyme Induction

Orally administered drugs which are absorbed in the intestine are transported via the portal vein to the liver where they undergo metabolism and then the resulting metabolites enter the general circulation. Generally, metabolic reactions transform drugs into more polar or water-soluble forms to facilitate excretion. Induction of Phase I reactions catalyzed by the cytochrome P450 enzyme plays an important role in the metabolism of drugs (Table 19.2). However, some Phase II metabolic transformations can also render a drug more toxic. Therefore, it is clear that herbal supplements that affect the cytochrome P450 enzyme activity can have a significant effect on the pharmacodynamics or the effect of therapeutic drugs on the body.

TABLE 19.2 Drug Metabolized by Various Isoenzymes of Cytochrome P450 Mixed Function Oxidase Family of Enzymes

Isoenzyme	Drugs*
CYP1A2	Amitriptyline, caffeine, clomipramine, clozapine, cyclobenzaprine, fluvoxamine, haloperidol, mexiletine, naproxen, olanzapine, acetaminophen, propranolol, ropivacaine, tacrine, theophylline, tizanidine, verapamil, R-warfarin, zileuton, zolmitriptan
CYP2B6	Bupropion, cyclophosphamide, efavirenz, methadone, sorafenib
CYP2C8	Amodiaquine, cerivastatin, paclitaxel, repaglinide, sorafenib, torsemide
CYP2C9	Diclofenac, ibuprofen, naproxen, piroxicam, tolbutamide, glipizide, glyburide, glibenclamide, amitriptyline, gluoxetine, rosiglitazone, tamoxifen, S-warfarin
CYP2C19	Omeprazole, pantoprazole, rabeprazole, diazepam, phenytoin, phenobarbital, amitriptyline, carisoprodol, citalopram, chloramphenicol, clomipramine, indomethacin, moclobemide, nelfinavir, nilutamide, primidone, progesterone, proguanil, propranolol, teniposide
CYP2D6	Amitriptyline, clomipramine, desipramine, fluoxetine, imipramine, paroxetine, propafenone, timolol, haloperidol, perphenazine, thioridazine, aripiprazole, atomoxetine, chlorpheniramine, chlorpromazine, codeine, debrisoquine, dexfenfluramine, dextromethorphan, donepezil, duloxetine, encainide, flecainide, fluvoxamine, lidocaine, metoclopramide, mexiletine, minaprine, nebivolol, oxycodone, perhexiline, phenacetin, phenformin, promethazine, propranolol, sparteine, tramadol, venlafaxine, tamoxifen
CYP2E1	Enflurane, halothane, isoflurane, methoxyflurane, sevoflurane, chlorzoxazone, theophylline
CYP3A/5	Metabolize majority of drugs, including **macrolides** (clarithromycin, erythromycin, telithromycin, etc.), **benzodiazepines** (alprazolam, diazepam, midazolam, triazolam, etc.), **immunosuppressants** (cyclosporine, tacrolimus, sirolimus, etc.), **antiretrovirals** indinavir, nelfinavir, ritonavir, saquinavir, etc.), **antihistamines** (astemizole, chlorpheniramine, terfenadine, etc.), **calcium channel blockers** (amlodipine, diltiazem, felodipine, nifedipine, verapamil, etc.), **cholesterol lowering drugs** (atorvastatin, lovastatin, simvastatin), **steroids** (hydrocortisone, progesterone, dexamethasone, etc.) and many other drugs including but not limited to caffeine, dapsone, fentanyl, finasteride, gleevec, quinine, risperidone, sildenafil, terfenadine

*Although many drugs are listed under various isoenzymes, this list is not complete. For more information, consult a pharmacology textbook and see also the source cited below.
Adapted from: Flockhart DA. Drug Interactions: Cytochrome P450 Drug Interaction Table. Indiana University School of Medicine (2007). http://medicine.iupui.edu/clinpharm/ddis/table.aspx.

PHARMACOKINETIC INTERACTIONS INVOLVING HERBAL SUPPLEMENTS

According to 2008 data, sales of herbal supplements in the United States accounted for an estimated US$4800 million, and the top 10 herbal supplements sold in the US were cranberry, soy, garlic, saw palmetto, ginkgo, echinacea, milk thistle, St John's wort, ginseng and black cohosh [8]. Among the most commonly used herbal supplements and dietary components in the United States, St John's wort and grapefruit have the most significant reported drug interactions in regard to pharmacokinetics and pharmacodynamics. The evidence surrounding other herbs is either weak or contradictory, and requires further investigation.

Drug Interactions with St John's Wort (*Hypericum perforatum*)

St John's wort demonstrates several characteristics of herbal supplements that contribute to problems associated with their use. Primarily used as an antidepressant or anxiolytic by way of inhibition of serotonin reuptake, St John's wort may cause side effects including photosensitization with erythema, itching and a demyelinating neuropathy, and may inhibit iron absorption [9]. The intended effect can cause "serotonin excess", with accompanying dry mouth, dizziness and confusion [9]. Numerous case reports have described that co-administration with serotonin reuptake inhibitors exacerbate this serotonin excess to include headache, diaphoresis and agitation, and may also cause serotonin syndrome [10–15].

Several active components have been isolated from St John's wort, and such compounds may be divided into at least six different categories, including naphthodianthrones (hypericin and pseudohypericin), flavonoids (quercetin, heperoside, rutin), biflavones, tannic acid, phenylpropanes and hyperforin [16]. These active ingredients influence a variety of different functions, and the actions of some constituents are diametrically opposed to those of others. Naphthodianthrones are cleared from plasma slowly with a plasma half-life of approximately 25 hours for pseudohypericin and approximately 40 hours for hypericin, and these are thought to be responsible for phototoxicity in high doses. Hyperforin is a ligand for the pregnane X receptor that regulates expression of CYP3A4 monooxygenase [17].

St John's wort has been shown to be a potent inducer of the cytochrome P450 enzymes CYP3A4, CYP2E1 and CYP2C19 [18, 19], as well as an enhancer of P-gp expression [20], which facilitate drug metabolism and efflux, respectively, and consequently reduce effective drug levels in the plasma. This potent induction of cytochrome P450 by St John's wort has been well demonstrated in a recent study where it inhibited the activity of ritonavir, a potent inhibitor of CYP3A, and led to reduction of midazolam plasma levels [21]. A case study reported significant interactions between St John's wort and cyclosporine leading to acute heart transplant rejection [22], while another clinical study reported similar decreases in renal transplant patients [23]. Furthermore, administration of St John's wort to healthy volunteers reduced tacrolimus plasma concentrations [24]. Clinical trials have demonstrated interactions between St John's wort and oral contraceptives, leading to breakthrough bleeding, follicular growth and possible ovulation [25–27]. Co-administration of St John's wort to opioid addict patients led to significant decreases in methadone and possible withdrawal syndrome [28]. Other drugs reported to be affected by St John's wort cytochrome P450 and P-gp inducing activity include digoxin [29], talinolol [30], ivabradine [31], verapamil [32], warfarin [33], indinavir [34], gliclazide [35], simvastatin [36], atorvastatin [37], omeprazole [38], oxycodone [39], irinotecan [40] and imatinib [41, 42], thus possibly increasing the risk of atrial fibrillation and flutter, cardiac arrhythmias, tachycardia, HIV drug resistance and treatment failure, hyperglycemia, cardiovascular disease, dyspepsia, chronic pain, and cancer progression. Furthermore, a past study has shown that plasma levels of the antifungal drug voriconazole increase and then significantly decrease after short- (10 hours) and long- (15 days) term administration of St John's wort, respectively, in CYP2C19 wild-type individuals as compared to deficient individuals [43]. In a similar manner, fexofenadine maximum plasma concentration was increased after a single dose of St John's wort followed by a decrease with long-term (2 weeks) treatment, presumably through a P-gp dependent manner [44].

These studies indicate that pharmacokinetic mechanisms exhibited by St John's wort may be complex and require further study. Nevertheless, given the considerable evidence outlined above, it is advised that healthcare professionals become aware of these potential drug interactions and that patients should refrain from using St John's wort. Indeed, the Food and Drug Administration issued a public health advisory in 2000 outlining its potential for harm.

Drug Interactions with Grapefruit (*Citrus paradisi*)

Grapefruit is a popular dietary component among North Americans. The active chemical compounds in grapefruit include flavones, isoflavones, flavonols, furanocoumarins and anthocyanidin, which have been found to have antioxidant, anti-inflammatory and antimicrobial activities. The flavonoids of interest include naringin, quercetin and kaempferol. Naringin composes about 10% of the dry weight of grapefruit, and is responsible for its taste and odor. It is hydrolyzed to naringenin by intestinal flora. Furanocoumarins, such as bergomattin, and flavonoids, such as naringin, may play the most active roles in the effects of grapefruit on plasma drug levels [45–49]. In light of its popularity, grapefruit has been associated with increased bioavailability of many drugs.

Clinical studies have found that grapefruit increases the oral bioavailability of the calcium channel blockers felodipine, nifedipine and pranidipine [46, 50, 51]. Later studies found that the increase in felodipine and nifedipine may not be due to naringin or quercetin [52, 53], but instead to inter-individual differences in naringin metabolism by intestinal flora [54]. The interaction between grapefruit juice and increase in plasma levels of calcium channel blockers such as felodipine and amlodipine was clinically significant, since patients experienced increased heart rate, decreased diastolic blood pressure, and headaches [55, 56]. Grapefruit juice was also found to increase the plasma levels of 17β-estradiol and its metabolite estrone in ovariectomized women on hormone replacement therapy [57]. Grapefruit juice also may affect cyclosporine pharmacokinetics in transplant patients [58–60] and patients with autoimmune disease [61]. Slight inhibition of cyclosporine metabolism, but not prednisone, for a brief period just after grapefruit ingestion, likely due to inhibition of intestinal cytochrome P450 enzymes, has been reported [58]. Initial observations of grapefruit juice-induced increase in felodipine may have depended on the route of administration where drug levels were affected by oral intake as compared to intravenous injection [62].

TABLE 19.3   Drugs whose Bioavailability is Increased by Grapefruit Juice

Calcium channel blockers and cardioprotective agents	Felodipine [46, 50], nifedipine [50], pranidipine [51], nimodipine [74], amiodarone [75], verapamil [76, 77], talinolol [71], aliskirin [72]
HMG-CoA reductase inhibitors	Atorvastatin [78], lovastatin [79], simvastatin [80–82]
Immunosuppressants	Cyclosporine [58–60], tacrolimus
Psychoactive drugs	Midazolam [83, 84], triazolam [84–87], quazepam [86], diltiazem [88], carbamazepine [89], buspirone [90]
Antimicrobial agents	Clarithromycin [91], saquinavir [92], primaquine [93], itraconazole [94, 95], halofantrine [96]
Oral contraceptives	Estradiol [57]
Others	Cisapride [97], sildenafil [98], budesonide [99], nilotinib [100], oxycodone [101], fexofenadine [70]

Grapefruit juice increases the plasma levels of many drugs which are likely metabolized by intestinal CYP3A4 activity (Table 19.3). Furthermore, grapefruit juice did not affect metabolism of quinine, which is mainly metabolized by CYP3A4 in the liver, thus supporting the view that grapefruit affects intestinal cytochrome P450 [63]. However, while a single intake of grapefruit juice may alter intestinal CYP3A4 [55, 62, 64], further investigations have found that repeated consumption may proceed to inhibit hepatic CYP3A4 [65, 66]. In contrast, grapefruit juice did not affect the pharmacokinetics or hemodynamics, such as elevated heart rate or blood pressure, of caffeine [67], which is a CYP1A2 substrate.

While inhibition of CYP3A4 delays drug metabolism and consequently increases plasma levels of affected drugs, grapefruit juice may also affect drug transport. In regard to drug efflux, grapefruit juice did not significantly affect digoxin pharmacokinetics, and thus is unlikely to be an important inhibitor of P-gp function [68]. However, one *in vitro* study has demonstrated impaired uptake of the antihistamine fexofenadine in epithelial cells transfected with OATP1A2 [69]. The possible role of grapefruit juice as an inhibitor of OATP was further extended in clinical studies [70–72]. Indeed, this pathway of inhibition by grapefruit juice may play an important role in regard to drugs, such as fexofenadine, that are not metabolized by either hepatic or intestinal CYP3A4 [73].

Drug Interactions with Echinacea (*Echinacea* spp.)

Widely used for their immunomodulatory properties, echinacea preparations are taken for respiratory tract infections such as colds, coughs and bronchitis. Echinacea extracts are prepared from plants belonging to the Asteraceae Family and *Echinacea* genus, including *E. purpurea*, *E. angustifolia* and *E. pallida*. These extracts consist of mainly lipophilic alkylamides (alkamides), which have not only been shown to exhibit anti-inflammatory properties [102], but may also affect drug metabolism by affecting cytochrome P450 activity.

A small clinical study of 12 healthy volunteers demonstrated that co-administration of echinacea significantly reduced the clearance of caffeine (CYP1A2 substrate) and tolbutamide. Although echinacea did not affect oral clearance of midazolam (CYP3A substrate), after intravenous administration of midazolam the area under the concentration–time curve of midazolam was reduced [103]. Another clinical study of 13 volunteers reported significant reductions in orally administered midazolam levels after treatment with echinacea for 28 days [104]. However, another similar clinical study reported no clinically significant interactions between echinacea and CYP1A2, CYP2D6, CYP2E1 or CYP3A4 activity [105]. A follow-up study confirmed that echinacea does not affect the activity of CYP2D6 in healthy volunteers [106]. To add to the confusion, a recent randomized controlled trial reported significantly reduced levels of S-warfarin, which has five times the potency of R-warfarin, after echinacea administration in healthy male subjects without affecting hemostasis [107]. In separate *in vitro* studies, echinacea extracts inhibited the activity of OATP-B [108] and P-gp [109] in epithelial cells, thus indicating that further studies should also focus on interactions associated with drug absorption.

Clearly, the conflicting results reported by different clinical studies indicate that further investigation of the interaction potential of echinacea extracts on drug pharmacokinetics is needed. Given the lack of case studies describing echinacea–drug interactions, it may be safe to suggest that serious health threats are unlikely. Nevertheless, significant differences in phenolic content have been found in commercial echinacea preparations [110], thus caution is advised in light of the contradictory findings regarding interactions with cytochrome P450 activity and lack of clinical studies focusing on drug transporters.

Drug Interactions with Ginkgo (*Gingko biloba*)

Ginkgo is intended to stimulate memory [111] and improve circulation. Inhibition of platelet activating factor receptor leading to hemorrhage is its most common unwanted effect. The pharmacologically active components are ginkgolides A, B and C, and bilobabides [112]. Case reports have indicated possible risks of spontaneous hemorrhage due to synergy with several platelet-inhibiting drugs and non-steroidal anti-inflammatory drugs (NSAIDs). A small study demonstrated that ginkgolides inhibited weal and flare responses to platelet-activating factor in healthy volunteers, and platelet aggregation in platelet-rich plasma [113]. A 70-year-old man was reported to suffer from spontaneous hyphema associated with ginkgo extract intake [114]. A 71-year-old man died of a intracerebral hemorrhage while taking ibuprofen for 4 weeks having also taken *Gingko biloba* extract for 2 years [115]. In a similar manner, a 78-year-old woman developed apraxia induced by an intracerebral hemorrhage while taking *Gingko biloba* in conjunction with chronic warfarin therapy [116]. In addition to possible interactions associated with hemostasis, a 26-year-old man complained of priapism associated with concurrent use of risperidone and ginkgo [117].

Further evidence of possible drug interactions involving *Gingko biloba* is supported by three *in vitro* studies that have shown inhibition of CYP3A4 and P-gp activity, net digoxin flux in intestinal epithelial cells [118], intestinal and hepatic glucuronidation of mycophenolic acid [119], and CYP2B6-mediated hydroxylation of the antidepressant bupropion induced by *Gingko biloba* [120]. Conversely, a clinical trial reported no changes to bupropion basic pharmacokinetic parameters in 14 healthy volunteers [121]. In regard to drug efflux, a clinical study confirmed *in vitro* evidence that repeated ginkgo administration for 14 days led to significantly increased talinolol (a P-gp substrate) plasma concentrations in healthy volunteers [122, 123]. Indeed, there has been conflicting evidence provided by studies assessing the role of ginkgo in affecting drug metabolism.

Contrary to case reports mentioned earlier, a small randomized controlled study concluded that *Gingko biloba* did not enhance clopidogrel antiplatelet activity [124]. Another small randomized controlled study reported no significant changes to plasma concentrations of warfarin enantiomers and clotting status in healthy subjects taking ginkgo for 7 days [125]. Given that CYP2C9 metabolizes warfarin, it is worth noting that levels of tolbutamide and diclofenac, which are metabolized by this enzyme, were not affected after ginkgo administration in healthy individuals [126]. Furthermore, a clinical study determined that CYP1A2, CYP2D6, CYP2E1 and CYP3A4 activities were not affected in healthy volunteers given *Gingko biloba* for 28 days [19]. A later study demonstrated that ginkgo induced CYP2C19, reduced the bioavailability of omeprazole and increased the production of its hydroxylated metabolites [127]. Indeed, a case report described fatal seizures and subtherapeutic levels of phenytoin, which is separately metabolized by CYP2C9 and CYP2C19, in an individual self-medicating with ginkgo [128]. A recent clinical study demonstrated that diazepam (another CYP2C19 substrate) metabolism was unaffected in healthy subjects taking ginkgo extracts orally for 28 days [129]. Finally, a recent study determined that administration of *Gingko biloba* extracts to mice led to significant alterations in the levels of drug metabolizing enzymes, as shown by gene microarray studies [130]. The conflicting evidence regarding drug interactions induced by ginkgo supplementation may be explained by the role of product quality and long-term intake.

Drug Interactions with Ginseng

The intended effects of ginseng are elevated energy, enhanced immune function and antioxidant activity. A variety of different ginseng products are available in the market, including Siberian ginseng (*Eleutherococcus senticosus*), American ginseng (*Panax quinquefolium*) and Korean ginseng (*Panax ginseng*). Siberian ginseng is composed of a heterogeneous group of eleutherosides, and studies assessing its impact on drug interactions have found no clinically relevant changes in CYP3A4 and CYP2D6 activity [131]. American ginseng root extracts are standardized to polysaccharides and were found not to affect the pharmacokinetics of zidovudine [132] or indinavir [133]; however, a double-blind randomized controlled trial reported reduced warfarin plasma levels and subsequent reduction in the International Normalization Ratio (INR) [134].

In contrast to American ginseng, Korean ginseng extracts are generally standardized to ginsenosides, which are large triterpenoid saponins, and Rb-1-2 and Rg1 are considered to be the most abundant and active compounds. In doses greater than 15 g/day, a ginseng abuse syndrome consisting of insomnia, hypertonia and edema has been reported [9]. Breast pain and post-menopausal bleeding has also been associated with ginseng use [9]. It increases clearance of ethanol by induction of both alcohol dehydrogenase and aldehyde dehydrogenase activity. *In vitro* studies have determined that ginseng may also stimulate glucose transport and induce hypoglycemia [135]. This alteration in glucose transport may partly explain the increased clearance of albendazole sulfoxide, which is the active metabolite of the anti-helminthic albendazole [136]. Two case studies have reported possible interactions between ginseng and phenelzine, including induction of mania and full return of depression in a 42-year-old woman [137], and insomnia and tremulousness in a 64-year-old woman [138]. Another case report has described the role of *P. ginseng* from an energy drink cocktail in altering imatinib efflux or metabolism via P-gp or CYP3A4, leading to hepatotoxicity [139]. However, an *in vitro* study has shown that Korean ginseng did not affect CYP3A4 activity [140]. Further clinical studies demonstrated that administration of Korean ginseng for 28 days did not have any effect on the activity of CYP1A2, CYP2D6, CYP2E1 or CYP3A4 [19]. A separate study reported a clinically insignificant reduction in CYP2D6 activity by Korean ginseng [141]. In contrast to American ginseng, administration of Korean ginseng for 14 days did not affect plasma levels of warfarin enantiomers and associated platelet aggregation and INR in healthy volunteers [33].

In summary, studies to date suggest that Korean ginseng has minimal effects on drug metabolism. However, further studies are necessary to strengthen this view. In addition, a past survey identified considerable differences in ginsenoside content between *P. ginseng* preparations [110].

Drug Interactions with Garlic (*Allium sativum*)

Garlic is often used for its antioxidant, lipid-lowering or antihypertensive properties. Its primary unintended effect is platelet dysfunction with hemorrhage. The effects of garlic are due to sulfur-containing compounds, including aliin, allicin and saponins. *In vitro* studies demonstrated that allicin exhibited a concentration-dependent inhibition of ritonavir efflux when tested on MDR1 (P-gp)-transfected epithelial cells and inhibited CYP3A4 activity [142]. Separate *in vitro* studies reported reduced efflux of saquinavir, while conversely increasing efflux of darunavir in hepatocytes after treatment with aged garlic extracts [143]. However, a clinical study indicated that ritonavir pharmacokinetics was not altered by garlic extracts taken for 4 days [144]. An additional clinical study has determined that longer supplementation of garlic for 20 days led to significant decreases in saquinavir [145]. Further animal studies have shown that oral administration of garlic extracts in rabbits can reduce plasma levels of isoniazid, a CYP2E1 substrate [146]. In addition, administration of garlic oil to healthy volunteers for 28 days resulted in a decrease in CYP2E1 activity [19, 141]. Case reports have suggested possible interactions between garlic and warfarin leading to bleeding episodes [147, 148]. In contrast to these case reports, clinical studies failed to demonstrate a significant effect of garlic on warfarin pharmacokinetics or pharmacodynamics [149, 150], but did demonstrate decreased potency in patients expressing wild-type VKORC1 (vitamin K epoxide reductase subunit 1) gene [150]. The significance of this information is that concurrent administration of garlic and CYP2E1 substrates may lead to significant drug interactions. Further caution is advised, since it is possible that longer-term intake of garlic may interfere with antiretroviral therapy.

Drug Interactions with Saw Palmetto (*Serenoa repens*)

Saw palmetto is reported to inhibit dihydrotestosterone binding to androgen receptors and 5α-reductase activity. This is intended to exert an anti-androgenic effect on benign prostatic hyperplasia. The main active phytochemicals include steroids, flavonoids, tannin, oils and resins. Saw palmetto has been shown to potently inhibit CYP2C9, CYP2D6 and

CYP3A4 *in vitro* [151]. Conversely, a clinical study reported no significant effect on CYP1A2, CYP2D6, CYP2E1 or CYP3A4 activity during saw palmetto supplementation for 28 days [105]. In a similar manner, treatment with saw palmetto for 14 days did not alter the metabolism and pharmacokinetics of dextromethorphan (CYP2D6 activity) or alprazolam (CYP3A4 activity) [152]. Although no unintended effects have been reported with saw palmetto, further clinical studies are required to determine whether it affects intestinal drug transporters.

Drug Interactions with Kava (*Piper methysticum*)

Kava is used as a sedative and anxiolytic. It may also induce extrapyramidal effects such as dyskinesia and torticollis, as well as induce hepatotoxicity, which led to the Food and Drug Administration to issue a public health advisory in 2002. Case reports have described reduced efficacy of levodopa due to interactions with kava, leading to exacerbation of Parkinson's disease in a 76-year-old woman [153]. Another case study described a 54-year-old man with lethargy and disorientation while taking the benzodiazepine alprazolam and kava [154].

The active phytochemicals found in kava are called kavalactones, which were found to inhibit CYP2C9, CYP2C19, CYP2D6 and CYP3A4 activities *in vitro* [155, 156]. A more comprehensive *in vitro* study demonstrated that CYP1A2, CYP2C8, CYP2C9, CYP2C19, CYP2D6 and CYP3A4 activities were inhibited in a dose-dependent manner [157]. Conversely, a clinical study determined that kava consumption only inhibited CYP2E1, but not CYP1A2, CYP2D6 or CYP3A4/5, activity [158]. Furthermore, kava supplementation for 14 days did not significantly affect digoxin pharmacokinetics, and thus is unlikely to affect P-gp function [159]. In light of these clinical studies and case reports kava should not be taken with a drug that is a CYP2E1 substrate, and caution is advised while taking dopaminergic drugs and benzodiazepines.

Drug Interactions with Ginger (*Zingiber officinale*)

Ginger is usually taken for nausea and dyspepsia. Its rhizomes contain gingerols (zingerone, zingeberol) and their shogaol derivatives from the drying process, terpenoids, alkanes, paradols and diarylheptanoids. *In vitro* studies have demonstrated that gingerols inhibit serotonin release and subsequent platelet aggregation [160]. A case report described a 76-year-old woman who presented with hematuria and gingival bleeding after taking non-steroidal anti-inflammatory drugs (NSAIDs) while on her regimen of hydrochlorothiazide, warfarin and acetaminophen in addition to self-supplementation with ginger root and powder [161]. However, another clinical study determined that pre-treatment with ginger for 7 days followed by co-administration with warfarin for another 7 days did not affect warfarin pharmacokinetics, INR or platelet aggregation [125].

The role of ginger in enhancing gastric emptying and the associated effect on the pharmacokinetics of extended release drug formulations remains controversial. One clinical study reported no effect of ginger on gastric emptying in healthy volunteers [162], while another study reported delayed gastric emptying in intensive care patients [163]. Conversely, other studies have demonstrated increased gastric emptying in healthy volunteers [164] and in patients with functional dyspepsia [165]. These discrepancies are likely due to different ginger preparations and dose.

Ginger may affect the minimal inhibitory concentration and exhibit synergy with antibiotics, since it was shown that treatment with gingerols increased bacterial membrane permeability and facilitated aminoglycoside entry [166]. In addition, ginger extracts exhibited synergistic action with clarithromycin against *Helicobacter pylori* [167] and were shown to inhibit P-gp function *in vitro* [168].

Drug Interactions with Valerian (*Valeriana officinalis*)

Valerian is taken for its sedative and anxiolytic effects. Active compounds include flavonones, alkaloids and sesquiterpenes. *In vitro* experiments have demonstrated that the flavonone 6-methylapigenin and the sesquiterpene valerenic acid can bind to gamma hydroxybutyric acid (GABA) (A) receptors [169, 170] and thus positively enhance benzodiazepine action. In regard to pharmacokinetics, an *in vitro* study demonstrated that valerian can increase CYP2D6 and CYP3A4 activity [171]. Conversely, the same authors contradicted their earlier findings and determined that valerian inhibited CYP3A4 activity while demonstrating the clinically irrelevant inhibition of digoxin efflux as a measure of P-gp activity at a high dose [118]. Regardless of these findings *in vitro*, a clinical study indicated that pre-treatment with valerian for 14 days did not significantly affect CYP2D6 and CYP3A4 activity in healthy volunteers [172]. Another clinical study demonstrated no changes to CYP1A2, CYP2D6, CYP2E1 or CYP3A4/5 activity after valerian treatment for 28 days [158].

It is unlikely that clinically relevant drug interactions will occur after concomitant use of valerian. However, given that valerian may affect P-gp activity, clinical studies are warranted to investigate this possibility. Although there are no clinically reported adverse effects, it should be recalled that valerian acts through GABA receptors and may counter the symptoms of benzodiazepine withdrawal.

Drug Interactions with Goldenseal (*Hydrastis canadensis*)

Taken for diuretic, laxative, hemostatic and immune enhancement effects, goldenseal may also produce paralysis, oxytocic effects, edema and hypertension. Active components of goldenseal include the alkaloids berberine and hydrastine. Goldenseal has been shown to inhibit CYP2C8, CYP2C9, CYP2C19, CYP2D6 and CYP3A4 activities *in vitro* [173–177]. Moreover, clinical studies demonstrated significant inhibition of CYP3A4/5 and CYP2D6 in healthy volunteers taking goldenseal for 14 or 28 days [106, 158, 178]. In contrast, a separate clinical study demonstrated no effects on the pharmacokinetics of the antiretroviral drug indinavir, a CYP3A4 substrate, in healthy volunteers taking goldenseal for 14 days [179], thus indicating possible differences in supplement composition. The ability of goldenseal to inhibit drug metabolism was further explored by another *in vitro* study which demonstrated significant reduction in the formation of carboxylated active metabolites of the antiviral pro-drug oseltamivir by carboxylesterase-1 [180]. In regard to drug transport, a separate clinical study found no changes to digoxin pharmacokinetics, thus indicating no impact on P-gp activity [159]. Given that goldenseal–drug interactions have been reported in clinical studies, caution is advised when monitoring drugs which are metabolized by CYP3A4/5 and CYP2D6.

Drug Interactions with Green Tea (*Camellia sinensis*)

Green tea is taken for its anti-inflammatory and anticancer properties. The antioxidant properties of green tea are maintained through dehydration of the leaves, and the main active component is the flavanol epigallocatechin gallate. Catechins from green tea extract have been found to inhibit the expression of CYP1A expression *in vitro* [181, 182]. Further studies in rats have determined that repeated administration of green tea extracts can alter midazolam levels, depending on the route of administration. Increased plasma levels of midazolam were found after oral administration, while the opposite was found after intravenous administration due to decreased intestinal CYP3A4 and increased hepatic CYP3A4 expression and activity, respectively [183]. In contrast, clinical studies have determined that administration of green tea extracts to healthy volunteers for 14 days did not affect either CYP3A4 or CYP2D6 [184]. Furthermore, another clinical study demonstrated no clinical effects on CYP1A2, CYP2D6, CYP2C9 and CYP3A4 activity after 4 weeks of green tea catechin administration [185]. Green tea extracts have been found to potently inhibit intestinal sulfotransferase SULT1A1 and hepatic SULT1A3 activities *in vitro* [186,187], but these observations have yet to be verified in humans.

Green tea and its components have been found to exhibit synergy with a number of agents with respect to antitumorigenic properties *in vitro* and *in vivo* [188]. Although these findings may suggest synergistic mechanisms, inhibition of efflux pumps may play a key role in maintaining high concentrations of co-administered drugs. Theanine, which is a major amino acid in green tea and is also a glutamate analog, was shown to interfere with glutamate transport, which in turn inhibited doxorubicin efflux from tumor cells *in vitro* [189, 190]. Further studies have revealed the role of green tea catechins in inhibiting P-gp function, leading to accumulation of doxorubicin in tumor xenografts *in vivo* [191]. Similarly, several components of green tea were found to inhibit P-gp function *in vitro*, which would lead to increased bioavailability of co-administered drugs [192]. Green tea extracts have also been found to enhance uptake of cationic organic compounds [193] and significantly inhibit OATP *in vitro* [108]. While results from clinical studies do not seem to indicate significant effects on cytochrome P450 enzymes, the role of green tea in altering P-gp activity warrants further investigation. Potential synergistic effects of green tea extracts with cancer therapeutics may be due to selective inhibition of P-gp and drug efflux pumps as seen *in vitro*, and these observations need to be verified with further clinical studies.

Drug Interactions with Curcumin (*Curcuma longa*)

Also known as turmeric, curcumin has anti-inflammatory, antispasmodic, and antioxidant effects. The major natural phenolic compounds found in the rhizomes are the curcuminoids. In regard to drug metabolism, curcumin does not affect CYP3A4 expression in human hepatocytes and intestinal cells *in vitro* [194, 195]. Similarly, another study has found no effect on CYP3A4 expression in human intestinal epithelial cells by curcumin; however, it was found to inhibit CYP3A4 activity [196]. Further studies have determined significant competitive inhibition of human recombinant CYP1A2, CYP2B6 and CYP3A4, and a non-competitive type of inhibition of CYP2C9 and CYP2D6 [197]. Similarly, curcuminoid extracts competitively inhibited CYP3A activity as opposed to the non-competitive inhibition on CYP2C9 and CYP2C19 activities, and lesser impact on CYP1A2, CYP2D6 and CYP2E1 activities [198]. In contrast, curcumin at any concentration did not appreciably inhibit CYP2C8/9, CYP2D6 or CYP3A4 activity in human hepatocytes *ex vivo* [199]. However, a recent clinical study has determined that administration of curcumin for 14 days to healthy volunteers inhibits CYP1A2 function but enhances CYP2A6 activity [200].

Many *in vitro* studies have demonstrated synergistic effects with other drugs [201]. In addition to possible synergistic effector pathways, curcumin may be altering drug transport to potentiate the effects of co-administered drugs. Indeed, curcumin and its active curcuminoids have been found to significantly inhibit multi-drug resistance protein MRP-1 and MRP-2 efflux pumps *in vitro* [202–205]. Lending further support to these findings, other studies have found that curcumin inhibits P-gp in multi-drug resistant cell lines [205–208]. Further studies in mice have determined that curcumin inhibited P-gp function by reducing sulfasalazine efflux [209]. In contrast, a clinical study has demonstrated diminished talinolol (a P-gp substrate) plasma levels, after a single dose in healthy volunteers given curcumin for 6 days [210]. This unexpected activity may have been due to metabolism of curcumin and insufficient duration and dose of curcumin to observe a specific inhibitory effect on P-gp function [210].

Although multiple studies *in vitro* have led to mixed conclusions regarding the role of curcumin in affecting cytochrome P450 activity, one clinical trial determined mixed results where CYP1A2 function was upregulated as opposed to CYP2A6 activity which was reduced. Further clinical studies resulted in an unexpected decrease in P-gp substrate, but this may have been due to the study design. Clearly, more clinical studies are needed to further investigate the role of curcumin in drug metabolism and absorption.

Drug Interactions with Black Cohosh (*Actaea racemosa*)

Used for its antirheumatic and antispasmodic properties, black cohosh is also well known to prevent uterine contractions and reduce the frequency and intensity of hot flashes associated with menopausal disorders. Black cohosh was found to inhibit CYP2B6, CYP2C19 and CYP2E1 in isolated human hepatic microsomes [177]. Another study confirmed the inhibition of CYP2C19 by black cohosh extracts *in vitro* [211]. A separate study reported inhibition of recombinant CYP3A4 *in vitro* [212]. Another study extended these findings to include the inhibition of CYP1A2, CYP2D6 and CYP2C9, in addition to CYP3A4, in cultured hepatocytes [213]. In contrast, a later study demonstrated no effects on human hepatic microsomal CYP3A4 activity [140]. Further support for these data was shown by following administration of black cohosh for 14 days to healthy volunteers; there was a lack of significant effect on CYP3A [214] or CYP2D6 [106] activity. A further study by the same authors demonstrated weak inhibition of CYP2D6 when black cohosh was administered to healthy individuals for 28 days; however, this was considered to be clinically irrelevant [158].

Investigations into the role of black cohosh in drug transport have demonstrated that black cohosh significantly inhibits estrone uptake in epithelial cells, thus suggesting possible inhibition of OATP [108]. Black cohosh may act synergistically with other therapeutics, as shown by enhancement of cytotoxicity of doxorubicin (a P-gp substrate) and docetaxel in murine breast cancer cells [215]. However, a clinical study has determined that administration of black cohosh to healthy volunteers for 14 days did not affect digoxin pharmacokinetics, thus indicating no effect on P-gp function [216]. Although many *in vitro* studies have demonstrated the role of black cohosh in affecting cytochrome P450 enzymes and drug transport proteins, follow-up clinical studies have shown no effect. Further clinical studies investigating the effect of black cohosh on other cytochrome P450 enzymes are needed to confirm the minimal drug interactions.

Drug Interactions with Milk Thistle (*Silybum marianum*)

Milk thistle is taken for its beneficial properties in treating hepatitis and liver cirrhosis. The antioxidant action of milk thistle confers further protection against hepatotoxicity during chemotherapy. Active ingredients of milk thistle seeds are found in silymarin, which is a mixture of the flavolignans silibinin (silybin), isosilibilin, silichristin and silidianin.

Silibinin was shown to significantly inhibit recombinant CYP3A4 and CYP2C9 activities [217] and downregulate CYP3A4 expression *in vitro* [218]. However, silibinin did not alter CYP3A4 activity in intestinal epithelial cells [142]. In support of this observation, a clinical study composed of healthy volunteers taking milk thistle for 3 weeks demonstrated no significant changes to the pharmacokinetics of indinavir [219], a substrate of CYP3A4. In a similar manner, separate clinical studies reported no effects on indinavir plasma levels after administration of silymarin for 14 days [220] or 28 days [221] in healthy individuals. These findings were further confirmed with another clinical study which demonstrated no effect on midazolam or irinotecan pharmacokinetics, and thus CYP3A4 activity, in healthy subjects taking milk thistle for 14 days [214, 222]. Furthermore, pre-treatment with silymarin did not affect the pharmacokinetics of a single dose of nifedipine, a CYP3A4 substrate [223]. Moreover, another clinical study demonstrated no effects on CYP2D6 activity after administration of milk thistle for 14 days [106]. A more extensive study demonstrated that administration of milk thistle to healthy subjects for 28 days did not affect CYP1A2, CYP2D6, CYP2E1 or CYP3A4 activity [105]. However, in another study milk thistle extracts were shown to inhibit CYP2C8 but not CYP1A2, CYP2C9, CYP2C19, CYP2D6, CYP2E1 and CYP3A4 in human hepatic microsomes [176]. Conversely, an *in vitro* study demonstrated inhibition of warfarin hydroxylation by CYP2C9, which may pose a risk for adverse bleeding events [224]. Finally, an *in vitro* study indicated possible interactions between milk thistle extract and CYP2C8 and CYP2C9, but that interactions are unlikely for CYP2C19, CYP2D6 and CYP3A4 [225].

In regard to cellular drug transport, silibinin did not alter P-gp mediated efflux of ritonavir in intestinal epithelial cells [142]. This finding was confirmed in a clinical study which reported no changes in digoxin pharmacokinetics and thus P-gp function after administration of milk thistle for 14 days [216]. The general consensus among *in vitro* and clinical trials indicates minimal impact on cytochrome P450 enzymes and drug transport by milk thistle. However, the role of milk thistle in inhibiting CYP2C8 and CYP2C9, which more specifically may affect warfarin metabolism, warrants further investigations in clinical studies.

CONTAMINATION OF HERBAL SUPPLEMENTS

In order to predict the effects of supplements on therapeutic drug monitoring, it is necessary to possess an understanding of the production process to predict the presence of adulterants, contaminants and toxins. Conflicting evidence from clinical trials regarding drug–herb interactions may be due to differences in herbal production. To control any variations, some clinical studies administered the purified active components of the herbal supplement in question. However, given the lack of standardized manufacturing processes, variations in the compositions of herbal supplements are likely to cause different effects and increase the confusion regarding the outcomes of many research studies. A study utilized high-performance liquid chromatography or gas chromatography to report considerable differences in the compositions of commercially available herbal supplements [110]. In addition, a number of herbal medicines have been found to induce hepatotoxicity through direct action or due to contamination with toxic compounds [226]. The induction of hepatotoxicity can alter drug metabolic pathways, which can further lead to potential drug interactions. With the lack of standardized practices, the induction of hepatotoxicity due to contaminants, and the increased likelihood of herbal supplements being taken in combinations, the threat of potential drug interactions remains very high.

ANALYTICAL INTERFERENCES CAUSED BY SOME HERBAL SUPPLEMENTS

While herbal supplements may cause unexpected changes to drug pharmacokinetics due to alterations of cytochrome P450 activity and drug transport proteins, they can also cause direct interferences to laboratory methods through immunological mechanisms. To date, traditional Chinese medicines have been shown to cross-react with antibodies against digoxin in a number of commercial assays. A more detailed discussion of this phenomenon is provided in Chapter 11 of this book. Briefly, Chan Su, which is prepared from secretions from Chinese toads, is used for its cardioprotective effects in a similar manner to digoxin. Indeed, both Chan Su and digoxin exhibit structural similarities which form the basis of the direct interference seen with immunoassays, particularly with fluorescence polarization immunoassays as compared to microparticle enzyme-based methods [227]. It was found that since Chan Su strongly binds to serum proteins, in contrast to digoxin, measuring free digoxin obtained with ultrafiltration will overcome this limitation with some immunoassays [227]. In a similar manner, Dan Shen, which is prepared from the roots of *Salvia miltiorrhiza*, is another Chinese medicine used for its cardioprotective effects. Given its structural similarity to digoxin, Dan Shen also exhibits direct interferences with fluorescence polarization detection, but not microparticle enzyme-based immunoassays [228].

CONCLUSIONS

While it is clear that studies have extensively demonstrated drug interactions induced by supplements such as St John's wort and grapefruit, the role of other supplements in this

TABLE 19.4 Clinically Based Evidence on Herbal Supplement Interference with Drug Bioavailability

Herbal supplement	Impact on biotransformation	Affected drugs
St John's wort (*Hypericum perforatum*)	*Inducers:* CYP3A4 [19, 21, 24, 31, 32, 36, 38–40, 42], CYP2E1 [19], CYP2C19 [38, 43], P-gp [20, 24, 29, 30, 44]	Midazolam [19, 21], chlorzoxazone [19], cyclosporine A [23], tacrolimus [24], norethindrone [25, 26], ethinyl estradiol [25, 26], 3-ketodesogestrel [27], methadone [28], digoxin [29], talinolol [30], ivabradine [31], verapamil [32], warfarin [33], indinavir [34], gliclazide [35], simvastatin[36], atorvastatin [37], omeprazole [38], oxycodone [39], irinotecan [40], imatinib [41, 42], voriconazole [43], fexofenadine [44]
Echinacea (*Echinacea* spp.)	*Inhibitor:* CYP1A2 [103] *Inducer:* hepatic CYP3A4 [103]	Caffeine [103], intravenous midazolam [103]
Ginkgo (*Ginkgo biloba*)	*Inhibitor:* P-gp [122, 123] There is conflicting clinical evidence regarding alterations to cytochrome P450 by ginkgo; further studies will need to assess the role of product quality and long-term ginkgo intake	Talinolol [122, 123]
Ginseng (*Panax* spp.)	American ginseng (*Panax quinquefolium*): reduction in INR [134]	Warfarin [134]
Garlic (*Allium sativum*)	*Inhibitor:* CYP2E1 [19, 141] Studies assessing longer-term intake of garlic may further shed light on possible interferences to other cytochrome P450 enzymes; clinical studies have yet to determine effects on P-gp	Saquinavir [145], chlorzoxazone [19, 141]
Saw palmetto (*Seronoa repens*)	To date, no significant effect on CYP1A2, CYP2D6, CYP2E1 or CYP3A4 activities.	
Kava (*Schisandra sphenanthera*)	*Inhibitor:* CYP2E1 [158]	Chlorzoxazone [158]
Ginger (*Zingiber officinale*)	To date, studies have not demonstrated any changes to cytochrome P450 enzyme activity; however, the role of ginger in enhancing gastric emptying, which will affect the pharmacokinetics of delayed release drugs, remains controversial and discrepancies are likely due to different ginger preparations and dose	N/A

Herb	Notes	Examples
Valerian (*Valeriana officinalis*)	To date, clinical studies have demonstrated no changes to CYP1A2, CYP2D6, CYP2E1 or CYP3A4/5 activity.	N/A
Goldenseal (*Hydrastis canadensis*)	*Inhibitor*: CYP2D6 [106, 158, 178] Conflicting reports of inhibition of CYP3A4 likely indicate differences in goldenseal preparations	Debrisoquin [106, 158, 178]
Grapefruit (*Citrus paradisi*)	*Inhibitor*: CYP3A4 [55, 62–66] While a single intake of grapefruit juice may alter intestinal CYP3A4, repeated consumption may proceed to inhibit hepatic CYP3A4 *Inhibitor*: OATP [70–73]	Felodipine [46, 50, 51, 55, 62], nifedipine [46, 50, 51], pranidipine [46, 50, 51], amlodipine [56], 17-β-estradiol [57], estrone [57], cyclosporine [58–61], prednisone [58]
Green tea (*Camellia sinensis*)	Conflicting reports may be due to decreased intestinal CYP3A4 and increased hepatic CYP3A4 expression and activity [183] Additional clinical studies are needed to verify inhibition of P-gp and OATP	Midazolam [183] May exhibit synergistic effects with anticancer agents by inhibiting drug efflux
Curcumin (*Curcuma longa*)	*Inhibitor*: CYP1A2 [200] *Inducer*: CYP2A6 [200] *Inducer*: P-gp [210] Unexpected activity on P-gp may need to be verified with known profiles of inter-subject variation in metabolism and longer-duration and higher doses of curcumin	Caffeine [200], talinolol [210]
Black cohosh (*Actaea racemosa*)	To date, black cohosh has been found not to significantly inhibit CYP1A2, CYP2D6, CYP2E1, CYP3A4 and P-gp	N/A
Milk thistle (*Silybum marianum*)	To date, no effect on CYP1A2, CYP2C9, CYP2D6, CYP2E1 and CYP3A4 has been identified	N/A

phenomenon warrants further investigation. Clinically important drug—herb interactions are summarized in Table 19.4. Inter-subject variability, dosing, timing, and lack of standardized practices in the production of herbal supplements may be responsible for the conflicting results between some studies. Clearly, more research focusing on the effects of herbal supplements on drug bioavailability, metabolism and excretion is needed. In addition to clinical studies, further elucidation of the molecular mechanisms behind drug—herb interactions will assist in identifying the root cause of discrepant results obtained from therapeutic drug monitoring. Further knowledge gained in this field will prevent an unnecessary drain on resources. Indeed, awareness by the clinical team is needed, and should be considered in the case of spurious results from the laboratory. Although laboratory personnel typically do not have access to the clinical history of the patient, they should consider the possibility of herbal interferences in the case of analytical interferences regarding therapeutic drug monitoring.

References

[1] Eisenberg DM, Davis RB, Ettner SL, et al. Trends in alternative medicine use in the United States, 1990—1997: results of a follow-up national survey. J Am Med Assoc 1998;280:1569—75.

[2] Eisenberg DM, Kessler RC, Foster C, et al. Unconventional medicine in the United States. Prevalence, costs, and patterns of use. N Engl J Med 1993;328:246—52.

[3] Bronstein AC, Spyker DA, Cantilena LR, et al. 2009 Annual Report of the American Association of Poison Control Centers' National Poison Data System (NPDS): 27th Annual Report. Clin Toxicol 2010;48:979—1178.

[4] Colalto C. Herbal interactions on absorption of drugs: Mechanisms of action and clinical risk assessment. Pharmacol Res 2010;62:207—27.

[5] König J. Uptake transporters of the human OATP family. Drug Transporters 2011;201:1—28.

[6] Kim RB. Organic anion-transporting polypeptide (OATP) transporter family and drug disposition. Eur J Clin Invest 2003;33:1—5.

[7] Cascorbi I. P-glycoprotein: tissue distribution, substrates, and functional consequences of genetic variations. Drug Transporters 2011;201:261—83.

[8] Cavaliere C, Rea P, Blumenthal M. Herbal supplement sales experience slight increase in 2008. HerbalGram, J Am Bot Assoc 2009;82:58—61.

[9] Miller LG. Herbal medicinals: selected clinical considerations focusing on known or potential drug—herb interactions. Arch Intern Med 1998;158:2200—11.

[10] Spinella M, Eaton LA. Hypomania induced by herbal and pharmaceutical psychotropic medicines following mild traumatic brain injury. Brain Inj 2002;16:359—67.

[11] Dannawi M. Possible serotonin syndrome after combination of buspirone and St John's wort. J Psychopharmacol 2002;16:401.

[12] Bonetto N, Santelli L, Battistin L, Cagnin A. Serotonin syndrome and rhabdomyolysis induced by concomitant use of triptans, fluoxetine and hypericum. Cephalalgia 2007;27:1421—3.

[13] Lantz MS, Buchalter E, Giambanco V. St John's wort and antidepressant drug interactions in the elderly. J Geriatr Psychiatry Neurol 1999;12:7—10.

[14] Gordon JB. SSRIs and St. John's wort: possible toxicity? Am Fam Physician 1998;57:950—3.

[15] Barbenel DM, Yusufi B, O'Shea D, Bench CJ. Mania in a patient receiving testosterone replacement post-orchidectomy taking St John's wort and sertraline. J Psychopharmacol 2000;14:84—6.

[16] Butterweck V. Mechanism of action of St John's wort in depression: what is known? CNS Drugs 2003;17:539—62.

[17] Moore LB, Goodwin B, Jones SA, et al. St John's wort induces hepatic drug metabolism through activation of the pregnane X receptor. Proc Natl Acad Sci 2000;97:7500—2.

[18] Obach RS. Inhibition of human cytochrome P450 enzymes by constituents of St John's wort, an herbal preparation used in the treatment of depression. J Pharmacol Exper Therapeut 2000;294:88—95.

[19] Gurley BJ, Gardner SF, Hubbard MA, et al. Cytochrome P450 phenotypic ratios for predicting herb–drug interactions in humans. Clin Pharmacol Ther 2002;72:276–87.

[20] Hennessy M, Kelleher D, Spiers JP, et al. St Johns wort increases expression of P-glycoprotein: implications for drug interactions. Br J Clin Pharmacol 2002;53:75–82.

[21] Hafner V, Jager M, Matthee AK, et al. Effect of simultaneous induction and inhibition of CYP3A by St John's wort and ritonavir on CYP3A activity. Clin Pharmacol Ther 2009;87:191–6.

[22] Ruschitzka F, Meier PJ, Turina M, et al. Acute heart transplant rejection due to Saint John's wort. Lancet 2000;355:548–9.

[23] Bauer S, Stormer E, Johne A, et al. Alterations in cyclosporin A pharmacokinetics and metabolism during treatment with St John's wort in renal transplant patients. Br J Clin Pharmacol 2003;55:203–11.

[24] Hebert MF, Park JM, Chen Y-L, et al. Effects of St John's wort (*Hypericum perforatum*) on tacrolimus pharmacokinetics in healthy volunteers. J Clin Pharmacol 2004;44:89–94.

[25] Murphy PA, Kern SE, Stanczyk FZ, Westhoff CL. Interaction of St John's wort with oral contraceptives: effects on the pharmacokinetics of norethindrone and ethinyl estradiol, ovarian activity and breakthrough bleeding. Contraception 2005;71:402–8.

[26] Hall SD, Wang Z, Huang S-M, et al. The interaction between St John's wort and an oral contraceptive. Clin Pharmacol Ther 2003;74:525–35.

[27] Pfrunder A, Schiesser M, Gerber S, et al. Interaction of St John's wort with low-dose oral contraceptive therapy: a randomized controlled trial. Br J Clin Pharmacol 2003;56:683–90.

[28] Eich-Höchli D, Oppliger R, Golay KP, et al. Methadone maintenance treatment and St John's wort. Pharmacopsychiatry 2003;36:35–7.

[29] Johne A, Brockmoller J, Bauer S, et al. Pharmacokinetic interaction of digoxin with an herbal extract from St John's wort (*Hypericum perforatum*). Clin Pharmacol Ther 1999;66:338–45.

[30] Schwarz UI, Hanso H, Oertel R, et al. Induction of intestinal P-glycoprotein by St John's wort reduces the oral bioavailability of talinolol. Clin Pharmacol Ther 2007;81:669–78.

[31] Portolés A, Terleira A, Calvo A, et al. Effects of *Hypericum perforatum* on ivabradine pharmacokinetics in healthy volunteers: an open-label, pharmacokinetic interaction clinical trial. J Clin Pharmacol 2006;46: 1188–94.

[32] Tannergren C, Engman H, Knutson L, et al. St John's wort decreases the bioavailability of *R*- and *S*-verapamil through induction of the first-pass metabolism. Clin Pharmacol Ther 2004;75:298–309.

[33] Jiang X, Williams KM, Liauw WS, et al. Effect of St John's wort and ginseng on the pharmacokinetics and pharmacodynamics of warfarin in healthy subjects. Br J Clin Pharmacol 2004;57:592–9.

[34] Piscitelli SC, Burstein AH, Chaitt D, et al. Indinavir concentrations and St John's wort. Lancet 2000;355:547–8.

[35] Xu H, Williams KM, Liauw WS, et al. Effects of St John's wort and CYP2C9 genotype on the pharmacokinetics and pharmacodynamics of gliclazide. Br J Pharmacol 2008;153:1579–86.

[36] Sugimoto K, Ohmori M, Tsuruoka S, et al. Different effects of St John's wort on the pharmacokinetics of simvastatin and pravastatin. Clin Pharmacol Ther 2001;70:518–24.

[37] Andrén L, Andreasson Å, Eggertsen R. Interaction between a commercially available St John's wort product (Movina) and atorvastatin in patients with hypercholesterolemia. Eur J Clin Pharmacol 2007;63:913–6.

[38] Wang L-S, Zhou G, Zhu B, et al. St John's wort induces both cytochrome P450 3A4-catalyzed sulfoxidation and 2C19-dependent hydroxylation of omeprazole. Clin Pharmacol Ther 2004;75:191–7.

[39] Nieminen TH, Hagelberg NM, Saari TI, et al. St John's wort greatly reduces the concentrations of oral oxycodone. European Journal of Pain 2010;14:854–9.

[40] Mathijssen RHJ, Verweij J, de Bruijn P, et al. Effects of St John's wort on irinotecan metabolism. Journal of the National Cancer Institute 2002;94:1247–9.

[41] Smith P, Bullock JM, Booker BM, et al. The influence of St John's wort on the pharmacokinetics and protein binding of imatinib mesylate. Pharmacotherapy 2004;24:1508–14.

[42] Frye RF, Fitzgerald SM, Lagattuta TF, et al. Effect of St John's wort on imatinib mesylate pharmacokinetics. Clin Pharmacol Ther 2004;76:323–9.

[43] Rengelshausen J, Banfield M, Riedel K-D, et al. Opposite effects of short-term and long-term St John's wort intake on voriconazole pharmacokinetics. Clin Pharmacol Ther 2005;78:25–33.

[44] Wang Z, Hamman MA, Huang SM, et al. Effect of St John's wort on the pharmacokinetics of fexofenadine. Clin Pharmacol Ther 2002;71:414–20.

[45] Kakar SM, Paine MF, Stewart PW, Watkins PB. 6'7'-Dihydroxybergamottin contributes to the grapefruit juice effect. Clin Pharmacol Ther 2004;75:569–79.

[46] Goosen TC, Cillie D, Bailey DG, et al. Bergamottin contribution to the grapefruit juice–felodipine interaction and disposition in humans. Clin Pharmacol Ther 2004;76:607–17.

[47] Paine MF, Widmer WW, Hart HL, et al. A furanocoumarin-free grapefruit juice establishes furanocoumarins as the mediators of the grapefruit juice–felodipine interaction. Am J Clin Nutr 2006;83:1097–105.

[48] Bailey DG, Dresser GK, Leake BF, Kim RB. Naringin is a major and selective clinical inhibitor of organic anion-transporting polypeptide 1A2 (OATP1A2) in grapefruit juice. Clin Pharmacol Ther 2007;81:495–502.

[49] Paine MF, Widmer WW, Pusek SN, et al. Further characterization of a furanocoumarin-free grapefruit juice on drug disposition: studies with cyclosporine. Am J Clin Nutr 2008;87:863–71.

[50] Bailey DG, Spence JD, Munoz C, Arnold JM. Interaction of citrus juices with felodipine and nifedipine. Lancet 1991;337:268–9.

[51] Hashimoto K, Shirafuji T, Sekino H, et al. Interaction of citrus juices with pranidipine, a new 1, 4-dihydropyridine calcium antagonist, in healthy subjects. Eur J Clin Pharmacol 1998;54:753–60.

[52] Bailey DG, Arnold JM, Munoz C, Spence JD. Grapefruit juice–felodipine interaction: mechanism, predictability, and effect of naringin. Clin Pharmacol Ther 1993;53:637–42.

[53] Rashid J, McKinstry C, Renwick AG, et al. Quercetin, an *in vitro* inhibitor of CYP3A, does not contribute to the interaction between nifedipine and grapefruit juice. Br J Clin Pharmacol 1993;36:460–3.

[54] Fuhr U, Kummert AL. The fate of naringin in humans: a key to grapefruit juice–drug interactions? Clin Pharmacol Ther 1995;58:365–73.

[55] Lundahl J, Regardh CG, Edgar B, Johnsson G. Relationship between time of intake of grapefruit juice and its effect on pharmacokinetics and pharmacodynamics of felodipine in healthy subjects. Eur J Clin Pharmacol 1995;49:61–7.

[56] Josefsson M, Zackrisson AL, Ahlner J. Effect of grapefruit juice on the pharmacokinetics of amlodipine in healthy volunteers. Eur J Clin Pharmacol 1996;51:189–93.

[57] Schubert W, Cullberg G, Edgar B, Hedner T. Inhibition of 17 beta-estradiol metabolism by grapefruit juice in ovariectomized women. Maturitas 1994;20:155–63.

[58] Hollander AA, van Rooij J, Lentjes GW, et al. The effect of grapefruit juice on cyclosporine and prednisone metabolism in transplant patients. Clin Pharmacol Ther 1995;57:318–24.

[59] Brunner LJ, Pai KS, Munar MY, et al. Effect of grapefruit juice on cyclosporin A pharmacokinetics in pediatric renal transplant patients. Pediatr Transplant 2000;4:313–21.

[60] Hermann M, Asberg A, Reubsaet JL, et al. Intake of grapefruit juice alters the metabolic pattern of cyclosporin A in renal transplant recipients. Intl J Clin Pharmacol Ther 2002;40:451–6.

[61] Ioannides-Demos LL, Christophidis N, Ryan P, et al. Dosing implications of a clinical interaction between grapefruit juice and cyclosporine and metabolite concentrations in patients with autoimmune diseases. J Rheumatol 1997;24:49–54.

[62] Lundahl J, Regardh CG, Edgar B, Johnsson G. Effects of grapefruit juice ingestion–pharmacokinetics and haemodynamics of intravenously and orally administered felodipine in healthy men. Eur J Clin Pharmacol 1997;52:139–45.

[63] Ho PC, Chalcroft SC, Coville PF, Wanwimolruk S. Grapefruit juice has no effect on quinine pharmacokinetics. Eur J Clin Pharmacol 1999;55:393–8.

[64] Lundahl JU, Regardh CG, Edgar B, Johnsson G. The interaction effect of grapefruit juice is maximal after the first glass. Eur J Clin Pharmacol 1998;54:75–81.

[65] Lilja JJ, Kivisto KT, Backman JT, Neuvonen PJ. Effect of grapefruit juice dose on grapefruit juice–triazolam interaction: repeated consumption prolongs triazolam half-life. Eur J Clin Pharmacol 2000;56:411–5.

[66] Greenblatt DJ, von Moltke LL, Harmatz JS, et al. Time course of recovery of cytochrome P450 3A function after single doses of grapefruit juice. Clin Pharmacol Ther 2003;74:121–9.

[67] Maish WA, Hampton EM, Whitsett TL, et al. Influence of grapefruit juice on caffeine pharmacokinetics and pharmacodynamics. Pharmacotherapy 1996;16:1046–52.

[68] Becquemont L, Verstuyft C, Kerb R, et al. Effect of grapefruit juice on digoxin pharmacokinetics in humans. Clin Pharmacol Ther 2001;70:311–6.

[69] Dresser GK, Bailey DG, Leake BF, et al. Fruit juices inhibit organic anion transporting polypeptide-mediated drug uptake to decrease the oral availability of fexofenadine. Clin Pharmacol Ther 2002;71:11–20.

[70] Dresser GK, Kim RB, Bailey DG. Effect of grapefruit juice volume on the reduction of fexofenadine bioavailability: possible role of organic anion transporting polypeptides. Clin Pharmacol Ther 2005;77:170–7.

[71] Schwarz UI, Seemann D, Oertel R, et al. Grapefruit juice ingestion significantly reduces talinolol bioavailability. Clin Pharmacol Ther 2005;77:291–301.

[72] Tapaninen T, Neuvonen PJ, Niemi M. Grapefruit juice greatly reduces the plasma concentrations of the OATP2B1 and CYP3A4 substrate aliskiren. Clin Pharmacol Ther 2010;88:339–42.

[73] Banfield C, Gupta S, Marino M, et al. Grapefruit juice reduces the oral bioavailability of fexofenadine but not desloratadine. Clin Pharmacokinet 2002;41:311–8.

[74] Fuhr U, Maier-Bruggemann A, Blume H, et al. Grapefruit juice increases oral nimodipine bioavailability. Intl J Clin Pharmacol Ther 1998;36:126–32.

[75] Libersa CC, Brique SA, Motte KB, et al. Dramatic inhibition of amiodarone metabolism induced by grapefruit juice. Br J Clin Pharmacol 2000;49:373–8.

[76] Ho PC, Ghose K, Saville D, Wanwimolruk S. Effect of grapefruit juice on pharmacokinetics and pharmacodynamics of verapamil enantiomers in healthy volunteers. Eur J Clin Pharmacol 2000;56:693–8.

[77] Fuhr U, Muller-Peltzer H, Kern R, et al. Effects of grapefruit juice and smoking on verapamil concentrations in steady state. Eur J Clin Pharmacol 2002;58:45–53.

[78] Lilja JJ, Kivisto KT, Neuvonen PJ. Grapefruit juice increases serum concentrations of atorvastatin and has no effect on pravastatin. Clin Pharmacol Ther 1999;66:118–27.

[79] Kantola T, Kivisto KT, Neuvonen PJ. Grapefruit juice greatly increases serum concentrations of lovastatin and lovastatin acid. Clin Pharmacol Ther 1998;63:397–402.

[80] Lilja JJ, Kivisto KT, Neuvonen PJ. Grapefruit juice–simvastatin interaction: effect on serum concentrations of simvastatin, simvastatin acid, and HMG-CoA reductase inhibitors. Clin Pharmacol Ther 1998;64:477–83.

[81] Lilja JJ, Kivisto KT, Neuvonen PJ. Duration of effect of grapefruit juice on the pharmacokinetics of the CYP3A4 substrate simvastatin. Clin Pharmacol Ther 2000;68:384–90.

[82] Lilja JJ, Neuvonen M, Neuvonen PJ. Effects of regular consumption of grapefruit juice on the pharmacokinetics of simvastatin. Br J Clin Pharmacol 2004;58:56–60.

[83] Andersen V, Pedersen N, Larsen NE, et al. Intestinal first pass metabolism of midazolam in liver cirrhosis – effect of grapefruit juice. Br J Clin Pharmacol 2002;54:120–4.

[84] Kupferschmidt HH, Ha HR, Ziegler WH, et al. Interaction between grapefruit juice and midazolam in humans. Clin Pharmacol Ther 1995;58:20–8.

[85] Hukkinen SK, Varhe A, Olkkola KT, Neuvonen PJ. Plasma concentrations of triazolam are increased by concomitant ingestion of grapefruit juice. Clin Pharmacol Ther 1995;58:127–31.

[86] Sugimoto K, Araki N, Ohmori M, et al. Interaction between grapefruit juice and hypnotic drugs: comparison of triazolam and quazepam. Eur J Clin Pharmacol 2006;62:209–15.

[87] Culm-Merdek KE, von Moltke LL, Gan L, et al. Effect of extended exposure to grapefruit juice on cytochrome P450 3A activity in humans: comparison with ritonavir. Clin Pharmacol Ther 2006;79:243–54.

[88] Christensen H, Asberg A, Holmboe AB, Berg KJ. Coadministration of grapefruit juice increases systemic exposure of diltiazem in healthy volunteers. Eur J Clin Pharmacol 2002;58:515–20.

[89] Garg SK, Kumar N, Bhargava VK, Prabhakar SK. Effect of grapefruit juice on carbamazepine bioavailability in patients with epilepsy. Clin Pharmacol Ther 1998;64:286–8.

[90] Lilja JJ, Kivisto KT, Backman JT, et al. Grapefruit juice substantially increases plasma concentrations of buspirone. Clin Pharmacol Ther 1998;64:655–60.

[91] Cheng KL, Nafziger AN, Peloquin CA, Amsden GW. Effect of grapefruit juice on clarithromycin pharmacokinetics. Antimicrob Agents Chemother 1998;42:927–9.

[92] Kupferschmidt HH, Fattinger KE, Ha HR, et al. Grapefruit juice enhances the bioavailability of the HIV protease inhibitor saquinavir in man. Br J Clin Pharmacol 1998;45:355–9.

[93] Cuong BT, Binh VQ, Dai B, et al. Does gender, food or grapefruit juice alter the pharmacokinetics of primaquine in healthy subjects? Br J Clin Pharmacol 2006;61:682–9.

[94] Lilja JJ, Backman JT, Laitila J, et al. Itraconazole increases but grapefruit juice greatly decreases plasma concentrations of celiprolol. Clin Pharmacol Ther 2003;73:192–8.

[95] Gubbins PO, McConnell SA, Gurley BJ, et al. Influence of grapefruit juice on the systemic availability of itraconazole oral solution in healthy adult volunteers. Pharmacotherapy 2004;24:460–7.

[96] Charbit B, Becquemont L, Lepere B, et al. Pharmacokinetic and pharmacodynamic interaction between grapefruit juice and halofantrine. Clin Pharmacol Ther 2002;72:514—23.

[97] Kivisto KT, Lilja JJ, Backman JT, Neuvonen PJ. Repeated consumption of grapefruit juice considerably increases plasma concentrations of cisapride. Clin Pharmacol Ther 1999;66:448—53.

[98] Jetter A, Kinzig-Schippers M, Walchner-Bonjean M, et al. Effects of grapefruit juice on the pharmacokinetics of sildenafil. Clin Pharmacol Ther 2002;71:21—9.

[99] Seidegard J, Randvall G, Nyberg L, Borga O. Grapefruit juice interaction with oral budesonide: equal effect on immediate-release and delayed-release formulations. Pharmazie 2009;64:461—5.

[100] Yin OQ, Gallagher N, Li A, et al. Effect of grapefruit juice on the pharmacokinetics of nilotinib in healthy participants. J Clin Pharmacol 2010;50:188—94.

[101] Nieminen TH, Hagelberg NM, Saari TI, et al. Grapefruit juice enhances the exposure to oral oxycodone. Basic Clin Pharmacol Toxicol 2010;107:782—8.

[102] Woelkart K, Marth E, Suter A, et al. Bioavailability and pharmacokinetics of *Echinacea purpurea* preparations and their interaction with the immune system. Intl J Clin Pharmacol Ther 2006;44:401—8.

[103] Gorski JC, Huang S-M, Pinto A, et al. The effect of echinacea (*Echinacea purpurea* root) on cytochrome P450 activity *in vivo*. Clin Pharmacol Ther 2004;75:89—100.

[104] Penzak SR, Robertson SM, Hunt JD, et al. *Echinacea purpurea* significantly induces cytochrome P450 3A activity but does not alter lopinavir—ritonavir exposure in healthy subjects. Pharmacotherapy 2010;30:797—805.

[105] Gurley BJ, Gardner SF, Hubbard MA, et al. *In vivo* assessment of botanical supplementation on human cytochrome P450 phenotypes: *Citrus aurantium, Echinacea purpurea*, milk thistle, and saw palmetto. Clin Pharmacol Ther 2004;76:428—40.

[106] Gurley BJ, Swain A, Hubbard MA, et al. Clinical assessment of CYP2D6-mediated herb—drug interactions in humans: effects of milk thistle, black cohosh, goldenseal, kava kava, St John's wort, and echinacea. Mol Nutr Food Res 2008;52:755—63.

[107] Abdul MIM, Jiang X, Williams KM, et al. Pharmacokinetic and pharmacodynamic interactions of echinacea and policosanol with warfarin in healthy subjects. Br J Clin Pharmacol 2010;69:508—15.

[108] Fuchikami H, Satoh H, Tsujimoto M, et al. Effects of herbal extracts on the function of human organic anion-transporting polypeptide OATP-B. Drug Metab Dispos 2006;34:577—82.

[109] Hansen TS, Nilsen OG. *Echinacea purpurea* and P-glycoprotein drug transport in Caco-2 cells. Phytother Res 2009;23:86—91.

[110] Krochmal R, Hardy M, Bowerman S, et al. Phytochemical assays of commercial botanical dietary supplements. Evid Based Complement Alternat Med 2004;1:305—13.

[111] Kleijnen J, Knipschild P. *Ginkgo biloba* for cerebral insufficiency. Br J Clin Pharmacol 1992;34:352—8.

[112] Kleijnen J, Knipschild P. *Ginkgo biloba*. Lancet 1992;340:1136—9.

[113] Chung KF, Dent G, McCusker M, et al. Effect of a ginkgolide mixture (BN 52063) in antagonising skin and platelet responses to platelet activating factor in man. Lancet 1987;1:248—51.

[114] Rosenblatt M, Mindel J. Spontaneous hyphema associated with ingestion of *Ginkgo biloba* extract. N Engl J Med 1997;336:1108.

[115] Meisel C, Johne A, Roots I. Fatal intracerebral mass bleeding associated with *Gingko biloba* and ibuprofen. Atherosclerosis 2003;167:367.

[116] Matthews Jr MK. Association of *Gingko biloba* with intracerebral hemorrhage. Neurology 1998;50:1933—4.

[117] Lin YY, Chu SJ, Tsai SH. Association between priapism and concurrent use of risperidone and *Gingko biloba*. Mayo Clin Proc 2007;82:1289—90.

[118] Hellum BH, Nilsen OG. *In vitro* inhibition of CYP3A4 metabolism and P-glycoprotein-mediated transport by trade herbal products. Basic Clin Pharmacol Toxicol 2008;102:466—75.

[119] Mohamed MF, Frye RF. Inhibition of intestinal and hepatic glucuronidation of mycophenolic acid by *Gingko biloba* extract and flavonoids. Drug Metab Dispos 2010;38:270—5.

[120] Lau AJ, Chang TK. Inhibition of human CYP2B6-catalyzed bupropion hydroxylation by *Gingko biloba* extract: effect of terpene trilactones and flavonols. Drug Metab Dispos 2009;37:1931—7.

[121] Lei HP, Ji W, Lin J, et al. Effects of *Gingko biloba* extract on the pharmacokinetics of bupropion in healthy volunteers. Br J Clin Pharmacol 2009;68:201—6.

[122] Fan L, Tao GY, Wang G, et al. Effects of *Gingko biloba* extract ingestion on the pharmacokinetics of talinolol in healthy Chinese volunteers. Ann Pharmacother 2009;43:944—9.

[123] Fan L, Mao XQ, Tao GY, et al. Effect of *Schisandra chinensis* extract and *Gingko biloba* extract on the pharmacokinetics of talinolol in healthy volunteers. Xenobiotica 2009;39:249–54.

[124] Aruna D, Naidu MU. Pharmacodynamic interaction studies of *Gingko biloba* with cilostazol and clopidogrel in healthy human subjects. Br J Clin Pharmacol 2007;63:333–8.

[125] Jiang X, Williams KM, Liauw WS, et al. Effect of ginkgo and ginger on the pharmacokinetics and pharmacodynamics of warfarin in healthy subjects. Br J Clin Pharmacol 2005;59:425–32.

[126] Mohutsky MA, Anderson GD, Miller JW, Elmer GW. *Gingko biloba*: evaluation of CYP2C9 drug interactions *in vitro* and *in vivo*. Am J Ther 2006;13:24–31.

[127] Yin OQ, Tomlinson B, Waye MM, et al. Pharmacogenetics and herb–drug interactions: experience with *Gingko biloba* and omeprazole. Pharmacogenetics 2004;14:841–50.

[128] Kupiec T, Raj V. Fatal seizures due to potential herb–drug interactions with *Gingko biloba*. J Anal Toxicol 2005;29:755–8.

[129] Zuo XC, Zhang BK, Jia SJ, et al. Effects of *Gingko biloba* extracts on diazepam metabolism: a pharmacokinetic study in healthy Chinese male subjects. Eur J Clin Pharmacol 2010;66:503–9.

[130] Guo L, Mei N, Liao W, et al. *Gingko biloba* extract induces gene expression changes in xenobiotics metabolism and the Myc-centered network. OMICS, J Integr Biol 2010;14:75–90.

[131] Donovan JL, DeVane CL, Chavin KD, et al. Siberian ginseng (*Eleutheroccus senticosus*) effects on CYP2D6 and CYP3A4 activity in normal volunteers. Drug Metab Dispos 2003;31:519–22.

[132] Lee LS, Wise SD, Chan C, et al. Possible differential induction of phase 2 enzyme and antioxidant pathways by american ginseng, *Panax quinquefolius*. J Clin Pharmacol 2008;48:599–609.

[133] Andrade AS, Hendrix C, Parsons TL, et al. Pharmacokinetic and metabolic effects of American ginseng (*Panax quinquefolius*) in healthy volunteers receiving the HIV protease inhibitor indinavir. BMC Complement Altern Med 2008;8:50.

[134] Yuan CS, Wei G, Dey L, et al. Brief communication: American ginseng reduces warfarin's effect in healthy patients: a randomized, controlled trial. Ann Intern Med 2004;141:23–7.

[135] Hasegawa H, Matsumiya S, Murakami C, et al. Interactions of ginseng extract, ginseng separated fractions, and some triterepenoid saponins with glucose transporters in sheep erythrocytes. Planta Med 1994;60:153–7.

[136] Merino G, Molina AJ, Garcia JL, et al. Ginseng increases intestinal elimination of albendazole sulfoxide in the rat. Comp Biochem Physiol C Toxicol Pharmacol 2003;136:9–15.

[137] Jones BD, Runikis AM. Interaction of ginseng with phenelzine. J Clin Psychopharmacol 1987;7:201–2.

[138] Shader RI, Greenblatt DJ. Phenelzine and the dream machine – ramblings and reflections. J Clin Psychopharmacol 1985;5:65.

[139] Bilgi N, Bell K, Ananthakrishnan AN, Atallah E. Imatinib and *Panax* ginseng: a potential interaction resulting in liver toxicity. Ann Pharmacother 2010;44:926–8.

[140] Wanwimolruk S, Wong K, Wanwimolruk P. Variable inhibitory effect of different brands of commercial herbal supplements on human cytochrome P-450 CYP3A4. Drug Metabol Drug Interact 2009;24:17–35.

[141] Gurley BJ, Gardner SF, Hubbard MA, et al. Clinical assessment of effects of botanical supplementation on cytochrome P450 phenotypes in the elderly: St John's wort, garlic oil, *Panax ginseng* and *Gingko biloba*. Drugs Aging 2005;22:525–39.

[142] Patel J, Buddha B, Dey S, et al. *In vitro* interaction of the HIV protease inhibitor ritonavir with herbal constituents: changes in P-gp and CYP3A4 activity. Am J Ther 2004;11:262–77.

[143] Berginc K, Trontelj J, Kristl A. The influence of aged garlic extract on the uptake of saquinavir and darunavir into HepG2 cells and rat liver slices. Drug Metab Pharmacokinet 2010;25:307–13.

[144] Gallicano K, Foster B, Choudhri S. Effect of short-term administration of garlic supplements on single-dose ritonavir pharmacokinetics in healthy volunteers. Br J Clin Pharmacol 2003;55:199–202.

[145] Piscitelli SC, Burstein AH, Welden N, et al. The effect of garlic supplements on the pharmacokinetics of saquinavir. Clin Infect Dis 2002;34:234–8.

[146] Dhamija P, Malhotra S, Pandhi P. Effect of oral administration of crude aqueous extract of garlic on pharmacokinetic parameters of isoniazid and rifampicin in rabbits. Pharmacology 2006;77:100–4.

[147] Burnham BE. Garlic as a possible risk for postoperative bleeding. Plast Reconstr Surg 1995;95:213.

[148] German K, Kumar U, Blackford HN. Garlic and the risk of TURP bleeding. Br J Urol 1995;76:518.

[149] Macan H, Uykimpang R, Alconcel M, et al. Aged garlic extract may be safe for patients on warfarin therapy. J Nutr 2006;136:793S–5S.

[150] Mohammed Abdul MI, Jiang X, Williams KM, et al. Pharmacodynamic interaction of warfarin with cranberry but not with garlic in healthy subjects. Br J Pharmacol 2008;154:1691–700.

[151] Yale SH, Glurich I. Analysis of the inhibitory potential of *Gingko biloba, Echinacea purpurea*, and *Serenoa repens* on the metabolic activity of cytochrome P450 3A4, 2D6, and 2C9. J Altern Complement Med 2005;11:433–9.

[152] Markowitz JS, Donovan JL, Devane CL, et al. Multiple doses of saw palmetto (*Serenoa repens*) did not alter cytochrome P450 2D6 and 3A4 activity in normal volunteers. Clin Pharmacol Ther 2003;74:536–42.

[153] Schelosky L, Raffauf C, Jendroska K, Poewe W. Kava and dopamine antagonism. J Neurol Neurosurg Psychiatry 1995;58:639–40.

[154] Almeida JC, Grimsley EW. Coma from the health food store: interaction between kava and alprazolam. Ann Intern Med 1996;125:940–1.

[155] Mathews JM, Etheridge AS, Black SR. Inhibition of human cytochrome P450 activities by kava extract and kavalactones. Drug Metab Dispos 2002;30:1153–7.

[156] Mathews JM, Etheridge AS, Valentine JL, et al. Pharmacokinetics and disposition of the kavalactone kawain: interaction with kava extract and kavalactones *in vivo* and *in vitro*. Drug Metab Disp 2005;33:1555–63.

[157] Unger M, Frank A. Simultaneous determination of the inhibitory potency of herbal extracts on the activity of six major cytochrome P450 enzymes using liquid chromatography/mass spectrometry and automated online extraction. Rapid Commun Mass Spectrom 2004;18:2273–81.

[158] Gurley BJ, Gardner SF, Hubbard MA, et al. *In vivo* effects of goldenseal, kava kava, black cohosh, and valerian on human cytochrome P450 1A2, 2D6, 2E1, and 3A4/5 phenotypes. Clin Pharmacol Ther 2005;77:415–26.

[159] Gurley BJ, Swain A, Barone GW, et al. Effect of goldenseal (*Hydrastis canadensis*) and kava kava (*Piper methysticum*) Supplementation on digoxin pharmacokinetics in humans. Drug Met Disp 2007;35:240–5.

[160] Koo KL, Ammit AJ, Tran VH, et al. Gingerols and related analogues inhibit arachidonic acid-induced human platelet serotonin release and aggregation. Thromb Res 2001;103:387–97.

[161] Lesho EP, Saullo L, Udvari-Nagy S. A 76-year-old woman with erratic anticoagulation. Cleveland Clin J Med 2004;71:651–6.

[162] Phillips S, Hutchinson S, Ruggier R. *Zingiber officinale* does not affect gastric emptying rate. A randomised, placebo-controlled, crossover trial. Anaesthesia 1993;48:393–5.

[163] Shariatpanahi ZV, Taleban FA, Mokhtari M, Shahbazi S. Ginger extract reduces delayed gastric emptying and nosocomial pneumonia in adult respiratory distress syndrome patients hospitalized in an intensive care unit. J Crit Care 2010;25:647–50.

[164] Wu KL, Rayner CK, Chuah SK, et al. Effects of ginger on gastric emptying and motility in healthy humans. Eur J Gastroenterol Hepatol 2008;20:436–40.

[165] Hu ML, Rayner CK, Wu KL, et al. Effect of ginger on gastric motility and symptoms of functional dyspepsia. World J Gastroenterol 2011;17:105–10.

[166] Nagoshi C, Shiota S, Kuroda T, et al. Synergistic effect of [10]-gingerol and aminoglycosides against vancomycin-resistant enterococci (VRE). Biol Pharm Bull 2006;29:443–7.

[167] Nostro A, Cellini L, Di Bartolomeo S, et al. Effects of combining extracts (from propolis or *Zingiber officinale*) with clarithromycin on *Helicobacter pylori*. Phytother Res 2006;20:187–90.

[168] Nabekura T, Kamiyama S, Kitagawa S. Effects of dietary chemopreventive phytochemicals on P-glycoprotein function. Biochem Biophys Res Commun 2005;327:866–70.

[169] Khom S, Baburin I, Timin E, et al. Valerenic acid potentiates and inhibits GABA(A) receptors: molecular mechanism and subunit specificity. Neuropharmacology 2007;53:178–87.

[170] Wasowski C, Marder M, Viola H, et al. Isolation and identification of 6-methylapigenin, a competitive ligand for the brain GABA(A) receptors, from *Valeriana wallichii*. Planta Med 2002;68:934–6.

[171] Hellum BH, Hu Z, Nilsen OG. The induction of CYP1A2, CYP2D6 and CYP3A4 by six trade herbal products in cultured primary human hepatocytes. Basic Clin Pharmacol Toxicol 2007;100:23–30.

[172] Donovan JL, DeVane CL, Chavin KD, et al. Multiple night-time doses of valerian (*Valeriana officinalis*) had minimal effects on CYP3A4 activity and no effect on CYP2D6 activity in healthy volunteers. Drug Metab Disp 2004;32:1333–6.

[173] Budzinski JW, Foster BC, Vandenhoek S, Arnason JT. An *in vitro* evaluation of human cytochrome P450 3A4 inhibition by selected commercial herbal extracts and tinctures. Phytomedicine 2000;7:273–82.

[174] Foster BC, Vandenhoek S, Hana J, et al. *In vitro* inhibition of human cytochrome P450-mediated metabolism of marker substrates by natural products. Phytomedicine 2003;10:334–42.

[175] Chatterjee P, Franklin MR. Human cytochrome p450 inhibition and metabolic-intermediate complex formation by goldenseal extract and its methylenedioxyphenyl components. Drug Metab Dispos 2003;31:1391–7.

[176] Etheridge AS, Black SR, Patel PR, et al. An *in vitro* evaluation of cytochrome P450 inhibition and P-glycoprotein interaction with goldenseal, *Gingko biloba*, grape seed, milk thistle, and ginseng extracts and their constituents. Planta Med 2007;73:731–41.

[177] Sevior DK, Hokkanen J, Tolonen A, et al. Rapid screening of commercially available herbal products for the inhibition of major human hepatic cytochrome P450 enzymes using the N-in-one cocktail. Xenobiotica 2010;40:245–54.

[178] Gurley BJ, Swain A, Hubbard MA, et al. Supplementation with goldenseal (*Hydrastis canadensis*), but not kava kava (*Piper methysticum*), inhibits human CYP3A activity *in vivo*. Clin Pharmacol Ther 2008;83:61–9.

[179] Sandhu RS, Prescilla RP, Simonelli TM, Edwards DJ. Influence of goldenseal root on the pharmacokinetics of indinavir. J Clin Pharmacol 2003;43:1283–8.

[180] Liu R, Tam TW, Mao J, et al. The effect of natural health products and traditional medicines on the activity of human hepatic microsomal-mediated metabolism of oseltamivir. J Pharm Pharm Sci 2010;13:43–55.

[181] Williams SN, Shih H, Guenette DK, et al. Comparative studies on the effects of green tea extracts and individual tea catechins on human CYP1A gene expression. Chem Biol Interact 2000;128:211–29.

[182] Williams SN, Pickwell GV, Quattrochi LC. A combination of tea (*Camellia senensis*) catechins is required for optimal inhibition of induced CYP1A expression by green tea extract. J Agric Food Chem 2003;51:6627–34.

[183] Nishikawa M, Ariyoshi N, Kotani A, et al. Effects of continuous ingestion of green tea or grape seed extracts on the pharmacokinetics of midazolam. Drug Metab Pharmacokinet 2004;19:280–9.

[184] Donovan JL, Chavin KD, Devane CL, et al. Green tea (*Camellia sinensis*) extract does not alter cytochrome P450 3A4 or 2D6 activity in healthy volunteers. Drug Metab Dispos 2004;32:906–8.

[185] Chow HH, Hakim IA, Vining DR, et al. Effects of repeated green tea catechin administration on human cytochrome P450 activity. Cancer Epidemiol Biomarkers Prev 2006;15:2473–6.

[186] Nishimuta H, Tsujimoto M, Ogura K, et al. Inhibitory effects of various beverages on ritodrine sulfation by recombinant human sulfotransferase isoforms SULT1A1 and SULT1A3. Pharm Res 2005;22:1406–10.

[187] Nagai M, Fukamachi T, Tsujimoto M, et al. Inhibitory effects of herbal extracts on the activity of human sulfotransferase isoform sulfotransferase 1A3 (SULT1A3). Biol Pharm Bull 2009;32:105–9.

[188] Suganuma M, Saha A, Fujiki H. New cancer treatment strategy using combination of green tea catechins and anticancer drugs. Cancer Sci 2011;102:317–23.

[189] Sadzuka Y, Sugiyama T, Suzuki T, Sonobe T. Enhancement of the activity of doxorubicin by inhibition of glutamate transporter. Toxicol Lett 2001;123:159–67.

[190] Sugiyama T, Sadzuka Y, Tanaka K, Sonobe T. Inhibition of glutamate transporter by theanine enhances the therapeutic efficacy of doxorubicin. Toxicol Lett 2001;121:89–96.

[191] Liang G, Tang A, Lin X, et al. Green tea catechins augment the antitumor activity of doxorubicin in an *in vivo* mouse model for chemoresistant liver cancer. Intl J Oncol 2010;37:111–23.

[192] Wang EJ, Barecki-Roach M, Johnson WW. Elevation of P-glycoprotein function by a catechin in green tea. Biochem Biophys Res Commun 2002;297:412–8.

[193] Monteiro R, Calhau C, Martel F, et al. Modulation of MPP+ uptake by tea and some of its components in Caco-2 cells. Naunyn Schmiedebergs Arch Pharmacol 2005;372:147–52.

[194] Raucy JL. Regulation of CYP3A4 expression in human hepatocytes by pharmaceuticals and natural products. Drug Metab Dispos 2003;31:533–9.

[195] Graber-Maier A, Buter KB, Aeschlimann J, et al. Effects of *Curcuma* extracts and curcuminoids on expression of P-glycoprotein and cytochrome P450 3A4 in the intestinal cell culture model LS180. Planta Med 2010;76:1866–70.

[196] Hou XL, Takahashi K, Kinoshita N, et al. Possible inhibitory mechanism of *Curcuma* drugs on CYP3A4 in 1α, 25 dihydroxyvitamin D3 treated Caco-2 cells. Intl J Pharm 2007;337:169–77.

[197] Appiah-Opong R, Commandeur JN, van Vugt-Lussenburg B, Vermeulen NP. Inhibition of human recombinant cytochrome P450s by curcumin and curcumin decomposition products. Toxicology 2007;235:83–91.

[198] Volak LP, Ghirmai S, Cashman JR, Court MH. Curcuminoids inhibit multiple human cytochromes P450, UDP-glucuronosyltransferase, and sulfotransferase enzymes, whereas piperine is a relatively selective CYP3A4 inhibitor. Drug Metab Dispos 2008;36:1594–605.

444 CHIN & BASKIN

[199] Mach CM, Chen JH, Mosley SA, et al. Evaluation of liposomal curcumin cytochrome p450 metabolism. Anticancer Res 2010;30:811—4.

[200] Chen Y, Liu WH, Chen BL, et al. Plant polyphenol curcumin significantly affects CYP1A2 and CYP2A6 activity in healthy, male Chinese volunteers. Ann Pharmacother 2010;44:1038—45.

[201] Strimpakos AS, Sharma RA. Curcumin: preventive and therapeutic properties in laboratory studies and clinical trials. Antioxid Redox Signal 2008;10:511—45.

[202] Wortelboer HM, Usta M, van der Velde, et al. Interplay between MRP inhibition and metabolism of MRP inhibitors: the case of curcumin. Chem Res Toxicol 2003;16:1642—51.

[203] Wortelboer HM, Usta M, van Zanden JJ, et al. Inhibition of multidrug resistance proteins MRP1 and MRP2 by a series of alpha, beta-unsaturated carbonyl compounds. Biochem Pharmacol 2005;69:1879—90.

[204] Chearwae W, Wu CP, Chu HY, et al. Curcuminoids purified from turmeric powder modulate the function of human multidrug resistance protein 1 (ABCC1). Cancer Chemother Pharmacol 2006;57:376—88.

[205] Limtrakul P, Chearwae W, Shukla S, et al. Modulation of function of three ABC drug transporters, P-glyco-protein (ABCB1), mitoxantrone resistance protein (ABCG2) and multidrug resistance protein 1 (ABCC1) by tetrahydrocurcumin, a major metabolite of curcumin. Mol Cell Biochem 2007;296:85—95.

[206] Chearwae W, Anuchapreeda S, Nandigama K, et al. Biochemical mechanism of modulation of human P-glycoprotein (ABCB1) by curcumin I, II, and III purified from Turmeric powder. Biochem Pharmacol 2004;68:2043—52.

[207] Bansal T, Awasthi A, Jaggi M, et al. Pre-clinical evidence for altered absorption and biliary excretion of iri-notecan (CPT-11) in combination with quercetin: possible contribution of P-glycoprotein. Life Sci 2008;83:250—9.

[208] Ampasavate C, Sotanaphun U, Phattanawasin P, Piyapolrungroj N. Effects of *Curcuma* spp. on P-glycoprotein function. Phytomedicine 2010;17:506—12.

[209] Shukla S, Zaher H, Hartz A, et al. Curcumin inhibits the activity of ABCG2/BCRP1, a multidrug resistance-linked ABC drug transporter in mice. Pharm Res 2009;26:480—7.

[210] Juan H, Terhaag B, Cong Z, et al. Unexpected effect of concomitantly administered curcumin on the phar-macokinetics of talinolol in healthy Chinese volunteers. Eur J Clin Pharmacol 2007;63:663—8.

[211] Ho SH, Singh M, Holloway AC, Crankshaw DJ. The effects of commercial preparations of herbal supplements commonly used by women on the biotransformation of fluorogenic substrates by human cytochromes P450. Phytother Res. 2011;25:983—9.

[212] Tsukamoto S, Aburatani M, Ohta T. Isolation of CYP3A4 inhibitors from the black cohosh (*Cimicifuga race-mosa*). Evid Based Complement Alternat Med 2005;2:223—6.

[213] Huang Y, Jiang B, Nuntanakorn P, et al. Fukinolic acid derivatives and triterpene glycosides from black cohosh inhibit CYP isozymes, but are not cytotoxic to Hep-G2 cells *in vitro*. Curr Drug Saf 2010;5:118—24.

[214] Gurley B, Hubbard MA, Williams DK, et al. Assessing the clinical significance of botanical supplementation on human cytochrome P450 3A activity: comparison of a milk thistle and black cohosh product to rifampin and clarithromycin. J Clin Pharmacol 2006;46:201—13.

[215] Rockwell S, Liu Y, Higgins SA. Alteration of the effects of cancer therapy agents on breast cancer cells by the herbal medicine black cohosh. Breast Cancer Res Treat 2005;90:233—9.

[216] Gurley BJ, Barone GW, Williams DK, et al. Effect of milk thistle (*Silybum marianum*) and black cohosh (*Cimicifuga racemosa*) supplementation on digoxin pharmacokinetics in humans. Drug Metab Dispos 2006;34:69—74.

[217] Sridar C, Goosen TC, Kent UM, et al. Silybin inactivates cytochromes P450 3A4 and 2C9 and inhibits major hepatic glucuronosyltransferases. Drug Metab Dispos 2004;32:587—94.

[218] Budzinski JW, Trudeau VL, Drouin CE, et al. Modulation of human cytochrome P450 3A4 (CYP3A4) and P-glycoprotein (P-gp) in Caco-2 cell monolayers by selected commercial-source milk thistle and goldenseal products. Can J Physiol Pharmacol 2007;85:966—78.

[219] Piscitelli SC, Formentini E, Burstein AH, et al. Effect of milk thistle on the pharmacokinetics of indinavir in healthy volunteers. Pharmacotherapy 2002;22:551—6.

[220] DiCenzo R, Shelton M, Jordan K, et al. Coadministration of milk thistle and indinavir in healthy subjects. Pharmacotherapy 2003;23:866—70.

[221] Mills E, Wilson K, Clarke M, et al. Milk thistle and indinavir: a randomized controlled pharmacokinetics study and meta-analysis. Eur J Clin Pharmacol 2005;61:1—7.

[222] van Erp NP, Baker SD, Zhao M, et al. Effect of milk thistle (*Silybum marianum*) on the pharmacokinetics of irinotecan. Clin Cancer Res 2005;11:7800–6.

[223] Fuhr U, Beckmann-Knopp S, Jetter A, et al. The effect of silymarin on oral nifedipine pharmacokinetics. Planta Med 2007;73:1429–35.

[224] Brantley SJ, Oberlies NH, Kroll DJ, Paine MF. Two flavonolignans from milk thistle (*Silybum marianum*) inhibit CYP2C9-mediated warfarin metabolism at clinically achievable concentrations. J Pharmacol Exper Ther 2010;332:1081–7.

[225] Doehmer J, Weiss G, McGregor GP, Appel K. Assessment of a dry extract from milk thistle (*Silybum marianum*) for interference with human liver cytochrome-P450 activities. Toxicol in Vitro 2011;25:21–7.

[226] Navarro VJ. Herbal and dietary supplement hepatotoxicity. Semin Liver Dis 2009;29:373–82.

[227] Dasgupta A, Biddle DA, Wells A, Datta P. Positive and negative interference of the Chinese medicine Chan Su in serum digoxin measurement. Elimination of interference by using a monoclonal chemiluminescent digoxin assay or monitoring free digoxin concentration. Am J Clin Pathol 2000;114:174–9.

[228] Wahed A, Dasgupta A. Positive and negative *in vitro* interference of Chinese medicine Dan Shen in serum digoxin measurement. Elimination of interference by monitoring free digoxin concentration. Am J Clin Pathol 2001;116:403–8.

Index

Note: Page numbers followed by *f* indicate figures, *t* indicate tables and *b* indicate boxes.

Rifabutin, therapeutic range, 208t
Rifampin
  therapeutic drug monitoring, 213–214
  therapeutic range, 208t
RMSE, *see* Root mean squared error
Root mean squared error (RMSE), 111
Rotonavir, therapeutic drug monitoring, 385
Rufinamide
  pharmacology, 251t
  structure, 250f
  therapeutic drug monitoring, 256–257

S

St John's wort, drug interactions, 422–423
Saliva, advantages and disadvantages for drug
    monitoring, 33t
Saquinavir, therapeutic drug monitoring, 386t
Saw palmetto, drug interactions, 427–428
Seizure, *see* Anticonvulsants
Selective serotonin reuptake inhibitors,
    see Antidepressants
Serotonin receptor HTR2A, antidepressant
    metabolism polymorphisms, 283–284
Serotonin syndrome, 278
Serotonin transporter, antidepressant metabolism
    polymorphisms, 284
Sertraline
  pharmacokinetics, 279t
  therapeutic range, 6t–8t
Serum
  advantages and disadvantages for drug monitoring,
    33t
  plasma specimen comparison, 39–41
  separator collection tube effects on drug monitoring,
    41–44, 42t
Sex differences
  drug response and metabolism, 14–15, 16t
  warfarin dose, 169
Single Molecule Real Time (SMRT) DNA sequencing,
    153
Sirolimus
  biomarkers in solid organ transplantation,
    see Immunosuppressants
  overview, 335–338
  structure, 326f
  therapeutic drug monitoring
    challenges, 337
    immunoassays, 336
    liquid chromatography/mass spectrometry,
      107
  therapeutic range, 6t–8t
SMRT DNA sequencing, *see* Single Molecule Real Time
    DNA sequencing

Solid phase microextraction (SPME), free drug
    concentration determination, 85, 90, 93
Sotalol
  therapeutic drug monitoring, 237
  therapeutic range, 221t–222t
Southern blot, 123
Specimens, *see also specific specimens*
  advantages and disadvantages by type for drug
    monitoring, 33t
  collection site influence on drug levels, 37–38
  free drug concentration determination, 96
  sample preparation steps, 44–45
  tampering in opioid drug tests, 408–409
  volume influence on drug levels, 38–39
Spironolactone
  digoxin immunoassay interference, 227–228
  structure, 228f
SPME, *see* Solid phase microextraction
SRM, *see* Standardized reference material
Standard two-stage (STS) approach, 108
Standardized reference material (SRM), 50–53
Statins, personalized medicine, 133
Stripentol
  pharmacology, 251t
  structure, 250f
  therapeutic drug monitoring, 257
STS approach, *see* Standard two-stage approach
Sulfonamides, therapeutic drug monitoring, 210

T

Tacrolimus
  biomarkers in solid organ transplantation,
    see Immunosuppressants
  dose adjustment using pharmacokinetic models,
    115–117
  overview, 333–335
  structure, 326f
  therapeutic drug monitoring
    challenges, 334–335
    immunoassays, 333
    liquid chromatography/mass spectrometry,
      334
  therapeutic range, 6t–8t
Tamoxifen, pharmacogenetics, 302–305, 304f
Tazobactam, *see* Piperacillin/tazobactam
T cell, immunosuppression biomarkers
  global markers
    ATP concentration in CD4+ cells, 355–359, 358t,
      359t
    CD30 in serum, 364–366
    interferon-γ in alloreactive T cells, 359–360
    lymphocyte proliferation, 363–364
    T cell activation surface markers, 360–362